# FUNDAMENTALS
# OF RESPIRATORY THERAPY

# FUNDAMENTALS OF RESPIRATORY THERAPY

## DONALD F. EGAN, M.D., F.C.C.P.

Medical Director, Eastern North Carolina Hospital,
Wilson, North Carolina

**Third edition**

*with 227 illustrations*

THE C. V. MOSBY COMPANY

Saint Louis   1977

**Third edition**

**Copyright © 1977 by The C. V. Mosby Company**

All rights reserved. No part of this book may be reproduced in
any manner without written permission of the publisher.

Previous editions copyrighted 1969, 1973

Printed in the United States of America

Distributed in Great Britain by Henry Kimpton, London

The C. V. Mosby Company
11830 Westline Industrial Drive, St. Louis, Missouri 63141

**Library of Congress Cataloging in Publication Data**

Egan, Donald F          1916-
   Fundamentals of respiratory therapy.

   First ed. published in 1969 under title: Fundamentals
of inhalation therapy.
   Bibliography: p.
   Includes index.
   1. Inhalation therapy.   I. Title.   [DNLM:
1. Inhalation therapy.   WB342 E28f]
RM161.E37   1977        615'.836        76-25810
ISBN 0-8016-1503-8

TS/CB/B   9   8   7   6   5   4   3   2   1

# PREFACE

Since publication of the second edition of *Fundamentals of Respiratory Therapy*, three events have occurred that are of great importance to respiratory therapists and therapy. First, in April of 1973 the standards of hospital respiratory therapy services, as proposed by the Joint Commission on Accreditation of Hospitals, were accepted and are now in operation. Brief though they are and lacking substance in many sections, the standards nevertheless represent a large step toward protecting the patient with pulmonary problems and giving much needed support to respiratory therapy and its technical and medical personnel. If hospitals are to maintain high accreditation, respiratory therapy must be recognized and accepted as a legitimate health source, not just a counterbalance to other hospital services that are fiscal liabilities. We all know that no dramatic overnight change will take place, and it will be a few years yet before the full objectives of the standards are realized. Still, overcoming inertia and making a start is a major achievement, and it is reassuring to know that some people of influence in our field have foresight and the willingness to act.

Second, perhaps the most stabilizing event in the recent history of respiratory therapy was the birth of the National Board for Respiratory Therapy. Certainly, housing the therapist and technician credentialling procedures under one roof makes the greatest of sense. It is most impressive that, despite the misunderstandings, suspicions, charges, and countercharges attending the emergence of the original technician certification program, the concept of the NBRT was able to flourish on reason and not founder on emotionalism. A mature move that should be easily recognized as such, creation of the NBRT will give added professionalism and credibility to both personnel levels involved. Credit is due those who worked to bring the Board to fruition, as many of us are aware of the obstacles with which they contended. Still, this is the kind of action that counts and that identifies a structure built on a strong foundation.

Third, and more representative of a trend than of a specific event is the growing criticism of the scientific validity of much of respiratory therapy. This is a topic deserving of an in-depth scholarly essay, and I recognize that a superficial treatment may tend to belittle its importance. It is important—very important. Many of the complaints against respiratory therapy are more than justified. I can recall no other facet of medicine that has so permeated hospital patient care, involved such critically ill patients, subjected these patients to physiological alterations as significant, and done this with such a positive economic impact, all with as meager a scientific background, as has respiratory therapy. This does not mean that all respiratory therapy is invalid or that much of it is not well founded, but we do know that many of the things we do are empirical or based on the somewhat nebulous support of "clinical observation." Many of the users are convinced of the value of respiratory therapy, but it remains for us who are responsible for it to demonstrate why it is effective or to delete those procedures, if any, that are no more useful than no therapy at all.

These developments were noted as a means of stressing that with growth and maturity comes increased responsibility. The stature of the respiratory therapist in the hospital should be enhanced, as his services now count toward his hospital's accreditation standing. His registration or certification will have more prestige as hospital co-workers and administrators become better acquainted with the credentialling mechanism. Accordingly, the registered therapist and the certified technician will be expected to demonstrate a more professional attitude. In the face of current criticism, the therapist's deportment must be above reproach, and his technical expertise confidence-inspiring.

It was with these considerations in mind, and as an attempt to meet their implied needs, that a host of notes, sketches, observations, and opinions were brought together, hopefully in harmony, to produce this third edition of *Fundamentals of Respiratory Therapy*. The objective of the work was to compact as much currently relevant essential material about respiratory therapy as possible into one book. On this third go-around, I have affirmed that while writing a text is very hard work, attempting to keep it updated is no easier. Respiratory therapy continues to grow, but I do not believe at quite the frenetic pace of the mid-sixties to early seventies. At the same time, literature pertinent to respiratory therapy has been sounding greater depths, slowly diminishing the wrench-and-bolt dominance of the recent past. This burdens an author with an increasing load of reading, reviewing, and judgmental weighing of material to decide what to remove from the old text and what to include in the new.

In this edition the section on basic sciences has been augmented, especially with a review of some aspects of chemistry with which it is felt the respiratory therapist should be familiar. In no way are the few pages devoted to chemistry intended to supplant a standard text or a well-taught course on the subject. Many therapists and students, however, are afraid of chemistry, perhaps from a past experience in which they found no relevance between it and their needs. I would hope that some of these might be stimulated to pursue its study further and reap the rich harvest of a good background of scientific knowledge. Concepts of some of the currently popular techniques such as positive end-expiratory pressure and intermittent mandatory ventilation have been explained and illustrated and a miscellany of comments made and opinions expressed on preclinical and clinical topics. For example, the abbreviation for gram has been changed from *gm* to *g*, conforming to standards described in *Units of Weights and Measure*, by L. J. Chisholm of the U.S. Department of Commerce/National Bureau of Standards, Miscellaneous Publication 286, 1967.

Reference is also made to terminology changes recommended by a special joint Committee of the American College of Chest Physicians and the American Thoracic Society.[32] These should be of interest to all in the field.

Some changes from the previous edition may involve only a sentence or two, but each was made for a specific purpose, and it is felt that this edition is just about as current as is possible at this time in basics and essentials. Like its predecessors, the third edition is directed primarily toward the respiratory therapy student and the therapist and technician reviewing for credentialling examinations. It should also be of help to nurses involved in respiratory care, to house staff and pulmonary fellows, and last, but not least, to the nonpulmonary specialist attending physician who wishes to be sure that his patients with respiratory diseases are properly managed. To all, happy reading.

**Donald F. Egan**

# CONTENTS

1  GASES, THE ATMOSPHERE, AND THE GAS LAWS, 1

2  SOLUTIONS AND IONS, 39

3  VENTILATION, 79

4  BLOOD GASES AND ACID-BASE BALANCE, 117

5  CARDIOVASCULAR SYSTEM, 156

6  CLINICAL CARDIOPULMONARY PATHOLOGY, 182

7  AEROSOL AND HUMIDITY THERAPY, 213

8  GAS THERAPY, 269

9  MECHANICAL VENTILATION, 322

10  RESPIRATORY THERAPY MANAGEMENT OF VENTILATORY FAILURE, 388

11  CHRONIC CARE AND REHABILITATION OF RESPIRATORY FAILURE, 468

12  THE ORGANIZATION, STAFFING, AND SERVICES OF A RESPIRATORY CARE DEPARTMENT, 487

APPENDIXES

1  Systems of measurements and equivalents, 504
2  Physiologic and selected physical abbreviations and symbols, 506
3  Altitude and depth characteristics of atmosphere, 507
4  Factors to convert gas volumes from ATPS to BTPS, 508
5  Temperature correction of barometric reading, 509

6  Factors to convert gas volumes from ATPS to STPD, 510
7  Factors to convert gas volumes from STPD to BTPS at given barometric pressures, 511
8  Low-temperature characteristics of selected gases and water, 511
9  Selected elements and radicals: symbols, approximate atomic weights, valances, 512
10  Calculation of $P_{CO_2}$ from H—H equation, 512
11  Relation of arterial oxygen saturation to capillary unsaturation, 513
12  Alveolar air equation, 514
13  Breathing nomogram, 515

ANSWERS TO EXERCISES, 516

REFERENCES, 517

# FUNDAMENTALS
## OF RESPIRATORY THERAPY

**Chapter 1**

# GASES, THE ATMOSPHERE, AND THE GAS LAWS

A gas, which may not be seen, cannot be felt, and has no inherent confining bound-aries, almost invokes an impression of nothingness until we become aware of the tremendous activity of its components and its great flexibility. It can be compressed, can expand, can produce heat, can cool, and can be liquefied. From its behavior, we can infer that a gas consists of much empty space, with its substance in minute particle form, and it is with the general relationship between such space and particles that we will be concerned.

## MOBILITY OF GASES

As a start, let us recall that all matter is composed of *atoms*, the characteristics of which differentiate the many elements that comprise our world. In chemical reactions it is atoms that combine with like or different atoms, separate from yet others, or re-group into new combinations. Compounds are made from such joining of atoms, the resulting products possessing characteristics distinctly different from those of their constituents.

The smallest particle of a substance that retains all of its properties is referred to as a *molecule*. This may consist of one or several atoms, but at least as many as are represented in the chemical formula of the substance. The term *gram molecular weight (gmw)* is frequently encountered in chemistry, and it is the weight in grams equal to the molecular weight of a substance, or the sum of all the atomic weights in its molecular formula. It must be noted, however, that not all substances have true mo-lecular structures, depending upon the type of bonding which holds together the atoms. Those classified as *ionic compounds* are essentially mixtures of fixed propor-tions of minute electrically charged particles called ions, without any basic molecular structure. Atomic bonding and further details of ions will be discussed in Chapter 2. Because the expression, gram molecular weight, is inappropriate for ionic compounds, we speak of *gram formula weight (gfw)*, which has the same meaning and is calculated in the same manner as gram molecular weight. It is proper to use either molecular weight or formula weight for substances that form molecules, but only formula weight is acceptable for ionic compounds.[1]

It is possible to differentiate between molecular and ionic substances by inspection of their formulas, but it is not our purpose to delve into such details of chemistry. Our interest is only to make use of those principles of chemistry that relate to our needs of this book. Actually, the problem is partially solved for us, since gases, which are our chief concern, do consist of molecules. Throughout the text, then, when referring to the structure or chemistry of gases, we will use the terms *molecules* and *gram molecular weights* as needed, but for all other substances we will use the unit of *gram formula weight*.

Thus the substance of gases consists of aggregates of small molecular particles that are in constant motion, called *kinetic activity*. The density with which atoms and molecules are packed determines the solidity or fluidity of all matter. Substances with a high density of particles are solids, while those with easily mobile particles are fluids. Gases and liquids fall into this second category. It should not be supposed that the atoms or molecules of solids cannot move, for they respond to such stimuli as vibrations, bending, stretching, and temperature. Fluidity, however, implies the easy flowing of particles over one another and the ability to conform readily to the confines of a container. Mercury, although a metal, can thus be described as fluid.

Particles that make up the substance of gases are minute in size, within the range of $10^{-8}$ to $10^{-7}$ cm in diameter, with weights varying from $10^{-23}$ to $10^{-20}$ g. The kinetic theory tells us that these particles are in *constant rapid* motion, following completely random paths, and that their speed is phenomenal. Hydrogen particles move $1.84 \times 10^5$ cm/sec (greater than 1 mile per second), and oxygen $4.6 \times 10^4$ cm/sec (one third of a mile per second).[2] During this intense activity the particles "collide" with one another and with the surface of enclosing containers. Actually, the particles probably repulse one another before physical contact, but the forces involved can best be visualized in the mind as collisions. The average number of collisions per second for each molecule of hydrogen is $1 \times 10^{10}$, for oxygen $4.6 \times 10^9$, and for carbon dioxide $6.2 \times 10^9$. The *mean free path* of gas molecules describes the average distance traveled by the molecules between collisions. Again, for hydrogen this distance is $1.66 \times 10^{-5}$ cm, for oxygen $8.8 \times 10^{-6}$ cm, and for carbon dioxide $5.8 \times 10^{-6}$ cm.[3] Very fine particles of an insoluble substance such as carbon or metal dust suspended in water, if viewed under a microscope, can be seen to move about in an erratic random manner. This is called *Brownian movement* and is produced by the kinetic activity of water molecules striking the suspended material.

To view the phenomenon of kinetic activity in familiar quantitative terms, let us imagine oxygen molecules in a pure sample of that gas to be the size of Ping-Pong balls. We can see them, in the mind's eye, in large numbers bouncing off walls, ceiling, floor, and each other, never stopping and never settling to the floor. Considering the relative sizes of oxygen molecules and Ping-Pong balls, the mean free path, and the average number of collisions of the molecules, the Ping-Pong balls would travel an average distance of 40 feet between collisions. This gives us some concept of the great distance between molecules in relation to their size as well as the mass of "nothingness" that makes up a gas.

## PRESSURE AND TEMPERATURE OF GASES

All gases exert pressure, whether free in the atmosphere, enclosed in a container, or dissolved in a liquid such as blood. In physiology this pressure is frequently referred to as the *tension* of a gas. Gas pressure is dependent upon molecular kinetic activity and is the result of molecular bombardment upon any confining surface, be it a steel cylinder or the earth's surface, and we may consider such pressure as the striking force of molecules attempting to escape. In addition, the force of the earth's gravity, by its effect on the molecular masses of the gas, augments the gas pressure against the dependent confining surface of a gas volume. Thus, in a container of gas, although the travel of molecules is random in all directions, pressure in the bottom of the vessel is somewhat higher than elsewhere, as the force of molecular impingement is aided by gravity. The amount of pressure exerted by a gas depends on the *number* of particles present and the *frequency* of their collisions. The frequency, in turn, is related to the *velocity* of the gas particles, since the greater the speed of travel, the greater will be the number of collisions per unit of time, the greater the force of collisions, and the greater the gas tension.

Gas particle velocity is not a constant value but is directly related to gas temperature, and as temperature rises the kinetic activity accelerates, molecular collisions increase in number, and the pressure of the gas rises. Conversely, with dropping temperature molecular activity declines, particle velocity and collision frequency drop, and pressure is lowered. The familiar increase in automobile tire pressure while driving on a hot pavement is an example of the relationship between gas tension and temperature. This relationship between molecular activity and temperature can be graphically illustrated by a special temperature scale, which the student will put to practical use when he studies the gas laws. We will describe the concept of *absolute temperature* and the two subscales by which it is calibrated. There is a temperature at which all molecular activity ceases, a theoretical value arrived at by projection and calculation, which, although closely approximated, has not actually been attained. If we are interested in the relative kinetic behavior of gases at various temperatures, a point of no activity produces a logical zero on which to build a scale. This is called *absolute zero* ($0°_{abs}$) and is the origin of the absolute temperature scale. If it is calibrated in Celsius temperature units, it is called the *Kelvin scale* (K), and if in Fahrenheit units, the *Rankine scale* (R).

### Kelvin scale

In Celsius units, molecular activity stops at about $-273°$ C. Therefore $0°$ K $= -273°$ C, and $0°$ C $= 273°$ K, since $0°$ C is 273 temperature units above $0°$ K. When used as symbols in formulas, Celsius temperatures are often designated by a small $t$ and absolute temperatures by a capital $T$ or a capital $K$. A simple equation to keep in mind is $°K = °t + 273$. In other words, to convert Celsius degrees to Kelvin, add 273. Thus:

$$25°\ C = 25 + 273 = 298°\ K$$
$$37°\ C = 37 + 273 = 310°\ K$$
$$-15°\ C = -15 + 273 = 258°\ K$$

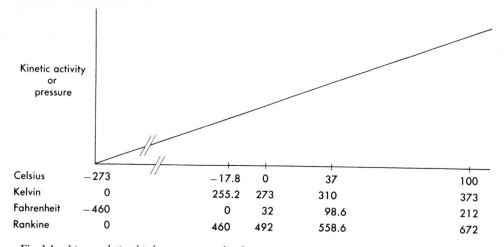

| | | | | | |
|---|---|---|---|---|---|
| Celsius | −273 | −17.8 | 0 | 37 | 100 |
| Kelvin | 0 | 255.2 | 273 | 310 | 373 |
| Fahrenheit | −460 | 0 | 32 | 98.6 | 212 |
| Rankine | 0 | 460 | 492 | 558.6 | 672 |

**Fig. 1-1.** Linear relationship between gas molecular activity, or pressure, and temperature. Comparable readings of the four scales are indicated for five temperature points.

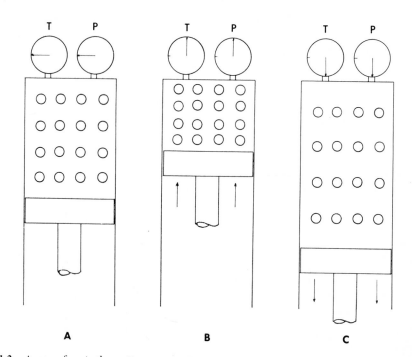

**Fig. 1-2.** A mass of gas in the resting state exerts a given pressure at a given temperature, in cylinder **A.** In **B,** as the piston compresses the gas, the molecules are crowded closer together, and the increased energy of molecular collisions is reflected in a rise of both temperature and pressure. Conversely, retraction of the piston in **C** allows the gas to expand, and the temperature and pressure drop as molecular interaction decreases.

**Rankine scale**

Used frequently in engineering but rarely in medical science, the Rankine scale is based on Fahrenheit units. Since $-273°$ C $= -460°$ F (refer to formulas to convert between Celsius and Fahrenheit scales), then $0°$ R $= -460°$ F, and $°R = °F + 460$. Fig. 1-1 is a scalar representation of the relation between gaseous kinetic activity, or pressure, and five commonly used temperatures of the four related scales.

Because of the relatively great distances between molecules, gases possess the quality of *compressibility*. When pressure is exerted on a gas, the molecules can be brought closer together as their intervening spaces are narrowed. Conversely, if the container of a volume of gas enlarges, the gas therein *expands* to accommodate the new volume, and its molecules range further apart. Fig. 1-2 illustrates the relationship between compression and expansion of a given mass of gas molecules and corresponding temperature and pressure changes. Because the tremendous energy of molecular collision is expended as heat, compression of a gas produces *heat* as well as a buildup of pressure among the molecules. As compression brings the molecules closer together, the frequency of collisions increases, and both heat and pressure increase. Thus the heat of compression may be considered as a means of dissipating the great increase in kinetic energy that accompanies compression. It should be apparent that expansion of a gas produces a drop in temperature as molecular collision frequency decreases. Cooling of expansion is utilized in refrigerating systems and is part of the natural phenomenon of cooling through expansion of large air masses.

## MOLAR VOLUME OF GASES

One of the major principles of physics and chemistry is *Avogadro's law* (Count Amadeo Avogadro, 1776-1856), which tells us that equal volumes of all gases at the same temperature and pressure contain the same number of molecules or, conversely, that at constant temperature and pressure equal numbers of molecules of all gases occupy the same volume. Further, it has been established that the weights of all atoms in grams corresponding to their atomic weights, the weights of all molecules in grams corresponding to their molecular weights, and the weights of ions of all nonmolecular compounds in grams corresponding to the formula weights of the compounds always contain the same number of their respective particles, $6.02 \times 10^{23}$. This is known as *Avogadro's number*. Although these quantities are often referred to as "gram atomic weights," "gram molecular weights," and "gram formula weights," they are each technically known as a *mole*. To put it another way, any quantity of matter that contains $6.02 \times 10^{23}$ atoms, molecules, or ions is called a mole. Later we will discuss physiologically active substances in concentrations so small that it will be more convenient to refer to them in terms of *thousandths of a mole*, or *millimole (mM)*. Just as moles are the weights of substances in grams equal to atomic weights (gaw), molecular weights (gmw), or formula weights (gfw), so are millimoles the weights of substances in milligrams equal to atomic weights (mgaw), molecular weights (mgmw), or formula weights (mgfw).

The volume occupied by one mole of a gas (1 gram molecular weight; $6.02 \times 10^{23}$ molecules) is the *molar volume*. It is important because it will allow us to calculate

**Table 1-1.** *Molar volume of selected gases under standard conditions**

| Gas | Symbol | Molar volume in liters |
|---|---|---|
| "Ideal gas" | | 22.414 |
| Ammonia | $NH_3$ | 22.094 |
| Carbon dioxide | $CO_2$ | 22.262 |
| Carbon monoxide | CO | 22.402 |
| Chlorine | $Cl_2$ | 22.063 |
| Helium | He | 22.426 |
| Hydrogen | $H_2$ | 22.430 |
| Hydrogen chloride | HCl | 22.248 |
| Nitrogen | $N_2$ | 22.402 |
| Oxygen | $O_2$ | 22.393 |
| Sulfur dioxide | $SO_2$ | 21.888 |

*Modified from Pimental, G. C., editor: Chemistry, an experimental science, San Francisco, 1963, W. H. Freeman Co., Publishers.

densities of gases and gas mixtures and to convert values for dissolved gases from volumes percent to moles per liter, a topic to be considered in some detail later. It is customary, for the sake of uniformity in comparing values, to measure molar volumes under what are termed *standard conditions,* a temperature of 0° C and an ambient pressure of 1 atmosphere. This is an artificial situation, however, since we do not ordinarily handle gases in the difficult environment of zero degree Celsius. When molar volumes are measured under common ambient conditions, then calculated to what they would be at standard (a technique known as "correcting a gas volume," which we will discuss shortly), we find that the natural intermolecular behavior of each gas causes its molar volume to deviate from the universal low pressure value. Table 1-1 compares molar volumes of several gases corrected from ambient to standard or measured directly at standard conditions.

If the student refers to the subject of molar gas volumes in the average chemistry textbook, he will probably find only the value 22.4 $\ell$/mole given for all gases. Actually, for most purposes this is usually adequate, and we see in Table 1-1 that it is representative of the molar volumes of oxygen, nitrogen, and carbon monoxide, gases with which we will be concerned as we continue our study. Even carbon dioxide, a most important respiratory gas, has a value rounded off to 22.3 $\ell$/mole, close to the universal normal. As a summary and general statement let us say that under standard conditions of a temperature of 0° C and a pressure of 1 atm, moles of all gases occupy *22.4 liters.* In this text the only exception will be found in a calculation involving carbon dioxide (p. 136), where the molar volume used for that gas is the more accurate one of *22.3 liters.*

## DENSITY OF GASES

Before considering the density of gases specifically, we will need some definitions. We must learn the relationship between the widely used physical terms *mass, weight,* and *density.* The word *mass* refers to the substance of an object, the quantity of matter it contains, and the number and nature of its molecules, and is characterized by

**Table 1-2.** *Examples of gas densities (D) under standard conditions*

$$D\ O_2 = \frac{gmw}{22.4} = \frac{32}{22.4} = 1.43\ g/\ell \qquad\qquad D\ He\ = \frac{gmw}{22.4} = \frac{4}{22.4} = 0.1785\ g/\ell$$

$$D\ N_2 = \frac{gmw}{22.4} = \frac{28}{22.4} = 1.25\ g/\ell \qquad\qquad D\ CO_2 = \frac{gmw}{22.4} = \frac{44}{22.4} = 1.965\ g/\ell$$

having inertia and by being subject to the pull of gravity. *Weight* is the gravitational pull of the earth upon a body; thus the greater the mass, the greater the weight. Mass is thereby proportional to weight and is measured in arbitrary units as weight, against such standards as the kilogram and the pound. It should be noted that weight varies with the position of mass relative to the surface of the earth, decreasing both toward the earth's center and away from its surface. The *inertia* of a body, that quality of mass which requires force to start it in motion from a resting state or to change its velocity once in motion, remains unchanged no matter where it is located.

*Density* may be defined as the amount of mass per unit volume of a body, the concentration of its molecules, and is usually employed as *weight density.* Density is thus the *weight of a body per unit volume* and in our field of interest is most often described in grams per cubic centimeter for solids and liquids, and grams per liter for gases. Other units, such as pounds per cubic foot, can also be used. A mass weighing 15 g and measuring 3 cc has a density of 5 g/cc. A ton of feathers and a ton of bricks weigh the same, but the obvious difference in the volumes of similar weights of these substances makes for widely differing densities. *Specific gravity* is a variation of density measurement whereby the density of solids and liquids is calibrated against the density of water used as a standard of unity, and gases against oxygen or hydrogen. A liquid with specific gravity of 1.5, for example, has a density half again as great as that of water. Specific gravity values of gases play a negligible role in pulmonary physiology, whereas gas densities are of great importance.

Since density equals weight divided by volume, the density of any gas can readily be calculated by dividing its *gram molecular weight* by the universal molar volume of 22.4 liters. The quotient is expressed as *grams per liter.* Examples of gas densities are shown in Table 1-2.

Densities of gas mixtures are easily calculated if the percentage composition of the mixture is known. Given the following mixed gases:

Gas A = 10%
Gas B = 60%
Gas C = 30%

$$D = \frac{(0.10 \times gmw\ A) + (0.60 \times gmw\ B) + (0.30 \times gmw\ C)}{22.4}$$

Calculate the density of a mixture of 30% hydrogen bromide (HBr) and 70% ethylene ($C_2H_4$):

$$D = \frac{(0.3 \times 81) + (0.7 \times 28)}{22.4} = \frac{43.9}{22.4} = 1.955\ g/\ell$$

*Exercise 1-1.* Calculate densities of the following, rounding off at three decimal places:

(a) $C_2H_2$ (acetylene)  
(b) $NH_3$ (ammonia)  
(c) $SiF_4$ (silicon fluoride)  
(d) CO (carbon monoxide)  
(e) $SO_2$ (sulfur dioxide)  

(f) 5% $CO_2$ + 95% $O_2$  
(g) 80% He + 20% $O_2$  
(h) 70% He + 30% $O_2$  
(i) 25% $CH_4$ + 75% $C_4H_{10}$  
(j) 3% $SO_2$ + 15% $N_2$ + 82% $O_2$  

## COMPOSITION OF THE ATMOSPHERE

The atmosphere upon which we, as oxygen-breathing creatures, are completely dependent is a mixture of many gases plus water vapor. The elements composing the atmosphere, with the exception of water vapor, which will be discussed separately later, have the approximate concentrations shown in Table 1-3.

The atmosphere is divided into two major segments, three subsegments, and several layers, each with certain physical and/or chemical properties,[4] outlined in Table 1-4:

1. The first major segment is the *inner atmosphere*, extending from the earth's surface to an altitude of about 600 miles; it is composed of the following subsegments called spheres:

   a. The *troposphere* extends from the earth's surface to an outer border called the tropopause, an average distance of some 8 miles up but varying with the latitude of the earth. It is higher over the equator than over the poles.

**Table 1-3.** *Approximate composition of the atmosphere*

| Element | Percent | |
|---|---|---|
| Nitrogen ($N_2$) | 78.08 | |
| Oxygen ($O_2$) | 20.95 | 99.99% |
| Argon (Ar) | 0.93 | |
| Carbon dioxide ($CO_2$) | 0.03 | |
| Neon (Ne) | $1.8 \times 10^{-3}$ | |
| Helium (He) | $5.0 \times 10^{-4}$ | |
| Krypton (Kr) | $1.0 \times 10^{-4}$ | |
| Hydrogen ($H_2$) | $1.0 \times 10^{-4}$ | 0.01% |
| Xenon (Xe) | $1.0 \times 10^{-5}$ | |
| Ozone ($O_3$) | $1.0 \times 10^{-5}$ | |
| Radon (Rn) | $6.0 \times 10^{-18}$ | |

**Table 1-4.** *Summary of atmospheric divisions*

| Atmosphere | Strata | Approximate height in miles |
|---|---|---|
| Free space | | Above 1200 |
| Outer | Exosphere | 600-1200 |
| | Ionosphere | 50-600 |
| | Stratosphere | 8-50 |
| Inner | Troposphere | 0-8 |

The troposphere is characterized by decreasing temperatures with altitude, reaching a low of approximately $-55°$ C ($-67°$ F), and has much turbulence.

b. The *stratosphere* continues from 8 to about 50 miles above the earth. The first layer of the stratosphere, from 8 to 15 miles up, is one of constant temperature around $-55°$ C ($-67°$ F) and has little turbulence. The next layer, from 15 to 30 miles, shows an increase in temperature, reaching a high of $10°$ C ($50°$ F). The third and last layer of the stratosphere, from 30 to 50 miles, has a sharp temperature drop to $-72°$ C ($-100°$ F), and there is a return of turbulence. At approximately 50 miles of altitude the stratopause separates the stratosphere from the next sphere.

c. The *ionosphere* reaches from a distance of 50 miles outward to a distance of 600 miles. Here there are several layers of ions, resulting from photochemical reactions between solar ultraviolet radiation and atmospheric molecules. The ionosphere is important as a reflector for the electromagnetic waves of radio communication. Temperatures in this sphere soar up to $2000°$ C ($3600°$ F), but because the density of the air molecules is so low in this region, such temperatures have little meaning in our usual concept of temperature. As with the other spheres, a boundary called the ionopause delineates the end of the ionosphere.

2. The second major segment is the outer atmosphere, which is also called the *exosphere*. This region extends from the 600-mile limit to about 1200 miles from earth, where it blends with the vacuum of *free space*. It is a marginal area where molecular collisions become progressively more rare.

The gravitational pull of the earth on atmospheric gas molecules produces the greatest density of molecules close to its surface, a density that decreases steadily outward to the vacuum of free space. It is speculated, however, that despite decreasing density, the percentage composition of the atmosphere, as described earlier, remains fairly constant to a height of at least some *60 miles*. Beyond this limit, with a decrease in mass air movement to keep the gases well mixed, there is a separation of the elements on the basis of their molecular weights. This phenomenon, called diffusion separation, disrupts the composition of the air as we know it on earth.

## MEASUREMENT OF AIR PRESSURE

In cardiopulmonary physiology and therapy of cardiopulmonary diseases, we are constantly dealing with the principles of gas pressure, and it is vitally important that the student clearly understand this aspect of gas physics. Pressure, in any context, is defined as a *force* applied to a specific *surface area*. For our purposes such force is usually expressed as grams per square centimeter ($g/cm^2$) or pounds per square inch ($lb/in^2$) (psi). The force exerted by gases is a result of their kinetic molecular bombardment already discussed, and in a mixture of gases such as air this force is the sum of molecular activity of all the constituent gases. If we visualize the atmospheric mantle enveloping the earth, described above, we can understand that the molecular activity of atmospheric gases will exert a force against the surface of the earth. To view it another way, we can see that the many miles of atmosphere rest upon the earth as an object rests upon a table, exerting a force of pressure on the earth's surface. It is of physiologic as well as meteorologic importance to be able to measure the force exerted by the air upon the earth.

Air pressure is measured indirectly by means of a barometer (*baros*, Greek, "weight"; *metron*, "measure"). Basically, a barometer consists of an evacuated glass tube approximately 37 inches tall with an inside diameter of 0.25 inch, closed at the top, and with its lower end immersed in a reservoir of mercury in a flexible container. The pressure of the atmosphere on the mercury reservoir forces the mercury up the vacuum tube, a distance above the reservoir surface relative to the atmospheric force, and the height of the column of mercury in the glass tube is measured in both inches and centimeters (Fig. 1-3). This procedure balances the pressure of the atmosphere against a column of mercury in a vacuum, and if the weight per surface area of the mercury can be calculated, this value will equal the pressure of the air.

A principle of physics tells us that the *pressure* exerted by a column of fluid is equal to the height of the column times the density of the fluid. Thus:

(1)  Pressure (P) in g/cm² = Height in cm × Density in g/cm³

$$P = cm \times \frac{g}{cm^3}$$

$$= g/cm^2$$

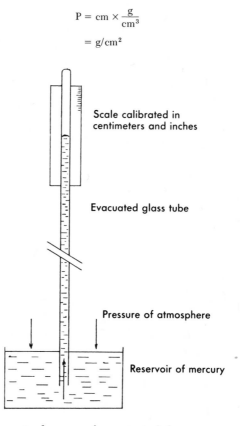

Scale calibrated in centimeters and inches

Evacuated glass tube

Pressure of atmosphere

Reservoir of mercury

**Fig. 1-3.**  The major components of a mercury barometer include a mercury reservoir, into which is inverted the open end of an evacuated glass tube, and a scale, by which the height of the mercury column can be read in inches and centimeters above the surface of the reservoir. The atmospheric pressure, acting on the surface of the mercury reservoir, is balanced by the weight of the column of mercury in the tube.

or

(2) Pressure (P) in lb/in$^2$ = Height in inches × Density in lb/in$^3$

$$P = \text{inches} \times \frac{\text{lb}}{\text{in}^3}$$

$$= \text{lb/in}^2$$

Because of shifting air currents and the mobility of huge masses of air, atmospheric density varies over different areas of the earth's surface and is reflected in constantly changing pressures as measured at the surface. Nevertheless, it has been demonstrated that at sea level the average atmospheric pressure will support a column of mercury 76 cm (760 mm), or 29.9 inches high. If we also know that mercury has a density of *13.6 g/cm*$^3$ (i.e., is 13.6 times as heavy as water), or *0.491 lb/in*$^3$, then we can easily calculate the atmospheric pressure ($P_B$) by the formulas just given.

(1) P in g/cm$^2$ = 76 × 13.6 = 1034 g/cm$^2$
(2) P in lb/in$^2$ = 29.9 × 0.491 = 14.7 lb/in$^2$

These two values, 1034 g/cm$^2$ and 14.7 lb/in$^2$, are used as standards and are called *1 atmosphere of pressure* (1 atm). It is evident, however, that for recording air pressure there is no need to calculate the actual g/cm$^2$ or lb/in$^2$ but only to record the height of the mercury column. Thus pressure might be reported as 77.2 cm (772 mm) or 30.4 inches Hg. In effect, this means that the atmospheric pressure is of such a magnitude that it is able to hold up a column of mercury 772 mm, or 30.4 inches, high. Their dynamic implications are exactly the same as actual force per surface area values of 1050 g/cm$^2$ and 14.9 lb/in$^2$.

Mercury is used as the agent for measuring the air pressure because its density is such that at ordinary pressures it assumes a height which is easy and convenient to read. It would be possible, although not practical, to construct a barometer of water. At 1 atm pressure (76 cm Hg, or 29.9 inches Hg) water, which is 13.6 times lighter than mercury, would rise to a height of *33.9 feet*. However, when very small pressures are being measured, expressing the pressure in terms of *centimeters of water* may be more convenient than in centimeters or millimeters of mercury. For example, a pressure of 2 cm Hg *(20 mm Hg)* is the same as 27.2 cm $H_2O$ (2 × 13.6). A pressure gauge calibrated in centimeters of water would be easier to read than one calibrated in centimeters or millimeters of mercury. In physiologic work the student will become accustomed to thinking and speaking in terms of both millimeters of mercury and centimeters of water. Inches of mercury or water are rarely used.

A device called an *aneroid barometer* is frequently used because of its convenient small size. It consists of a sealed evacuated metal box with a flexible, spring-supported top that responds to changes in atmospheric pressure, schematically illustrated in Fig. 1-4. Motion of its top is magnified by levers to activate a geared pointer, which indicates the pressure on a scale calibrated against a mercury barometer. Less precise than a mercury instrument, the aneroid barometer is practical for nonscientific or domestic use.

To complete the study, we should consider that method of measuring pressure which uses the *dyne*, frequently encountered in meteorology and physics. A dyne is defined as a unit of *force* that, when acting upon a 1 g mass, gives to the mass an *ac-*

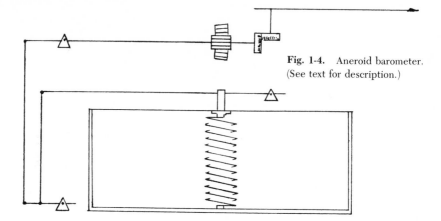

**Fig. 1-4.** Aneroid barometer. (See text for description.)

*celeration of 1 cm/sec/sec*, or *1 cm/sec²*. It is a fact of basic physics that a freely falling 1 g mass (under the influence of gravity) will accelerate, or continuously pick up speed, 980.7 cm/sec for every second it falls. It thus accelerates 980.7 cm/sec/sec, or 980.7 cm/sec². This can be thought of as a force of 1 g acting on itself (1 g force acting on 1 g mass), producing an acceleration of 980.7 cm/sec², and therefore an acceleration of 1 cm/sec² of a 1 g mass would be produced by a force of 1/980.7 of a gram. A dyne is thus equal to a force exerted by 1/980.7 g, or $1.02 \times 10^{-3}$ g, and this is practically the equivalent of a milligram. For easy visualization, then, a dyne can be considered as the amount of force that would be exerted by a *milligram weight*.

The meteorologist often expresses air pressure in dynes, using his own terms of *barye, bar,* and *millibar* (mb). To understand this system, note the following relationships:

$$1 \text{ atm} = \text{Height of Hg} \times \text{Density of Hg} = 76 \times 13.6 = 1034 \text{ g/cm}^2$$

or

$$1 \text{ atm} = 1034 \text{ g/cm}^2 \div 1.02 \times 10^{-3} \text{ (or } 1034 \times 980.7) = 1.014 \times 10^6 \text{ dynes/cm}^2$$

The meteorologic units of pressure are defined as follows:

| | |
|---|---|
| 1 barye | $= 1 \text{ dyne/cm}^2$ |
| 1 bar | $= 10^6 \text{ dynes/cm}^2 = 10^6 \text{ baryes}$ |
| 1 millibar (mb) | $= 10^3 \text{ dynes/cm}^2 = 10^{-3} \text{ bar} = 10^3 \text{ baryes}$ |

Thus 1 standard atmosphere of pressure = 1034 g/cm² = $1.014 \times 10^6$ dynes/cm² = 1.014 bars = 1014 millibars. In meteorology, atmospheric pressure is most frequently expressed as *millibars*. Millibars can be approximately converted to g/cm² by multiplying by 1.02. In summary, then, the pressure of 1 atm can be expressed as follows:

760 mm (76 cm) Hg
29.9 inches Hg
33.9 feet $H_2O$
1034 g/cm²
14.7 lb/in²
$1.014 \times 10^6$ dynes/cm²
1014 millibars

*Exercise 1-2.* Calculate the following pressures to the nearest tenth:

(a)  752 mm Hg, in $g/cm^2$
(b)  31.4 inches Hg, in $lb/in^2$
(c)  766 mm Hg, in $lb/in^2$
(d)  28.4 inches Hg, in $g/cm^2$
(e)  30.7 inches Hg, in feet $H_2O$

(f)  1022 $g/cm^2$, in mm Hg
(g)  15.2 $lb/in^2$, in inches Hg
(h)  15 cm $H_2O$, in mm Hg
(i)  1018 mb, in mm Hg
(j)  766 mm Hg, in mb

In cardiopulmonary physiology the effect of gases is frequently considered in terms of their partial pressures. *Dalton's law of partial pressures* tells us that the total pressure of a gaseous mixture is equal to the sum of the partial pressures of the constituent gases and that the partial pressure of each gas in the mixture is the pressure it would exert if it occupied the entire volume alone. Thus each gas contributes its share of the total pressure of a mixture in proportion to its percentage of the mixture. A gas that comprises 25% of a mixture of gases therefore will exert a partial pressure of 25% of the total pressure. To simplify an illustration, *dry* air may be considered to consist of only two major gases, $O_2$ at 21% and $N_2$ at 79%. Assuming a normal atmospheric pressure of 760 mm Hg, we can show individual partial pressures as follows:

$$P_B \text{ (dry)} = 760 \text{ mm Hg}$$
$$P_{O_2} = 760 \times 0.21 = 160 \text{ mm Hg}$$
$$P_{N_2} = 760 \times 0.79 = \underline{600 \text{ mm Hg}}$$
$$760 \text{ mm Hg}$$

## HYPOBARISM AND HYPERBARISM

*Hypobarism* and *hyperbarism* refer to air pressures significantly below and above, respectively, the sea level normal of 760 mm Hg, or 1034 $g/cm^2$. They are of great importance in man's excursions into outer space and into the sea. Indeed, one aspect of medicine under current investigation is that of hyperbaric medicine, in which the patient is subjected to the effects of several atmospheres of pressure.

It is obvious that with increasing altitude there is decreasing atmospheric pressure. At any point above the earth there is less air beyond it to exert pressure than there is on the earth's surface. Conversely, as one descends into the earth, there is a longer column of air exerting pressure on every square centimeter or square inch of surface area, demonstrated by a rising barometric pressure. Increasing pressure is most dramatically exemplified by descent into the sea. Here, water pressure rather than air pressure surrounds the immersed body; but when man invades deep water for a prolonged stay, he must surround himself with protective air at a pressure sufficient to balance that of the water. Because water is heavy and not compressible, a state of hyperbarism is reached much more quickly than is hypobarism above the earth. As a guide, each 33 feet of seawater represents a pressure of 1 atm.

Since we are ultimately interested in the amount of oxygen available to the body cells and will soon learn of the relation between this availability and the pressure of oxygen partial pressure, let us consider the effect of changing atmospheric pressure on oxygen partial pressure. Assume a concentration of oxygen in dry air of 20.95% (this is expressed as the $F_{O_2}$, or fractional concentration of $O_2$). At a $P_B$ of 760 mm Hg, the $P_{O_2} = 760 \times 0.2095 = 159$ mm Hg. Although the $F_{O_2}$ of air at 25,000 feet is still 0.2095, the $P_B$ is only 282 mm Hg and the $P_{O_2}$ is thus 59 mm Hg. The important point to note is that, although the $F_{O_2}$ at sea level and at 25,000 feet is the same, the kinetic activity of oxygen at the high altitude is equal to that of a mixture containing only 7.8% oxygen on the ground. In contrast, at a depth of 66 feet into the sea the weight of water exerts a pressure equal to that of 3 atm, or 2280 mm Hg. Air breathed by a diver at this depth would also be subjected to this same pressure, and its $P_{O_2}$ would be 20.95% of 2280, or 477 mm Hg.

Appendix 3 is a table that compares some of the characteristics of dry air at altitudes up to 300,000 feet and, when subjected to pressure at various depths in the sea, to a low of 297 feet. Sea level values are outlined at $0$, with altitudes above and sea depths below. The air density values $(g/\ell)$ assume a sea level temperature of 15° C, at which temperature air has a density of 1.250 $g/\ell$. The relationship between gas density and temperature will be described in detail later. The column *Atm* indicates the fraction or multiple of 1 atm pressure found at the various levels of altitude and depth; *%$O_2$ Equiv* refers to percentages of oxygen in breathing mixtures at sea level that would have oxygen partial pressures equal to those recorded in the $P_{O_2}$ column. The student is not expected to memorize this table but to study it so that he will understand the wide environmental variation to which the body is subjected when it ventures from the surface of the earth. Some of the principles illustrated in the table will have important clinical meaning later.

***Exercise 1-3.*** Assuming a $F_{O_2}$ of 0.2095, calculate the following to the nearest tenth:

(a) The $P_{O_2}$ of dry air at a $P_B$ of 752 mm Hg
(b) The $P_{O_2}$ of dry air at 1068 mb, in mm Hg
(c) The $P_B$ in mm Hg with a $P_{O_2}$ of 140 mm Hg
(d) The $P_{O_2}$ of dry air at 50 ft of seawater
(e) The seawater depth with an $O_2$ equivalent of 100%

## HUMIDITY

The discussions so far have been concerned only with dry gases, but it is now time to consider the important role played by water in gas physics. Invisible moisture is present in the atmosphere in the form of a vapor, assuming the state and characteristics of a gas, and is sometimes referred to as "molecular water" to distinguish it from visible gross "particulate water," such as mist. In this state water particles are subjected to the same kinetic activity as other gases and, like them, exert their own partial pressure, called *vapor pressure*. Atmospheric conditions vary the amount of water vapor in the air, but molecular water is constantly entering the air whenever air is exposed to a water surface.

Water enters the atmosphere by vaporization. A volume of water, like a gas, is in constant molecular activity. The energy of some molecules near the surface causes them to escape into the surrounding air, just as long as there is room for them in the air mixture. Thus a steady flow of air across the water surface accommodates a continuing flow of escaping water molecules, and *evaporation* progressively reduces the water reservoir (Fig. 1-5, *A*). Another principle of physics provides that heat is required to produce the change in state from liquid to gas that occurs in vaporization; this heat is taken from the air immediately adjacent to the water supply, thereby cooling the air. It is this cooling of vaporization that is responsible for the summer cooling effects of large bodies of water. However, should a cover be placed over the water volume, the air thus trapped over the surface will be filled with all the water vapor molecules it can hold and will be described as *saturated with water vapor*. At this point, vaporization does not stop, but a state of equilibrium is established, in which for every molecule escaping from the water another molecule returns to the reservoir from the overlying saturated air (Fig. 1-5, *B*).

Two factors that influence vaporization are temperature and pressure. Vaporization is directly related to temperature, and this relationship can be viewed from two different directions. First, the warmer the air the more vapor it can hold. In other words, the *capacity* of air for water vapor increases with temperature. Thus, if warm air passes over a water surface, its greater capacity will permit an increased escape of molecules from the water per unit of time, and evaporation will be hastened. Second, if heat is applied to the volume of water, the kinetic activity of water molecules will be increased and more will escape the surface per unit of time (Fig. 1-5, *C*). If, in this instance, a cover is placed over the heated water, the increased kinetic energy of escaping molecules will force more of them into the trapped air, increasing the saturation of the air with a greater number of molecules under an increased pressure (Fig. 1-5, *D*). Water content of air, or any gas, and its degree of saturation are thus a function of temperature. The influence of pressure on vaporization is an inverse one and is mediated through its action at the water surface. It is convenient to visualize vaporization as the escape of water molecules from the surface against the opposition of adjacent air molecules. As the surrounding air pressure increases or decreases, vaporization will be correspondingly retarded or augmented.

The amount of water in a given mass of air (or any gas) can be recorded in one of three ways.

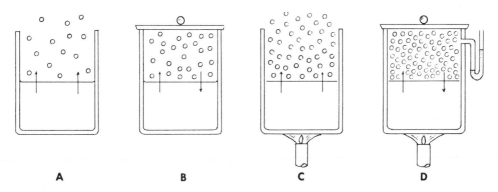

**A**          **B**          **C**          **D**

**Fig. 1-5.** The factors influencing vaporization of water are shown in these four sketches. In **A**, the kinetic activity of molecules at the surface carries the molecules into the surrounding air, and evaporation gradually reduces the reservoir. If the container is covered, as in **B**, vaporization does not stop but a state of equilibrium is reached when the air trapped in the container becomes saturated. At this point, water molecules leave and return to the reservoir in equal numbers. If the open container is heated, **C**, the increased molecular activity speeds the rate of vaporization. When the container is both covered and heated, **D**, more vapor will crowd into the trapped air, raising the vapor pressure as indicated by the attached manometer.

*Absolute humidity.* This is a measurement of the content or actual weight of water present in a given volume of air expressed in grams per cubic meter (or pounds per cubic foot or yard). Water may be physically extracted from a known air volume by an absorbing agent and weighed, or it may be computed by meteorologic data according to the techniques of the United States Weather Bureau.[5]

*Relative humidity.* Frequently used is a comparison of the *content* of water in a volume of air (absolute humidity) and the *amount* of water the air can hold at a given temperature if saturated, or its *capacity.* The ratio of *content/capacity* is the *relative humidity* (RH) and is reported as a percent. If air contains half the water, at a given temperature, that it has the capacity to contain, the RH equals 50%. Thus at room temperature, air has a capacity of approximately 18 g/m$^3$. If the water content is computed as 12 g/m$^3$, the air is thus 67% saturated and its RH equals 67%. Instruments called *hygrometers* allow direct and simple measurement of RH without the necessity of extracting and weighing water content of air samples.

*Water vapor pressure.* In contrast to other gases in a mixture, partial pressure of water vapor does not depend on its fractional concentration in the mixture but entirely upon temperature and relative humidity. Actual measurements of water vapor pressure in saturated air have been made over a wide range of temperature, and their values are available in handbooks of chemical data. The vapor pressure in gas less than saturated is the product of its saturated tension, at a given temperature, times the relative humidity, which must be specified. Thus at a stated temperature, vapor tension of a gas with 50% RH is one half that of saturated gas. It is important to understand that *for specific conditions of humidity and temperature, water vapor pressure is an absolute value, regardless of the concentrations of other gases present.* Therefore the partial pressure of other gases is calculated as the product of their fractional concentrations × [total atmospheric pressure − water vapor pressure (which must be computed first)]. In pulmonary physiology, for the most part, gases are considered either to be dry, with no water vapor pressure, or to be saturated. Appendix 4 is the reproduction of a part of a large table that lists the water vapor tensions of saturated gas within the usual physiologic range of our interest. The column to the right represents, at given temperatures, that portion of any atmospheric pressure due solely to water vapor. Thus at 25° C, in a gas saturated with water and regardless of other gas concentrations, 23.8 mm Hg of the total $P_B$ is due to the action of water molecules. If the gas were a mixture under an atmospheric pressure of 760 mm Hg, and the fractional concentration of oxygen were 0.21, the oxygen partial pressure would be 0.21 (760 − 23.8) = 154.6 mm Hg. This principle will be used extensively in the next section.

The *dew point* of air is that temperature at which the air becomes saturated with its contained water vapor. Imagine a water content of air sufficient to comprise a relative humidity of 90% at a given temperature. Should the air temperature drop, the RH with the same content of water will increase, since at lower temperatures the water *capacity* of the air lessens. A temperature can be reached at which the water content now fully saturates the air, with a RH of 100%; at this point excess water vapor, which the air cannot hold, begins to condense as visible droplets on small objects such as blades of grass. This temperature is the dew point. This phenomenon is frequently observed on cooling iced beverage glasses in warm humid weather. As the temperature of the glass drops, the air adjacent to the glass also cools and finally at the dew point water in the air begins to condense on the glass surface.

When an air mass near the earth's surface reaches its dew point, excess water often precipitates as very fine but visible water particles, so light they remain suspended in air as mist or fog. When larger air masses at higher altitudes are chilled by cold air currents, excess water usually falls out as rain or snow. Urban and industrial contamination of air has produced a mixture of fog and smoke or other vapors, called *smog*, which has important public health significance. Smogs may be held close to the ground by a natural phenomenon called a *temperature inversion*, when the air, instead of showing a progressive cooling from the ground up, contains a layer of warm air at heights of from 300 to 3000 feet. In such a state the air is very quiet, with little or no currents to carry away its contaminants.

To prepare for the specific use (in physiologic calculations) of the characteristics of pressure and humidity just covered, the student must understand some conventions adopted in the interest of uniformity. The following definitions should be learned:

1. Standard temperature and pressure (STP) means 0° C and 760 mm Hg.
2. Body temperature (BT) means 37° C.
3. Ambient temperature or pressure (A) means the existing environmental temperature or pressure (as opposed to standard).
4. Saturated gas (S) means a volume of gas with a relative humidity of 100% at a given temperature.
5. Dry gas (D) means a volume of gas with *no* vapor in it.

The various abbreviations are usually grouped, the following being typical examples frequently used:

1. STPD means a volume of dry gas, at a temperature of 0° C and a $P_B$ of 760 mm Hg.
2. BTPS means a volume of gas saturated with water vapor, at 37° C and the ambient environmental $P_B$.
3. ATPS means a volume of gas saturated with water vapor at ambient temperature (room temperature) and pressure.

When reporting data on gases for physiologic evaluation, we use the following general rules:

1. Volumes of gases as they exist in the lungs are recorded as BTPS.
2. Gases that undergo chemical reaction in the body, such as those measured in blood samples, are recorded as STPD.
3. If saturated gas volumes are to be used in physiologic calculation, they are first corrected to what their volumes would be if dry; then after the calculation are corrected back to the saturated value. Techniques of such manipulation will be learned in the following pages.

## GAS LAWS

The physics of the natural laws governing gas behavior is a study of considerable depth, invoking many principles and theories that are beyond the scope of our needs in respiratory therapy. Our prime concern will be consideration of the so-called *gas laws*, which describe the relationships among the interdependent variables of temperature, pressure, volume, and mass of gases. These relationships are often referred to as the *ideal behavior* of gases because they are based on theoretical principles that are valid under limited conditions. Fortunately, however, these limitations apply to the usual physiologic ranges with which we have to contend. The *real behavior* of gases concerns deviations from those relationships that we would expect on the basis of the gas laws, under conditions outside the physiologic range. We will first describe the principles and use of the ideal gas laws and then consider some real characteristics of gases when they are exposed to extremes of temperature and pressure.

The ideal gas laws are widely used in chemistry, physics, and pulmonary physiology and in the latter are most frequently concerned with changes in gas volumes brought about by changes in temperature and pressure. The role played by humidity, we will see, is mediated through its effect on pressure. Clinical pulmonary physiology is vitally concerned with various segments of lung volumes and what happens to these volumes with environmental or pathologic changes. It is essential that an effective technician, whether he works in a laboratory or in clinical medicine, understands the fundamentals of the gas laws. In the following definitions and applications of the laws, "temperature" *always* means *absolute temperature* (T, or K, as described earlier).

Before describing the ideal gas laws in the traditional manner, memorizing the eponyms by which they are known, let us fix in our minds some relationships that will allow us to figure out the laws regardless of how they are named. For our purposes at this time, we will sidestep such details as molecular structure and chemical activity and consider that a given sample of any gas is characterized only by the four properties of temperature (T), pressure (P), volume (V), and mass (n, for number of molecules, generally expressed as weight or density). What we want to know is this—if any two of these factors are kept unchanged, and the third is varied, what will happen to the fourth? At this point we need to digress briefly and review the concept of the arithmetical *proportionality constant*, which we will designate as k.

The expression $AB = k$ tells us that, in a given circumstance, all numerical values given to factor A when multiplied by all values given to factor B must equal the same product, k. Thus, if *k* is specified as 12, and we know that $A = 4$, then B must equal 3 so that $4 \times 3 = 12$. If we wish to increase factor A to 6, we must reduce B to 2. The factors in this instances are called *variables* and are said to be *inversely related* to one another; in order for their product to remain constant, if one varies, the other must be changed proportionately in the *opposite* direction. Similarly, if several factors are involved, such as $ABCD = k$, and two remain fixed, the other two can vary inversely with one another. Thus $2 \times 4 \times 6 \times 8 = k$ could change to $4 \times 4 \times 6 \times 4 = k$. We can derive the general rule that when two variables are factors whose product is a constant, these variables are inversely related. In contrast, if two variables are expressed as a ratio with a constant quotient, $A/B = k$, we see that a change in one will necessitate a proportionate change in the other in the *same* direction. These variables are thus *directly related*.

Finally, inversely and directly related variables can easily be combined to show their dependency on one another. It should be evident that $AB/CD = k$ means that A and B are inversely related, C and D are inversely related, but both A and B are directly related to C and D. These relationships can be clearly demonstrated by the student if he will assign numerical values to the variables, determine the k, and then alter any two, keeping the remaining pair unchanged. In all instances the product-quotient must remain fixed at its original value.

The four properties of gases, noted above, are considered to be variables, even mass, whose role as a variable will be clarified later. The relationships among them, in a given sample of gas under specific baseline conditions, can be compactly expressed as:

$$PV/Tn = k$$

It is as if the substance of a gas is made up of these parameters, and although the total quantity of the sample (k) cannot be changed, the component properties can vary among themselves. As in the example of the above paragraph, the relations among the gas properties are clear. Pressure and volume vary inversely; temperature and mass vary inversely; pressure and volume each varies directly with temperature and mass. Now we can look at three sets of interrelationships among the gas variables which are known as the gas laws, and we can see that they are based on the above ratio, in each case with the elimination of those properties that are specified as unchanged.

**Boyle's law.** If temperature (T) and mass (n) remain unchanged, volume (V) varies *inversely* with the pressure (P). This means that, at a constant temperature and mass, as increasing pressure is *applied to* a given volume of gas, the volume decreases. Obviously, there must be a limit to the shrinkage of the gas volume because the mass of gas cannot simply disappear as the pressure increases. Actually, the increments in volume reduction become smaller as the units of pressure increase, until a point is reached at which this reciprocal relationship between pressure and volume no longer exists. At this point the ideal behavior of the gas ceases, and physical changes in the characteristics of the matter of the gas occur, which will be described later as the real behavior referred to earlier. It is apparent that the converse response of a volume of gas will accompany a reduction in pressure applied to it. These inverse relationships can be expressed as $PV = k$, eliminating T and n, since they do not vary in this instance and thus do not influence the relationships.

**Charles' law.** If pressure (P) and mass (n) are kept unchanged, volume (V) varies *directly* with changes in the absolute temperature (T). This means that if a mass of gas is kept under a constant pressure, as the absolute temperature of the gas is increased or decreased, its volume will increase or decrease accordingly. Again, as in Boyle's law, the mass of gas cannot be cooled into nothingness, and at a certain point the ideal behavior ceases and other factors come into play. This direct relationship between temperature and volume can be expressed as $V/T = k$, since for the quotient to remain stable, if one value changes, the other must change proportionately in the same direction.

**Gay-Lussac's law.** If volume (V) and mass (n) remain fixed, the pressure (P) *exerted by* a gas varies *directly* with the absolute temperature (T) of the gas. This means that if the volume of a mass of gas is kept unchanged, as the absolute temperature of the gas is increased or decreased, its pressure will increase or decrease accordingly. The linear relationship in Fig. 1-1 shows that, theoretically, with no pressure exerted by a gas at $0°$ K, changes in pressure are proportional to changes in absolute temperature values and are expressed as $P/T = k$. As might be expected, this relation is valid only in the limited *ideal* range.

When the gas laws are put to practical use, as described in the section below, we will be concerned with changes in volume, pressure, and temperature in a given gas sample with a fixed number of molecules. Therefore, since n will not be a variable in these circumstances, it can be disregarded, and the three gas laws just defined can be combined into the single simplified expression:

$$PV/T = k$$

If the student remembers this one ratio, though he may forget which proper name goes with which law, he can easily visualize the relationship between any pair of variables when the third is fixed.

## COMBINED GAS LAWS

When gas is subjected to changes in P, V, T, and n, singly or in combination, the total product-quotient of PV/Tn remains unchanged. In effect, these variables represent the *matter* of the gas, which is neither increased nor decreased but, rather, "redistributed" among the variables. This can be stated as follows:

$$\frac{P_1 V_1}{T_1 n_1} = \frac{P_2 V_2}{T_2 n_2}$$

The subscript 1 indicates a *before* value, and 2 an *after* value. Thus the products and quotients of the gas variables before a change in one or more of them must be the same after.

In pulmonary physiology, most of the time we will wish to know how much change there will be in a gas volume if it is subjected to changes in pressure and/or temperature. Since the total mass of gas will not be affected, as noted above, the quantity n can be eliminated from the gas equation, but careful analysis of gas problems is necessary to determine whether such a shortened version of the equation can be used. When the equation is now written as

$$\frac{P_1 V_1}{T_1} = \frac{P_2 V_2}{T_2}$$

it is apparent that, knowing five of the six factors, we can calculate the sixth by simple algebraic rearrangement to equate the unknown with the known data. We will know the original volume ($V_1$), the original pressure ($P_1$), the original temperature ($T_1$); we will also know the new pressure ($P_2$) and the new temperature ($T_2$). We will then rearrange the equation so that our unknown, the new volume ($V_2$), will equal all of our known values. Thus:

$$V_2 = \frac{V_1 \times P_1 \times T_2}{P_2 \times T_1}$$

By putting the known values in their places in the equation and carrying out the indicated arithmetic, we can easily solve the equation. This procedure is called *correcting* a gas volume for changes in pressure and temperature.

This is the form of the *combined gas laws* that is the basis for most of the gas volume calculations, and it should be *learned* well, not by rote memory but through an understanding of what the equation means. If we examine the equation, we can see that the new or corrected gas volume ($V_2$) is a *proportion* of the original volume ($V_1$) according to changes in P and T. In fact, the equation as written actually demonstrates Boyle's law:

$$V_1 \times \frac{P_1}{P_2}$$

and Charles' law:

$$V_1 \times \frac{T_2}{T_1}$$

the two gas laws dealing with volume change. We know, from Boyle's law, that if pressure on a gas is increased, its volume will decrease. In such an instance, $P_2$ will be greater than $P_1$, and in the above equation, since $V_1$ will be multiplied by a fraction *less* than 1, $V_2$ will be reduced. The student can see that the converse is also true and can in a similar manner see how the combined gas laws also uphold Charles' law.

**Exercise 1-4.** Set up the combined gas laws to solve for the following:

(a) $P_2$, (b) $T_1$, (c) $V_1$, (d) $T_2$

## CORRECTION OF DRY GAS VOLUMES

The following technique is suggested for the student to use in all gas volume calculations to avoid mistakes of omission. When proficiency has been reached, short-cuts to suit individual needs can be employed.

**Problem 1.** Given 100 ml of dry gas measured at 37° C and 760 mm Hg $P_B$, what would be its volume at 60° C?

*Solution:*

$V_1 = 100$             $V_2 = ?$

$P_1 = 760$            $P_2 = 760$

$t_1 = 37$             $t_2 = 60$

$T_1 = 37 + 273 = 310$      $T_2 = 60 + 273 = 333$

$$V_2 = \frac{V_1 P_1 T_2}{P_2 T_1} = \frac{100 \times 760 \times 333}{760 \times 310} = 107.4 \text{ ml}$$

(*Note:* Since $P_1 = P_2$, both *could* have been eliminated from the equation, but it is better for the beginner to include all data.)

**Problem 2.** Given 100 ml of dry gas measured at 37° C and 760 mm Hg $P_B$, what would be its volume at 800 mm Hg?

*Solution:*

$V_1 = 100$             $V_2 = ?$

$P_1 = 760$            $P_2 = 800$

$t_1 = 37$             $t_2 = 37$

$T_1 = 37 + 273 = 310$      $T_2 = 37 + 273 = 310$

$$V_2 = \frac{V_1 P_1 T_2}{P_2 T_1} = \frac{100 \times 760 \times 310}{800 \times 310} = 95 \text{ ml}$$

**Problem 3.** Given 100 ml of dry gas at 37° C and 760 mm Hg, what would be its volume at 60° C and 800 mm Hg?

*Solution:*

$$V_1 = 100 \qquad\qquad V_2 = ?$$
$$P_1 = 760 \qquad\qquad P_2 = 800$$
$$t_1 = 37 \qquad\qquad t_2 = 60$$
$$T_1 = 310 \qquad\qquad T_2 = 333$$

$$V_2 = \frac{V_1 P_1 T_2}{P_2 T_1} = \frac{100 \times 760 \times 333}{800 \times 310} = 102 \text{ ml}$$

**Exercise 1-5.** Convert the following dry gas volumes, as indicated (to 3 digits):

(a) 150 ml at 25° C and 752 mm Hg, to 0° C
(b) 2.5 liters at 18° C and 762 mm Hg, to 748 mm Hg
(c) 325 ml at 20° C and 770 mm Hg, to 37° C and 760 mm Hg
(d) 22.4 liters at 15° C and 730 mm Hg, to 5° C and 755 mm Hg
(e) 95 ml at 28° C and 784 mm Hg, to 20° C and 768 mm Hg

## CORRECTION OF GAS VOLUMES CONTAINING WATER VAPOR

Most physiologic gas volume calculations involve gases saturated with water vapor and require correction of volumes from the saturated to the dry state, or the reverse. The student will find it helpful to keep in mind that, since water vapor is in essence a space-occupying gas in a mixture of gases, its removal from a gas volume will shrink the volume and its addition will increase the volume. Thus, in the examples and exercises to follow, whenever a volume of gas saturated with water vapor is to have its volume calculated to what it would be in the dry state (corrected from saturated to dry), the dry volume will be smaller, *unless* other conditions of pressure and temperature counteract the shrinkage. Conversely, correcting from dry to saturated will give a larger volume.

At a fixed temperature, if a gas sample is in a container permitting it to respond to ambient pressure, it reaches a static volume where the pressure it exerts exactly balances the ambient. Water vapor added to dry gas will have two effects. First, the increased number of molecules will obviously enlarge the volume until the total molecular kinetic activity again equilibrates with ambient. Second, because water vapor exerts a pressure that is dependent only on temperature and relative humidity, and is independent of other gases with which it mixes, the partial pressures of the other gases will be accordingly reduced to maintain parity with ambient.

The effect of moisture in gas volume calculations is mediated through the partial pressure it exerts at a given temperature and saturation, rather than its quantitative amount or fractional concentration, and it slightly modifies the application of Boyle's law. The relevance of Boyle's law to this situation can be understood if we view it as follows. The law tells us that a gas volume varies inversely with the ambient pressure applied to it. Let us imagine some water vapor being instantaneously added to a sample of dry gas, with the temperature remaining constant. Because of the added water molecules, the kinetic activity, and thus the pressure, of the now wet gas will momentarily exceed the ambient that is applied to it. The volume will expand until molecular activity and pressure of the larger number of molecules finally decrease to equilibrate with ambient. Just prior to the addition of vapor molecules, the dry gas is in equilibrium with ambient pressure, and thus, in volume correction data, the initial pressure to be used is the ambient. As soon as vapor molecules are added, the pressure of the gas goes up, and this has the same effect on gas volume as if the ambient pressure went down a like amount. Thus the final pressure affecting gas volume is the ambient *minus* the vapor pressure, and in conformity with Boyle's law, volume increases.

For convenience, we might refer to the effective pressure in the gas data tabulation as being corrected for water vapor pressure and designate it as $P_c$. Thus, $P_c = (P - P_{1H_2O}$ at t), where P is the total effective pressure, t the temperature of the gas, and $P_{H_2O}$ the vapor pressure at t as listed in the right column of the table in Appendix 4, if we are dealing with gas saturated with water vapor. Boyle's law can now be expressed as follows:

$$V_2 = \frac{V_1 \times (P_1 - P_{1H_2O} \text{ at } t_1)}{(P_2 - P_{2H_2O} \text{ at } t_2)} = \frac{V_1 \times P_{1c}}{P_{2c}}$$

Let us assume that $V_1$ is dry gas, $V_2$ is water-saturated gas, and pressure and temperature remain unchanged. Because $V_1$ is dry, there will be no $P_{H_2O}$ to subtract from $P_1$. Thus $P_{1c}$ will be unchanged from $P_1$ and will be larger than $P_{2c}$, making $V_2$ larger than $V_1$. This is *expected*, since it is the same as adding moisture to a volume of gas, then calculating the new volume. Use of the *corrected pressure* in Boyle's law simultaneously adjusts for changes in both pressure and humidity. The format for arranging data as demonstrated above will be modified a bit to accommodate water vapor effect:

| | | | | |
|---|---|---|---|---|
| $V_1$ | = initial volume | | $V_2$ | = final volume |
| $P_1$ | = initial pressure | | $P_2$ | = final pressure |
| t | = initial temperature | | $t_2$ | = final temperature |
| $P_{1H_2O}$ | = partial pressure of water vapor at $t_1$ | | $P_{2H_2O}$ | = partial pressure of water vapor at $t_2$ |
| $P_{1c}$ | = corrected initial pressure | | $P_{2c}$ | = corrected final pressure |
| | = $P_1 - P_{1H_2O}$ | | | = $P_2 - P_{2H_2O}$ |
| $T_1$ | = $t_1 + 273$ | | $T_2$ | = $t_2 + 273$ |

$$V_2 = \frac{V_1 \times P_{1c} \times T_2}{P_{2c} \times T_1}$$

The following examples illustrate the ease with which the combined gas laws can make corrections for changes in any or all of the variables of pressure, temperature, and water vapor.

**Problem 1.** Given 100 ml of saturated gas at 760 mm Hg and 25° C, what would be its volume if dry at the same pressure and temperature?

*Solution:*

| | | | | |
|---|---|---|---|---|
| $V_1$ | = 100 | | $V_2$ | = ? |
| $P_1$ | = 760 | | $P_2$ | = 760 |
| $t_1$ | = 25 | | $t_2$ | = 25 |
| $P_{1H_2O}$ | = 23.8 | | $P_{2H_2O}$ | = 0 |
| $P_{1c}$ | = 736.2 | | $P_{2c}$ | = 760 |
| $T_1$ | = 298 | | $T_2$ | = 298 |

$$V_2 = \frac{V_1 P_{1c} T_2}{P_{2c} T_1} = \frac{100 \times 736.2 \times 298}{760 \times 298} = 96.8 \text{ ml}$$

**Problem 2.** Given 100 ml of saturated gas at 760 mm Hg and 25° C, what would be its volume saturated at the same pressure and 37° C?

*Solution:*

$$
\begin{array}{llll}
V_1 & = 100 & V_2 & = ? \\
P_1 & = 760 & P_2 & = 760 \\
t_1 & = 25 & t_2 & = 37 \\
P_{1H_2O} & = 23.8 & P_{2H_2O} & = 47 \\
P_{1c} & = 736.2 & P_{2c} & = 713 \\
T_1 & = 298 & T_2 & = 310
\end{array}
$$

$$
V_2 = \frac{V_1 P_{1c} T_2}{P_{2c} T_1} = \frac{100 \times 736.2 \times 310}{713 \times 298} = 107.5 \text{ ml}
$$

**Problem 3.** Given 100 ml of saturated gas at 754 mm Hg and 20° C, what would be its volume as dry gas at 764 mm Hg and 37° C?

*Solution:*

$$
\begin{array}{llll}
V_1 & = 100 & V_2 & = ? \\
P_1 & = 754 & P_2 & = 764 \\
t_1 & = 20 & t_2 & = 37 \\
P_{1H_2O} & = 17.5 & P_{2H_2O} & = 0 \\
P_{1c} & = 736.5 & P_{2c} & = 764 \\
T_1 & = 293 & T_2 & = 310
\end{array}
$$

$$
V_2 = \frac{V_1 P_{1c} T_2}{P_{2c} T_1} = \frac{100 \times 736.5 \times 310}{764 \times 293} = 102.1 \text{ ml}
$$

**Problem 4.** Given 100 ml of saturated gas at 754 mm Hg and 20° C, what would be its volume saturated at 764 mm Hg and 37° C?

*Solution:*

$$
\begin{array}{llll}
V_1 & = 100 & V_2 & = ? \\
P_1 & = 754 & P_2 & = 764 \\
t_1 & = 20 & t_2 & = 37 \\
P_{1H_2O} & = 17.5 & P_{2H_2O} & = 47 \\
P_{1c} & = 736.5 & P_{2c} & = 717 \\
T_1 & = 293 & T_2 & = 310
\end{array}
$$

$$
V_2 = \frac{V_1 P_{1c} T_2}{P_{2c} T_1} = \frac{100 \times 736.5 \times 310}{717 \times 293} = 108.5 \text{ ml}
$$

**Exercise 1-6.** Correct the following gas volumes to four digits:

(a) 250 ml, saturated at 750 mm Hg and 20° C, to saturated at 764 mm Hg and 25° C
(b) 1.75 liters, dry at 752 mm Hg and 26° C, to saturated at 770 mm Hg and 33° C
(c) 58 ml, saturated at 748 mm Hg and 21° C, to dry at 730 mm Hg and 30° C
(d) 430 ml BTPS at 766 mm Hg, to STPD
(e) 2.28 liters, saturated at 1006 mb and 72° F, to saturated at 1022 mb and 90° F

## CORRECTION OF BAROMETRIC READING

Because the barometer is composed of brass, it reacts by expansion and contraction to ambient temperature changes. Even more important, the column of mercury not only responds to atmospheric pressure changes but, like a large thermometer, is significantly affected by temperature. Thus, when we read the mercury level of a barometer, we see the effects of both pressure and temperature. For accuracy in assessing the effects of pressure on gas volume, we must correct our *observed* reading for changes in the mercury column due to temperature. A formula based upon expansion coefficients of brass and mercury at given temperatures is the basis for a table of correction factors prepared by the United States Weather Bureau and reproduced in part in Appendix 5 for the pressures and temperatures most frequently encountered. The table values are *subtracted* from the observed reading. At 30° C an observed barometric reading of 750 mm Hg would be corrected for temperature by subtracting 3.66 from 750 for a corrected reading of 746.34, rounded off usually to 746.3 or even 746, depending upon the degree of accuracy desired. For $P_B$'s between those tabulated, interpolation is used. Thus, the correction factor for 764 mm Hg at 25° C is 3.09 (factor for 760 mm Hg) + 0.4 of the difference between 3.09 and 3.13 (factor for 770 mm Hg). Since $0.4(3.13 - 3.09) = 0.4 \times 0.04$, or 0.016, the final factor is $3.09 + 0.016$, or 3.106, rounded off to 3.11. From a practical point of view, under usual circumstances the only temperature variations affecting barometric reading are those of the room housing the barometer. Since it is unlikely that the temperature of the average laboratory would exceed seasonal changes of 60° to 80° F (16° to 27° C), or the $P_B$ range 740 to 780 mm Hg, the correction factors would usually be between 1.9 and 3.4.

When given a problem in gas volume correction, the student may assume the barometric value to be a *corrected* one unless the data specify an *observed* reading. In fact, by custom in any circumstance in which $P_B$ is not specified, it is taken to be 760 mm Hg. However, suppose we are asked to correct a volume of a patient's exhaled air, at an *observed* $P_B$ of 753 mm Hg, with a room temperature of 21° C, to STPD. Our *first* step is to correct the observed pressure for room temperature effect and to record the corrected pressure as $P_1$ in our listed data. The 760 mm Hg of the STPD needs no correction because it is a *stated* value, not observed. Thus our data would read:

| | | | | |
|---|---|---|---|---|
| $V_1$ | = | | $V_2$ | = |
| $P_1$ | = 750.4 | | $P_2$ | = 760 |
| $t_1$ | = 21 | | $t_2$ | = 0 |
| $P_{1H_2O}$ | = 18.7 | | $P_{2H_2O}$ | = 0 |
| $P_{1c}$ | = 731.7 | | $P_{2c}$ | = 760 |
| $T_1$ | = 294 | | $T_2$ | = 273 |

On the other hand, to make a somewhat exaggerated example, if a volume of gas were collected under one set of observed $P_B$ and ambient temperature and we were asked to calculate its volume at a different observed $P_B$ and temperature, both $P_1$ and $P_2$ would be corrected values for their respective temperatures. If the principles of correction are understood, the student can reason out the proper calculation procedure for any combination of data, no matter how bizarre.

***Exercise 1-7.*** Set up the final formula to correct $V_1$ to $V_2$ according to the following conditions of observed pressures (correct $P_B$ to one decimal place):

(a) Dry, 730 mm Hg, 30° C to saturated, 730 mm Hg, 30° C
(b) Saturated, 750 mm Hg, 24° C to saturated, 760 mm Hg, 24° C
(c) Saturated, 744 mm Hg, 20° C to dry, 744 mm Hg, 25° C
(d) Dry, 756 mm Hg, 15° C to saturated 738 mm Hg, 22° C
(e) Dry, 766 mm Hg, 24° C to dry, 738 mm Hg, 30° C

## USE OF FACTORS IN GAS VOLUME CALCULATIONS

Factors are constant values, such as the product-quotients of data that are always present in a certain calculation. Thus, instead of doing the individual arithmetic for each calculation, we use prepared factors. In gas volume determinations, three frequently encountered computations are (1) correction from ATPS to BTPS, (2) correction from ATPS to STPD, and (3) correction from STPD to BTPS. For each of these there are factors available that materially reduce the amount of arithmetic needed, and because the student should understand the derivation of these short-cut agents, they will be described individually.

*Factors to correct volumes from ATPS to BTPS.* The values in the first column of Appendix 4, when multiplied by $V_1$, will in one simple step correct a gas volume from ATPS to BTPS. Actually, the factors give a very close approximation because, as the footnote to the table explains, all the factors are based on a $P_B$ of 760 mm Hg. Although the answer obtained using a factor might differ from one derived from detailed calculations, the discrepancy is usually small. Derivation of the factors can be illustrated by an example. Let us correct a volume of gas $(V_1)$ saturated at 760 mm Hg and 25° C, to saturated at 760 mm Hg and 37° C (ATPS to BTPS).

$$
\begin{array}{ll}
V_1 \;= & \qquad V_2 \;= \\
P_1 \;= 760 & \qquad P_2 \;= 760 \\
t_1 \;= 25 & \qquad t_2 \;= 37 \\
P_{1H_2O} = 23.8 & \qquad P_{2H_2O} = 47 \\
P_{1c} \;= 736.2 & \qquad P_{2c} \;= 713 \\
T_1 \;= 298 & \qquad T_2 \;= 310 \\
\end{array}
$$

$$
V_2 \;= \frac{V_1 P_{1c} T_2}{P_{2c} T_1} = \frac{V_1 \times 736.2 \times 310}{713 \times 298} = V_1 \times 1.075
$$

Note that the product-quotient for the pressure, temperature, and humidity corrections equals 1.075, the same value found in Appendix 4 corresponding to a gas temperature of 25° C. The student is urged to work out one or two more of these factors in a similar manner, to fix the principle in his mind. If, in the example above, $P_1$ were 752 mm Hg and $P_2$ were 758 mm Hg and the calculation were done by the detailed method, the value by which $V_1$ would be multiplied would be *1.066*. The decision concerning whether to sacrifice accuracy for expediency is usually determined by each individual or laboratory according to needs and objectives.

*Factors to correct volumes from ATPS to STPD.* Factors of Appendix 6, when multiplied by $V_1$, will correct $V_1$ from ATPS to STPD. It is emphasized that the barometric readings of the left column are *observed* values, *not* corrected for temperature. In other words, to use this table, we must use the direct reading from the barometer, since the factors *include* temperature adjustment. Let us correct a saturated gas volume at an observed $P_B$ of 770 mm Hg and a room temperature of 20° C to dry gas at 760 mm Hg and 0° C. The first step is to correct 770 mm Hg for 20° C to 767.5 mm Hg. Our data are thus:

$$
\begin{array}{ll}
V_1 \;= & \qquad V_2 \;= \\
P_1 \;= 767.5 & \qquad P_2 \;= 760 \\
t_1 \;= 20 & \qquad t_2 \;= 0 \\
P_{1H_2O} = 17.5 & \qquad P_{2H_2O} = 0 \\
P_{1c} \;= 750 & \qquad P_{2c} \;= 760 \\
T_1 \;= 293 & \qquad T_2 \;= 273 \\
\end{array}
$$

$$
V_2 \;= \frac{V_1 P_{1c} T_2}{P_{2c} T_1} = \frac{V_1 \times 750 \times 273}{760 \times 293} = V_1 \times 0.919
$$

The tabular factor for 770 mm Hg and 20° C is likewise 0.919.

***Factors to correct volumes from STPD to BTPS.*** Factors for this conversion are given in Appendix 7. With ambient pressure as the only variable to consider, the factor for correction to an ambient pressure of 750 mm Hg is derived as follows:

$$
\begin{array}{ll}
V_1 \quad = & V_2 \quad = \\
P_1 \quad = 760 & P_2 \quad = 750 \\
t_1 \quad = \quad 0 & t_2 \quad = \quad 37 \\
P_{1H_2O} = \quad 0 & P_{2H_2O} = \quad 47 \\
P_{1c} \quad = 760 & P_{2c} \quad = 703 \\
T_1 \quad = 273 & T_2 \quad = 310
\end{array}
$$

$$
V_2 \quad = \frac{V_1 P_{1c} T_2}{P_{2c} T_1} = \frac{V_1 \times 760 \times 310}{703 \times 273} = V_1 \times 1.227
$$

The tabular factor for 750 mm Hg is likewise 1.227.

## CALCULATIONS INVOLVING WEIGHT AND DENSITY OF GAS

Gas problems dependent upon variations in weight and density of gases are frequently encountered in chemistry and physics, although rarely in pulmonary physiology. Still, the student should learn how to use the general gas laws equation to solve such problems. It was indicated earlier that the $n$ in the gas laws equation refers to numbers of gas molecules, representing gas weight or density. When analyzing a problem involving weight or density, the student will find it helpful to remember that at $P_B$ of 760 mm Hg and 273° K, 1 gmw of a gas occupies 22.4 liters. With a little practice he will learn how to combine his data to get the desired information. The following examples will illustrate the handling of a few simple, typical problems.

***Problem 1.*** If the density of oxygen is 1.43 g/$\ell$ at 0° C and 1 atm, what is its density at 20° C and 720 mm Hg? (*Note:* Although volume is not mentioned, it is implied in the use of the term *density*, g/$\ell$. Thus $V_1$ equals $V_2$ and need not be considered.)

*Solution:*

$$
\begin{array}{ll}
V_1 = & V_2 = \\
P_1 = 760 & P_2 = 720 \\
T_1 = 273 & T_2 = 293 \\
n_1 = \quad 1.43 \text{ g}/\ell & n_2 = ?\text{ g}/\ell
\end{array}
$$

$$
n_2 = \frac{n_1 \times P_2 \times T_1}{P_1 \times T_2} = \frac{1.43 \times 720 \times 273}{760 \times 293} = 1.26 \text{ g}/\ell
$$

***Problem 2.*** What volume will be occupied by 2.35 g of $SO_2$ at 25° C and 750 mm Hg? (*Note:* The *before* values will be the volume occupied by 1 gmw at STP to permit the setting of a ratio.)

*Solution:*

$$
\begin{array}{ll}
V_1 = \quad 22.4 \text{ liters} & V_2 = ? \text{ liters} \\
P_1 = 760 & P_2 = 750 \\
T_1 = 273 & T_2 = 298 \\
n_1 = 64 \text{ g} & n_2 = \quad 2.35 \text{ g}
\end{array}
$$

$$
V_2 = \frac{V_1 \times P_1 \times T_2 \times n_2}{P_2 \times T_1 \times n_1} = \frac{22.4 \times 760 \times 298 \times 2.35}{750 \times 273 \times 64} = 0.910 \text{ liter}
$$

***Problem 3.*** How many grams of air will a 500-liter tank hold if it is filled to 3 atm at 15° C? Assume the gmw of air to be 29. (*Note:* $n_1$ = density $\times$ 500 = [29/22.4] $\times$ 500 = 647 g)

*Solution:*

$$V_1 = 500 \text{ liters} \qquad\qquad V_2 = 500 \text{ liters}$$
$$P_1 = \quad 1 \qquad\qquad P_2 = \quad 3$$
$$T_1 = 273 \qquad\qquad T_2 = 288$$
$$n_1 = 647 \text{ g} \qquad\qquad n_2 = ? \text{ g}$$

$$n_2 = \frac{n_1 \times P_2 \times T_1}{P_1 \times T_2} = \frac{647 \times 3 \times 273}{1 \times 288} = 1840 \text{ g}$$

In the interest of economizing on time and space, a detailed description of the *molar gas constant* will not be undertaken here. It is a numerical value of the constant of the ratio $PV/nT = k$, where n is in number of moles of gas and V is 22.4 liters at 1 atm and 273° K. For respiratory physiologic use of the gas laws, the molar gas constant is less meaningful than is the tabular system explained on the preceding pages. Once the present technique is mastered, however, the student may find it of interest to study the molar constant and increase his breadth of knowledge of this aspect of physics.

## PROPERTIES OF GASES AT EXTREME TEMPERATURES AND PRESSURES

Having covered the ideal gas laws in some detail, we understand the theoretical response of gases to changes in pressure, volume, temperature, and density; we will now consider variations from such relationships as gases are subjected to both low temperatures and high pressures, revealing their *real* characteristics. This will prepare the student for his exposure to the commercially prepared gases with which he will treat patients.

We are familiar with the tremendous kinetic activity of gaseous molecules, a force that permits a mass of gas to distribute itself in an increasing volume of space or, lacking the freedom of mobility, to keep up a steady pressure in its restraint. Opposing the kinetic action of the molecules is another force, called *van der Waals force*, which consists of an attraction between the molecules, tending to draw them together. Although it is independent of temperature, the effectiveness of van der Waals forces is related to both temperature and pressure. For example, at a high temperature the increased kinetic molecular activity far overshadows the van der Waals energy, rendering the latter relatively impotent, whereas at very low temperatures the resulting decrease in kinetic action makes the molecules much more responsive to mutual attraction. By the same token, low pressures exerted on a gas permit the molecules to move freely of their own kinetic volition with little influence by attractive forces, in contrast to the molecular crowding of high pressures, which permits greater increase in the van der Waals effect. In addition to the attractive force between gas molecules, another factor that influences the relation between pressure and volume is attributed to the space occupied by the molecules themselves. Under moderate to low pressures exerted on a given container full of gas, the total mass of matter of the wide-ranging molecules is but a negligible fraction of the total volume of the gas. As the volume is reduced by increasing pressure, however, the resulting molecular density, which is not compressible, comprises a proportionately larger portion of the overall gas volume, disturbing the volume response to pressure predicted by the ideal gas laws.

We can summarize these observations by generalizing that at very low temperatures and/or very high pressures gases deviate in their behavioral patterns as predicted by the classical gas laws because of the influence of the van der Waals intermolecular attractive force and the volume of compressed gas molecules. Our purposes do not justify pursuing the details of such phenomena further, since in clinical practice the simple ideal gas laws are sufficiently accurate. For those scientists and technicians whose work requires maximum precision, there is available a modification of Boyle's law that includes correction for the van der Waals effect and density of molecules; and handbooks of chemistry and physics have prepared tables of constants to facilitate such calculations for a wide variety of gases. We will, however, be interested in the effects of excessive temperatures and pressures on the *state* of gases, since those we use may be in liquid or solid forms as well as gaseous. The most familiar example of the three states of matter is that of water, which we know as a solid (ice), gas (vapor), and liquid. Before discussing the state of matter in relation to therapeutic gases, we must deviate slightly to describe and define some physical terms that will make it easier to understand the interesting characteristics of prepared gases. Although we are familiar with the concepts of gas pressure and temperature as functions of kinetic activity we have not learned the physical units by which heat (energy) is expressed.

## Units of heat

*Calorie (cal).* The quantity of heat required to raise the temperature of 1 g of water from 14.5° to 15.5° C is used as the standard and is called a *calorie*. In general use the definition simply describes the amount of heat necessary to raise the temperature of 1 g of water 1° C. For convenience, in dealing with large quantities the term *large calorie (Cal)* is sometimes used and is equal to 1000 calories. If it is desired to calculate the heat produced by a chemical reaction, for example, the ingredients are placed in the reaction chamber of an instrument called a *calorimeter*. The heat of the chemical reaction is absorbed by a carefully weighed mass of water surrounding the reaction chamber, and the temperature change in the water is precisely measured. The weight of water in grams multiplied by the Celsius rise in temperature calculates the total calories produced, which can then be expressed as so many calories per unit of weight of the reacting substances. The exact structure of a calorimeter is dependent upon the use to which it is put, but the principle always involves the transfer of heat to a measured mass of water.

*British thermal unit (Btu.)* This is the English measurement system counterpart of the calorie and is the amount of heat required to raise the temperature of 1 lb of water 1° F. One Btu is equal to 252 calories. Generally, science uses the calorie unit of heat expression, consistent with the use of other metric measurements, but engineering and commerce employ the Btu along with other elements of the English system. This unfortunate dichotomy of standards places a burden on the respiratory therapist, who must be familiar with both systems, for his work involves contact with scientific data and the metric system, on the one hand, and commercial gases and other equipment standardized in the English system, on the other.

*Heat capacity.* This refers to the number of calories required to raise the tempera ture of 1 g of a substance 1° C, or 1 lb of a substance 1° F. By definition, the heat capacity of water is 1 calorie in the metric system and 1 Btu in the English system.

*Specific heat.* This value is a *ratio* between the amount of heat required to raise the temperature of 1 g of a substance 1° C, or 1 lb of a substance 1° F, at a specific temperature, and the amount of heat required to raise the temperature of 1 g of water 1° C, or 1 lb of water 1° F, at the specified temperature. Numerically, specific heat is equal to heat capacity, in either of the systems, but because it is a ratio, it is a pure number with no inherent dimensions and has the same meaning in any system of units.

For example, the specific heat of hydrogen, measured at 1 atm and 21° C (70° F) is 3.41. This means that:

$$\frac{\text{Heat required to raise 1 g } H_2 \text{ 1° C, or 1 lb } H_2 \text{ 1° F, at a given temperature}}{\text{Heat required to raise 1 g } H_2O \text{ 1° C, or 1 lb } H_2O \text{ 1° F, at a given temperature}} = 3.41$$

Thus it takes 3.41 times as much heat to elevate the gas temperature as that of the water—3.41 calories for 1 g of gas as against 1 calorie for 1 g of water, or 3.41 Btu per pound of gas as against 1 Btu for 1 lb of water.

Because specific heat is among the data frequently provided for medical and commercial gases, special mention should be made of the two ways in which it can be measured. First, the specific heat can be calculated by heating a *constant volume* of a gas, in which case the heat energy applied is transformed into increasing molecular energy. Second, the heated gas may be kept at a *constant pressure*, as in a flexible container, and in this instance because the expanding gas performs work (uses up heat) in displacing the surrounding atmosphere, more energy is required to bring the gas to the specific temperature. Thus a gas has two specific heats, that of constant pressure $(C_p)$ being larger than that of constant volume $(C_v)$. In the example of hydrogen, cited above, 3.41 is the constant pressure value, whereas at constant volume its specific heat is 2.40.

Finally, among the specifications of a given gas, the specific heat may be listed as *Btu/(lb-mole)(°F)*, or less frequently as *cal/(g-mole)(°C)*. This merely gives the heat value for a pound-molecular weight, or a gram-molecular weight, rather than for a pound or a gram. If we wish to convert the figure to a simpler pound or gram relation, it need only be divided by the molecular weight of the gas. Expressed as pound mole or gram mole specific heat, hydrogen is 6.89, or 3.41 times 2.02 (molecular weight of hydrogen).

### Change of state

Because all matter can change its state under certain conditions, theoretically it should be considered as nonspecific or labile in its physical characteristics. However, our familiarity with the usual forms of matter, as we encounter them in daily activities, endows them with a fixed physical state. In respiratory therapy we deal with the so-called *permanent gases* because in our contact with them they are in the gaseous state. Yet these same gases can just as well be liquid or solid, depending upon the pressures or temperatures to which they are exposed, and in the interest of economy and ease of transportation and storage, it is often convenient to transform an otherwise "permanent" gas into the liquid or solid state. The therapist should understand the basic thermodynamics of changes of state of those substances he uses as therapeutic gases as well as he understands the function and performance of his mechanical equipment. This means that he must understand the terms and expressions used to describe the specifications of commerically prepared gases, so we will start with a basic term that will lead us into a sequential discussion of the thermal and pressure characteristics of the various states of matter.

If we were to consider the three states of a given substance and on the same graph were to plot individually the various combinations of temperature, in °C, and pressure, in atmospheres, at which the liquid form of the substance and its vapor could transform one into the other—the solid and the liquid, and the solid and the vapor (sublimation)—three lines would be generated that would intersect at one point. This plot of temperature and pressure is called the *triple point*. The significance of this point is that it is the only combination of temperature and pressure that allows the solid, liquid, and vapor forms of a given substance to exist in equilibrium with one another. Every substance has its own triple point, but Fig. 1-6 is a schematic noncalibrated example of the triple point of water. *AB* plots the boiling points of water at various pressures or, to look at it another way, the saturated vapor pressure at different temperatures. This emphasizes the relationship between increasing pressure and increasing boiling points of water. *AB* terminates at the so-called *critical point*, which will be described below. Segment *AD* represents the conditions for water to *sublime*, or to pass directly from the solid state (ice) to vapor, or back. *AC* relates the transition points between ice and liquid water, the melting (or freezing) points. The steepness of *AC* indicates the relatively small effect exerted by pressure on melting or freezing points. At any plot of pressure and temperature that falls within the confines of *CAB* water can exist *only* as a liquid. Similarly, below *DAB*, pressures are too low for water to be anything other than gaseous. However, it should be noted that if the temperature is above the triple point, an elevation of pressure would transform the vapor into a liquid, and if below this point, directly into ice. *DAC* delineates the pressure-temperature conditions necessary for the formation of ice. Thus at all points along each line two phases of matter exist in complete equilibrium, but only at the triple point do all three equilibrate simultaneously. It should be noted that if the pressure on a volume of water is reduced from 1 atm (760 mm Hg) to 0.0063 atm (4.8 mm Hg), the boiling point of water will drop from 100° C to almost 0° C; but because the reduced pressure slightly alters the melting point of ice (freezing point of water), the lines intersect at 0.01° C. Therefore, at a pressure of 4.8 mm Hg and a temperature of 0.01° C, ice, water, and water vapor coexist in equilibrium, not in a static state but actively, as molecules of the substance (water) transform themselves from one form to the other forms. To appreciate the wide variation in range of triple points, note that the value for Freon-14 is −184° C and 0.88 mm Hg, whereas that of krypton is −157° C and 548 mm Hg.

We will now consider the following specific changes in state: solid to liquid and reverse, liquid to vapor and reverse, and solid to vapor and reverse. The student must always bear in mind that such changes are made only at the expense of energy, this energy being supplied by heat that is either given or taken by the matter undergoing change.

*Solid to liquid and liquid to solid.* A solid will convert to its liquid form at a given temperature known as its *melting point.* The range of melting points is vast, as carbon has a melting point in excess of 3500° C and helium, less than −272.2° C. Melting is little affected by pressure, as noted in the example of water in Fig. 1-6. In order to energize molecules from the fixed immobile (but not motionless) state of a solid into the more freely mobile fluid state, heat is required, which may be applied to the substance or may be extracted by the substance from its surroundings. Thus, with a melting point high above ambient, much heat must be applied to melt a mass of lead, but ice will extract heat from the atmosphere to fuel its transformation into liquid.

The heat needed to melt a substance is referred to as the *heat of fusion* (sometimes called the latent heat of fusion) and is defined as the calories required to change 1 g of the substance, or the Btu to change 1 lb of the substance, from the solid to the liquid state without changing its temperature. It is called *latent* because at a specific temperature, the melting point, the energy of the applied heat is utilized to effect the molecular change from solid to fluid and does not change the temperature of the mass. Only after the change of state has taken place does continued heat elevate the temperature of the newly formed liquid. Fig. 1-7 depicts the melting point of a solid mass to which heat is being applied. The solid is heated from *A* to *B*, with a simultaneous rise in temperature, but at *B* liquefaction begins and from *B* to *C* the temperature of the matter does not vary as the heat energy is utilized in the physical change. After melting is complete, at *C*, continued heat raises the temperature of the liquid from *C* to *D*. The temperature at *BC* is the melting point of the substance. Although pressure has little influence on melting, for the sake of uniformity scientific tables often report heats of fusion at the triple points. Thus the latent heat of fusion of ice is 80 cal/g, calcium chloride 54 cal/g, oxygen 3.3 cal/g, and argon 6.7 cal/g to give some idea of the diversity of energy needed for this change in state.

Freezing is the reverse of melting, with the conversion of a liquid form into solid. Because considerable energy is utilized in transforming a solid into liquid, this "stored" energy is released during the process of freezing so that, in a sense, freezing is a heating process in that the freezing liquid must give up heat (by being exposed to cold) as its molecules assume the stable configuration of a solid mass. Thus for pure substances freezing and melting points are concurrent. In common usage the transition point between solid and liquid forms is called the freezing point, for matter that is usually in liquid state, and the melting point, for matter that is usually in solid state; i.e., water freezes at 0° C, whereas lead melts at 327° C.

*Liquid to vapor and vapor to liquid.* These interchanges of physical states are the most relevant to our interest in therapeutic gases, and we have already considered in some detail the mechanism of simple evaporation as the escape of molecules from a liquid surface to mix with the ambient gases immediately adjacent to the surface. Maximum change of state from liquid to vapor (vaporization), however, occurs through the phenomenon of boiling, which differs significantly from evaporation. In the latter, water molecules diffuse into and become a part of ambient gases, whereas the vapor released by boiling escapes with sufficient force to displace, by pushing back, the surrounding gas. Also, whereas simple evaporation is purely a surface activity, boiling

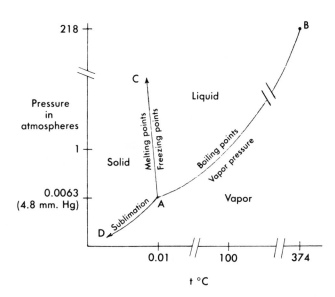

**Fig. 1-6.** The intersection of the three lines at *A* represents the *triple point* of water. Thus, at a temperature of 0.01° C and a pressure of 4.8 mm Hg, the three states of water (ice, liquid, and vapor) exist in equilibrium. The graphs show the temperature-pressure relationships of boiling, freezing, and sublimation of water.

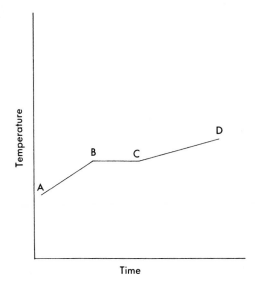

**Fig. 1-7.** *Heat of fusion* is illustrated by the temperature-time graph. Heat applied to a solid raises its temperature from *A* to *B;* at *B*, the solid begins to liquefy (melt). From *B* to *C*, the applied heat is utilized to accomplish the change in state, and the temperature of the substance does not rise further until liquefaction is complete, *C* to *D*.

produces large bubbles of vapor throughout the depth of the liquid, which rise to the surface to escape. Boiling occurs at the *boiling point*, a temperature at which the vapor pressure of a liquid equals the pressure exerted on the liquid by the weight of the atmosphere, and is influenced by two important factors. First, the boiling point is directly related to this force with which the atmosphere rests on the liquid surface, since the weight of the air molecules retards the escape of vapor molecules. The greater the pressure applied by ambient molecules the greater must be the kinetic energy of the fluid molecules to escape against the pressure, energy that can only come from increasing heat. On the other hand, lower ambient pressures allow the easier escape of molecules, and boiling can occur at much lower temperatures. Second, dissolved substances exert a cohesive force that increases the bonding among the molecules so that greater heat energy is required to free them into the vapor state, elevating the boiling point. Although we are accustomed to associate the phenomenon of boiling with high temperatures, such as water at 100° C (212° F), the boiling points of the liquid state of substances we call gases have exceedingly low values. For example, whereas tungsten boils at 5900° C. neon boils at −246° C, ozone at −112° C, and oxygen at −183° C.

Just as energy is needed to liquefy a solid, so is it required to vaporize a liquid, and this energy is called the *heat of vaporization* (sometimes the latent heat of vaporization, or simply the latent heat). It is defined as the calories required to vaporize 1 g of a liquid, or the Btu to vaporize 1 lb of a liquid, at its normal boiling point. When water is put on a stove to boil, its temperature rises steadily until the boiling point is reached, and then it maintains a constant temperature even though heat continues to enter it. This undetectable or "latent" heat reflects the energy necessary to release the forces holding together water molecules, freeing them to become vapor. It is interesting to note that the heat of vaporization for water is 540 cal/g, at 100° C, considerably higher than the heat of fusion of ice. This pointedly demonstrates that more energy is required to free water molecules into the vapor state than to rearrange them from the solid to the liquid state.

The therapist will often see the latent heat (of vaporization) listed in the specifications of commercial gases as Btu/lb-mole. For example, the latent heat of methane ($CH_4$, mol wt 16.04) is given as 3519 Btu/lb-mole, at its normal boiling point of −258.6° F (−126° C). This means that to convert 16.04 lbs of methane (1 lb-mol wt) from a liquid to a gas, 3519 Btu of heat must be supplied, and since *latent heat* refers to the heat required to change 1 lb or 1 g of substance, the above value can be reduced to the basic units of both the English and metric systems as follows:

(1) $\dfrac{\text{Btu/lb-mole}}{\text{gmw}} = \text{Btu/lb}$ $\qquad\qquad\qquad \dfrac{3519}{16.04} = 219 \text{ Btu/lb}$

(2) Because 1 Btu = 252 calories and 1 lb = 454 g

$\dfrac{\text{Btu/lb-mole} \times 252}{454} = \text{Btu/lb-mole} \times 0.554$

$\qquad\qquad\qquad\qquad = \text{cal/g-mole}$ $\qquad\qquad 3519 \times 0.554 = 1950 \text{ cal/g-mole}$

(3) $\dfrac{\text{Btu/lb-mole} \times 0.554}{\text{gmw}} = \text{cal/g}$ $\qquad\qquad \dfrac{3519 \times 0.554}{16.04} = 122 \text{ cal/g}$

For every liquid there is a temperature above which the kinetic energy of the molecules is so great that the attractive forces cannot maintain them in a liquid state. This temperature is called the *critical temperature*. Because there is no pressure able to maintain the molecules of the matter in a liquid state above this temperature, the critical temperature is the highest temperature at which a substance can exist as a liquid. If an evacuated sealed tube partially filled with liquid is heated, vapor will escape into the vacuum. The density of the vapor will steadily increase as that of the liquid substance decreases, and when the critical temperature of the liquid is reached, the densitites of both vapor and the remaining liquid will be equal and the two phases of matter will become identical without a line of demarcation between them. Further elevation of the temperature will transform the entire mass into vapor. The pressure exerted by the vapor within the evacuated tube at the critical temperature is the *critical pressure*, and on a plotted vapor pressure–temperature curve, the two values identify what is known as the *critical point*. Each substance has its own critical point, at which the gas phase is in equilibrium with the liquid phase and the two are not visibly separated. Attention is drawn to point *B* on the graph of the triple point, Fig. 1-6. This represents the critical point of water, at a pressure of 218 atm and a temperature of 374° C. Here the densities of the liquid and vapor phases are indistinguishable, the two are in equilibrium, and beyond this temperature no pressure alone can revert the mass to liquid. Compare the high values for water with the critical values of the gases in Table 1-5.

The terms *gas* and *vapor* are often erroneously used interchangeably, but the concept of critical temperature will help us to differentiate between them. Gas is a substance with a critical temperature so low that at the usual ambient conditions of temperature and pressure it cannot exist as a liquid with a surface exposed to atmosphere. If the temperature of a gas is above its critical value, it cannot be compressed into a liquid by a pressure of any magnitude. Such substances are referred to as *permanent gases*. On the other hand, vapor is the gaseous state of a substance which also exists *simultaneously* in a liquid *or* solid state. Oxygen therefore is a permanent gas, since it has no solid or liquid phase with its gaseous under ambient conditions. Water is both a liquid and a gas at room temperature and 1 atmosphere of pressure, and thus its gaseous phase is a vapor. Vapor may also be described as molecular emanations from a substance with a critical temperature so high that it exists as a liquid at 1 atmosphere of pressure. Appendix 8 lists the critical temperatures of several gaseous and vaporous substances.

Although we have described the critical points of matter in terms of the stability of liquids, it should be evident that they apply as readily to the transition of gas to

**Table 1-5.** *Critical points of three gases*

|  | °C | °F | atm |
|---|---|---|---|
| Helium | −267.9 | −450.2 | 2.3 |
| Oxygen | −118.8 | −181.1 | 49.7 |
| Carbon dioxide | 31.1 | 87.9 | 73 |

liquid. To effect a change of state from gas to liquid, we must cool the gas below its critical temperature and then compress it. Theoretically, it is possible to liquefy a gas by cooling alone, dropping its temperature below the substance's boiling point, but under no circumstances is it possible to liquefy it by pressure alone if its temperature is above its critical point. The further below its critical temperature a gas can be cooled, the less pressure is needed to liquefy it. Thus it can be seen that any gas whose critical temperature is above ambient can be liquefied by pressure alone because allowing the gas to equilibrate with ambient temperature actually keeps it below its critical temperature. Carbon dioxide has a critical temperature slightly above normal room temperature, 31° C, with a corresponding critical pressure of 73 atm, but at room temperature of 21.5° C, less than 60 atm of pressure are needed to convert the gas to liquid.

Only those gases whose critical temperatures are above ambient can be kept in the liquid state for everyday use at room temperature, and they must be under pressure in strong storage cylinders. The anesthetic gases cyclopropane and nitrous oxide, along with carbon dioxide, are commercially supplied as tanked liquids, and Table 1-6 compares their critical points with the approximate pressures at which they are kept at room temperature to maintain their liquid state. There are many industrial gases that are converted to the liquid state for ease of mass transportation, and with critical temperatures above ambient, they need only be kept under sufficient pressure to assure their liquid form. With release of pressure the liquid reverts immediately to gas.

Oxygen presents a more complicated problem, but because of its widespread medical and industrial use, carriage and storage are greatly facilitated by keeping it in the liquid state. In contrast to the three gases illustrated above, oxygen has a low critical temperature of −118.8° C (−181.1° F), and we know that no pressure will be able to keep it in liquid form above that value. In the manufacture of oxygen, large quantities of filtered air are subjected to tremendous pressures of up to 200 atm. This, of course, produces much heat, and the compressed gas is passed through heat exchangers and then subjected to a pressure drop of 5 atm. The rapid cooling brings the oxygen in the air below its boiling point of −183° C (−297° F), and it liquefies. If oxygen can be kept in an insulated container so that its temperature does not exceed its boiling point, it will remain liquid at atmospheric pressure. Should higher temperatures be necessary, then it must be subjected to increasing pressures; but at no time can it be allowed to exceed its critical temperature of −118.8° C, for then it will convert immediately to

**Table 1-6.**   *Pressures needed to maintain liquid state of gases at room temperature*

| Gas | Critical temperature | | Critical pressure | | Approximate pressure in commercial cylinder at room temperature | |
| --- | --- | --- | --- | --- | --- | --- |
| | °C | °F | atm | psi | atm | psi |
| Cyclopropane | 125 | 257 | 54.2 | 797 | 5.4 | 79 |
| Nitrous oxide | 36.5 | 97.7 | 71.8 | 1054 | 50.6 | 745 |
| Carbon dioxide | 31.1 | 87.9 | 73.0 | 1071 | 57.0 | 838 |

gas. Reference will again be made to this fact in the discussion of therapeutic gases.

*Solid to vapor and vapor to solid.* Although it may not be readily apparent, solid matter, as well as liquid, can vaporize, and at any given temperature solids have definite vapor pressures. The strong odor given off by naphthalene (mothballs) is ample evidence of the escape of vapor from a solid. The direct transition from the solid to the gaseous state is called *sublimation*, and because a change of state is involved, energy is transferred. The heat, in calories per gram or Btu per pound, required to convert 1 g or 1 lb, respectively, of a solid into a vapor is called the *heat of sublimation*. Sublimation somewhat resembles boiling because it occurs when the vapor pressure of the solid equals that of the opposing ambient pressure and because increasing and lowering the ambient pressure directly displaces the subliming point. If temperature is below the melting point of a substance, a drop in pressure causes it to sublime; if the temperature is above the melting point, pressure drop produces boiling. At exactly $0°$ C the vapor pressure over ice is 4.6 mm Hg, and if a vacuum less than this pressure is applied to the ice, the ice will sublime directly into water vapor.

Carbon dioxide is an interesting example of sublimation. If the gas is cooled to its critical point of $-57°$ C, it will freeze and the vapor will equilibrate with the solid at a pressure of 5.1 atm, an unusually high level compared with other permanent gases, most of which are considerably subatmospheric. When solid carbon dioxide is exposed to the atmosphere, the drop in pressure from 5.1 to 1 atm causes the solid state to sublime directly into vapor. We are all familiar with the behavior of commercially prepared solid carbon dioxide, popularly called "dry ice," as it gradually disappears when exposed to ambient conditions, leaving no trace of moisture. On the other hand, if solid carbon dioxide is subjected to pressures in excess of 5.1 atm and allowed to warm above $-57°$ C, it will melt into a liquid without boiling.

It is possible to produce carbon dioxide snow by suddenly releasing the compressed liquid from a commercial tank. A rush of very cold vapor will emerge, carrying with it fine snowlike particles of solidified carbon dioxide. The rapid vaporization of the liquid in the tank requires heat, and in a sense the liquid steals this heat from itself, freezing part of the material so that the remainder may vaporize.

We can relate the heat energy involved in sublimation to the energies of fusion and vaporization, already described, in the following way. Consider that a given mass of matter is progressing through changes of state from solid to liquid to vapor. We know that the step from solid to liquid utilizes energy, which we call heat of fusion; the conversion of liquid to vapor requires heat of vaporization. Even though the direct transformation from solid to vapor eliminates the liquid phase, the same total energy is required, and the heat of sublimation is thus equal to the sum of heats of fusion and vaporization.

In summary, we can say that all matter can theoretically exist in three physical states or forms, depending upon specific conditions of pressure and temperature. Those substances that we commonly refer to as gases are in the vaporous state because ambient pressure and temperature cannot maintain them as liquids or solids, and we have discussed the physical conditions that permit their conversion to the latter forms. It should be evident now why the ideal gas laws are not applicable to conditions of extreme pressure and temperature. The clear-cut relationships between pressure, temperature, and volume described by the laws break down as the factors of intermolecular force, molecular mass, and change of state influence the behavior of gases subjected to these extremes. This does not diminish the practical clinical value of the gas laws, but understanding the deviations from the laws permits us to see how matter can be manipulated and modified to serve specific purposes. The table in Appendix 8 compares some of pressure-temperature characteristics of a few selected gases and water so the student can see the tremendous range of values that distinguish one type of matter from another. In all probability, data such as these will play no direct role in the therapist's clinical duties, but it is hoped that, knowing something of the nature of the substances that he handles in his daily activities, his work will be a bit more meaningful.

# Chapter 2

# SOLUTIONS AND IONS

An understanding of some of the characteristics of solutions and ions is necessary to appreciate many of the chemical phenomena of physiology. Especially is this true of respiratory gas transport and acid-base balance, which are so important to us. It is assumed that the student is already familiar with the names of elements, atomic weights, valence, and simple chemical reactions through previous exposure to basic science. Nevertheless, this is felt to be a most appropriate place to pause briefly and review such timely topics as the structure of atoms, atomic stability, atomic bonding, and ionic and covalent compounds, even though we will have to confine ourselves to the most superficial incursion into these basics of chemistry. It is hoped that recall will be stimulated in those students who have had formal courses in chemistry and that those to whom chemistry is foreign will enjoy at least a general understanding of the material, and perhaps be encouraged to pursue further independent study.

## ATOMIC STRUCTURE

The classic definition of an atom describes it as the smallest particle of an element that can take part in a chemical change. For all practical purposes it can be thought of as the ultimate in the breakdown or degradation of matter, the final indivisible particle. We know this is not true, of course, because atoms can be fragmented, but extraordinary effort is required and it does not occur in usual chemical reactions. An element is a substance composed of one kind of atom, and a compound is a substance consisting of two or more different kinds of atoms. It is the constituent atoms that impart to matter its great variety of characteristics, through a myriad of combinations of the 105 different atoms presently identified. We will take a brief look at atomic architecture and acquaint ourselves with those structures most relevant to our needs.

*Components of an atom.* An atom can be visualized as an infinitesimally miniature orbital system, much like our sun and planets, with a central *nucleus* surrounded by peripheral smaller particles called *electrons*, circling it mostly in pairs but with a few as singles. The composition of the nucleus and the number of orbiting electrons are different and unique for each of the different kinds of atoms. It is estimated that the diameters of atoms range from $1 \times 10^{-8}$ cm to $5 \times 10^{-8}$ cm. The nucleus is the largest part of an atom, with a diameter approximately $10^{-13}$ cm, and while it may contain many kinds of matter referred to as particles, only two comprise all of its mass. *Protons* are particles with positive electrical charges and give to the nucleus overall electrical positivity, while *neutrons*, as the name implies, have no electrical charge. Protons and neutrons have about the same mass of $1.67 \times 10^{-24}$ g and are responsible for the weight of the atom. Other unstable nuclear components such as positrons, mesons, hyperons, and neutrinos, contribute nothing to the mass or chemical characteristics of atoms and are of interest only to the nuclear scientist. For our purposes we can consider atomic nuclei as consisting solely of protons and neutrons, although there is one atom that has no neutrons. *Electrons* are particles of matter with a mass of some $9.1 \times 10^{-28}$ g and are negatively charged, as opposed to the nuclear protons. Because of their lightness, electrons have no influence on atomic weight.

Fig. 2-1 diagrams the structure of the two simplest and lightest atoms, hydrogen and helium. Note that hydrogen is the atom referred to above with no neutrons in its nucleus so that, essentially, hydrogen consists only of one proton and one electron, the latter represented by an orbiting dot in the sketch. Mention will be made of this later in the chapter. Helium has double the number of electrons and protons of hydrogen and includes two neutrons in its nucleus.

More typical of an "average" atom is the metal potassium (Fig. 2-2). Its mass is composed of nineteen protons and twenty neutrons, with its electrons arranged in pairs and one single concentrically about the nucleus. The student is urged to let his imagination see the sketch in three dimensions, with the large circles extended into spheres, surrounding a spherical nucleus, representing orbits of electrons whirling rapidly around the nucleus. In the resting, or inactive, ground state the atom is electrically neutral. Since the nucleus of an atom of a given element has its own characteristic number of protons, it must have the same number of orbiting electrons to maintain electrical neutrality. The potassium atom therefore has nineteen electrons distributed among four orbits.

*Electron orbits.*   The orbits are known as *electron shells*, or *principal energy levels*. The simplest of the atoms, hydrogen and helium, have but one electron shell each, while the nineteen most complex atoms have seven. The principal energy levels

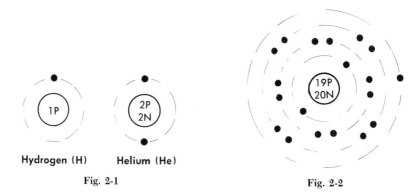

Hydrogen (H)       Helium (He)

Fig. 2-1                          Fig. 2-2

**Fig. 2-1.** Atomic structure of hydrogen and helium. Hydrogen has no neutrons and only one orbiting electron and one proton. Helium is heavier with two protons and two neutrons.

**Fig. 2-2.** Atomic structure of potassium. The significance of the single outer orbiting electron will be clarified later.

are designated both by numbers 1 through 7 and by capital letters K through Q. To accommodate increasing numbers of electrons among the larger, more complex atoms, the principal energy shells may have one to four *subshells,* identified by lower case letters s, p, d, and f. Fig. 2-3 diagrams one half of one of the large atoms, demonstrating all seven electron shells and the number of subshells in each. Principal levels 1(K) and 7(Q) have only one orbit each for their electrons, while levels 4(N) and 5(O) have four sublevels, like separate floors in a large building. Level 2(L) has two subshells and levels 3(M) and 6(P) each has three subshells. Space limitations prevent

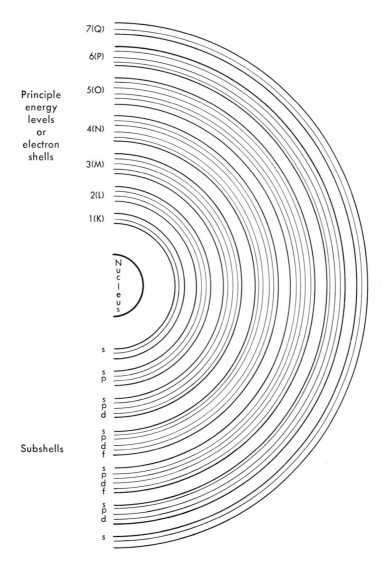

**Fig. 2-3.** Imaginary section through one of the large atoms showing the maximum number of available shells and subshells for orbiting electrons. Placing all orbits on the same plane is an inaccurate simplification for the sake of illustration, as is the deliberate omission of overlapping of shells 3 through 7.

exposition of further details in Fig. 2-3, but even the subshells contain subordinate orbits, or electron pathways known as *orbitals*, each limited to a maximum of *one pair* of electrons. Single, or unpaired, electrons may occupy an orbital of incompletely filled subshells. Subshell s has only one orbital, p has three, d has five, and f has seven orbitals. These illustrations and descriptions oversimplify reality for the sake of explaining general principles. Actually, the electron shells are not all spherical in shape, and there are overlaps among principal levels 3 through 7. For example, subshell 3d falls between subshells 4s and 4p, and subshell 4d is found between 5s and 5p. Such spatial arrangements of the electrons relate to internal energies of the atom and help to explain the progressive sequence of increasing atomic complexity. For our purposes we will continue with the simplest view of atomic structure that we can.

The pattern of electron spacing among all the different kinds of atoms is summarized in Table 2-1. The maximum number of electrons that can be accommodated in each subshell and orbital is shown on the left, while in the center is the total for each principal level, and on the right are the cumulative totals. These figures are *possible* maximal numbers of electrons, but all shells and subshells that contain electrons are not necessarily filled. Another view of electron distribution is given in Table 2-2, which is a section from a larger table of all 105 elements, showing the location of electrons in principal levels and sublevels. For the sake of space economy this segment includes only the first thirty-six elements and the last and most complex element for comparison. Provisions for the electron orbits of the remaining eighty-six elements are clear, however. Designations of principal energy levels, subshells, and maximum numbers of electrons per subshell are given at the top of the table. The *atomic numbers* (Z) refer to the numbers of both nuclear protons and orbiting electrons of each element and provide a practical sequence of listing the elements.

In summary, a rough mental image of a large atom might see it as a marble, representing the nucleus, dense with protons, neutrons, and other particles, suspended in the center of a hollow rubber ball, and this pattern of construction continued until a total of seven increasingly larger balls have been used, each symbolizing an electron shell. Within the walls of these rubber balls, tiny specks of paired and occasional

**Table 2-1.**   *Electron distribution among subshells and principal shell*

| Maximum number electrons per subshells | | | Maximum number electrons per principal shell | | | |
|---|---|---|---|---|---|---|
| Subshell | Orbitals | Electrons | Shell | Subshells | Electrons | Total electrons |
| s | 1 | 2 | 1(K) | s | 2 | 2 |
| p | 3 | 6 | 2(L) | sp | 8 | 10 |
| d | 5 | 10 | 3(M) | spd | 18 | 28 |
| f | 7 | 14 | 4(N) | spdf | 32 | 60 |
| | | | 5(O) | spdf | 32 | 92 |
| | | | 6(P) | spd | 18 (11)* | 110 (103) |
| | | | 7(Q) | s | 2 | 112 (105) |

*Maximum number of electrons actually in level 6(P) of the known elements is 11 (2-6-3). Other numbers in parentheses are based on this figure.

single electrons can be seen whirling in orbitals of the one to four different levels, or subshells. Regardless of the size or complexity of an atom, for our purposes we are interested only in the outermost orbiting electrons. These are known as *valence electrons* and are responsible for the bonding of atoms into crystals, molecules, and compounds.

   *Atomic stability.* If we could endow atoms with the quality of volition, we could say that every atom wishes to achieve a state of *stability*. Basically, atomic stability exists when the *outermost energy level* of a given atom contains just eight

**Table 2-2.** *Electronic configurations of the atoms*

| Atomic number (Z) | Element | (K) s | (L) s | (L) p | (M) s | (M) p | (M) d | (N) s | (N) p | (N) d | (N) f | (O) s | (O) p | (O) d | (O) f | (P) s | (P) p | (P) d | (Q) s |
|---|---|---|---|---|---|---|---|---|---|---|---|---|---|---|---|---|---|---|---|
| 1 | H | 1 | | | | | | | | | | | | | | | | | |
| 2 | He | 2 | | | | | | | | | | | | | | | | | |
| 3 | Li | 2 | 1 | | | | | | | | | | | | | | | | |
| 4 | Be | 2 | 2 | | | | | | | | | | | | | | | | |
| 5 | B | 2 | 2 | 1 | | | | | | | | | | | | | | | |
| 6 | C | 2 | 2 | 2 | | | | | | | | | | | | | | | |
| 7 | N | 2 | 2 | 3 | | | | | | | | | | | | | | | |
| 8 | O | 2 | 2 | 4 | | | | | | | | | | | | | | | |
| 9 | F | 2 | 2 | 5 | | | | | | | | | | | | | | | |
| 10 | Ne | 2 | 2 | 6 | | | | | | | | | | | | | | | |
| 11 | Na | 2 | 2 | 6 | 1 | | | | | | | | | | | | | | |
| 12 | Mg | 2 | 2 | 6 | 2 | | | | | | | | | | | | | | |
| 13 | Al | 2 | 2 | 6 | 2 | 1 | | | | | | | | | | | | | |
| 14 | Si | 2 | 2 | 6 | 2 | 2 | | | | | | | | | | | | | |
| 15 | P | 2 | 2 | 6 | 2 | 3 | | | | | | | | | | | | | |
| 16 | S | 2 | 2 | 6 | 2 | 4 | | | | | | | | | | | | | |
| 17 | Cl | 2 | 2 | 6 | 2 | 5 | | | | | | | | | | | | | |
| 18 | Ar | 2 | 2 | 6 | 2 | 6 | | | | | | | | | | | | | |
| 19 | K | 2 | 2 | 6 | 2 | 6 | | 1 | | | | | | | | | | | |
| 20 | Ca | 2 | 2 | 6 | 2 | 6 | | 2 | | | | | | | | | | | |
| 21 | Sc | 2 | 2 | 6 | 2 | 6 | 1 | 2 | | | | | | | | | | | |
| 22 | Ti | 2 | 2 | 6 | 2 | 6 | 2 | 2 | | | | | | | | | | | |
| 23 | V | 2 | 2 | 6 | 2 | 6 | 3 | 2 | | | | | | | | | | | |
| 24 | Cr | 2 | 2 | 6 | 2 | 6 | 5 | 1 | | | | | | | | | | | |
| 25 | Mn | 2 | 2 | 6 | 2 | 6 | 5 | 2 | | | | | | | | | | | |
| 26 | Fe | 2 | 2 | 6 | 2 | 6 | 6 | 2 | | | | | | | | | | | |
| 27 | Co | 2 | 2 | 6 | 2 | 6 | 7 | 2 | | | | | | | | | | | |
| 28 | Ni | 2 | 2 | 6 | 2 | 6 | 8 | 2 | | | | | | | | | | | |
| 29 | Cu | 2 | 2 | 6 | 2 | 6 | 10 | 1 | | | | | | | | | | | |
| 30 | Zn | 2 | 2 | 6 | 2 | 6 | 10 | 2 | | | | | | | | | | | |
| 31 | Ga | 2 | 2 | 6 | 2 | 6 | 10 | 2 | 1 | | | | | | | | | | |
| 32 | Ge | 2 | 2 | 6 | 2 | 6 | 10 | 2 | 2 | | | | | | | | | | |
| 33 | As | 2 | 2 | 6 | 2 | 6 | 10 | 2 | 3 | | | | | | | | | | |
| 34 | Se | 2 | 2 | 6 | 2 | 6 | 10 | 2 | 4 | | | | | | | | | | |
| 35 | Br | 2 | 2 | 6 | 2 | 6 | 10 | 2 | 5 | | | | | | | | | | |
| 36 | Kr | 2 | 2 | 6 | 2 | 6 | 10 | 2 | 6 | | | | | | | | | | |
| 105 | Ha | 2 | 2 | 6 | 2 | 6 | 10 | 2 | 6 | 10 | 14 | 2 | 6 | 10 | 14 | 2 | 6 | 3 | 2 |

electrons. Unfortunately, this description cannot be dogmatically applied to all 105 elements, since many of the more complex atoms have electron distributions that do not follow such a simple scheme. Nevertheless, the outer orbit octet principle applies to many of those which will be of interest to us in our study of physiology and which are found among the thirty-six elements listed in Table 2-2. In keeping with our policy of simple descriptions, we will confine our discussion to clear-cut examples, and only briefly note relevant exceptions.

Reference to Table 2-2 shows us that subshells s and p, in any principal level but K, must be filled with their allocated electrons to be stable and that until stability is reached, no electrons may occupy a more peripheral subshell. A major exception to this rule involves energy level K, which has but one subshell. Here stability is reached with only two electrons, filling subshell s. Thus an atom with two electrons in its one and only energy level (K), or eight electrons in the most peripheral of any of the other six levels, is a satisfied and stable atom, with no desire for chemical interaction. There are only six elements whose atoms are naturally stable, rendering them very chemically inactive. They are the so-called *inert gases* helium (two electrons), neon, argon, krypton, xenon, and radon. The first four of these are in Table 2-2 as Z-2, Z-10, Z-18, and Z-36, while the remaining two are larger atoms, Z-54 and Z-86.

All atoms, other than those of the inert gases, have varying degrees of chemical activity, which is a reflection of their attempts to reach stability by giving electrons to, by accepting electrons from, or by sharing electrons with other atoms. For example, atoms with one, two, or three valence electrons (such as Z-11, sodium; Z-12, magnesium; Z-13, aluminum) tend to release them, emptying the outer orbits and letting the next lower shells satisfy electronic stability. In contrast, those with five, six, or seven valence electrons (such as Z-15, phosphorus; Z-16, sulfur; Z-17 chlorine) tend to accept three, two, or one electrons to reach stable octets. Atoms with four valence electrons (such as Z-6, carbon; Z-14, silicon) can either release or accept four electrons. Some atoms neither donate nor accept electrons but reach stability by sharing them with other atoms. Finally, because the outer subshells of the inert gases are filled, there are no valence electrons available for either exchange or sharing.

**Valence.** The term *valence* is an expression of atomic combining capacity and refers to the number of electrons able to participate in exchange or sharing during chemical reactions. In current textbooks there is increasing use of the term *oxidation number*, which, although not a true synonym of valence, has the same implication as valence in atomic bonding and the same numerical value. Valence is designated by positive and negative sign superscripts following elemental symbols, as $Na^+$, and $S^=$. We have already indicated that atoms at rest are electrically neutral, with equal numbers of positive nuclear protons and negative orbiting electrons. In a chemical reaction, if one atom releases electrons to another to reach stability, the first atom will be left with more positive protons than negative electrons, and will thus have a net positive charge. Electron donors such as potassium, $K^+$, and calcium, $Ca^{++}$, are said to have positive valences, or oxidation numbers, equal to the number of freed electrons. Atoms accepting electrons, on the other hand, become negatively charged and have negative valences, or oxidation numbers, equal to the number of electrons received, such as chlorine, $Cl^-$, and oxygen, $O^=$. When atoms share electrons, valence signs are usually those the atoms have in other combinations where they exchange electrons. Finally, elements that donate electrons in a reaction are said to be *oxidized*, or to undergo *oxidation*, while those which are electron acceptors are *reduced*, or undergo *reduction*. An element that is itself oxidized reduces another and is called a *reducing agent;* the converse is true for an *oxidizing agent.*

Most of the relatively simple atoms of elements Z-1 through Z-20 are so common and familiar that their *usual* valences are well known to chemistry students. Indeed, one can estimate such valences by inspecting the electron distribution from Table 2-2. Even among these elements, however, there are valences unexpected from the electron configuration. For example, nitrogen not only has multiple valence values but also multiple valence signs, as $+5$, $+3$, $-3$. Such inconsistencies apparently arise from the orientation of electrons within subshell orbitals, rendering their exchange susceptible to various chemical, thermal, and pressure influences. On the other hand, manganese, Z-25, has possible valences of $+2$, $+3$, $+4$, $+6$, $+7$. Here as with many of the other larger atoms, there are unfilled subshells (i.e., 3d) proximal to the outermost s and p orbits. This changes the combining characteristics from simple to more complex than we can delve into here. Chemical reactions of these atoms may involve electrons in the *next* to outermost shell, as well as the valence electrons. At no time, however, can the valence number exceed 7. The serious chemist must learn many chemical and combining characteristics of all the elements with which he works, so that he will be able to determine which oxidation number is appropriate for a specific element in a given reaction. Fortunately, for our use the common values will suffice, and in general these will be the first valence numbers given for the elements listed in the table of Appendix 9.

## ATOMIC BONDING

A chemical bond is a force that holds atoms together in crystals or molecules. We will describe the two major kinds of atomic bonding, *ionic* and *covalent*.

*Ionic (electrovalent) bonding.* It is in this type of union between and among atoms that the electron exchange (donation and acceptance), described above, takes place. When electrons are gained or lost, we know that the involved atoms are left with either increased positive or negative charges. These charged atoms are called *ions;* those with positive charges ($Na^+$) are *cations*, and those with negative charges ($F^-$) are *anions*. The symbols for ions and the valence designation of elements are thus the same.

Fig. 2-4 illustrates the electron exchange between potassium and chlorine to form the salt potassium chloride (KCl). Note that only the valence electrons in the outermost shells are depicted, since they alone participate in any bonding examples we might use, and we know that all inner energy levels are filled. Although potassium has one more energy level than does chlorine, the major difference in electron distribution lies in the outermost shells. Here, potassium has one electron, and chlorine, seven. If potassium donates its electron to chlorine (is oxidized and reduces chlorine), potassium's M shell, with eight electrons, becomes its outermost, and the atom

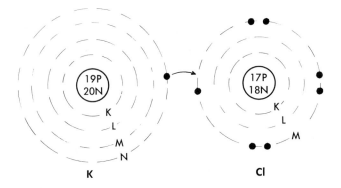

**Fig. 2-4.** Ionic bonding of K to Cl by the transfer of a single electron from K to Cl. (See text for further details.)

achieves stability. The loss of the electron converts the potassium atom into an ion, leaving it with nineteen nuclear protons to eighteen orbiting electrons, giving it a net ionic charge, valence, and oxidation number of $+1$. When the chlorine atom accepts the single electron from potassium (is reduced and oxidizes potassium), the electron octet of chlorine's M shell is completed and it is stabilized. Chlorine is now an ion with eighteen electrons to seventeen protons and a $-1$ electrical charge, valence, and oxidation number.

Electrovalent bonding is characteristic of the highly reactive elements with strong electropositivity and negativity that need to lose or gain one to three electrons to reach stability. Metals are in this group, as are such negative valence elements as fluorine, chlorine, oxygen, and sulfur, among many others. There are criteria for identifying ionically bonding elements, but they are beyond our present scope. Some elements, such as fluorine, chlorine, and oxygen as examples, can participate in both ionic and covalent bonding, depending upon the nature of specific reactions.

Ionic compounds do not form true molecules. Instead, myriads of cations and anions are held together in aggregates called crystals and referred to as giant molecules, or macromolecules. In aqueous solution, crystals break down into their constituent ions, a process called *dissociation*, a phenomenon that will be discussed in some detail very soon.

*Covalent bonding.* Electrons are shared in pairs, rather than exchanged, in covalent bonding and compounds. This type of union is formed between elements with less contrasting properties than those of ionic compounds, between two atoms of the same element, and between hydrogen and carbon in the thousands of organic compounds of which they are major ingredients. The elementary gases $H_2$, $N_2$, $O_2$, $Cl_2$, $Br_2$, and $I_2$ are covalent compounds, as are HCl, $H_2O$, $NH_3$, $SO_2$, $SO_3$, $CH_4$, to cite a few common substances among many others.

In contrast to the crystalline structure of ionic compounds, atoms covalently bonded form molecules, the smallest intact units of matter capable of independent existence. Their formulas are molecular formulas that can be used to calculate true gram molecular weight. Because ionic compounds have no molecular form and dis-

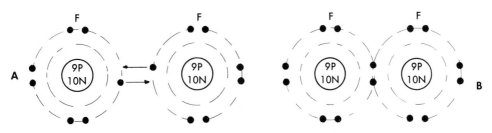

**Fig. 2-5.** Single bond, single element, symmetrical, nonpolar covalent bonding joins two atoms of elemental fluorine (**A**) into a molecule of fluorine gas (**B**), each atom sharing an electron from the other.

sociate into their ultimate particles, ions, they have only empirical formulas, which express the ratios of their combined elements and from which gram formula weights can be derived. This was briefly noted at the beginning of the text.

There are two varieties of covalent bonds, *nonpolar* and *polar*. The term *polar*, as used here, refers to the distribution of electrical charges throughout the covalent molecule. If positive and negative charges are evenly spread about a particle so that neither dominates any area, the particle is said to be nonpolarized, or *nonpolar*. In contrast, a particle on which positive charges gather predominately in one region, and negative charges in another, is considered polarized (possessing positive and negative poles), or *polar* in nature. The net electrical activity of both particles may actually be neutral, but because of local concentrations of opposing charges, the polarized particle is much more responsive to electrical influences surrounding it than is the relatively inert nonpolar particle.

Polarization of covalent molecules is dependent upon three factors. First, molecules that are symmetrically constructed with spatially well-balanced atoms tend to have a uniform spread of electrical charges, without polarization, while those with less symmetry are apt to concentrate their charges into poles. Second, the nuclei of some atoms have a greater attraction for electrons than do the nuclei of others and gather most of the electrons in their vicinity. This creates an area, or pole, of negativity that must be countered by an opposing positive pole. Third, when one atom is endowed with a larger number of electrons than is its partner or partners, the ensuing imbalance creates molecular polarity. Let us now consider some examples of the covalent bond.

*Nonpolar covalent bonding.* Fig. 2-5 illustrates the simple covalent union of two atoms of fluorine into a molecule of fluorine gas, with the formula $F_2$. Each atom needs but one electron to build a stable octet in its outer shell. The atoms compromise, in a sense, by combining their single electrons into a pair shared by both, creating a diatomic molecule. This is an example of a single bond, single element, symmetrical, nonpolar covalent compound. Fig. 2-6, on the other hand, demonstrates the structure of methane ($CH_4$), a multiple bond, dissimilar element, symmetrical, nonpolar covalent compound.

In contrast to ionic compounds, nonpolar covalent substances have no ions into which they can dissociate in water solution, nor do they form ions easily in solution because of their electrically neutral status.

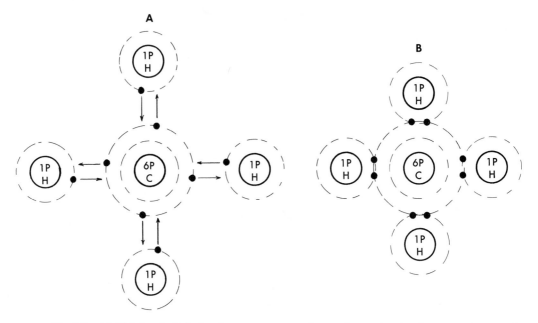

**Fig. 2-6.** Multiple bond, dissimilar element, symmetrical, nonpolar covalent bonding joins one atom of C with four atoms of H (**A**), to make the organic compound, methane, $CH_4$ (**B**).

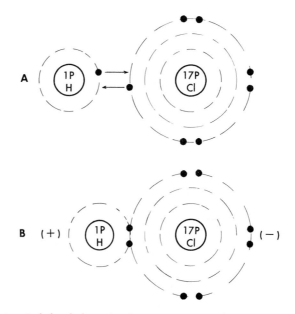

**Fig. 2-7.** **A,** HCL is a single bond, dissimilar element, asymmetrical, covalent bonded compound. **B,** It forms dipoles, with areas of opposing electrical charges. (See text for explanation).

*Polar covalent bonding.* By definition, polar covalency implies opposing molecular regions of electrical charges. Molecules so unbalanced are referred to as *dipoles*, possessing two poles. Fig. 2-7 shows us that hydrogen chloride (HCl) is such a dipole, or a polar covalent compound. The predominance of electrons about the chloride atom compared with the hydrogen gives a negativity to the chloride portion of the molecule, leaving the hydrogen end generally positive. The polarity is indicated in the sketch by the charge signs at each pole of the molecule.

One atom of oxygen holds two atoms of hydrogen in double, polar, covalent bonding to make a molecule of water. Fig. 2-8 illustrates the characteristic structure of a water molecule whereby the hydrogen atoms diverge from one another at an angle of 105°. This gives distinct polarity to the molecule, with negativity at the oxygen end and positivity about the hydrogens.

Generally speaking, and in contrast to nonpolar substances, polar molecules *ionize* in aqueous solution. This means that the molecules break into ions that are formed when the molecules dissolve, as opposed to the dissociation into ions already present in ionic compounds, as noted above. In terms of ion formation, polar covalent compounds are intermediate between the strong ion production of electrovalent substances, and the negligible activity of those with nonpolar covalent bonds. Even within the polar group there is considerable variation, the cited examples representing extremes. Hydrochloric acid readily forms many ions in a water solution, while water itself generates very few. However, we will soon learn that these few are of great importance.

With this quick refresher as a starting point, let us familiarize ourselves first with characteristics and types of solutions, then electrolytes and ions, and finally acidity and alkalinity. To understand solutions we need to know the systems of measuring quantities of substances going into solution, especially systems based on molecular, equivalent, and milliequivalent weights. Experience has shown this to be a problem area for many students, so we will begin with a discussion of gram equivalent weights.

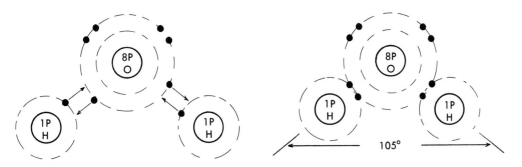

**Fig. 2-8.** The water molecule is a double covalent, polar compound, with two atoms of hydrogen attached to one atom of oxygen at an angle of 105 degrees to one another.

## EQUIVALENT WEIGHTS

Weights of reacting substances that have equal chemical power are referred to as *equivalents, equivalent weights,* or *chemical equivalents.* Thus if A reacts chemically with B, one equivalent of A will react exactly with one equivalent of B, and there will be no excess of reactants remaining. The same is true, of course, of identical fractions or multiples of chemical equivalents.

There are two magnitudes of equivalent weight measurements, related to one another in the ratio of 1:1000. Thus the term *equivalent* is a general one, and in specific uses the proper unit must be stated. The two levels of equivalents are the *gram equivalent weight (gEq)* and the *milligram equivalent weight, or milliequivalent (mEq).* A gram equivalent weight is related to a milligram equivalent weight as a gram is related to a milligram. Thus 1 gram equivalent equals 1000 milliequivalents. To avoid confusion, we will follow the usual format of defining and describing chemical equivalents in terms of the gram equivalent weight since the milliequivalent is merely a convenience modification of the former, and we will discuss it separately a little farther on.

### Gram equivalent weight

The gram equivalent weight of a substance is its quantitative chemical reacting unit and is defined as *the gram mass that contains, replaces, or reacts with (directly or indirectly) the Avogadro number, or 1 mole, of hydrogen atoms.* This does sound pretty stilted and formidable but as the student learns to use equivalents, he will see much more clearly what they mean. Before getting into their use, let us consider how equivalent weight values are calculated for elements and radicals, acids, bases, and salts. Definitions of acids, bases, and salts will be considered further on in this chapter.

***Equivalent weight of an element or radical.*** The equivalent weight of an element or a radical is the weight in grams that can combine with or replace in a chemical reaction 1 gram atomic weight (1 mole) of hydrogen or *other* monovalent elements. For example:

1. In hydrochloric acid (HCl), one atom of chlorine combines with one atom of hydrogen. In terms of moles or gram atomic weights this means that 35.5 g of Cl (atomic weight of Cl) combines with 1 g of H (gram atomic weight of H). Therefore the equivalent weight of Cl is the same as its gram atomic weight, 35.5 g.

2. One atom of S combines with two atoms of H in hydrogen sulfide ($H_2S$), which means that 32 g of S (1 mole) combines with 2 g of H (2 moles). Consistent with the terms in the definition of a gEq, then, 0.5 gram atomic weight of S combines with, or is chemically "equivalent" to, 1 atomic weight of H. The gram equivalent weight of S is thus 0.5 its gram atomic weight, or 16 g.

3. The formula of sulfuric acid ($H_2SO_4$) shows us that one sulfate group ($SO_4$) combines with two atoms of H. Thus 0.5 gram formula weight, or 0.5 mole of sulfate, is the equivalent of 1 mole of H atoms. The equivalent weight of $SO_4$ is 0.5 its gram formula weight, or 48 g.

4. These samples demonstrate that the numerical value of the gEq of an element

or radical is simply its gram atomic, or gram formula, weight divided by its valence, with a disregard for the valence sign. If an element has more than one valence, the valence must either be specified or apparent from the element's observed chemical combining properties. Thus with a valence of $+1$ the gEq of Na is its gram atomic weight of 23 g; the gEq of $Cu^{++}$ is its atomic weight divided by 2, or 31.7 g; the gEq of $Br^{\equiv}$ is its atomic weight divided by 3, or 26.6 g.

*Equivalent weight of an acid.* This is the weight in grams of the acid that contains 1 gram atomic weight (1 mole) of *replaceable* hydrogen. If the reader is doubtful of the meaning of replaceable hydrogen, it is suggested that he consult a chemistry textbook for a detailed explanation. Perhaps, however, a few examples will suffice as a review.

1. If we consider the unbalanced equation of the following reaction, $HCl + Na \rightarrow NaCl + H$, we see that the single H atom of HCl is replaced by Na. We can therefore conclude that 1 mole of HCl contains 1 mole of replaceable H, and that, by definition, the gram equivalent weight of HCl is the same as its gram formula weight, or 36.5 g.

2. The two hydrogen atoms of sulfuric acid ($H_2SO_4$) are both considered replaceable. Thus if 1 mole of the acid contains 2 moles of replaceable hydrogen, for the ratio to conform to the definition given above, 0.5 mole of acid must contain 1 mole of replaceable H. The gram equivalent weight of $H_2SO_4$ is therefore 0.5 its gram formula weight, or 49 g.

3. Carbonic acid ($H_2CO_3$) has two hydrogen atoms, but in reactions under physiological conditions, which will be dealt with later in the text, only one is considered replaceable. This is illustrated in the reaction $H_2CO_3 + Na \rightarrow NaHCO_3 + H$. Only one hydrogen atom is released, the other remaining "bound." Thus, despite the presence of two H atoms, 1 mole of acid contains only 1 mole of replaceable H, and the gram equivalent weight of $H_2CO_3$ is its gram formula weight, or 62 g.

4. As a general rule, the gEq of an acid can be calculated by *dividing its gram formula weight by the number of H atoms in its formula.* Exceptions to this rule are those acids whose hydrogen atoms are not completely replaceable, or are variably replaceable according to specific reactions. The major exceptions in our area of interest are carbonic acid, illustrated above, and phosphoric acid ($H_3PO_4$), an important physiological buffer. Equivalent weights of both are determined by the conditions of their chemical reactions.

*Equivalent weight of a base.* As might be guessed, the equivalent weight of a base is the weight of the base in grams that contains 1 gram formula weight (1 mole) of *replaceable* hydroxyl radicals. Like the acids just described, the gEq of a base is calculated by *dividing its gram formula weight by the number of OH groups in its formula.* There are some bases with incomplete replaceability of their hydroxyls, but none really concerns us at this time.

*Equivalent weight of a salt.* The equivalent weight of a *normal* salt (one that does not contain irreplaceable H or OH from the reacting acids or bases as described above) is the gram weight that contains 1 gEq of either of its components. Only one needs to be analyzed, since of necessity the other will have the same chemical equivalency.

1. For example, we know that the gEq of Cl is 1 gram atomic weight, or 35.5 g. Since a mole of the salt, NaCl, contains 1 gram atomic weight, or 1 gEq, of Cl, the equivalent weight of NaCl is its gram formula weight, 58.5 g.

2. Because Na is a monovalent element, we know that its gEq is 1 gram atomic weight. In the formula of the salt, $Na_2SO_4$, the subscript 2 tells us that there are 2 gram atomic weights of Na per mole of the salt. If 1 mole of $Na_2SO_4$ has 2 gEq of Na, then 0.5 mole would contain 1 gEq. The gram equivalent weight of $Na_2SO_4$ therefore is 0.5 its formula weight, or 71 g.

3. The gram equivalent weight of a normal salt can easily be calculated by *dividing its gram formula weight by the total of either positive or negative valence.* The total valence is the valence of a given element multiplied by the subscript of that element or radical as it appears in the formula of the salt. Thus the gram equivalent weight of ferric oxide ($Fe_2O_3$) is 159.8 ÷ 6, or 26.6 g.

4. For a *complex* salt such as an acid, basic, or double salt, the gEq must be calculated for a specific element or radical of the salt. The gEq of the components of sodium dihydrogen phosphate ($NaH_2PO_4$) are:

| | |
|---|---|
| For $Na^+$ | gfw of salt ÷ 1 |
| $H^+$ | 2 |
| $PO_4^=$ | 3 |

*Exercise 2-1.* Assuming complete replaceability of H and OH, calculate the equivalent weights of the following:

| | |
|---|---|
| (a) HBr | (f) KOH |
| (b) $H_3PO_4$ | (g) $Zn(OH)_2$ |
| (c) $HNO_2$ | (h) $Al(OH)_3$ |
| (d) $H_3AsO_4$ | (i) $NH_4OH$ |
| (e) $H_2S$ | (j) $Mg(OH)_2$ |

*Exercise 2-2.* Calculate the gram equivalent weights of the following:

(a) $MgF_2$
(b) $CaCl_2$
(c) $Na_3PO_4$
(d) $Ca_3(PO_4)_2$
(e) $Al(OH)_2Cl$

*Converting gram weight to equivalent weight.* To determine the number (or fraction) of gram equivalent weights in a given weight of a substance, *the gram weight of the substance is divided by its calculated equivalent weight.* Thus 58.5 of NaCl divided by its gEq of 58.5 g = 1 gEq, whereas 29.25 g of NaCl divided by 58.5 g = 0.5 gEq. Or, 407.8 g of $AgNO_3$ divided by 169.9 = 2.4 gEq.

Finally it should be pointed out that an equivalent of a compound, or a fraction or multiple thereof, contains the same degree of equivalency of each of its components. For example:

(1) 1 gEq NaCl $\quad = \dfrac{23 + 35.5}{1} = \quad$ 58.5 g

$\quad$ 1 gEq Na $\quad = \dfrac{23}{1} \quad = $ 23.0 g

$\quad$ 1 gEq Cl $\quad = \dfrac{35.5}{1} \quad = \underline{35.5 \text{ g}}$
$$\qquad\qquad\qquad\qquad\qquad\qquad 58.5 \text{ g}$$

(2) 2 gEq $Na_2CO_3 = \dfrac{2[23(2) + 60]}{2} = \quad$ 106.0 g

$\quad$ 2 gEq Na $\quad = \dfrac{2(23)}{1} \quad = $ 46.0 g

$\quad$ 2 gEq $CO_3 \quad = \dfrac{2(12 + 48)}{2} = \underline{60.0 \text{ g}}$
$$\qquad\qquad\qquad\qquad\qquad\qquad 106.0 \text{ g}$$

Thus if we wished 2 gEq of sodium and could disregard other ingredients, we could measure out 117.0 g of NaCl, 106.0 g of $Na_2CO_3$, or 109.3 g of $Na_2PO_4$.

***Exercise 2-3.*** Calculate the number of gEq's in the stated quantities of the following compounds:

(a) 62 g $MgF_2$
(b) 50 g $CaCl_2$
(c) 120 g $Na_3(PO_4)$
(d) 10 g $Ca_3(PO_4)_2$
(e) 1.5 kg $CuCl_2$

## Milligram equivalent weight

When referring to small amounts of chemically reacting substances, especially as found in physiological chemistry, it is often convenient to use the terms *milligram equivalent, or milliequivalent weight (mEq)*. A milliequivalent is 0.001 of a gram equivalent weight and is expressed in milligrams instead of grams. Just as a gram consists of 1000 milligrams, so 1 gEq is equal to 1000 mEq. It should be restated here that the terms *equivalent* or *equivalent weight* are general ones, without specification of units of measurement. They apply equally to scales of grams and milligrams. For example, we know that the gram equivalent weight of NaCl is 58.5 g, but we can also say that its milliequivalent weight is 58.5 mg. In other words, the equivalent weight of NaCl is 58.5, and it is up to us to apply gram or milligram units as occasions warrant. Thus, because 58.5 g NaCl are 1 gEq, 58.5 mg are actually 0.001 gEq, but to minimize the awkwardness of decimal fractions the small amount is much better called 1 mEq. Again, to show the relationship, 0.5 gEq can be called 500 mEq if desired, and 1340 mEq can be 1.34 gEq.

As a guide only, when calculating equivalents, if weights of substances are given in grams, equivalents are probably better expressed in gram equivalent weights, and if in milligrams, in milliequivalent weights. Also, if specified weights of substances, when given in or converted to *grams*, are numerically greater than their equivalent weights, the results should be given in gram equivalents, and if they are less, given in milliequivalents. The following examples may be helpful.

(1) Convert 150 mg of calcium chloride ($CaCl_2$) to equivalents:

    (a) 1 gEq = gfw ÷ 2 = 55.5 g   *or*
        1 mEq = mgfw ÷ 2 = 55.5 mg

    (b) 150 mg = 0.150 g

therefore

    (c) 0.150 g ÷ 55.5 g = 0.0027 gEq (awkward)   *or*
        150 mg ÷ 55.5 mg = 2.7 mEq (better)

(2) Convert 45 g MgO to equivalents:

    (a) 1 gEq = gfw ÷ 2 = 20.2 g   *or*
        1 mEq = mgfw ÷ 2 = 20.2 mg

    (b) 45 g = 45,000 mg

therefore

    (c) 45,000 mg ÷ 20.2 mg = 2,228 mEq (awkward)   *or*
        45 g ÷ 20.2 g = 2.23 gEq (better)

*Exercise 2-4.* Convert the following to the proper corresponding weights or equivalents:

    (a) 5.3 g $Na_2CO_3$
    (b) 6.8 mg $CaSO_4$
    (c) 1.2 g $CuCl_2$
    (d) 2.3 mEq $AlBr_3$
    (e) 9.5 mEq $AgNO_3$

**Use of equivalent weights**

The importance of the equivalent weight as a chemical unit of measurement is its use in calculating quantities of substances reacting with one another and the products of such reactions. Consider the following (note that it is more meaningful to depict water as a 1:1 compound of a hydrogen atom and a hydroxyl group, HOH, than a 2:1 of hydrogen and oxygen, as in $H_2O$—to be clarified later):

$$Ca(OH)_2 + 2HNO_3 \longrightarrow Ca(NO_3)_2 + 2HOH$$

| | Ca(OH)₂ | 2HNO₃ | Ca(NO₃)₂ | 2HOH |
|---|---|---|---|---|
| Number of moles | 1 | 2 | 1 | 2 |
| Gram formula weight | 74 | 2 × 63 | 164 | 2 × 18 |
| | 74 | 126 | 164 | 36 |
| | | (200) | | (200) |

This balanced equation, with equal weights of substances on both sides, shows us the quantities and proportions of both reactants and products involved in the reaction. It can be simplified, however, by obviating the need to balance it with coefficients as above, yet still show the proportion of ingredients that will exactly react. Let us rewrite the equation, entering only 1 equivalent for each substance, and the corresponding gram equivalent weights.

$$Ca(OH)_2 + HNO_3 \longrightarrow Ca(NO_3)_2 + HOH$$

| | Ca(OH)₂ | HNO₃ | Ca(NO₃)₂ | HOH |
|---|---|---|---|---|
| Number of equivalents | 1 | 1 | 1 | 1 |
| Gram equivalent weights | 37 | 63 | 82 | 18 |
| | | (100) | | (100) |

By writing the equation in terms of equivalent weights, balancing it is unnecessary, and we see that the proportions of reactants and products are the same as above. Single equivalent weights were used in this example for simplicity, but it should be apparent that any fraction or multiple could just as well have been used, in either gram or milligram equivalent units.

In medicine it has become customary to refer quantitatively to certain essential substances that are highly reactive in the body in terms of their equivalent weights. This is especially true of such elements as sodium, potassium, and chlorine and the bicarbonate radical $HCO_3^-$, which are in small enough quantities to be measured in milliequivalents. To the physiologist the number of chemically reactive units (mEq) present in the blood is more meaningful than just bulk weight in milligrams. Since the therapist will have occasion to note certain laboratory data of his patients, the method of reporting the above elements by the laboratory should be explained.

In the hospital clinical laboratory these blood chemicals (also known as *electrolytes*, to be described later) are quantitatively measured in *milligrams per 100 ml of blood*, customarily referred to as *mg %*. We will use the modern designation of *mg/dl*, dl being the abbreviation of deciliter, one tenth of a liter, or 100 ml. These values are then converted by the technician into the corresponding *equivalent weights* and reported as so many milliequivalents per *liter* of blood, or *mEq/ℓ*. Transposition between mEq/ℓ and mg/dl is easily accomplished as follows:

$$(1) \quad mEq \quad = \quad \frac{mg}{equiv\ wt}$$

$$mEq/\ell = \frac{mg/dl \times 10}{equiv\ wt}$$

$$(2) \quad mg \quad = mEq \times equiv\ wt$$

$$mg/dl \quad = \frac{mEq/\ell \times equiv\ wt}{10}$$

Thus, if in a blood sample there were 322 mg/dl of sodium, it would be reported as

$$\frac{322 \times 10}{23} = 140\ mEq/\ell$$

As a check, $140\ mEq/\ell = \dfrac{140 \times 23}{10}$ or 322 mg/dl.

In hospital medical practice, electrolyte replacement is commonplace therapy. This is accomplished by the intravenous infusion of solutions in which the electrolyte content is stated in milligrams per 100 ml of solution, and as milliequivalents per liter. A typical example is a solution known as Lactated Ringer's Injection (Hartmann's solution), the label of which lists its ingredients as shown in Table 2-3.

Table 2-4 lists the equivalents of electrolytes more accurately, as calculated from milligram percentage, using the formula above for converting to mEq/ℓ.

Equivalents, of course, can be calculated for any volume of solution. As an example, one oral preparation lists its potassium chloride content as 3 g for each 15 ml (tablespoonful) dose. Each dose thus provides 40.2 mEq of both potassium and chloride.

**Table 2-3.**  *Concentrations of ingredients listed on label of Ringer's solution container*

|  | mg/dl |  | Approximate mEq/ℓ |
|---|---|---|---|
| NaCl | 600 | Na | 130 |
| NaC$_3$H$_5$O$_3$ (Na lactate) | 310 | Cl | 109 |
| KCl | 30 | C$_3$H$_5$O$_3$ | 28 |
| CaCl$_2$ | 20 | K | 4 |
|  |  | Ca | 3 |

**Table 2-4.**  *Calculated milliequivalents (mEq) of ingredients of lactated Ringer's solution*

|  | Na | Cl | Lactate | K | Ca |
|---|---|---|---|---|---|
| NaCl | 102.6 | 102.6 |  |  |  |
| NaLac | 27.7 |  | 27.7 |  |  |
| KCl |  | 4.0 |  | 4.0 |  |
| CaCl$_2$ |  | 3.6 |  |  | 3.6 |
| Total mEq/ℓ | 130.3 | 110.2 | 27.7 | 4.0 | 3.6 |

*Exercise 2-5.*  Convert the following to the corresponding mEq/ℓ or mg/dl:

(a)  296 mg/dl Na
(b)  82 mEq/ℓ Cl
(c)  23 mg/dl K
(d)  9 mg/dl Ca
(e)  26 mEq/ℓ HCO$_3$

## DEFINITION OF A SOLUTION

A solution is an intimate mixture of two substances, with one so evenly dispersed throughout the other that the mixture is homogeneous. The substance being dissolved, or going into solution, is called the *solute* and the medium in which it is dissolved is called the *solvent*. The ease with which a solute mixes with a solvent is a measure of its solubility. The four factors influencing solubility are:

1. *Nature of the solute.* The degree to which all substances go into solution in a given solvent is a physical characteristic of matter, with wide variability.
2. *Nature of the solvent.* As with solutes, solvents vary widely in their ability to incorporate substances into solutions.
3. *Temperature.* In general, the solubility of most solid solutes increases with temperature; the solubility of gases, however, varies inversely with temperature.
4. *Pressure.* Solubility varies directly with pressure.

A solution is described as *dilute* if it has a relatively small amount of solute in proportion to solvent. Fig. 2-9 shows three different states of a solution. In Fig. 2-9, A, the solution is considered dilute because it has relatively few solute particles. A *saturated* solution is one with the maximum amount of solute that can be held by a given volume of solvent at a constant temperature, in the presence of an excess of

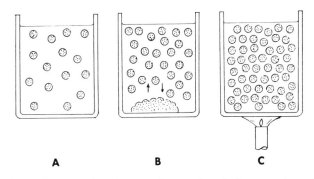

**Fig. 2-9.** In the dilute solution, **A,** the solute particles are relatively few in number, whereas in the saturated solution, **B,** the solvent contains all the solute it can hold in the presence of an excess of solute. Heating the solution, **C,** dissolves more solute particles, which may remain in solution if gently cooled, creating a state of supersaturation.

solute. In such a mixture the dissolved solute is in equilibrium with the undissolved solute. Saturated solutions are usually prepared by adding a known excess of solute to the solvent, allowing the excess to remain in contact with the solution. Fig. 2-9, *B,* is a saturated solution, and the excess solute is depicted as an undissolved mass at the bottom of the container. Although there is more solute in contact with solvent than the latter can accommodate at a fixed temperature, the excess must not be thought of as completely inert. Particles of solute precipitate into the solid state at the same rate that new molecules leave the supply of solute and go into solution. This is the state of equilibrium that characterizes a saturated solution. A solution is said to be *supersaturated* when it contains more solute in solution than does a saturated solution at the same temperature and pressure. If a saturated solution is heated, upsetting the solute equilibrium and allowing more solute to go into solution, and the remaining undissolved solute is filtered and the solution allowed to cool gently, then the solution will contain an excess of dissolved solute. Solution *C* in Fig. 2-9 can be considered the result of applying heat to the solution *B*, driving the remainder of the excess solute into solution. The additional dissolved particles may remain in solution, even after cooling to the temperature of the original saturated state, if extreme care is taken. Such a supersaturated solution is unstable, and the excess of dissolved solute may be precipitated out of solution by such physical stimuli as shaking or vibrating, or by adding to the solution a small amount of the solid solute.

Most of the solutions of physiologic importance in the body are *dilute* in nature, and it is of interest that solutes in dilute solution demonstrate many of the properties of gases. This behavior is due to the relatively large distances between the molecules of solute in dilute concentrations, and it is hoped that the student may be stimulated to learn, through independent study, how the principles of the gas laws apply to liquids. We will concern ourselves only with brief descriptions of four of the major characteristics of solutions:

1. *Vapor pressure depression.* The vapor pressure of a solution is less than that of the pure solvent. This is attributed to interference with the escape of solvent molecules by solute molecules, at the liquid surface.

2. *Boiling point elevation.* The boiling point of a solution is higher than that of the pure solvent, and its elevation is directly proportional to the number of solute particles in a given weight of solvent.

3. *Freezing point depression.* The freezing point of a solution is lower than that of the pure solvent, and its depression is directly proportional to the number of solute particles in a given weight of solvent.

4. *Osmotic pressure.* This will be discussed separately, a few paragraphs later.

## QUANTITATIVE CLASSIFICATION OF SOLUTIONS

1. *Ratio solution.* The relationship of the solute to the solvent is expressed as a proportion (1:100, parts per thousand, etc.). This is used quite frequently in describing concentrations of pharmaceuticals.

2. *Weight per volume solution (W/V).* Often erroneously referred to as a "percent solution," the W/V solution is the one most commonly used in pharmacy and medicine for solids dissolved in liquids. It is calibrated in *weight of solute per volume of solution as grams of solute per 100 ml of solution.* Thus, although 50 g of glucose in 1 liter of solution is not a true percent relationship, since a weight cannot be a percent of a volume, it is customarily called a 5% (W/V) solution. In contrast, a liquid dissolved in a liquid is measured as volumes of solute to volumes of solution.

3. *Percent solution (%).* Used in chemistry, a percent solution is calibrated as *weight of solute per weight of solution.* Thus 5 g of glucose dissolved in 95 g of water is true percent solution, since the glucose is 5% of the total solution weight of 100 g.

4. *Molal solution (m).* Less frequently used in physiological chemistry than are the two types to be described below, a molal solution contains *1 mole of solute per kilogram of solvent (or 1 millimole per gram of solvent).* Thus a 1 m solution of NaCl contains 58.5 g (1 gram formula weight) dissolved in 1000 *g of solvent.* It is of value when stability of precise concentrations of moles are desired over a wide temperature range. Volumes of liquid vary with temperature changes as do gases, although of course to only a fraction of the magnitude of gas volume changes. With its solvent measured in weight, the concentration of a molal solution is independent of temperature. For a specific solution at all temperatures a given *weight* of the solvent, regardless of its *volume*, will contain the same number of moles.

    a. What is the molality of a solution with 162.4 g of $FeCl_3$ dissolved in 500 g of water?

        (1) 1 m solution = 162.4 g (1 gfw)/1000 g $H_2O$
        (2) 162.4 g/500 g = 324.8 g/1000 g
        (3) 324.8 g ÷ 162.4 g = 2 gfw/1000 g
        (4) Solution = *2 molal (2 m)*

    b. How much $K_2SO_4$ must be dissolved in 250 g water to make a 0.75 m solution?

        (1) 1 m solution = 174.2 g (1 gfw)/1000 g $H_2O$
        (2) 0.75 m solution = 174.2 × 0.75 = 130.65 g/1000 g
        (3) 130.65 g/1000 g = 32.66 g/250 g
        (4) 32.66 g/250 g $H_2O$ = 0.75 m

5. *Molar solution (M).* Chemically and physiologically the molar solution and the

normal solution, to be described next, are the most important of all solutions. A molar solution has *1 mole of solute per liter of solution (or 1 millimole per milliliter of solution)*. A 1 M solution of NaCl thereby contains 58.5 g (1 gram formula weight) *per liter of solution;* a 0.5 M solution has 29.25 g/$\ell$ of solution; a 2 M solution has 117 g/$\ell$ of solution, etc. The solute is measured into a container, and the solvent is added to the total solution volume desired. The molar solution is chemically important because equal volumes of solutions of equal molarity contain the same number or fractions of solute moles.

a. What is the molarity of a solution with 1.07 g $NH_4Cl$ dissolved in 100 ml of solution?

    (1) 1 M solution = 53.5 g (1 gfw)/1000 ml solution
    (2) 1.07 g/dl = 10.7 g/1000 ml
    (3) 10.7 g ÷ 53.5 g = 0.2 gfw/1000 ml
    (4) Solution = *0.2 molar (0.2 M)*

b. In what volume of solution must 41 g $Ca(NO_3)_2$ be dissolved to make a 3 M solution?

    (1) 1 M solution = 164 g (1 gfw)/1000 ml solution
    (2) 3 M solution = 164 g × 3 = 492 g/1000 ml
    (3) 492 g/1000 ml = 41 g/83.3 ml
    (4) 41 g dissolved in *83.3 ml* solution = 3 M solution

6. *Normal solution (N)*. Widely used in chemistry and biochemistry, the normal solution has *1 gram equivalent weight of solute per liter of solution (or 1 milligram equivalent weight per milliliter of solution)*. Accordingly, 1 gfw of HCl, ½ gfw of $H_2SO_4$, ⅓ gfw of $AlF_3$, and ⅙ gfw of $Al_2(SO_4)_3$, each dissolved in *1 liter of solution*, make 1 N solutions of the respective solutes. For all *monovalent* solutes, normal and molar solutions are one and the same because the equivalent weights of such solutes equal their gram formula weights. Equal volumes of solutions of the same normality contain chemically equivalent amounts of their solutes. If the solutes react chemically with one another, then equal volumes of the solutions will react completely, and neither substance will remain in excess. Solutions of known normality are often used as *standard solutions* in an analytical process known as titration for determining the concentrations of other solutions.

a. What is the normality of a solution with 39.75 g of $Na_2CO_3$ dissolved in 250 ml of solution?

    (1) 1 N solution = 53 g (1 gEq = 1 gfw ÷ 2) /1000 ml solution
    (2) 39.75 g/250 ml = 159 g/1000 ml
    (3) 159 g ÷ 53 g = 3 gEq/1000 ml
    (4) Solution = *3 normal (3 N)*

b. What weight of $K_3PO_4$ must be dissolved in 5 ml of solution to make a 1.5 N solution?

    (1) 1 N solution = 70.8 g (1 gEq = 1 gfw ÷ 3)/1000 ml solution   *or*
                 70.8 mg (1 mEq = 1 gEq ÷ 1000)/ml solution
    (2) 1.5 N solution = 70.8 × 1.5 = 106.2 g/1000 ml   *or*
                  70.8 × 1.5 = 106.2 mg/ml

(3)  106.2 g/1000 ml = 0.531 g/5 ml    *or*
106.2 mg/ml = 531 mg/5 ml
(4)  *0.531 g* dissolved in 5 ml solution = 1.5 N solution    *or*
*531 mg* dissolved in 5 ml solution = 1.5 N solution

(*Note:* 0.531 g and 531 mg are exactly the same. This exercise demonstrates that either gEq or mEq units can be used, the choice depending upon which is more consistent with the magnitudes of measurements involved.)

**Exercise 2-6.** Calculate the following:

(a) How many grams of solute are there in 300 ml of a 3% (W/V) solution?
(b) What volume will contain 70 mg of solute of a 7% (W/V) solution?
(c) How many grams of solute and solvent are needed for 250 g of a 10% solution?
(d) What weight of water is needed to dissolve 13 g of $BaCl_2$ to make a 0.25 m solution?
(e) What is the molarity of a solution with 16 g of $CH_3OH$ (methyl alcohol) in 200 ml of solution?
(f) How many milliliters of 0.1 M $AgNO_3$ solution contain 8.5 g of solute?
(g) How many grams of $C_{12}H_{22}O_{11}$ (cane sugar) are there in 50 ml of a 3 M solution?
(h) What is the normality of a solution with 13.25 g of $Na_2CO_3$ in 500 ml of solution?
(i) How many milliliters of 2 N solution of $AlCl_3$ contain 8.9 g?
(j) How many milligrams of $Al_2(SO_4)_3$ are there in 10 ml of 0.2 N solution?

## OSMOTIC PRESSURE

One of the physical characteristics of solutions that has great physiologic significance is *osmotic pressure*. This is a measurable force produced by mobility of the solvent particles under certain conditions. Imagine a thin porous sheet so constructed as to permit the passage through it of molecules of solvent but not solute. Such a structure is called a *semipermeable membrane*. Should such a membrane be placed so as to divide a solution into two compartments, molecules of solvent would pass freely through it from one side to the other (Fig. 2-10, *A*). However, the number of molecules that pass (or diffuse) in one direction must be equaled by the number passing in the opposite direction to maintain an equal ratio between solute and solvent particles (which determines the concentration of the solution) on both sides of the membrane.

Let us now put a solution on one side of the semipermeable membrane and pure solvent on the other. Solvent molecules will move through the membrane, but only in one direction, from the pure solvent to the solution and will continue to move until the supply of solvent is exhausted. The force driving the solvent molecules through the membrane is termed *osmotic pressure* and can be measured by connecting the expanding column of the solution to a manometer (Fig. 2-10, *B* and *C*). This pressure can be considered as a force that tries to distribute solvent molecules so there will be the same ratio between solute and solvent particles, thus the same concentration, on both sides of the membrane. Or it may be convenient to visualize osmotic pressure as the attractive force of solute particles in a concentrated solution. If we modify the conditions by placing a 50% solution on one side of the membrane and a 30% solution on the other, again the solvent molecules will penetrate the barrier from the dilute to the concentrated side (Fig. 2-10, *D* and *E*). The greater number of solute particles per solvent molecules in the concentrated solution attract solvent molecules away from the smaller concentration of solute particles in the dilute solution, and mi-

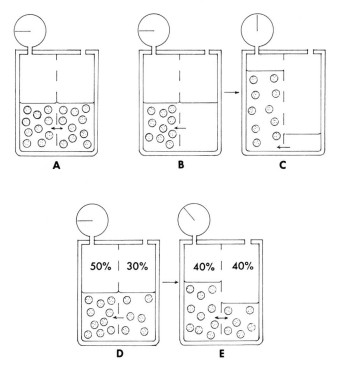

**Fig. 2-10.** Osmotic pressure is illustrated by the solutions in the above five containers. The containers are divided into two compartments by semipermeable membranes that permit the passage through them of solvent molecules but not solute (dotted circles). The numbers of solute particles represent relative concentrations of the solutions, and since they are fixed in number and are confined by the membranes, volume changes are a function of the diffusible solvent, movements of which are indicated by the arrows through the membranes. The arrows between containers **B** and **C**, and **D** and **E**, indicate progressive sequences of osmotic pressure. (See text for further description.)

gration of solvent molecules will continue until the attractive force (osmotic pressure) of solute is equal on both sides of the membrane. Such an equilibrium implies an equal ratio of solute/solvent particles in both compartments, or an equal concentration of 40%. At this point solvent particles move equally in both directions.

Osmotic pressure is directly proportional to the concentration of solute and will be twice as strong in a 2% solution as in a 1%. Thus, for a given *amount* of solute, the osmotic pressure is inversely proportional to the volume, an application of Boyle's law to liquids. Also, osmotic pressure varies directly with temperature, increasing $1/273$ for each degree Celsius.

Body cell walls are semipermeable membranes, and through the action of osmotic pressure the distribution of water throughout the body is kept within physiologic ranges. The term *tonicity* refers to the relative degree of osmotic pressure exerted by a solution. In a very general way the average body cellular fluid has a tonicity equal to that of a 0.9% NaCl solution, often referred to as physiologic saline. For comparative purposes any other solution with similar tonicity is called *isotonic,* one with greater tonicity *hypertonic,* and one with less *hypotonic.* Some cell walls possess *selective permeability,* allowing the passage not only of water but of specific solutes, and through this mechanism nutrients and physiologically active substances are distributed throughout the body.

## DILUTION CALCULATIONS

Often it is necessary to make a dilute solution from a stock preparation, and this can be done accurately if the concepts of solution concentrations are understood. Such dilution problems usually involve medications and are based on the pharmacologic weight/volume percent principle defined earlier. Diluting a solution increases its volume without changing the *amount* of solute it contains but reduces its concentration. Therefore the amount of solute in a given sample after dilution is the same as was present in the smaller original volume. It should be clear that the amount of solute present in a sample of a solution can be expressed as *volume* times *concentration.* For example, the amount of solute in 50 ml of a 10% solution (10 g/dl) is $50 \times 0.1 = 5$ g. In diluting a solution, then, the initial volume times the initial concentration equals the final volume times the final concentration. This may be simplified as

$$V_1 C_1 = V_2 C_2$$

and when three of the data are known, the fourth can be calculated.

1. Given 10 ml of a 2% solution, dilute to a concentration of 0.5%. This requires finding the new volume.

$$V_1 C_1 = V_2 C_2$$

$$V_2 = \frac{V_1 C_1}{C_2} = \frac{10 \times 2}{0.5} = 40 \text{ ml}$$

Thus 30 ml added to 10 ml of 2% solution make 40 ml of 0.5% solution.

2. If 50 ml of water are added to 150 ml of a 3% solution, calculate the new concentration.

$$V_1 C_1 = V_2 C_2$$

$$C_2 = \frac{V_1 C_1}{V_2} = \frac{150 \times 3}{200} = 2.25\%$$

3. Given 50 ml of $\frac{N}{3}$ solution, dilute it to $\frac{N}{10}$ concentration. Here, concentration is given as normality, but it can be used as well as percent.

$$V_1 C_1 = V_2 C_2$$

$$V_2 = \frac{V_1 C_1}{C_2} = \frac{50 \times 0.333}{0.1} = 167 \text{ ml}$$

*Exercise 2-7.* Calculate the following:

(a) To what volume would 15 ml of a 6% solution be diluted to make a 4% solution?

(b) How much water would be added to 65 ml of a 3% solution to make 2.5%?

(c) What was the concentration of 25 ml of solution, if the addition of 14 ml of water produced a 6.5% solution?

(d) How much 3 M solution is needed to make 12 ml of 0.2 M solution?

(e) If 92.75 mg of $Na_2CO_3$ are dissolved in 0.5 ml of water, what would be the normality of the solution after the addition of 0.67 ml of water?

## OTHER "SOLUTIONS"

Two types of liquid mixtures that are considered with solutions but which do not have specific characteristics of solutions are *colloids* and *suspensions*. Colloids (sometimes called *dispersions* or *gels*) consist of large molecules, or clumps of molecules, that are able to attract and hold large numbers of water molecules. Egg white, glue, soap, and gelatin are common examples. Colloid solutions are cloudy or opalescent, exert only slight osmotic pressure, and have little effect on boiling or freezing points. *Suspensions*, of which clay in water is a typical example, consist of large particles that are merely suspended in a liquid vehicle without the intimate relationship between solvent and solute found in solutions. Dispersion of the suspended particles depends on physical agitation, and when the mixture is allowed to stand, the particles settle out.

## ELECTROLYTES AND IONS

One of the most important cardiopulmonary functions is the stability of acid-base balance, to be discussed in detail later; but to understand its fundamentals, the student must first understand the principles of electrolytes and ions. Indeed, the mechanism for regulation of acidity and alkalinity of the body and the transportation of respiratory gases to and from the tissues are so intimately related that neither can be fully intelligible without knowledge of the other. We will now consider some of the terms to be used later in our study of physiology.

Any substance in *aqueous* solution capable of carrying an electric current is called an *electrolyte;* nonconductors are called *nonelectrolytes*. In general, solutions of ionic or electrovalent compounds, which include many of the common chemically active inorganic substances, are good conductors of electricity. Nonpolar covalent compounds, however, have a wide range of conductivity, from the highly conductive hydrogen chloride to the barely conductive carbonic acid.

Nonelectrolytes and electrolytes differ also in their effects on the freezing and boiling points of water. Any substance dissolved in water will lower the freezing point and raise the boiling point. If the solute is a true nonelectrolyte, a 1 molal solution will depress the water's freezing point $1.86°$ C and elevate its boiling point $0.52°$ C. In contrast, a 1 molal solution of an electrolyte alters these points two to four times more than does the nonelectrolyte. The effect of solute on solvent freezing and boiling is a function of concentration of solute particles. The more particles of solute per weight of solvent the greater the displacement of freezing and boiling temperatures. Thus there must be more particles of solute per weight of solvent in an electrolyte solution than in a nonelectrolyte solution of equal molality.

Recall that solutions of the same molality have the same number of moles (gram molecular or gram formula weights) of solute in the same *weight* of solvent. For example, a 1 m solution of simple sugar, glucose $(C_6H_{12}O_6)$, a nonpolar covalent substance composed of molecules, will contain 1 gram molecular weight of sugar, or $6.02 \times 10^{23}$ molecules, per kilogram of water. This concentration of molecular particles lowers the freezing point of water $1.86°$ C and elevates its boiling point $0.52°$ C. A 1 m solution of sodium chloride, on the other hand, depresses the freezing point and elevates the boiling almost twice as much as does the sugar. This means that the salt solution must have a larger number of particles in solution than does the sugar, or more than $6.02 \times 10^{23}$ particles per kilogram of water. Because sodium chloride is an electrovalent compound, in solution 1 mole does not form $6.02 \times 10^{23}$ molecules of NaCl, as the sugar does, but breaks down into a larger number of the smaller sodium and chloride ions. It is the larger number of these small ions that exerts a greater influence on the freezing and boiling of water than does the smaller number of larger sugar molecules.

In relation to other subject matter, we have already made several references to ions, but because their role in the physiology of health and disease is so important, we will now spend a little time describing their origins and relationships to ionic, polar covalent, and nonpolar covalent compounds. Our interest is only in aqueous solutions because water is the physiological solvent, and we will discuss the important function played by water dipoles in ion production.

## Ion formation

The principle of ion formation includes the following three tenets: (1) electrolytes in solution exist as ions; (2) ions are atoms or groups of atoms that carry electric charges; (3) water solutions of electrolytes contain equal numbers of positive (cations) and negative (anions) ions. Let us consider solutions of the three types of compounds noted above and see how they contribute to ion formation.

*Ionic (electrovalent) solutions.* Lacking molecular structure, ionic compounds exist as an orderly arrangement of their constituent ions in masses called crystals. It is important to note that ions are present in such compounds even in the dry undissolved state. The process of dissolving consists of separating crystals into individual ions. The ions are thus freed from their mutual bonds and immediately distribute themselves uniformly throughout the solvent. This phenomenon is referred to as *ionic dissociation*, or just plain *dissociation*, since the ions released are existing ions already present in the solute rather than newly formed. Dissociation is the opposite of association, the breaking down of substances into their component parts, in this instance the dissociation of crystals into ions.

The prototype of ionic or electrovalent dissociation in aqueous solution is that of sodium chloride, shown as follows:

$$Na^+Cl^- \, (s) \longrightarrow Na^+ \, (aq) + Cl^- \, (aq)$$

where s = solid state (g = gas; l = liquid); aq = "in water"; charge signs in the compound formula indicate ions existing in the solid crystalline state, before dissolving; arrow indicates complete dissociation into ions. For the sake of simplicity this equation may be written:

$$NaCl \longrightarrow Na^+ + Cl^-$$

Solutions of sodium chloride contain equal numbers of Na and Cl ions to maintain electrical equilibrium. Calcium chloride ($CaCl_2$), in contrast, produces twice as many anions as cations, but the total charges remain equal:

$$Ca^{++}Cl_2^- \longrightarrow Ca^{++} + Cl^- + Cl^-$$

It was originally thought that the role of water as a solvent was purely passive, providing a uniform medium in which electrolytic dissociation could somehow spontaneously occur. The dipole water molecule is now recognized as being critically important in this phenomenon, participating in solute dissociation, and regulating the degree to which ions are produced. For the moment we will direct our attention to the first of these functions, and take up the second later.

Fig. 2-11 schematically represents the dissociation of sodium chloride. A crystalline mass of Na and Cl ions rests on the bottom of the container. Water molecular dipoles are separating the crystalline ions through the electrical attraction of their polar charges. Negative oxygen poles of water molecules draw away from the crystal the positive Na ions, while positive hydrogen poles relate similarly to Cl ions. As the ions diffuse throughout the solvent, each is loosely held by an escort of several water molecules surrounding it and facing it with appropriate oppositely charged poles. The number of water dipoles associated with a particular ion depends on the size and charge of the ion, and Fig. 2-11 is not intended to be quantitatively accurate. An ion thus associated with water dipoles is said to be *hydrated*. Hydration is a kinetic state, as water molecules continually interchange from ion to ion and between ions and the solvent mass.

Generally, ionic compounds are strong electrolyes, strength in this text being a function of the degree of electrical conductivity. Conductivity, in turn, depends on the number of ions formed, and thus the larger the concentration of ions made available by a solute the stronger electrolyte it is. A little further below we will discuss quantitative aspects of ion production.

***Polar covalent solutions.*** We know that molecular covalent compounds have no inherent ions of their own. In solution, however, through action similar to that described for the dissociation of sodium chloride, water dipoles can break the covalent bonds of polarized molecules and produce ions. In this circumstance ions are made from molecules in water solution where none existed before, and such a phenomenon is called *ionization*, as differentiated from ionic dissociation, discussed above. We

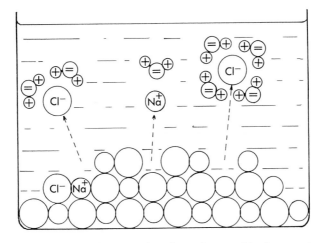

**Fig. 2-11.** NaCl is shown as a crystalline mass of ions being dissociated by the attraction of water dipoles. (See text for a more detailed description.)

will consider ionization of a strong covalent electrolyte, a weak covalent electrolyte, and the very special condition of ionization of water.

*Ionization of a strong polar covalent electrolyte.* Hydrogen chloride is a good example of a strong covalent electrolyte. In the pure liquid state from compression and cooling of the gas, or when dissolved in an organic nonpolar covalent solvent such as benzene, HCl does not conduct electricity, thus demonstrating lack of ions of its own, but when dissolved in water, it becomes an active electrolyte. The dramatic change in properties after HCl dissolves must be attributed to some function of water solvent molecules. Fig. 2-12 illustrates the fundamental reaction between HCl molecules and water dipoles. Fig. 2-12, *A*, shows the negative pole of a water molecule reacting with the positive pole of an HCl molecule. The effect is seen in Fig. 2-12, *B*, where the water dipole, through electrical attraction, has pulled away the hydrogen from the chloride atom, leaving the chloride with the shared electrons, thereby creating a chloride anion and a hydrogen cation. Ionization has been accomplished. Hydrogen ions, however, cannot exist alone in solution but only in combination with a dipole water molecule as indicated in Fig. 2-12, *C*. The hydrated hydrogen ion becomes a group of three atoms with an overall net electrical charge of +1. It is called a *hydronium ion*. In terms of chemical action the hydronium ion is the hydrogen ion, with the same meaning as the notation, $H^+$. For convenience the latter is more commonly used in chemical equations involving hydrogen ions, and we shall use it almost exclusively in the remainder of this text. Note that the simple hydrogen ion $H^+$ is actually

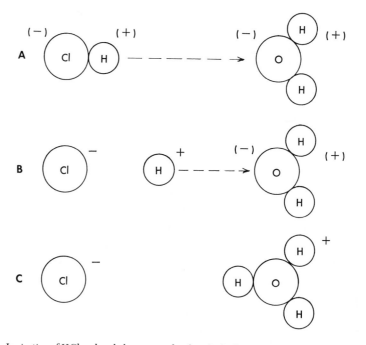

**Fig. 2-12.** Ionization of HCl molecule by a water dipole. The hydrogen atom is separated from the chloride by the negative pole of a water molecule. (See text for details.)

a proton. From Fig. 2-1 it can be seen that when a hydrogen atom loses its electron to become an ion, the only electrical charge left is the single nuclear proton. The hydronium ion therefore is actually a hydrated proton.

The ionization of HCl depicted in Fig. 2-12 can be expressed chemically as follows:

$$HCl\ (g) + H_2O\ (l) \longrightarrow H_3O^+\ (aq) + Cl^-\ (aq)$$

or more simply

$$HCl \longrightarrow H^+\ (aq) + Cl^-\ (aq)$$

or simply

$$HCl \longrightarrow H^+ + Cl^-$$

Observe that the formula for HCl is written without charge signs, as opposed to $Na^+Cl^-$, to demonstrate its molecular rather than ionic structure. Finally, the student should understand that the process of ionization changes the nature of the substance ionized. Hydrogen chloride, as a gas or a solute in a nonpolar solvent, is transformed into hydrochloric acid when ionized in an aqueous solution. It then acquires properties characteristic of acids, some of which will be reviewed shortly.

*Ionization of a weak polar covalent electrolyte.* Many of the organic compounds of the body are weak electrolytes and play important roles in maintaining healthy homeostasis. In fact, the mechanism of acid-base balance, an understanding of which is so important to us in the management of pulmonary disease patients, is dependent upon the principles of low level ionization.

We will use acetic acid as an example of a weak electrolyte. It is an organic acid (the major ingredient of vinegar), with a formula that can be written two ways. As a simple statement of the relative number of atoms in the compound, it can be represented as $C_2H_4O_2$, but this gives no clues as to its structure. When written as $CH_3COOH$, it is consistent with the custom of recording organic acids with the anion first and the hydrogen cation last. Acetic acid thus consists of the *acetate ion*, $CH_3COO^-$, with a single negative oxidation number, and a hydrogen ion, $H^+$.

When we characterize acetic acid as a weak electrolyte, we imply that it has some but not much molecular polarity, and a strong covalent bond that is difficult for the water dipole to break. Its ionizing equation is:

$$CH_3COOH + H_2O \rightleftharpoons H_3O^+ + CH_3COO^-$$

or

$$CH_3COOH \rightleftharpoons H^+ + CH_3COO^-$$

Note the use of double arrows in this equation, an indication that the reaction can go in both directions simultaneously, a *reversible reaction*. While molecules of acetic acid are breaking down into ions (movement to the right), some of the ions are recombining into molecules (movement to the left). The arrows actually represent a state of equilibrium, whereby the number of molecules ionizing are equaled by the number re-formed from ions. Some degree of quantitation can be expressed by the equation's arrows. A single arrow to the right shows a complete reaction in that direction, with no equilibrium established between molecules and ions, but a conversion of all molecules to ions, leaving only ions to remain in solution. Thus $HCl \rightarrow H^+ + Cl^-$ means full ionization of HCl, the sign of a strong electrolyte. The reaction $Na^+Cl^- \rightarrow Na^+ + Cl^-$ similarly shows complete dissociation of the electrovalent salt into its component ions, also indicating a strong electrolyte. In general, less than complete ionization is often shown by two arrows of equal length, but a known very weak electrolyte can be clearly identified by unequal arrows as used above for acetic acid. This means the compound has a stronger tendency to remain molecularly bound than to ionize.

Weak electrolytes exist in aqueous solution mostly as molecules with only a few ions. Fig. 2-13 nonquantitatively compares the degree of ionization of acetic acid with that of hydrochloric acid and emphasizes the larger number of particles, disregarding size, in a strong than in a weak electrolyte.

*Ionization of water.* Water is one of the weakest electrolytes, yet upon its seemingly negligible amount of ionization depend physiological acid-base balance and our system of recording it. For reasons as yet unclear, attraction between a rare pair of water dipoles can develop a bond uniting the oxygen of one and a hydrogen of the other that is stronger than the internal covalent bond of the second molecule. Fig. 2-14 illustrates the union of two water molecules and then their separation into *hydronium* and *hydroxide (OH$^-$)* ions according to the reaction:

$$H_2O + H_2O \;\rightleftharpoons\; H_3O^+ + OH^-$$

or

$$H(OH) + H(OH) \;\rightleftharpoons\; HH(OH)^+ + OH^-$$

or better yet

$$HOH \;\rightleftharpoons\; H^+ + OH^-$$

The hydronium ion so formed is exactly like that generated in the ionization of hydrogen chloride, described earlier. Note that the formula for water can be written in two ways, as we showed above for acetic acid. The formula $H_2O$ indicates that a molecule consists of two hydrogen atoms linked to one oxygen atom; HOH indicates the same thing, but in addition emphasizes the two ions that derive from a very few of the molecules. The latter is the preferred notation, especially in an ionization equation, while the more common $H_2O$ will continue to be used in other circumstances.

Similarly, the hydronium ion in the second equation is written $HH(OH)^+$ to be consistent with the HOH of water and to underscore its ionic structure. This is not an official notation and is used here only for emphasis. In general, we will refer to the hydrogen ion simply as $H^+$.

The ionization equation, with its unequal arrows, indicates the weakness of water as an electrolyte. Nonetheless, because some ionization does occur, water may be thought of as a very dilute aqueous solution of hydrogen and hydroxide ions, or a solution of these two ions in molecular water.

*Nonpolar covalent solutions.* An even distribution of charges gives to nonpolar covalent compounds an electrical symmetry that prevents polarity. It creates strong internal molecular bonding that successfully resists the attraction of water solvent dipoles. A nonpolarized molecule may be seen as presenting a defensive perimeter on which any given point is electrically neutral because of surrounding balanced charges. In a sense, water dipoles can find no handgrip by which to pull apart the solute molecules. Methane, diagrammed in Fig. 2-6, is a good example of a nonpolar covalent substance. Solutions of these compounds, then, produce no ions, conduct no electrical current, and are *nonelectrolytes*.

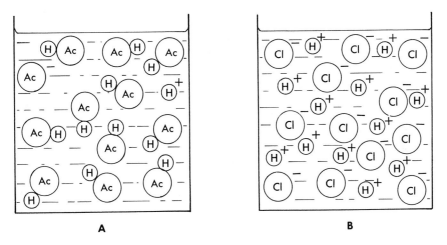

**Fig. 2-13.** In **A,** the weak electrolyte, acetic acid, exists almost entirely as intact molecules, with only one cation and one anion each illustrated. In contrast, the strong electrolyte, HCl, in **B** is completely ionized.

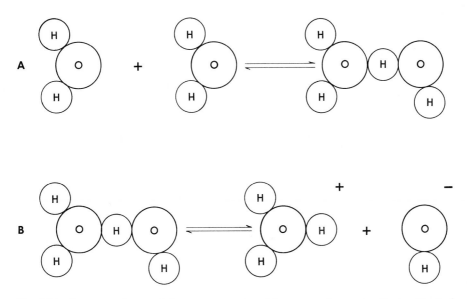

**Fig. 2-14.** Ionization of water. **A** depicts a rare union of the oxygen of one water dipole with a hydrogen atom of another. In **B** the two dipoles separate into hydronium and hydroxide ions. See text for description of ion formation.

## IONIC CHARACTERISTICS OF ACIDS, BASES, AND SALTS
### Acids

There are two definitions of an acid. The older Arrhenius* description states that an acid is a compound whose aqueous solution contains hydrogen ions. Such substances consist of a hydrogen atom or atoms *covalently* bonded to a negative valence nonmetal or radical, which gives the acid its name. By definition, then, an acid must be an electrolyte that produces hydrogen ions and anions. More consistent with modern chemical views is the Brønsted-Lowry definition, which simply calls an acid *any* compound that is a *proton donor*. This includes substances other than those we recognize as traditional acids. For example, the ammonium ion $NH_4^+$ qualifies as an acid, since it can release a proton ($H^+$) in the following reaction, which produces ammonia gas ($NH_3$):

$$NH_4Cl + NaOH \longrightarrow NH_3 + NaCl + HOH$$

The Na and Cl ions are called *spectator ions* because they are not involved in the proton transfer, which is the important event of this reaction. By eliminating them, we can write the equation ionically and demonstrate the acidity of the ammonium ion:

$$NH_4^+ + OH^- \longrightarrow NH_3 \, (g) + HOH$$

The ammonium ion donated a hydrogen ion (proton) to the reaction, and it was accepted by the hydroxyl ion ($OH^-$), converting the former into ammonia gas and the latter into water. There really is very little difference between the two acid definitions, and our use of the term *acid* in this text will generally refer to compounds that are readily seen to be sources of H ions in solution.

In Chapter 1, under the discussion of equivalent weight, we used the term *replaceable hydrogen* in relation to acids. We can now use *ionizable hydrogen* for practical purposes as synonymous with the former but a little more specific for our present use. Let us consider two levels of acid complexity.

*Acids with single ionizable hydrogen.* Simple compounds such as the following ionize into one cation and anion each:

$$\begin{array}{lll} HCl & \longrightarrow & H^+ + Cl^- \\ \text{(Hydrochloric acid)} & & \text{(Chloride ion)} \\ HBr & \longrightarrow & H^+ + Br^- \\ \text{(Hydrobromic acid)} & & \text{(Bromide ion)} \\ HNO_3 & \longrightarrow & H^+ + NO_3^- \\ \text{(Nitric acid)} & & \text{(Nitrate ion)} \end{array}$$

*Acids with multiple ionizable hydrogens.* All of the potential hydrogen ions in an acid may not be made available at once but in stages. More will be said of this in the next section, but for now let us understand that the degree of ionization tends to increase as an electrolyte solution becomes more dilute. Concentrated sulfuric acid ionizes only one of its two hydrogen atoms per molecule:

$$H_2SO_4 \longrightarrow H^+ + HSO_4^-$$
$$\text{(Bisulfate, or acid sulfate, ion)}$$

---

*Svante August Arrhenius (1859-1927), Swedish chemist and physicist.

With further dilution, second stage ionization occurs:

$$H_2SO_4 \longrightarrow H^+ + H^+ + SO_4^=$$
$$\text{(Sulfate ion)}$$

Similarly, three stages of phosphoric acid ionization can be summarized as follows:

$$H_3PO_4 \longrightarrow H^+ + H_2PO_4^-$$
$$\text{(Dihydrogen phosphate ion)}$$
$$H^+ + H^+ + HPO_4^=$$
$$\text{(Monohydrogen, or biphosphate, ion)}$$
$$H^+ + H^+ + H^+ + PO_4^{\equiv}$$
$$\text{(Phosphate ion)}$$

The greater the concentration of hydrogen ions, the more acid or the stronger acid is the solution. Acids characteristically have a sour taste. They react with metals to produce hydrogen gas, and with bases to form salts and water.

## Bases

The Arrhenius definition of a base describes it as a compound whose aqueous solution contains hydroxyl ions and which destroys the properties of dissolved acids with which it is mixed. Such compounds are called *hydroxides* and consist of metals, or the metal equivalent, ammonium cation $(NH_4^-)$, *ionically* bound to a hydroxyl ion or ions. The student might already anticipate that a Brønsted-Lowry base is any compound that *accepts a proton*, including among the bases many substances other than hydroxides. Let us examine examples of bases in the two classifications of hydroxides and nonhydroxides.

*Hydroxide bases.* In aqueous solution the following are typical dissociations of hydroxide bases:

$$Na^+OH^- \longrightarrow Na^+ + OH^-$$
$$K^+OH^- \longrightarrow K^+ + OH^-$$
$$Ca^{++}(OH^-)_2 \longrightarrow Ca^{++} + 2OH^-$$

Inactivation of an acid, as part of the definition of a base, is accomplished by a hydroxide through the reaction of its $OH^-$ with the acid's $H^+$ (proton acceptance by the base), forming water:

$$NaOH + HCl \longrightarrow NaCl + HOH$$

*Nonhydroxide bases.* We will limit ourselves to aqueous solutions of two common substances in this group.

*Ammonia.* In the description of acids we demonstrated how ammonium ion can be called an acid by donating a proton and becoming ammonia. Ammonia doubly qualifies as a base by reacting with water to produce $OH^-$:

$$NH_3 + HOH \rightleftharpoons NH_4^+ + OH^-$$

and by neutralizing $H^+$ directly:

$$NH_3 + H^+ \rightleftharpoons NH_4^+$$

In both instances $NH_3$ accepted a proton to become $NH_4^+$.

*Carbonates.* The reactions of this group, of which sodium carbonate will be the example, are very relevant to some of our interests in pulmonary physiology. The carbonate ion, $CO_3^=$, can react with water to produce $OH^-$. First,

$$Na_2CO_3^= \rightleftharpoons 2Na^+ + CO_3^=$$

then

$$CO_3^= + HOH \rightleftharpoons \underset{\text{(Bicarbonate ion)}}{HCO_3^-} + OH^-$$

The carbonate ion accepted a proton ($H^+$) from water, became the bicarbonate ion, and produced an hydroxyl ion. The carbonate ion can also directly react with $H^+$ to inactivate it as follows:

$$CO_3^= + H^+ \rightleftharpoons HCO_3^-$$

Bases have a bitter taste, and most of them feel slippery or soapy. The soluble hydroxides or carbonates of sodium and potassium are sometimes referred to as *alkalis*. Finally, bases react with acids to form salts and water.

### Salts

The most common of compounds, salts, are composed of metal or ammonium ions electrovalently joined to anions other than the hydroxyl. There are many ways of producing salts, but the simplest and most instructive for our current discussion is by the reaction between an acid and a base, as noted in the descriptions of these last two compounds:

$$HCl + NaOH \longrightarrow NaCl + HOH$$

There are three classifications of salts, which depend on the degree of hydrogen and hydroxyl replacement from the parent acids and bases.

*Normal salt.* A normal salt is a compound formed by the complete replacement of hydrogen ions from its antecedent acid as follows:

$$H^+Cl^- + Na^+OH^- \longrightarrow Na^+Cl^- + H^+OH^-$$
$$H^+NO_3^- + K^+OH^- \longrightarrow K^+NO_3^- + H^+OH^-$$

*Acid salt.* An acid salt results from only partial replacement of hydrogen ions from the related acid, leaving some "acidity" (hydrogen ion or ions) in the salt:

$$\underset{\text{(Carbonic acid)}}{H_2^+CO_3^=} + Na^+OH^- \longrightarrow \underset{\text{(Sodium bicarbonate)}}{Na^+HCO_3^-} + H^+OH^-$$

Sodium bicarbonate can also be called sodium acid carbonate because of its H atom, although we will soon be getting to know it as a physiological base for reasons we hope will be clear at the proper time. Right now, because of the importance of this salt, we will take some liberties with the above equation to emphasize a point. Both H atoms in $H_2CO_3$ may ionize under proper conditions, but in the physiological environment of the human body, the illustrated single hydrogen ionization is the only reaction possible. To underscore the ions involved, carbonic acid can be rewritten to show it composed of only one hydrogen ion and the univalent *bicarbonate ion, $HCO_3^-$*. The reaction will look like this:

$$H^+HCO_3^+ + Na^+OH^- \longrightarrow Na^+HCO_3^- + H^+OH^-$$

From our point of view, this version of carbonic acid is more reasonable than was the first, and it clarifies the origin of the very important bicarbonate ion.

**Basic salt.** A basic salt contains an unreplaced hydroxyl ion from the base generating it, such as:

$$Ca^{++}(OH^-)_2 + H^+Cl^- \longrightarrow Ca^{++}(OH^-)Cl^- + H^+OH^-$$
$$\text{(Calcium hydroxide)} \qquad\qquad \text{(Basic calcium hydroxide)}$$

There are no basic salts that are significant in our areas of interest in pulmonary physiology.

## MEASUREMENT OF ELECTROLYTIC ACTIVITY
### Electrolytic equilibrium

The physiologically active chemical compounds of the body are, for the most part, weak electrolytic covalent substances, and their ionic behavior can be stated as follows:

1. A proportion of the molecules in an aqueous solution of a weak covalent electrolyte ionize, and the remainder of the molecules persist intact. At a given temperature and concentration, equilibrium is maintained between the ions and the un-ionized molecules.
2. After the establishment of ionic equilibrium, the *product* of the *molar* concentration (moles per liter) of the ions divided by the *molar* concentration of the un-ionized molecules is a *constant* value at a given concentration of solution and temperature. This is a special type of *equilibrium constant* called an *ionization constant*, or K. It cannot be emphasized too strongly that such a relationship exists *only* with aqueous solutions of *weak* electrolytes.

### Degree of dissociation or ionization

We pointed out earlier that the strength of an electrolyte depends upon the percentage of its solute that dissociates if it is ionic or ionizes if it is covalent. An important bit of datum therefore, in evaluating the electrolytic strength of a substance, is its percent of ion production. Handbooks of chemistry and other sources provide this information, always specifying the molar concentrations of the solutions and the temperature at which the values are valid. To give the student some idea of the range of numbers involved, Table 2-5 lists the percentages of three strong and three weak electrolytes that produce ions in 0.1 M solutions at a temperature of 25° C. NaOH is the only electrovalent compound in the group, and we can say of it that 90% *dissociates* into Na and OH ions. Of HCl we can say that 90% of its molecules *ionize* into H and Cl ions. In contrast, only 0.01% (0.0001) of molecules of boric acid $(H_3BO_3)$ ionize.

**Table 2-5.**  *Percent ion formation of 0.1 M solutions at 25° C* *

| NaOH | 90% | $CH_3COOH$ | 1.33% |
|------|-----|------------|-------|
| HCl | 90% | $H_2CO_3$ | 0.207% |
| $HNO_3$ | 90% | $H_3BO_3$ | 0.0076% |

*Based on new data since last edition.

**Table 2-6.** *Influence of concentrations of sodium chloride (NaCl) solution on freezing point depression of water**

| Aqueous molal NaCl concentration | Depression of freezing point (° C) per mole of NaCl |
|---|---|
| 1.00 | 3.37 |
| 0.10 | 3.48 |
| 0.010 | 3.60 |
| 0.0010 | 3.66 |
| 0.00010 | 3.72 |

*Data from Metcalf, H. C., et al.: Modern chemistry, New York, 1966, Holt, Rinehart & Winston, Inc., and Boylan, P. J., et al.: Elements of chemistry, Boston, 1962, Allyn & Bacon, Inc.

Theoretically, because electrovalent compounds such as sodium chloride, sodium hydroxide, and silver nitrate are 100% ionic in their crystalline forms, they should undergo 100% ionic dissociation in aqueous solution. The same is true of the strong covalent acids. Electrical conductivity measurements of such solutions, and less than maximal alteration of freezing and boiling points of water, indicate that 100% ion production is not always realized. The term *apparent degree of dissociation,* or *ionization,* as opposed to *actual* is used for values such as those in Table 2-5.

The reason for this discrepancy is found in the effect of solute dilution on dissociation and ionization. It was noted earlier that the water dipole influences the degree of ion production and, more recently, that solute concentration is important in determining equilibrium constants. In a concentrated solution there may not be enough water molecules to separate and hydrate the large number of ions of electrovalent compounds or to ionize polar covalent molecules. The closely packed ions of a concentrated solution tend to interfere with each other's activities, and they act as relatively small numbers of groups rather than large numbers of individual ions. Solvent freezing and boiling points are thus less affected than they would be by a larger number. Diluting a given electrolyte solution reduces interaction among ions and increases the apparent dissociation and ionization. This is one of the reasons for the multiple stages of ionization described and illustrated earlier for sulfuric and phosphoric acids. The student thus should note that diluting the concentration of a solute may increase the concentration of its ions. Table 2-6 demonstrates the effect on the freezing of water of increases in dissociation of sodium chloride by progressive tenfold molal dilution.

Let us make a quantitative comparison between a 0.1 M solution of HCl with 90% ionization and a 0.1 M solution of $H_2CO_3$ with 0.207% ionization. One liter of each solution will contain 0.1 mole, or 0.1 gmw, of its respective acid solute. Ninety percent of the HCl molecules, or 0.90 of 0.1 mole, 0.09 of a mole, dissociate into ions; 0.01 of a mole or gmw remains as intact molecules. Since each dissociating molecule produces one cation and one anion, the concentration, or number per liter of each, is the same as the concentration of the dissociating molecules. Thus we can summarize the ionic and molecular concentrations of the 0.1 M HCl solutions:

Concentration of H ions = 0.09 mole (or g-ion) per liter
Concentration of Cl ions = 0.09 mole (or g-ion) per liter
Concentration of HCl molecules = 0.01 mole (or g-mole) per liter

Of the 0.1 M solution of $H_2CO_3$, which dissociates into $H^+$ and $HCO_3^-$ (bicarbonate) ions, 0.00207 of 0.1 of a mole, or 0.000207 mole of the acid dissociates into ions; 0.9979 of 0.1 mole, or 0.09979 of a mole remains undissociated. Thus:

Concentration of H ions = 0.000207 mole (g-ion) per liter
Concentration of $HCO_3$ ions = 0.000207 mole (g-ion) per liter
Concentration of $H_2CO_3$ molecules = 0.09979 mole (g-mole) per liter

Furthermore, a 0.1 M solution contains $6.02 \times 10^{23} \times 0.1$, or $6.02 \times 10^{22}$ molecules per liter. Therefore, on the basis of the known percentage of molecules that ionize, the actual number of ions and molecules per liter can be computed as shown in Table 2-7.

Examples of ionization can be expressed in one equation, relating the ionized and un-ionized molecules with the constant. It must be remembered that this relationship holds only for weak electrolytes. The numerators of the following equations are in *molar* concentrations (moles, or gram-ionic, or gram-atomic weights per liter) of ions, and the denominators are in molar concentrations (moles or gram-molecular weights per liter) of un-ionized molecules of solute.

Brackets indicate concentrations of ions as well as of molecules and undissociated solute. Unless otherwise specified, the concentration implied is *moles per liter*. Thus $[H^+]$ means moles per liter of hydrogen ions, but the expression gram-ions per liter is occasionally encountered; $[HCO_3^-]$ means molar concentration of bicarbonate ions per liter: $[H_2CO_3]$ signifies moles per liter of un-ionized, intact carbonic acid molecules.

(1) Symbolic representation of an acid, HA:
$$\frac{[H^+][A^-]}{[HA]} = K$$

(2) Symbolic representation of a base, BOH:
$$\frac{[B^+][OH^-]}{[BOH]} = K$$

(3) Acetic acid:
$$\frac{[H^+][CH_3COO^-]}{[CH_3COOH]} = 1.8 \times 10^{-5}$$

(4) Carbonic acid:
$$\frac{[H^+][HCO_3^-]}{H_2CO_3} = 4.3 \times 10^{-7}$$

(5) Boric acid:
$$\frac{[H^+][H_2BO_3^-]}{H_3BO_3} = 5.8 \times 10^{-10}$$

**Table 2-7.** *Concentrations of ions and molecules in 0.1 M HCl and 0.1 M $H_2CO_3$*

| | $H^+$ per liter | Anions per liter | Undissociated molecules per liter |
|---|---|---|---|
| 0.1 M HCl | $5.418 \times 10^{22}$ | $5.418 \times 10^{22}$ | $6.02 \times 10^{21}$ |
| 0.1 M $H_2CO_3$ | $1.246 \times 10^{20}$ | $1.246 \times 10^{20}$ | $6.0074 \times 10^{22}$ |

### Calculation of ionization (equilibrium) constant

The actual calculation of an ionization constant will be demonstrated, using acetic acid ($CH_3COOH$). At 25° C, 1.33% of a 0.1 M solution of the acid undergoes ionization, and thus 98.67% of the molecules do not ionize. Slight though it is, the ionization of acetic acid is $CH_3COOH \rightleftharpoons H^+ + CH_3COO^-$.

1. Since 0.1 M solution of acetic acid contains 0.1 gmw of acid per liter, of which 1.33% ionizes, then $0.1 \times 0.0133$ or 0.00133 of a mole of acid per liter produces ions, and $0.1 \times 0.9867$ or 0.09867 of a mole per liter remains un-ionized.

2. Each molecule that ionizes produces two ions, $H^+$ and $CH_3COO^-$ (acetate ion), and the concentration of *each* is thus the same as that of the ionizing molecules, 0.00133 of a mole of ions per liter. Accordingly, the concentration of un-ionized molecules is 0.09867 of a mole of ions per liter.

3. By definition, K is equal to the ratio between the product of the molar ion concentrations and the molar concentration of the un-ionized molecules, or:

$$\frac{[H^+][CH_3COO^-]}{[CH_3COOH]} = K$$

$$\frac{0.00133 \times 0.00133}{0.09867} = K$$

$$K = 1.8 \times 10^{-5}$$

*Exercise 2-8.* Calculate the K of the following symbolic acid and base:

(a) 0.1 M HA, with 2.5% ionization
(b) 0.05 M BOH, with 1.9% dissociation

## Ionization constant of water

The ionization of *water* is the basis for a system of calibrating acidity and alkalinity that will be discussed below. Pure water produces the two ions $H^+$ and $OH^-$, and although its degree of ionization is very minute, it has an important ionization constant. In a sense, water consists of an aqueous solution of $H^+$ and $OH^-$, or it may be considered a solution of these two ions dissolved in molecular water. Its ion/molecule ratio can be expressed in the usual manner:

$$\frac{[H^+][OH^-]}{[HOH]} = K$$

However, the degree of ionization of water is so small, and the concentration of un-ionized molecules is proportionally so large, that any small change in the degree of ionization would not produce a detectable reciprocal change in the concentration of the un-ionized molecules. If one stood on a beach holding a dozen grains of sand in one hand, dropping six of them or adding six more to the hand from the beach would not noticeably affect the concentration of sand on the beach, but it would make a great difference to the concentration in the hand. So it is with un-ionized water molecules. There are so many of them in relation to the number that ionize into H and OH ions that should there be, from time to time, some variation in the number that do ionize, the effect on the large concentration of intact molecules [HOH] would be insignificant, but ionic concentrations $[H^+]$ and $[OH^-]$ would be greatly altered. Thus the molar concentration of molecular water, for all practical purposes, does not change and can be considered as another constant in the ratio. The ratio can be rewritten as:

$$\frac{[H^+][OH^-]}{K_2} = K_1$$

and

$$[H^+][OH^-] = K_1 K_2 = K_w$$

The dissociation constant of water, $K_w$ has been determined to be $1 \times 10^{-14}$. Therefore, if

$$[H^+][OH^-] = 10^{-14}$$

then, because there is one $H^+$ for each $OH^-$, the concentration of each ion is *$10^{-7}$ moles or gram ions per liter*. Pure water is as much acid as it is base, and it is thus *neutral* in action.

## DESIGNATION OF ACIDITY AND ALKALINITY

We have seen that pure water is neutral in its reaction, with equal $[H^+]$ and $[OH^-]$. Using this as a reference point, we can state that any solution having a *greater* $[H^+]$ than that of water is acid in its reaction or any solution with lesser $[OH^-]$ than that of water is also acidic. Similarly, a solution with a greater $[OH^-]$, or a lesser $[H^+]$, than that of water is basic in reaction. By agreement, the *hydrogen ion concentration* $[H^+]$ of pure water has been adopted as the standard by which to compare reactions of other solutions. Electrochemical techniques are used to measure the $[H^+]$ of unknown solutions and the degree of their acidity or alkalinity determined by variation of their $[H^+]$ above or below $1 \times 10^{-7}$. Thus a solution with a $[H^+]$ of $8.2 \times 10^{-4}$ has a *higher* $[H^+]$ than water and is acid; one with a $[H^+]$ of $3.6 \times 10^{-8}$ has less hydrogen ions than water and is alkaline. There are two related techniques for recording acidity and alkalinity of solutions, using the $[H^+]$ of water as the neutral standard:

*Nanomoles per liter of $[H^+]$.* The first method reports simply the actual measured molar concentration of H ions, which can then be compared to that of water. We know the $[H^+]$ of water is $1 \times 10^{-7}$ of a mole per liter, but this is an awkward expression to verbalize. Written as a decimal, it would be 0.0000001, or one ten millionth of a mole, also awkward. Being smaller than a millionth, a ten millionth falls into the next thousandth increment of the decimal system, the billionth (prefixed *nano*). Thus one ten millionth equals 100 billionths, and the H ion concentration of water can be designated as 100 nanomoles (nM) per liter. With this as a reference, any solution having a $[H^+]$ of 100 nM/$\ell$ is neutral, greater than 100 nM/$\ell$ acid, and less than 100 nM/$\ell$ alkaline. The degree of acidity or alkalinity is proportional to the distance of a given $[H^+]$ from the 100 nM/$\ell$ reference. This system of nomenclature is limited in its use because of the tremendous range of possible $[H^+]$, from the very acid to the very alkaline. It is not feasible to convert all $[H^+]$ values to nanomoles, since this does not eliminate all awkward numbers. The system is applicable to needs of cardiopulmonary physiology, however, because the range of H ion concentrations is very narrow and seldom exceeds values of 20 to 100 nM/$\ell$.

**pH.** Second, to simplify acid-base comparisons the principle of *pH* was developed. pH is the "hydrogen ion exponent," *the negative log of the hydrogen ion concentration, used as a positive number.* It is derived by converting the entire value for $[H^+]$ to a single negative exponent of 10 by calculating its logarithm. The $[H^+]$ of water is $1 \times 10^{-7}$, and since the log of $1 \times 10^{-7}$ is $-7$, the pH of water is 7. Note the following equations:

(1) $[H^+]$ of $8.2 \times 10^{-4}$
$pH = \log 8.2 \times 10^{-4} = \overline{4}.914 = -3.086 = 3.09$
(2) $[H^+]$ of $4.0 \times 10^{-8}$
$pH = \log 4.0 \times 10^{-8} = \overline{8}.602 = -7.398 = 7.40$
(3) $[H^+]$ of $6.7 \times 10^{-11}$
$pH = \log 6.7 \times 10^{-11} = \overline{11}.826 = -10.174 = 10.17$

It is obvious that any solution with a pH of 7 is neutral, corresponding to the $[H^+]$ of pure water. As the pH value *decreases* numerically below 7, because it is in reality a negative log, it represents an actual $[H^+]$ greater than 7 and therefore is acid. Conversely, pH values greater than 7 represent lower $[H^+]$ and are alkaline. The pH scale represents this graphically:

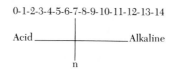

0-1-2-3-4-5-6-7-8-9-10-11-12-13-14

Acid _____|_____ Alkaline

n

The compactness of the pH scale is nicely illustrated if we compare its midpoint and two extremes with corresponding molar concentrations of H ions:

| pH | $[H^+]$ |
|----|---------|
| 0 | $10^0$ or 1.0 M/$\ell$ |
| 7 | $10^{-7}$ or 100 nM/$\ell$ |
| 14 | $10^{-14}$ or $10^{-5}$ nM/$\ell$ |

**Exercise 2-9.** Calculate the pH of the following to two decimals:

(a) $[H^+] = 7.6 \times 10^{-5}$
(b) $[H^+] = 3.04 \times 10^{-2}$
(c) $[H^+] = 5.16 \times 10^{-12}$
(d) $[H^+] = 1.01 \times 10^{-8}$
(e) $[H^+] = 8.66 \times 10^{-10}$

**Exercise 2-10.** Calculate the $[H^+]$ of the following:

(a) pH = 3.21
(b) pH = 8.92
(c) pH = 5.01
(d) pH = 10.26
(e) pH = 6.66

# Chapter 3

# VENTILATION

The terms *ventilation* and *respiration* are frequently used interchangeably because they are generally synonymous, but to many there is a subtle difference between them. Ventilation may be considered as the mechanical movement of air into and out of the lung in a cyclic fashion, whereas respiration often refers to the exchange of oxygen and carbon dioxide in the lung and at the body cell. The primary function of the lung is respiration, to supply the body with oxygen and to remove the waste product of metabolism, carbon dioxide; but to fulfill this function the lung must have adequate ventilation. Thus we will begin our study of cardiopulmonary physiology with a consideration of the first need—aeration of the lung.

Ventilation is a cyclic activity, both automatic and voluntary, and it consists of two components—an inward flow of air, called *inhalation* or inspiration, and an outward flow, called *exhalation* or expiration. The physical forces responsible for this air movement constitute the mechanics of ventilation. The inhalation-exhalation cycle moves a volume of gas into and out of the respiratory tract, the *tidal volume* ($V_T$). As the student observes his own ventilatory pattern, he will note that both tidal volume and *rate of breathing* (f, for frequency per minute) vary with physical activity. The product of these two factors, and a physiologically important parameter to evaluate, is the *minute volume* ($V_E$). This is the amount of gas moved per minute, and although theoretically it should equal the tidal volume times the frequency, for practical reasons it is defined as the volume *exhaled* per minute (indicated by its symbol) and is measured by time-collecting exhaled respiratory gas. The relationships between tidal volume, minute volume, frequency, the nature of the airways through which the gas flows, and the physical forces responsible for gas movement are critical in determining the effectiveness of ventilation, and some of the important factors influencing them will be defined and discussed.

## DEAD SPACE (REBREATHED VOLUME)

The term *dead space* ($V_D$) will be used preferentially in this text simply because at this time it is the more common of the two. It may be superseded by *rebreathed volume* ($V_{RB}$) in the near future because, as will be indicated below, the latter is a more accurate expression.

It is of utmost importance that the respiratory therapist understand the concept of *dead space* and the role it plays in ventilation. Dead space is defined as that portion of the respiratory tract which is *ventilated but not perfused by the pulmonary circulation.* It should be recalled that *perfusion* refers to the end point in arterial blood flow, where capillaries and tissue cells come into intimate contact for mutual exchange of contents. A review of anatomy will remind the student that the respiratory tract is supplied by two circulations, the systemic and the pulmonary. The conducting airways of the bronchial tree are served by the systemic circulation, and the bronchial and bronchiolar cells (as any other body tissue) are perfused by branches of the bronchial arteries to maintain their viability and function. The alveoli, however, are perfused by capillaries of the pulmonary circulation, and it is here that pulmonary arterial blood bathes the alveolar cells and is but a fraction of a micron away from alveolar air. Only at this level can oxygen and carbon dioxide pass between air and blood. By definition, then, ventilatory dead space consists of the conducting airways down to the level of gas exchange and *any alveoli* that, for one reason or another to be considered later, receive less than their normal pulmonary capillary perfusion. It is thus evident that dead space does not contribute to respiration but constitutes a volume which must be filled by ventilation before air can reach perfused alveoli.

Dead space is of three types: *anatomic* ($V_D$ ant), *alveolar* ($V_D$ alv), and *physiologic* ($V_D$ phys). These are diagrammatically illustrated in Fig. 3-1.

1. *Anatomic dead space* consists of the purely conducting airways of the nose and mouth, pharynx, larynx, trachea, bronchi, and bronchioles to the respiratory level.

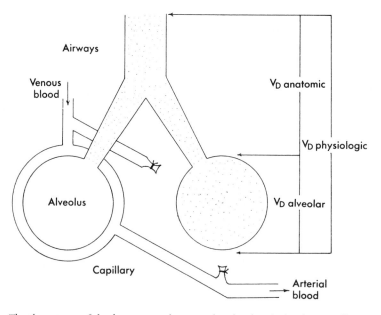

**Fig. 3-1.** The three types of dead space are shown in this sketch, which schematically represents two alveoli, their supporting airways, and capillaries. One alveolus is normally perfused and ventilated; but the capillary to the other is shown as if it were tied off and removed, so that the alveolus is freely ventilated but not perfused. The relationships of the dead spaces are indicated, as defined in the text.

2. *Alveolar dead space* is a less well-defined volume that consists of a variable number of alveoli whose perfusion is reduced or absent due, among other causes, to gravitational shifts in pulmonary blood flow distribution in the normal subject and to impaired flow in the diseased.
3. *Physiologic dead space* is the sum of the anatomic and alveolar dead spaces, and its description as "physiologic" implies that it is the functional dead space of ventilation.

Measurement of dead spaces can be performed in the cardiopulmonary laboratory by techniques that will not be discussed here. In theory, all alveoli should be perfused, with no alveolar dead space. Therefore physiologic and anatomic dead spaces should be identical and, as a rough guide, in the average adult should measure approximately between 150 and 160 ml. Should there be some alveoli with inadequate perfusion, a small alveolar dead space will exist that will increase the physiologic dead space.

Two points should be emphasized at this time. First, dead space is not dead at all because it is a functional volume that plays an important part in ventilation and is bounded by living tissue. Second, it is a volume that is rebreathed. Let us suppose the volume of air exhaled by a subject is 500 ml and his dead space is 150 ml. Of the 500 ml of air exhaled, the first 150 ml come from the upper portion of the respiratory tract, the conducting airways, or dead space, and the remaining 350 ml from the alveoli. At the end of exhalation, then, airways are not empty but contain 150 ml of air that have been moved up from the alveoli. With the next inhalation this 150 ml volume of dead space air, which has already been breathed, will be the first of the inspired air to be drawn back down into the alveoli and rebreathed. The student will later find this principle of rebreathed volumes of critical importance in the management of patients on mechanical ventilators.

## CLASSIFICATION OF VENTILATION

Types of ventilation may be classified according to the two categories of physiologic and clinical ventilation. *Physiologically*, we can consider *total ventilation*, or *minute volume* ($\dot{V}_E$), *dead space ventilation* ($\dot{V}_D$), and *alveolar ventilation* ($\dot{V}_A$). For safe and effective management of patients in ventilatory failure, the respiratory therapist must clearly understand the differences between and the importance of each of these types:

1. *Total ventilation* refers to the amount of air moved into and out of the entire respiratory tract in liters per minute in the resting state. Normally ranging from 5 to 10 $\ell$/min, this volume gives only a rough estimation of ventilatory efficiency, since it does not indicate how much air is reaching alveoli.
2. *Dead space ventilation* is the minute volume in liters that ventilates the physiologic dead space.
3. *Alveolar ventilation* is the minute volume in liters that ventilates all the perfused alveoli and obviously is the difference between the total and dead space ventilation. Usually it is between 4 and 5 $\ell$/min.

Functionally, only the alveolar ventilation is of importance, since it determines how much air will be available for gas exchange. Perhaps it is already evident that a patient's breathing pattern can be so disturbed that, with a rapid rate and a small tidal volume, a large total volume of air may be moved which does little more than ventilate the dead space, leaving only a small amount to reach the alveoli.

*Clinically,* in the resting state we note *normal ventilation, hypoventilation,* and *hyperventilation:*

1. *Normal ventilation* is that amount of minute ventilation which provides adequate alveolar ventilation at a normal rate and with a minimum of effort. We will see later that disruption of easy ventilation by disease, even with satisfactory alveolar aeration, can produce some of man's most serious physical disability.

2. *Hypoventilation* is that state of impaired breathing whereby the alveoli are inadequately ventilated to fulfill the body's gas exchange needs. Hypoventilation may be the result of either a *pathologic increase in dead space* (as from pulmonary distention, or increased ventilation/perfusion ratios, to be described later) or a *reduction in alveolar minute volume* (as from abnormally small tidal volumes, or retarded breathing frequency). Table 3-1 illustrates theoretical exaggerated examples, with volumes measured in milliliters. To compensate for an increased $V_D$, the patient must increase either rate or tidal volume, and in each instance the additional muscular effort is disabling. From a practical point of view, conditions causing a reduced ventilatory rate usually do not permit voluntary compensation by increasing the tidal volume, although sometimes a patient with restricted volumes can manage a compensatory rate increase. Again, this is possible only to a certain degree and is also physically strenuous. We will see later that the patient with this defect, by virtue of his underlying

**Table 3-1.** *Types of hypoventilation and their compensation*

| | *Normal* | *Hypoventilation due to increased $V_D$* | *Compensation* | |
|---|---|---|---|---|
| $V_T$ | 450 | 450 | 450 | 600 |
| $V_D$ | 150 | 300 | 300 | 300 |
| f | 15 | 15 | 30 | 15 |
| $\dot{V}_E$ | 6750 | 6750 | 13,500 | 9000 |
| $\dot{V}_D$ | 2250 | 4500 | 9000 | 4500 |
| $\dot{V}_A$ | 4500 | 2250 | 4500 | 4500 |

| | *Normal* | *Hypoventilation due to reduced tidal volume* | *Compensation* |
|---|---|---|---|
| $V_T$ | 450 | 225 | 225 |
| $V_D$ | 150 | 150 | 150 |
| f | 15 | 15 | 60 |
| $\dot{V}_E$ | 6750 | 3375 | 13,500 |
| $\dot{V}_D$ | 2250 | 2250 | 9000 |
| $\dot{V}_A$ | 4500 | 1125 | 4500 |

disease, is usually unable to compensate at all. The respiratory therapist will find that the treatment of hypoventilation will be one of his most demanding responsibilities.

3. *Hyperventilation* is an overaeration of the alveoli beyond physiologic needs due to an increase in tidal volume or rate or both and may be voluntary or involuntary. It can upset respiratory stability and impair circulation, but it is especially important for the therapist to note that hyperventilation is often induced by certain respiratory therapy procedures, a point that will be strongly emphasized later during discussions on techniques.

## ACTION OF VENTILATORY MUSCLES[6-8]
### Movements of the thoracic cage

At this time the student should review the anatomy of the thorax, paying particular attention to the relationships between the skeletal parts, the shape of the ribs, and the thoracic musculature. The thorax is somewhat like a cone, with a wide base bounded by the diaphragm and a narrow opening at the top called the *operculum*. The latter is bounded by the first ribs and the manubrium of the sternum. For pur-

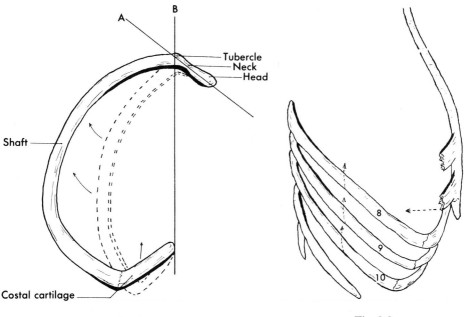

**Fig. 3-2**                                        **Fig. 3-3**

**Fig. 3-2.** The two axes about which the vertebrosternal ribs rotate during ventilation are indicated by lines *A* and *B*. The former passes through the length of the rib head and neck; the latter follows an A-P direction from the tip of the coastal cartilage to the tubercle. The rib undergoes a compound movement from its starting position (dotted outline), the shaft swinging upward and laterally about axis *B*, and the anterior end moving upward about axis *A*.

**Fig. 3-3.** The vertebrochondral ribs, *8* to *10*, have laterosuperior movement like ribs 2 to 7, but elevation of their anterior ends retracts the lower end of the sternum, shortening the A-P diameter of the thorax in that plane.

poses of discussion the ribs are grouped into three categories—the *first rib*, the *vertebrosternal ribs* (2 to 7), and the *vertebrochondral ribs* (8 to 10):

1. The *first rib* moves about the axis of its neck, raising and lowering the sternum. Although the motion is slight, it produces some increase in the anteroposterior (A-P) diameter of the chest. During quiet breathing this action is not utilized, but it becomes important under conditions of stress.

2. The six *vertebrosternal ribs* (2 to 7) play an important role in ventilation. In contrast to the first rib, these move about two axes simultaneously, the axis of the rib neck and the axis between the angle of the rib and its sternal junction (Fig. 3-2). As they rotate about the axes of their necks (*A*, in Fig. 3-2), their sternal ends rise and fall, thus increasing the A-P thoracic diameter. This action is referred to as the "pump handle motion." At the same time these ribs move about the longer axes from their angles to the sternum (*B*, in Fig. 3-2), leading to an up-and-down motion of the middle segments of the ribs. This, called a "bucket handle" motion, produces an increase and decrease in the transverse diameter of the chest. Thus the compound action of these ribs increases and decreases both A-P and transverse diameters smoothly and synchronously.

3. The *vertebrochondral ribs* (8 to 10) have rotation patterns similar to the vertebrosternal group. However, elevation of the anterior ends of these ribs produces a backward movement of the lower end of the sternum, with *reduction* in thoracic A-P diameter (Fig. 3-3). Outward rotation of the middle portions of the ribs increases the transverse diameter, as do the vertebrosternal ribs.

There are some who do not believe the ribs rotate about their neck axes but rather *abduct* by a sliding motion. Ribs 11 and 12 are not included in any of the above groups, since they do not participate in changing the contour of the chest but instead act as muscular insertion points.

### Diaphragm

The diaphragm is one of the two major ventilatory muscles, which, by its location and action, is best able to vary the volume of the thorax to produce the pressure changes needed for ventilation. It arises from three locations, the lumbar vertebrae, the costal margin, and the xiphoid, its fibers converging to interlace into a broad connective tissue sheet called the *central tendon*. The configuration of this muscle is that of a tent or a dome, dividing the chest from the abdomen. It is pierced by several structures, such as the esophagus, the aorta, many nerves, and the vena cava and receives its motor innervation from the *phrenic nerves*. Although the diaphragm is a single anatomic structure, the union of its central tendon with the fibrous pericardium functionally divides its dome into two "leaves." For convenience these are often referred to as the right and left diaphragms, or hemidiaphragms. With the liver immediately below it, the right dome is about 1 cm higher than the left, in the resting position, at the end of a quiet exhalation; and although the movements of both leaves are usually synchronous, because each has its own nerve supply, each may function independently of the other.

The mechanical action of the diaphragm is twofold:

1. Contraction draws down the central tendon, flattening its contour, increasing the volume of the thorax, and lowering intrathoracic pressure. As the diaphragm descends, intra-abdominal pressure increases and the muscles of the abdominal wall relax, allowing the upper abdomen to balloon outward. Splinting or rigidity of the abdominal wall interferes with diaphragmatic descent.

2. Contraction of the costal fibers of the diaphragm *raises* and *everts* the costal margin if the dome is intact and intra-abdominal pressure is normal. As the abdominal pressure increases during inspiration, this pressure acts as a fulcrum against which continued contraction of the diaphragmatic fibers pull up and out on the costal margin. In Fig. 3-4 the descending diaphragm is opposed by increasing intra-abdominal pressure. This pressure finally stabilizes the central portion of the disphragm so that the force of continued contraction is expended as traction on the costal attachments of the diaphragm. Because of the springlike tension of the ribs and the contour of the thorax at this level, the costal margin is pulled upward and outward, increasing the lateral diameter of the chest.

During inhalation therefore, as the diaphragm contracts, its dome descends and the costal margin of the chest moves outward so that the thorax enlarges both vertically and transversely. It is important to understand and visualize this combined action, since it is easily disturbed in pulmonary disease. Thus, if the diaphragm is abnormally low in position, not only is there a diminished vertical excursion (with a resulting reduction in tidal volume), but contraction of the costal fibers, instead of elevating the costal margin, may even pull in the lower chest boundary and narrow the thorax laterally. Fig. 3-4, *B*, shows an abnormal diaphragm, low in position and relatively flat in contour. Because of its starting position, it can descend very little on contraction, and

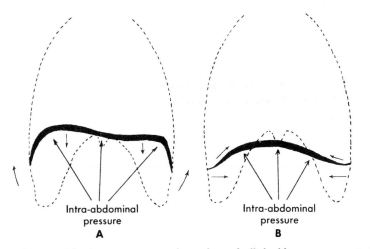

Intra-abdominal
pressure
**A**

Intra-abdominal
pressure
**B**

**Fig. 3-4.**  **A,** As the normal diaphragm contracts, it descends, gradually building up pressure in the abdomen until the intra-abdominal pressure acts as a fulcrum against which continued contraction everts the costal margin, enlarging the thorax further. **B,** Contraction of the diaphragm, which is abnormally low at the start of inspiration, can only pull in the costal margin, reducing the lower thoracic diameters.

with loss of its domed shape, contraction tends to pull its fibers centrally on a horizontal plane. This pulls in the costal margin and reduces the diameter of the chest. Much of the little gain in vertical diameter from the limited mobility of the diaphragm is negated by the simultaneous lateral shortening. The diaphragm takes no active part in exhalation and returns to its inspiratory resting position during the passive recoil of the thorax, to be explained later. During forced exhalation, as against resistance, the diaphragm does expel gas from the lung as it is pushed upward by intra-abdominal pressure generated by contracting abdominal muscles.

At rest the normal tidal movement of the diaphram is about 1.5 cm, and with deep breathing, 6 to 10 cm. With quiet breathing the excursions of both leaves of the diaphragm are about equal, but with a deep inspiration the right diaphragm may move more than the left. In the supine position the total diaphragmatic movement is the same as in the erect position. In a head-down, 45-degree supine tilt, however, the resting level of the diaphragm rises about 6 cm, causing a reduction of the functional residual capacity and the expiratory reserve volume. When the subject lies in a lateral position, his lower diaphragm tends to rise into the chest. Although the diaphragm is the principal ventilatory muscle and the only one used in normal quiet breathing, it is not essential for survival, as adequate ventilation is possible even when the diaphragm is completely paralyzed. It is estimated that, in the normal adult, each centimeter of vertical movement moves 350 ml of air; thus an excursion of 1.5 cm would effect a tidal volume of 525 ml. This figure does not include the additional increase in thoracic volume from expansion of the lower thorax, which, of course, would increase the tidal volume.

Affected by paralysis, the diaphragm (either or both leaves) tends to stay at the normal level at rest. During deep inhalation, howwever, it *rises* as other ventilatory muscles or one normal hemidiaphragm produce a fall in intrathoracic pressure. In quiet breathing the paralyzed leaf may remain immobile or move in either direction. The inspiratory balance of pressure above and below the diaphragm tends to make the paralyzed leaf rise, whereas outward movement of the lower ribs tends to stretch and flatten it, and its final course is the resultant of these two forces.

Finally, it should be noted that the diaphragm performs important functions other than ventilation. Because it is able to aid in generating high intra-abdominal pressure by remaining fixed while the abdominal muscles contract, the diaphragm greatly facilitates defecation, vomiting, coughing and sneezing, and parturition.

## Intercostal muscles

The intercostals, the second of the major ventilatory muscles, consist of two sets of muscles filling the gaps between the ribs; they are designated as *external* and *internal:*

1. The *external intercostal muscles* arise from the inferior edge of each rib from the rib tubercle to its costochondral junction. The fibers pass inferiorly and anteriorly to insert into the superior edge of the rib below. These muscles are thicker posteriorly than anteriorly and are thicker than the internal intercostals.
2. The *internal intercostal muscles* are located beneath the external intercostals and arise from the inferior edge of each rib from the anterior end of the inter-

costal space to the rib angles. The fibers pass inferiorly and posteriorly to insert into the superior edge of the rib below. This muscle group is divided into two functional parts:

a. *Interosseous* portion, located between the sloping parts of the ribs
b. *Intercartilaginous* portion, located where the costal cartilages slope superiorly and anteriorly

Although there is considerable controversy as to the exact mechanism by which the intercostal muscles function, it is well established that by contraction they elevate the ribs, thereby increasing the inspiratory chest volume. This function has been documented by noting its absence during paralysis of muscles. In addition, the muscles solidify and stabilize the chest wall and prevent intercostal bulging or retraction during intrathoracic pressure changes. It is believed that most of the ventilatory effect of the intercostals is produced by the external intercostals and the intercartilaginous portion of the internal intercostals. These muscles contract during inhalation and maintain contraction into early exhalation, by this action elevating the ribs. In the presence of flows up to 40 $\ell$/min the intercostals are quiet during most of exhalation. However, with flows in excess of 50 $\ell$/min the intercostals of the lower spaces contract toward the end of exhalation and also do the same during voluntary maximum exhalation. This action probably gives stability to the chest in the presence of powerful abdominal contraction. As noted above, intercostal contraction continues into early exhalation during quiet breathing, but it then fades as expiratory airflow rises to its maximum. This is not a true exhalation act of the intercostals, for if it were, the peak expiratory airflow would occur at once while lung recoil was also maximal. It is believed that this function of the intercostals is to retard airflow during early exhalation and to facilitate a smoother and less turbulent exhalation. Finally, it appears that contraction of the interosseous portion of the internal intercostals *depresses* the ribs; but the exact role they play in normal ventilation is not clear.

## Scalene muscles

The *anterior*, *medial*, and *posterior* scalene muscles, although individual structures, are considered as a functional unit. Primarily skeletal muscles of the neck, they are also *accessory muscles of ventilation* and play an important role in breathing. The scalenes arise from the transverse processes of the lower five cervical vertebrae and insert into the upper surface of the first rib (anterior and medial scalenes) and the second rib (posterior scalene).

Although the scalenes give support to the neck, we are interested in their ventilatory action. Basically, they elevate and fix firmly the first and second ribs. Their most important function is to aid inhalation under conditions of stress when the diaphragm and intercostal muscles are inadequate to fulfill respiratory needs; this may occur in normal subjects undergoing severe exertion or in patients with pulmonary disease. In a normal subject *static* inspiratory efforts (against a closed glottis or other obstruction, with no movement of air) bring the scalenes into play as intra-alveolar pressure drops; and when this pressure reaches $-10$ cm $H_2O$, scalenes are active in all subjects. During expiratory efforts the scalene muscles are inactive until intra-alveolar pressure reaches 40 cm $H_2O$, at which point they contract. It is felt that the expiratory function of the scalene muscles is to fix the ribs against the contraction of the abdominal muscles and to prevent herniation of the apex of the lung during coughing.

**Sternomastoid muscle**

Designed to rotate the head and support it, the sternomastoid is another accessory ventilatory muscle of importance. It arises by two heads from the manubrium of the sternum and the medial end of the clavicle. The heads fuse into a single body that courses superiorly and slightly posteriorly to insert into the mastoid process and occipital bone of the skull. This muscle is usually prominent on each side of the neck of most subjects and is especially noticeable with rotary movements of the head.

When functioning to mobilize the head, the sternomastoid pulls from its sterno-clavicular origin, rotating the head to the opposite side and turning it slightly upward. As a ventilatory muscle, however, when the subject fixes the head and neck with other skeletal muscles, the sternomastoid pulls from its skull insertions and elevates the sternum, increasing the A-P diameter of the chest. In all subjects it contracts when intra-alveolar pressures reach $-10$ cm $H_2O$ but has no action during exhalation. In the supine position most subjects during normal free breathing can attain a volume of 2.5 liters and a flow of 60 $\ell$/min without use of the sternomastoids. An interesting discrepancy should be noted. During natural, free breathing, normal subjects can move about 2.5 liters of air at intra-alveolar pressures varying from $-25$ to $-50$ cm $H_2O$ with the diaphragm and intercostals alone, and yet under static conditions an intra-alveolar pressure of $-10$ cm $H_2O$ brings the sternomastoid into play. This is not clearly understood.

In chronic pulmonary disease the sternomastoid becomes active in inhalation when the thorax becomes so inflated (elevated resting level) that the low diaphragm loses its efficiency. As the sternomastoids contract and pull up on the sternum, the ribs rotate about their neck axes but not about the rib angle–sternal junction axes. This produces an up-and-down motion with little side expansion. In extreme cases A-P expansion of the thorax may cause the lower ribs to become indrawn, partially negating the increase in chest volume.

**Pectoralis major muscle**

The third most important accessory ventilatory muscle, the pectoralis major, is a powerful bilateral anterior chest muscle with the primary function of pulling the upper arms into the body in a hugging motion. It is a large, fan-shaped muscle arising from the medial half of the clavicle, the anterior surface of the sternum and the first six costal cartilages, and a fibrous sheath enclosing muscles of the abdominal wall. The muscle fibers converge into a thick tendon that inserts into the upper part of the humerus. It is the pectoralis major that forms the anterior fold of the axilla, and in a muscular individual its outlines are plainly visible beneath the skin.

Like the other accessory ventilatory muscles, the pectoralis pulls in a direction opposite to that of its primary function. If the arms and shoulders are fixed, as by leaning on the elbows or firmly grasping a table, the pectoralis muscle can use its insertion as an origin and pull with great force on the anterior chest, lifting up ribs and sternum and increasing thoracic A-P diameter. The respiratory therapist will soon become accustomed to seeing patients with chronic pulmonary disease assume characteristic poses for maximum use of their pectoralis. In advanced cases most of the air moved may be the result of the action of this powerful muscle. It aids inhalation only, taking no part in exhalation.

### Abdominal muscles

Several muscles make up the abdominal wall, with the obvious purpose of providing support and safety to the abdominal contents. Some of them, however, play an indirect but important role in ventilation and can thus be considered as accessory ventilatory muscles. Four of these will be briefly identified:

1. The *external oblique* arises from the lower eight ribs; posterior fibers insert into the iliac crest, and the rest course obliquely down and forward to insert into a fibrous sheath (aponeurosis) with their counterparts from the other side; the lower edge forms the inguinal ligament in the groin.
2. The *internal oblique* arises from the iliac crest and the inguinal ligament; posterior fibers pass upward to insert into the last three ribs; the rest slope upward and forward to a fibrous aponeurosis.
3. The *transverse abdominal* arises from the costal cartilages of the lower ribs, iliac crest, and lateral part of the inguinal ligament; it passes horizontally forward to an aponeurosis.
4. The *abdominal rectus* arises from the pubic bones, passes upward in a sheath formed by the aponeuroses described above, and inserts into costal cartilages 5 to 7; it is often well defined in a muscular individual.

The abdominals are expiratory muscles with two important actions—to increase intra-abdominal pressure and to draw the lower ribs down and medially. In the relaxed supine position the abdominals are inactive during quiet breathing; and they are often inactive in the erect position. With increasing ventilation, they come into play when the expiratory flow reaches 40 $\ell$/min. At this level of gas velocity or in the presence of significant resistance to exhalation, or if exhalation is required beyond the preinspiratory resting level (as in inflating a balloon), the elastic recoil of the thorax does not have adequate force to remove enough air in the allotted time. In such circumstances, contraction of the powerful abdominals builds up strong intra-abdominal pressure and drives the diaphragm, like a piston, into exhalation. Contraction of these muscles also occurs at the end of voluntary maximum *inhalation* and is a factor limiting the extent of inhalation. In chronic pulmonary disease, especially in the presence of airway obstruction, effective use of the abdominals is often lost, and without this powerful generator of force to push the diaphragm into expiratory action, the patient is at a great disadvantage.

### Summary of ventilatory muscle action

There are other muscles that play varying roles in assisting ventilation and thus can qualify as accessory ventilatory muscles. Most of them are concerned with stabilizing the body to provide better leverage for muscles directly concerned with air movement. However, if the therapist thoroughly understands the function of the muscles just described above, he will have an adequate foundation for learning some of the therapeutic techniques to be taken up later. In summary, the function of the ventilatory muscles may be tabulated as follows:

1. *Quiet ventilation*
   a. Inspiration
      (1) Diaphragm in all subjects
      (2) Intercostals in most subjects
      (3) Scalenes in some subjects
   b. Expiration
      (1) Some persistence of contraction of inspiratory muscles early in expiration
2. *Moderately increased ventilation*
   a. For flows up to 50 ℓ/min, same as above
   b. For flows between 50 and 100 ℓ/min, sternomastoid action toward end of inspiration; increased abdominals and intercostals toward end of expiration
3. *Greatly increased ventilation*
   a. Above 100 ℓ/min all inspiratory accessories active, and abdominals active throughout expiration

## LUNG-THORAX RELATIONSHIP

Effective ventilation depends on cooperative but reciprocal action between the lung and the thorax, a relationship crudely illustrated by the balloon-in-a-box model in Fig. 3-5, the box representing the thorax, and the balloon the lungs. A review of anatomy will recall that, between the pleura-lined thoracic wall and the pleura-covered lung, there exists the *pleural* or *intrapleural space*. Although in the living subject the approximation of the two pleural surfaces, separated by only a thin film of moisture, makes the space more potential than real, it plays an important role in ventilation and for purposes of illustration is depicted in sketches as a true space.

The resting level or resting position of the chest is the configuration that it assumes at the end of a quiet effortless exhalation and is often referred to as the *end-expiratory position*, less frequently as the *preinspiratory level*. In Fig. 3-5, *A*, the relations of the lung and thorax are shown at the resting level. The airtight thoracic box encloses a

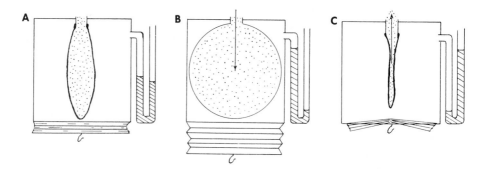

**Fig. 3-5.** Balloon-in-a-box model of the lung-thorax. **A,** In the resting position, a small negative pressure in the box keeps the balloon slightly distended with air. **B,** As the box expands by dropping its floor, its cavity becomes more negative, and air flows into the balloon. **C,** If the floor of the box is pushed higher than its usual resting level, positive pressure develops in the box, expressing additional air from the balloon but not emptying it.

small partial vacuum of about $-4$ cm $H_2O$, as indicated by the attached manometer, maintained by opposing elasticity of the lungs and thorax, to be described in more detail below. The pulmonary balloon is suspended in the box, and because it is exposed to and in equilibrium with atmospheric pressure, the surrounding subatmospheric intrathoracic pressure keeps it partially filled with air. Thus at the end of exhalation there is still a considerable amount of air in the lungs. The inspiratory flow of air into the lung is brought about by enlargement of the thoracic box through the effort of ventilatory muscles. Fig. 3-5, *B*, shows the accordion-like bottom of the box dropping, enlarging the volume of the box, and simulating the action of the diaphragm. The living thorax, a flexible structure, also expands laterally as muscles act on the ribs. Intrathoracic pressure drops further with this increase in volume of the sealed container, the pressure drop is transmitted into the balloon across its flexible wall, intraballoon (intra-alveolar) pressure momentarily becomes subatmospheric, and air flows into it. This difference between the higher atmospheric and lower alveolar pressures is called a *pressure gradient* ($\Delta P$). It is a "head of pressure" that allows fluid to flow from the high end of the gradient to the low. The concept of gradients is of great importance in cardiopulmonary physiology and will be extensively used later in this text. During quiet inhalation, intrapleural pressure drops only to about $-6$ cm $H_2O$, but a strong inspiratory effort against an obstruction, such as a closed glottis, can drop the pressure to $-50$ cm $H_2O$. Exhalation is a passive recoil of the elastic stretch of the lung balloon, made possible by a relaxation of the muscular forces acting on the thoracic box. Air flows from the lung until the resting level is reached to terminate the cycle. Exhalation can be continued below the resting level by bringing into play positive expiratory muscular forces. Principally, this invokes strong contractions of the abdominal muscles to force the diaphragm into the thorax, as illustrated in Fig. 3-5, *C*. With this maneuver the resting negative intrathoracic pressure is replaced by a positive pressure that, against strong resistance, may reach 70 cm $H_2O$.[9] Although more air is forced from the lungs, the latter can never be completely emptied.

We have described, in general terms, the basic factors responsible for airflow into and out of the lungs and will now consider some of the forces that both initiate and limit air movement. As referred to above, the ventilatory cycle is the net sum of the action of the opposing forces of the chest and lung, and we will use a different model to illustrate these points, emphasizing that we are not talking about another subject but viewing the same from a slightly different angle. The thorax (which in our context includes the diaphragm) consists of flexible ribs and muscles; and through the intrinsic elastic forces of its tissues, it tends to expand and enlarge, much as a bent bow is under stress to spring straight. Counteracting these chest forces are forces of the lung, whose elastic tissues are stretched and tend to contract and shrink. To understand how these two systems of elastic energy relate to one another, consider the lung-thorax complex as consisting of one set of *bowed flat* springs (thorax) exerting an expansile force tied to a *stretched coiled* spring (lungs) exerting a contractile force, each holding the other in check (Fig. 3-6). Expansion and contraction of the coiled spring represent increase and decrease, respectively, in lung volume. At the resting level the chest and lung forces are equal in opposite directions, momentarily in perfect balance, as each pre-

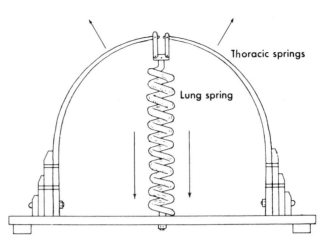

**Fig. 3-6.** The counteracting forces of the lungs and thorax are schematically represented by two sets of springs. In the resting position, the bowed flat thoracic springs are shown as held under bent tension by the coiled lung spring, itself partially stretched by the action. Arrows indicate the direction each spring tends to move to reach its own position of rest. From the lung-thorax resting position, the thorax can expand or contract, depending upon the action of the ventilatory muscles. These muscles can assist the thoracic springs to overcome the restraint of the lung spring, or they can compress the thoracic springs and assist the recoil of the lung spring.

vents the other from following its natural inclination. Although we refer to this brief static period as "resting," it must not be thought that expenditure of energy is wanting, any more than a temporary stalemate in a rope-pull contest can be considered free of physical activity. Indeed, in the airtight balloon-in-a-box structure of the lung-thorax, at the resting position each force is pulling against the other with power equal to that exerted by a 4 cm column of water, developing in the intervening intrapleural "space" a partial vacuum of the same magnitude. It is this intrapleural subatmospheric pressure that holds together the coiled lung spring and the flat, bowed thoracic springs, as the barrel and plunger of a capped syringe are held together by the subatmospheric pressure developing in the syringe barrel in response to attempts to separate the parts.

Inhalation can occur only when the resting level balance between the forces of the lung and thorax is broken by the addition of muscular energy to the elasticity of the thorax. In addition to the effect of diaphragmatic contraction on chest expansion, the intercostal and accessory ventilatory muscles, in a sense, take hold of the bowed "flat springs" of Fig. 3-6 and pull them outward to help them overcome the "coiled spring" of the lung. It is easy to imagine that the depth of inspiration is determined by the amount of chest force applied to overcome lung stretch and that this effort, in turn, is regulated by the mechanism of ventilatory control already discussed. At the end-inspiratory level necessary to satisfy immediate body gas needs, airflow stops and the chest and lung forces are again in momentary balance. At this point the muscles activating the thorax relax, and the elasticity of the stretched lung, along with the increased intra-abdominal pressure, passively returns the lung-thorax system to the resting level. Exhalation against resistance such as obstructive airway disease, in which

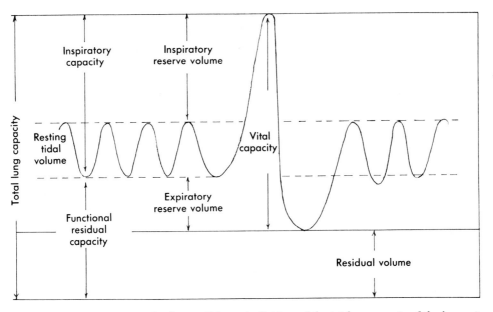

**Fig. 3-7.** Lung capacities and volumes. Volumetric divisions of the total gas capacity of the lungs. A capacity consists of two or more volumes. (See text for description.)

pulmonary passive recoil lacks the force to move air at a suitable rate, or exhalation below the resting level, as noted earlier and shown in Fig. 3-5, *C*, principally utilizes the abdominal muscles to generate the power necessary to deflate the lung. By employing a little imagination, we can visualize this effort as a force bowing the flat springs of Fig. 3-6. Against obstruction this active expiratory force helps the coiled spring to return the expanded thorax to the resting position. To expel air below the resting level, this force helps the coiled spring to flex the increasing resistance of the flat springs. Details of other factors influencing the function of the lung-thorax system, such as surface tension and bronchopulmonary diseases, will be discussed in the following sections.

This is an advantageous point at which to introduce the subject of lung volumes, since they depend on the lung-thorax relationship. Fig. 3-7 illustrates the volumetric divisions of the total capacity of the lung, and it should be observed that a designated capacity consists of two or more volumes. The lower dashed line identifies the end-expiratory resting level, and the upper line, the *tidal volume* ($V_T$) end-inspiration. Because the chest forces limit collapse of the lung at the end-expiratory resting level, air remains in the lung at this point and is called the *functional residual capacity* (FRC). Forced exhalation, as described above, can remove air below the resting level by "dipping into" the FRC. This extra air, so expelled, is the *expiratory reserve volume* (ERV). Even after the most strenuous expiratory effort, air still remains in the lung and cannot be removed voluntarily; this is known as the *residual volume* (RV). Thus the FRC is the sum of the ERV and the RV. If a subject inhales *maximally* from the resting level, then exhales *maximally*, he will move a quantity of air known as the *vital capacity* (VC), so called because all his ventilation is within its limits. Note that the VC consists of three volumes, the ERV, the $V_T$, and the *inspiratory reserve volume* (IRV). The last represents the available expansion of the lung-thorax, beyond resting needs, for exertion or any other demand for deep breathing. The *inspiratory capacity* (IC) measures the total inhalation potential from the resting level. Finally, the sum of the VC and the RV comprises the *total lung capacity* (TLC). All these values can be measured in the cardiopulmonary laboratory, by direct or indirect methods, and although our current interest in them will be confined to their relationship to physiology and disease, some rough guides to their actual values should be of interest to the student. There is great variability in lung volume measurements among individuals, depending upon size and physical conditioning, and between health and disease; but Table 3-2 gives some quantitative visualization for average normal adults.

In Fig. 3-6, if we separate the sets of springs, it is apparent that each set will follow its natural tendency—the thoracic flat springs will spring outward and the lung coiled spring will contract. The same phenomenon will occur if we break the vacuum-sealed intrapleural space, letting it equilibrate with the atmosphere. If the thorax (either side or both) is opened, it will actually expand to a larger volume and assume its own *thoracic resting position*. At the same time the lung, freed from its suction adherence to the thoracic wall, will collapse to a smaller volume than the RV of the intact system; but even when exposed to atmospheric pressure, the lung does not become completely airless and still contains a small amount of air called *minimal air*. Fig. 3-8 diagrammatically illustrates the effect of breaking the seal between thorax and lung. In *A*, the lung-thorax is at the resting level, where the lung contains the FRC. *B* depicts the results of equilibrating the intrathoracic space with atmospheric pressure by opening the intact thorax. The lung collapses to its smallest size, the minimal air volume, whereas the thorax enlarges to its unopposed thoracic resting position. *C* is a plot of the TLC against *A* and *B*, breaking the VC into increments of 20% each. The normal lung-thorax resting position is seen to be at approximately 30% of the VC, whereas with disruption of the system the minimal air level of the lung is about 40% of the RV and the thorax expands to its resting level of some 50% of the VC.

Finally, aiding the synchronous movement of lung and thorax is the force of *pleural traction*. In the normal intact lung-thorax complex, both visceral and parietal pleura are in contact during the entire breathing cycle, separated only by the thin film of fluid covering the pleural surfaces, mentioned above. The cohesive force of

**Table 3-2.** *Normal lung volumes*

| | |
|---|---|
| Vital capacity | 2.5 to 5.0 liters |
| Expiratory reserve volume | 0.8 to 1.2 liters |
| ERV/VC ratio | 0.25 to 0.40 |
| Functional residual capacity | 1.5 to 2.7 liters |
| Residual volume | 0.8 to 1.5 liters |
| Total lung capacity | 3.3 to 6.5 liters |
| RV/TLC ratio | 0.25 or less |

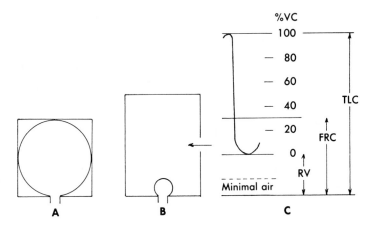

**Fig. 3-8.** The resting levels of the intact lung-thorax and the separated lung and thorax are plotted against the total lung capacity. In **A,** the intact system at its resting level contains the *FRC* and is expanded to about 30% of the *VC*. In **B,** the arrow indicates a break in the thoracic wall, exposing the lung to atmosphere and destroying the lung-thorax seal. The lung, containing the *minimal air,* collapses to a new resting level, which is about 40% of the *RV*, and the thorax expands to its own unopposed level of about 50% of the *VC*.

this fluid layer, working with the intra-alveolar pressure gradient, helps to hold together the pleural surfaces so that, as the thorax expands and contracts, the lung accompanies it smoothly. In a sense the lung is partially "dragged" into inflation by the thorax and is held firmly against the inner thoracic wall during exhalation.

## SURFACE TENSION AND VENTILATION

So far, the collapsing tendency of the lung springs has been attributed only to the elastic fibers in its structure. Augmenting this elastic recoil, however, is another factor that has assumed clinical importance—*surface tension* (ST); a brief review of the principles of surface tension will expedite understanding its role in ventilation.[10-12] Surface tension may be defined as the force exerted by molecules moving away from the surface and toward the center of a liquid, tending to make a sphere or a curved surface smaller. It occurs at an *interface* or junction between two substances, such as liquid and air, and is best illustrated in a relatively small drop of fluid. Molecules in the mass of a liquid are subjected to physical forces of mutual attraction and are so balanced that they can freely move in all directions. Those molecules on the surface, however, can be attracted only inwardly by their fellow molecules, and the pressure they exert can be likened to an elastic film tending to contract into a sphere. Fig. 3-9 illustrates the force of mass attraction between liquid molecules. Those molecules at the fluid-air interface have no molecules distally to attract them but are pulled only centrally. This tension over the surface of a drop of liquid keeps it intact in a spherical shape while falling in space or resting on a surface. Surface tension is measured in *dynes per linear centimeter across the surface* and may be visualized as the force (in dynes) necessary to produce a tear 1 cm long in the surface layer of a liquid, if one could grasp the surface in the hands and stretch it like a thin rubber sheet until it split. ST is a demonstrable phenomenon that permits an insect to walk on the surface of a pond

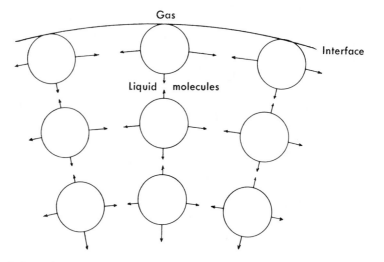

**Fig. 3-9.** The force of surface tension in a drop of liquid is shown by the action of its fluid molecules. Those molecules within the substance of the drop are mutually attracted to one another (arrows) and can move about randomly in a state of balance. Mass attraction can pull the molecules of the outermost layer inward only, creating a centrally directed force, called surface tension, which tends to contract the liquid into a sphere. Pressure within the drop is raised above atmospheric and is expressed by the formula of LaPlace, described in the text.

**Table 3-3.** *Examples of surface tension*

| *Substance* | *°C* | *ST in dynes/cm* |
|---|---|---|
| Water | 20 | 73 |
| Water | 37 | 70 |
| Tissue fluid | 37 | 50 |
| Whole blood | 37 | 58 |
| Plasma | 37 | 73 |
| Ethyl alcohol | 20 | 22 |
| Mercury | 17 | 547 |

and enables a needle to float in a glass of water. Surface tensions vary widely among substances and for the same substance vary inversely with temperature. Table 3-3 lists some examples of surface tension values.

The force of ST, like a fist compressing a ball, produces an increase in pressure within a drop of liquid above the ambient. Thus a pressure gradient, or difference in pressure ($\Delta P$), exists across the surface of the drop. The P within the drop, dependent on the specific ST and the radius of the drop, is expressed by the formula of LaPlace as:

$$P = \frac{2\ ST}{r}$$

where ST is in dynes/cm, r is the radius in centimeters, and P is in dynes/cm². The derivation of this formula is explained in any standard text of physics. Given a drop

$\uparrow pH$  $U \cdot meq$  $- - = 0.06314$ $0.06$ -7.

ICK wall   $k^+ < 5o$.

Aam.   $0 -$   37

$i \cdot n \cdot$   ④ ③

$15.46 - 5 \times 8$.
$1.35$
$0.9$   $14$   $21$

$17.5 \cdot 1$ $4$ $5.36$
$2 \frac{}{}$ $2.7$ $9$
$1.3.78$ $St$   $1.40$
$H \, conc : 1.33 \times 0.06314 + 0.01$ nag
$70.$
$St$

$803$
$90$

$070$:
$\frac{000}{000}$ $005$
$000$

$Obg_2$:

$$\left( \frac{cco_2 - cag_2}{cco_2 - cvo_2} \right)$$

Problem →

Q3 - -- FiO₂ - Try to wean.

(H) ↑ → Reduce hyperventilation
(H) ↑ → Extubation.

$$\frac{dS}{dt} = \overline{(1HO_2 - PaO_2)\,0.02} \quad 760^?$$

$$= 4.57\,(PAO_2 - PaO_2)\,0.002. \quad 12\cdots$$

$$1\cdots = 360\,Pa$$

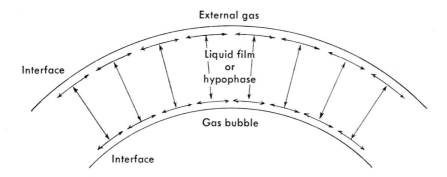

**Fig. 3-10.** A bubble is a volume of gas enclosed by a thin film of fluid, which has two surfaces. Thus, the forces of surface tension on both surfaces produce a pressure within the bubble twice that in a liquid drop of the same substance and radius.

with a radius of 2 mm and a ST of 60 dynes/cm, calculate the pressure inside the drop:

$$P = \frac{2 \times 60}{0.2 \text{ cm}} = \frac{120}{0.2} = 600 \text{ dynes/cm}^2$$

or

$$P = \frac{600 \text{ dynes/cm}^2}{980} = 6.13 \times 10^{-1} \text{ g/cm}^2$$

or

$$P = Ht \times D$$

$$\therefore Ht = \frac{P}{D} = \frac{6.13 \times 10^{-1}}{1} = 6.13 \times 10^{-1} \text{cm H}_2\text{O}$$

The principle regulating internal pressure of a drop applies equally to a gas bubble in a liquid mass. The gas in the bubble is subject to the same pressure as the center of a drop of the same radius if the substance of the drop has the same ST as the liquid surrounding the bubble. It makes no difference if fluid is surrounded by gas, or gas by fluid; if there is only a single interface, the same radius, and the same ST, the internal compression forces are the same.

In contrast is the effect of surface tension on an isolated bubble, which for purposes of description can be considered as a spherical volume of gas enclosed in a thin film of fluid, Fig. 3-10 shows that, thin though it is, the film contains a finite amount of liquid and is called the *hypophase*. Because ST is found only at an interface, and the bubble wall has two gas-fluid interfaces at its two surfaces, the compression force of ST on the enclosed gas is *twice* that exerted by a spherical drop of the same size and substance. Thus the STs of the two surfaces act together to compress the gas bubble. The pressure gradient across a bubble wall can also be expressed by LaPlace's law, with a modification:

$$P = \frac{4 \text{ ST}}{r}$$

where ST is the surface tension of the liquid in which the bubble is immersed and r is the radius of the bubble in centimeters. It is apparent that if the example in the pre-

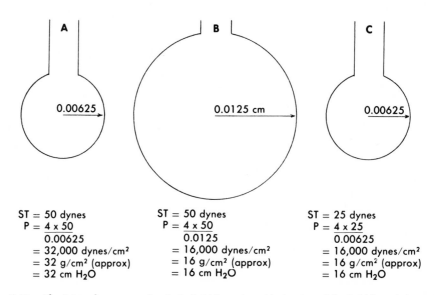

$$ST = 50 \text{ dynes}$$
$$P = \frac{4 \times 50}{0.00625}$$
$$= 32{,}000 \text{ dynes/cm}^2$$
$$= 32 \text{ g/cm}^2 \text{ (approx)}$$
$$= 32 \text{ cm } H_2O$$

$$ST = 50 \text{ dynes}$$
$$P = \frac{4 \times 50}{0.0125}$$
$$= 16{,}000 \text{ dynes/cm}^2$$
$$= 16 \text{ g/cm}^2 \text{ (approx)}$$
$$= 16 \text{ cm } H_2O$$

$$ST = 25 \text{ dynes}$$
$$P = \frac{4 \times 25}{0.00625}$$
$$= 16{,}000 \text{ dynes/cm}^2$$
$$= 16 \text{ g/cm}^2 \text{ (approx)}$$
$$= 16 \text{ cm } H_2O$$

**Fig. 3-11.** The internal pressure of a single bubble varies with the size of the bubble and the surface tension of its liquid film. An increase in radius from **A** to **B** drops the pressure, but **C** shows that the same pressure drop can accompany a reduction in surface tension, without changing bubble size.

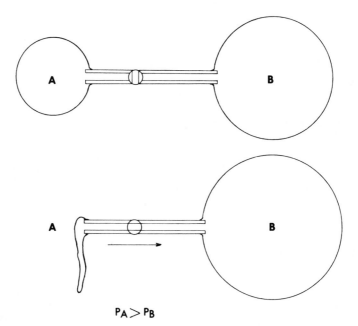

$$P_A > P_B$$

**Fig. 3-12.** When two bubbles of different sizes, **A** and **B**, but with the same surface tension, are allowed to communicate, the greater pressure in the smaller causes it to empty into the larger.

ceding paragraph were a bubble instead of a drop, the pressure would be double the calculated value.

From the foregoing it can be seen that for a given liquid the *smaller* the drop or bubble the *greater* will be the pressure from surface tension. When inflating a balloon, we must use maximum force to *start* inflation, to overcome the initial resistance, then progressively less, up to the capacity of the balloon. Similarly, it would require more pressure to inflate a small bubble than a large one because of the increased pressure of ST in the former. Fig. 3-11 illustrates changes in pressure in an isolated bubble accompanying changes in size and in ST. As the size of the bubble increases from *A* to *B*, the pressure drops, according to LaPlace's law. The bubble at *C* demonstrates that the pressure can remain unchanged if the ST is somehow lowered. Or, to view it differently, Fig. 3-12 shows that if two bubbles of different sizes are allowed to communicate, the smaller will empty into the larger because of the greater pressure in the former.

Bubbles massed together as a foam behave differently than when individually isolated.[13] Fig. 3-13 shows that bubbles in clumps lose their outer air-fluid surfaces and retain only single interfaces, resembling bubbles in a volume of liquid. As a consequence, the internal pressure in grouped bubbles is related to twice the surface tension (2 ST) of the surrounding liquid rather than four times (4 ST), as described above for single bubbles.

The ability to alter surface tension is a physical phenomenon of great importance to pulmonary physiology, and the principle involved will be discussed before we relate it to function. Certain substances can lower ST on contact with fluid surfaces and are called *surfactants*. Soaps and detergents are the most common examples. These agents weaken the molecular bonds at the surface, thus reducing the surface tension and lowering intrabubble pressure. Fig. 3-11, *C*, illustrates this effect. An air bubble in water shrinks and finally disappears under the stress of ST pressure as the pressure hastens the diffusion of air out of the bubble, but the addition of soap to the water, by lowering ST, prolongs or stabilizes the bubble. On the other hand, a surfactant such

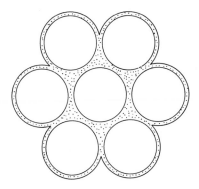

**Fig. 3-13.** The bubble in the center of the sketch illustrates that while an isolated bubble suspended in air can have two air-fluid interfaces, when it is clumped in a mass of foam, it retains only its inner interface. (See text for the significance of this.)

as a detergent, by reducing ST, disrupts and disperses small drops of water, making the water "wetter" and increasing its ability to penetrate deeper into fabrics and minute crevices for better removal of dirt.

Let us recall the microscopic structure of the lung, with its millions of alveoli, each one of which is in intimate contact with a thin film of intercellular fluid, and let us view it as a mass of tiny bubbles almost like a foam in interstitial fluid. It is easy now to imagine each of these "alveolar bubbles" as being subjected to forces of tissue fluid surface tension; and indeed, experimental and clinical evidence indicates that ST is an important factor in the mechanics of ventilation. The passive exhalation recoil of the "lung springs" to the resting position is due to alveolar ST acting with the elastic fibers of the lung. The effect of lung ST is to produce alveolar collapse, and reinflation by inhalation against the ST pressure would be very difficult were it not for the presence in the alveoli of a natural surfactant.

Pulmonary surfactant exists as a single molecule-thick film lining the alveolar walls. Chemically, it is a phospholipid, composed of fatty acids bound to lecithin, and it functions in a most remarkable fashion. Apparently there is a fixed amount of surfactant in each alveolus, and its ability to lower ST depends on a quantitative ratio between it and alveolar surface area. At the ventilatory resting level, because the alveoli are partially deflated, there is a relatively large amount of surfactant in relation to alveolar surface area. Surface tension is lowered, intrapulmonary pressure is lowered, and the alveoli can be easily inflated. As the alveoli distend with inhaled air, their stretched walls present an increasing surface area, the surfactant film becomes stretched and thinned, the ratio of surfactant to surface area falls, and the effect of surfactant decreases. During alveolar distention, the contractile force of ST gradually increases, and at end-inspiration, when muscular inspiratory effort ceases, the combination of ST and lung elasticity deflates the alveoli to their resting functional residual capacity, completing the breathing cycle. The "half-life" of surfactant is measured in hours (the length of time it takes for half a given mass to disappear in the metabolic process of deterioration), and if its natural replacement is impaired or it is pathologically destroyed faster than it can be replaced, alveolar collapse (atelectasis) rapidly develops.[14] Were it not for the action of pulmonary surfactant, inflating partially collapsed alveoli would require great physical effort and inhalation would be seriously handicapped. Indeed, in disease states characterized by absence of surfactant, the work of breathing is at times insurmountable. Finally, since at any given time all alveoli are not necessarily identical in size, smaller alveoli tend to empty into larger neighboring alveoli, in accordance with the principle illustrated in Fig. 3-12. This serious interference with even distribution of ventilation is prevented by surfactant, which through its varying ratio to surface area, maintains uniform pressure within all alveoli, regardless of size.

*Exercise 3-1.* Calculate the following:

(a) At the resting level, if lung ST is 30 dynes/cm, how many centimeters of water pressure are needed to start inflation of an alveolus with a diameter of 90 $\mu$?

(b) With a ST of 70 dynes/cm, what is the diameter of a bubble of foam that can be maintained by an inflating pressure of 9 mm Hg?

## ELASTIC RESISTANCE TO VENTILATION

When discussing the "springs" of the lung and thorax, we were describing the characteristic of *elasticity*, whereby an object that is stretched by a force tends to recoil to its original shape or position upon release of the force. The elasticity of the lung-thorax presents a resistance that must be overcome during inhalation, a resistance that often increases in disease. A measurement of elasticity, called *compliance*, can be made to evaluate the work of breathing; it gives an estimate of the "stiffness" of the lungs and thorax. Compliance is defined as the *volume change in the lung per unit of pressure change*, and its units are liter per centimeter of water. Measurements must be made under *static* conditions, or at points of *no airflow*, to eliminate other factors such as airflow resistance. It is evident that as the lungs *lose* their elasticity and become less compliant, or stiffer, the value of this ratio decreases. For a simple analogy, if a balloon contained 1 liter of air under a pressure of 15 cm $H_2O$ and it expanded to 1.5 liters after the pressure was raised to 20 cm $H_2O$, its compliance equals $\Delta V \div \Delta P$, or $0.5 \div 5$, or $0.1$ $\ell$/cm $H_2O$. The pressure-volume relationship of a simple spring is illustrated in Fig. 3-14, where there is a linear response of spring distance to force, up to the limit of stretch. The human ventilatory system, however, is composed of two sets of springs as previously illustrated in Fig. 3-6, and the lung-thorax compliance is obviously the net resultant of each. Thus ventilatory compliance can be considered as a triad of total compliance of lung and thorax ($C_{LT}$), compliance of the lung alone ($C_L$), and compliance of the thorax alone ($C_T$). It should be noted that the compliance of the lung-thorax is *less* than that of either lung or thorax alone; and the student who is acquainted with electrical terminology will recognize that the relationship between total compliance and its two constituents is expressed in the same inverse manner as electrical resistors in parallel:

$$\frac{1}{C_{LT}} = \frac{1}{C_L} + \frac{1^{15}}{C_T}$$

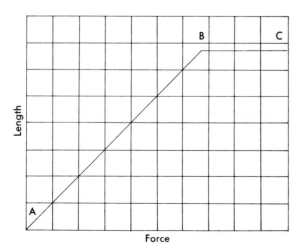

**Fig. 3-14.** The graph demonstrates compliance of a simple spring (increase in length/increase in force). With increasing force, the spring lengthens in a linear manner, from *A* to *B*, but at the point of maximum stretch further force produces no additional increase in length, *B* to *C*.

*Lung-thorax compliance* ($C_{LT}$) can be measured in one of three general ways: (1) The subject, completely relaxed voluntarily or from anesthesia or disease, is placed in a body respirator with his head outside at ambient pressure, and ventilation is controlled by the application of negative pressure to the surface of the body (Fig. 3-15). With the subject exhaling into a measuring device such as a spirometer and by varying the negative pressure and correlating this with the volume of air moved, the flexibility of the combined lungs and thorax in terms of liters of air moved per centimeter $H_2O$ pressure exerted can be calculated.[15] (2) A cuffed endotracheal tube placed in an anesthetized subject allows ventilation of the lungs at various delivered *positive* pressures. These values, with their corresponding tidal volumes measured in a spirometer, provide compliance data. Normal $C_{LT}$ by both these methods is about *0.1 ℓ/cm $H_2O$.* (3) A slightly different technique is the construction of a *relaxation-pressure curve.*[16] With a small pressure-transmitting plastic tube attached to a recording device and placed in his nose, the subject inhales a measured amount of air from a spirometer. Then, with tightly closed nose and mouth, he relaxes his ventilatory muscles, and the elastic recoil of lung and thorax produces an alveolar pressure recorded by the nasal tube. Repeated at different $V_E$ levels, a curve is produced. Compliance by this method is a bit higher than by the above two methods, about *0.12 ℓ/cm $H_2O$.* It should be noted that whether the ventilatory pressure is positive or negative makes no difference; for compliance depends upon the *absolute* pressure change for each volume change.

*Pulmonary compliance* ($C_L$) is calculated by measuring the *intrapleural pressure* at different levels of end-inspiratory volumes and plotting a pressure-volume curve that is generally linear in the ranges used. Since it is hazardous to invade the pleural cavity, a balloon-tipped catheter is swallowed until the balloon is at a midchest position. The balloon is attached to a pressure-recording device, and the soft-walled esophagus readily transmits surrounding intrapleural pressure to the balloon. The subject inhales to several different levels from a volume recorder (spirometer), and at the peak of each tidal volume (momentarily a static state with no airflow), the cor-

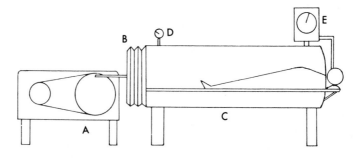

**Fig. 3-15.** This is a schematic representation of a subject in a body respirator. The motor, *A*, operates bellows, *B*, to create a rhythmic subatmospheric pressure in the cylindrical respirator, *C*, which is recorded by gauge, *D*. As the subject is ventilated by negative pressure applied to his body, his exhaled air is collected and measured in a meter, *E*. Volume change of the lung-thorax per unit of pressure applied can be determined.

responding pressure is noted. From these data, liters per centimeter of water can be calculated. An intraesophageal tube records negative intrapleural pressure of a spontaneously breathing subject, but the lungs of a relaxed unconscious or anesthetized subject can be inflated with a positive pressure and the same data obtained. Fig. 3-16 schematically represents the record of three breaths with their corresponding intraesophageal pressures, demonstrating a normal lung compliance of $0.2$ $\ell$/cm $H_2O$.

*Thoracic compliance* $(C_T)$ is determined indirectly by using the inverse relationship described above. If lung-thorax and lung compliances are determined simultaneously, their values can be used to calculate $C_T$. Thus, if $C_{LT} = 0.1$ $\ell$/cm $H_2O$ and $C_L = 0.2$ $\ell$/cm $H_2O$, then:

$$\frac{1}{C_{LT}} = \frac{1}{C_L} + \frac{1}{C_T} \qquad\qquad \frac{1}{C_T} = \frac{1}{0.1} - \frac{1}{0.2}$$

$$\frac{1}{0.1} = \frac{1}{0.2} + \frac{1}{C_T} \qquad\qquad C_T = 0.2 \ \ell/\text{cm } H_2O$$

**Exercise 3-2.** Calculate the thoracic compliance in the following example:

$$\begin{aligned}\textit{Given:} \quad & C_{LT} = 0.072 \ \ell/\text{cm } H_2O \\ & C_L = 0.12 \ \ell/\text{cm } H_2O \\ \textit{Calculate:} \quad & C_T\end{aligned}$$

## NONELASTIC RESISTANCE TO VENTILATION

The forces of ventilation must overcome not only elastic tissue tension but also the resistance offered by nonelastic tissue, such as muscle, cartilage, fat, abdominal contents, and the movement of large blood vessels and airways over one another. The inertia of these structures corresponds to the retarding effect of *friction* in any mobile system and modifies the ideal pressure-volume relationship previously described. The work involved in overcoming tissue friction can be illustrated simply as in Fig. 3-17, graphing the stretch of a spring hampered by friction. The uninhibited length response to increasing pressure without friction is recorded as a dashed line (similar to Fig. 3-14), whereas the response slowed by friction follows the solid line.

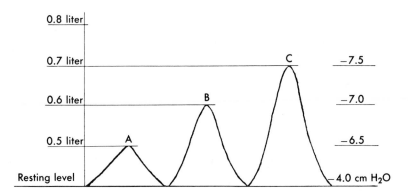

**Fig. 3-16.** From the resting level with an intrapleural pressure of $-4$ cm $H_2O$ to the static end-inspiratory point A, 0.5 liter of air moves with a pressure change of 2.5 cm $H_2O$. The same p-v relationships exist at B and C. Compliance calculated between any two points is $0.2$ $\ell$/cm $H_2O$.

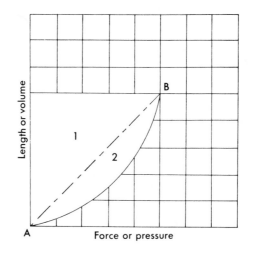

**Fig. 3-17.** Point *A* is the resting level, and *B* is end-inspiration. Dashed *A-B* represents the pressure-volume relationship of pure elastic resistance, and curved *A-B* the "drag" added by nonelastic friction. At *B*, where airflow momentarily ceases, nonelastic resistance is inactive because it is dependent upon movement. The curved line thus disappears, leaving only the elastic resistance of stretch. Areas *1* and *2* represent the work of overcoming elastic and nonelastic resistance, respectively.

The latter is curved, as a result of the drag of friction. Area 1 represents the amount of work done to overcome elasticity, and Area 2 the additional work to overcome friction.[17]

Fig. 3-17 demonstrates another important characteristic of nonelastic resistance. The tension of elasticity is *continuously* present, once force has been applied to a spring, whether the force is static or changing. In the lung-thorax, once distention has started, elasticity is present whether air is flowing or the lung is at a static breath-holding position. Nonelastic resistance is present *only* during movement, as when force is moving the spring or air is flowing in the lung, and is absent at static positions of no airflow. In Fig. 3-17, point *A* represents the resting position of no airflow and no distention of the lung; point *B* is the end-inspiratory pause with distention but no airflow. At *B*, therefore, only elastic resistance is active. The maximum effect of nonelastic resistance is noted where the two lines are most divergent, the period of greatest rate of airflow.

## AIRWAY RESISTANCE TO VENTILATION

Flow of gas through airways always encounters resistance that varies with characteristics of the gas and the conducting passages. Factors such as gas viscosity and turbulence, which modify flow, will be discussed below, but first we will look at the relationships between resistance, gas flow, and pressure. Resistance (R) is a ratio between the driving pressure responsible for gas movement and the flow of the gas, and it is measured in cm $H_2O/\ell$/sec. The pressure, in cm $H_2O$, is the so-called *transairway pressure*, or the *gradient* between the mouth (atmospheric) and the alveolar pressures. It produces the gas flow, which is calibrated in liters per second. During spontaneous inhalation, muscular energy lowers the intrathoracic and alveolar pressures, $P_A$, below atmospheric or mouth pressure, $P_m$, while during assisted breathing most ventilators drive gas under pressure into the airways so that $P_m$ exceeds $P_A$. In either instance there is a pressure gradient from mouth to alveoli allowing airflow into the lung. Thus it makes no difference whether the gradient is positive or negative, since it is the absolute difference that moves air. The relationships between resistance, pressure gradient, and flow are shown in this equation:

$$R = \frac{P_m - P_A}{\dot{V}} = \frac{\Delta P}{\dot{V}}$$

This means that if the resistance remains constant, the *difference* in pressure (pressure drop) from mouth to alveoli will increase if flow is increased and will decrease if flow is decreased.

Let us consider an airway as a tube, the proximal end of which is connected to a gas pressure source (atmosphere, mechanical ventilator), and the distal end closed by a flexible balloon (alveolus). At the moment gas flow starts into the tube, there will be a maximum pressure gradient from mouth to alveoli ($P_m - P_A$) with gas in the tube exerting decreasing lateral pressure down its length, but once gas moves into the alveolus, intraluminal and alveolar pressures will increase, gradually reducing the gradient. When flow stops (end-inspiration), if there is *time*, lateral and alveolar pressures will equilibrate with mouth pressure because at this moment, with no gas flow, pressure will be maximum and uniform throughout the system. The student should note that for the first time we are emphasizing the importance of time in ventilation, a factor that will assume major proportions in our later discussion of patient management.

The object of breathing, spontaneous or artificially supported, is to deliver a sufficient volume of air to the alveoli within an appropriate time period to satisfy body gas exchange needs. Thus emphasis is on gas volume per unit of time, or flow, and the pressure can be considered as a necessary adjunct to generate this flow. In the preceding equation, if we consider the resistance of a given tube to be constant, we can then look specifically at the critical relationship between pressure and flow. If flow is to be increased, for example, the $P_m - P_A$ difference must be widened, and this can be accomplished in one of two ways. (1) During spontaneous, unassisted breathing, $P_m$ corresponds to atmospheric pressure and can be considered another constant. $P_A$ thus becomes the variable pressure component that must be reduced to increase the gradient, and it is lowered by a more forceful inspiratory effort, generating a larger negative intrathoracic pressure. (2) When breathing is assisted by positive pressure applied to the airway, $P_m$ is the variable factor, and it must be increased to widen the gradient. The obvious conclusion is that gas flow across a conducting system can only be increased or decreased by increasing or decreasing the driving pressure correspondingly. Thus $R = P/\dot{V}$.

The normal airway resistance ranges from *0.6 to 2.4 cm $H_2O/\ell$ /sec*, measured at a standard flow rate of *0.5 $\ell$ /sec*. Suppose pulmonary disease so alters airways by partial obstruction that, to overcome the resistance, strong inspiratory efforts are needed, dropping the alveolar pressure to lower values and widening the mouth-alveolar gradient. The following examples compare the data of such a condition with the normal and illustrate the increase in resistance that such a gradient implies:

$$\textit{Normal:} \quad R = \frac{\Delta P}{\dot{V}} = \frac{1}{0.5} = 2 \text{ cm } H_2O/\ell/sec$$

$$\textit{Abnormal:} \quad R = \frac{\Delta P}{\dot{V}} = \frac{5}{0.5} = 10 \text{ cm } H_2O/\ell/sec$$

Specialized laboratory equipment is available to supply the data needed to calculate airway resistance. Flows are measured with a sensitive apparatus called a *pneumotachograph,* which converts gas velocity into pressure and transmits this pressure to a calibrated recorder, either photographic or electronic, from which final measurements are made. Precise alveolar pressures are best determined by a *body plethysmograph,* an airtight box in which the subject sits or reclines. As he breathes, the pressure changes in his alveoli are reciprocated in the space about him in the box and relayed to a suitable recorder.

Airway resistance is the result of friction among molecules of flowing gas and between the molecules and the wall of the conducting tube. The two physical gas characteristics contributing to resistance are *density* and *viscosity.* The former has been adequately described earlier, and we will now define and discuss the latter. Viscosity of a gas (or liquid) corresponds to friction of a moving solid and varies with individual gases, directly with temperature. The more viscous a gas the more resistive it is to motion or change of form. It can be visualized as a time-related force exerted by a moving plane surface over a stationary plane surface, expressed in dyne-seconds per square centimeter. A frictional force of 1 dyne over an area of 1 cm² for a distance of 1 cm and a period of 1 second is called a *poise.* It should be apparent that viscosity of liquids is greater than that of gases, and the values for both are small enough that they are expressed as fractions of poises. Viscosity of liquids is usually recorded as *centipoises* ($10^{-2}$ poises) and of gases as *micropoises* ($10^{-6}$ poises). A few examples in Table 3-4 illustrate the ranges of these values.

Although the student is not expected to be familiar with the details of this aspect of gas physics, analysis of the formula by which gas viscosity is calculated will reveal

**Table 3-4.**   *Examples of viscosity measurements*

|  | *Substance* | *° C* | *Poises* |
|---|---|---|---|
| Liquids | Water | 20 | $1.005 \times 10^{-2}$ |
|  | Alcohol, ethyl | 20 | $1.2 \quad \times 10^{-2}$ |
|  | Glycerine | 20 | $1490 \quad \times 10^{-2}$ |
|  | Oil, castor | 10 | $2420 \quad \times 10^{-2}$ |
| Gases | Air | 18 | $182.7 \times 10^{-6}$ |
|  | Carbon dioxide | 20 | $148 \quad \times 10^{-6}$ |
|  | Oxygen | 19 | $201.8 \times 10^{-6}$ |
|  | Helium | 20 | $194.1 \times 10^{-6}$ |

some relationships of great importance to the respiratory therapist. *Poiseuille's law* tells us that when gas flows through a tube:

$$n = \frac{\Delta P \pi r^4}{8 l \dot{V}}$$

where n is viscosity, $\Delta P$ is a pressure gradient in dynes per square centimeter between the two ends of the tube, r is the tube radius in centimeters, l is the tube length in centimeters, $\dot{V}$ is gas flow in cubic centimeters per second, and $\pi/8$ is a constant.

The importance of this formula to the general topic of ventilation is the information it gives when manipulated to our purposes. First let us rearrange the equation and equate the two important kinetic ventilatory factors, *pressure* and *flow*, to the others. (*Note:* Unless otherwise specified, our use of the term *pressure* means a pressure recorded on a gauge or other device that measures the pressure as above or below ambient atmospheric. Since this implies a "gradient," it is not necessary to use the symbol $\Delta P$, but merely P.)

$$P = \frac{n 8 l \dot{V}}{\pi r^4} \qquad\qquad \dot{V} = \frac{P \pi r^4}{8 l n}$$

If we are not interested in quantitative relationships but only in the general effects of changes in these parameters, one on the other, we can modify the equations by eliminating those factors that would not change significantly under the specified conditions. Pi and 8 are obvious constants; in a given subject the tubing length, l, representing the airways, is also generally a constant; since a subject breathes but one gas at a time, for any given circumstance gas viscosity is constant. It is important to note that tube radius, r, is not a constant because in disease airway patency is often a critical variable. Thus the above two equations can be rewritten as simple *proportionalities:*

$$P \cong \frac{\dot{V}}{r^4} \qquad\qquad \dot{V} \cong P r^4$$

Finally, these two can be combined into a single expression that clearly shows the reciprocal relationships between the three important variables:

$$\frac{P r^4}{\dot{V}} = k$$

In clinical pulmonary physiology one of the most frequently encountered conditions is that which involves narrowing of the airways through disease. The above ratio tells us that:

1. If the delivery pressure of gas ventilating the lung remains constant, the flow of the gas will vary directly with the *fourth power* of the radius of the airway. We see how a small change in bronchial caliber can effect a tremendous change in the amount of gas reaching alveoli per unit of time.
2. If the flow of the ventilating gas is to remain constant, the delivery pressure must vary inversely with the fourth power of the airway radius. Thus to maintain stable ventilation in the presence of narrowing airways, we may need great increases in driving pressure.

It might be of interest to the student to note that our use of Poiseuille's law merely reinforces the concept of pressure-flow relationship described at the beginning of this section, and quantitates it in terms of airway size. If we consider viscosity (n) as a form of resistance and transform Poiseuille's equation into a proportionality by eliminating the constants, then the two expressions of pressure-flow relationship we have so far encountered are very similar:

$$R = \frac{\Delta P}{\dot{V}} \qquad\qquad n \cong \frac{\Delta P}{\dot{V}}$$

In the respiratory tract there are three types of airflow patterns that are related to gas viscosity and density—*laminar, turbulent,* and *tracheobronchial* flow, illustrated in Fig. 3-18.

*Laminar flow* is a smooth unobstructed flow of gas through a tube of relatively uniform diameter, with few directional changes, and is found mostly in the trachea and main bronchi. Laminar flow is influenced principally by *viscosity* of the gas being moved, at low to moderate flows, and thus the relationships outlined earlier are pertinent in terms of the amount of air moved per unit of time or the pressure needed to move it. In respiratory physiology significant changes in inhaled gas viscosity are rarely of clinical importance. However, uniform narrowing of an airway reduces flow in proportion to the fourth power of the new radius or requires a similar increase in driving pressure to maintain a steady flow.

*Turbulent flow* is rough, with much eddy formation, like that of a stream running over a tortuous, rocky bed, and in the airways is generated by sudden changes in direction or acute reduction in diameter. Flow can also be turbulent, even in smooth

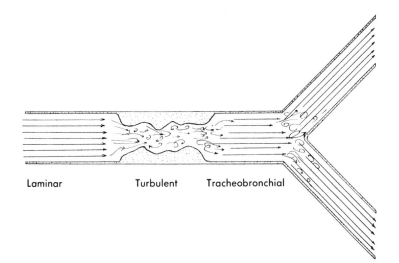

Laminar          Turbulent          Tracheobronchial

**Fig. 3-18.**  Three patterns of airflow are found in the respiratory tract. *Laminar* flow is straight and unobstructed, found in the large air passages. *Turbulent* flow is rough and swirling, the result of obstruction and sudden directional changes. *Tracheobronchial* flow is a combination of the two, found in the constantly branching and continuously narrowing airways. (Modified from Comroe, J. H., Jr., et al.: The lung, Chicago, 1962, Year Book Medical Publishers, Inc.)

passages, at high velocity. Ninety percent of the turbulence in the normal respiratory tract occurs in the irregular passages between the nose and trachea, but it is also found in the distal branchings of the small bronchi and bronchioles.[17] It is a factor of great clinical importance in all airways damaged by disease, especially where abnormal secretions, mucosal edema, or structural changes produce abrupt narrowing.

The influence of turbulence on ventilation is best explained by the *Bernoulli effect* (Daniel Bernoulli, 1700-1782), a natural phenomenon widely evident in our daily lives and the functional basis for much of the equipment used in respiratory therapy. Fig. 3-19, *A*, shows the fundamental relationships among pressure, gas flows and air passage restriction. The derivation of this inverse association of gas pressure and velocity, on which the Bernoulli effect depends, is detailed later in a discussion of the types of fluid energy. Fig. 3-19, *B*, illustrates a modification of the Bernoulli effect found in a *venturi* (Giovanni Venturi, 1746-1822). The venturi includes a dilatation of the gas passage just distal to an obstruction, and if the angulation of the funnel is not over 15 degrees, the gas pressure will be restored nearly to its prerestriction level. Widely used in fluid mechanics, venturis in respiratory therapy equipment are designed to draw in or "entrain" a second gas to mix

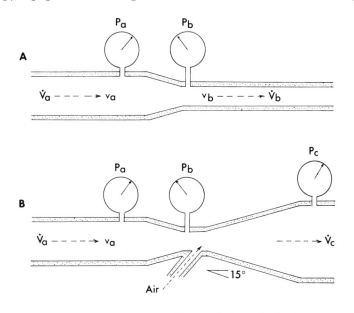

**Fig. 3-19.**  **A,** The Bernoulli effect demonstrates that the *pressure* exerted by a steady flow of gas or liquid in a conducting tube varies *inversely* as the *velocity* of the fluid. With an abrupt narrowing of the passage, since the volume of fluid per unit of time leaving ($\dot{V}_b$) must equal the time-volume entering the tube ($\dot{V}_a$), the linear motion of the fluid per unit of time (velocity, v) must increase as it traverses the stricture ($v_b > v_a$). Thus there is a pressure drop distal to the restriction ($P_b < P_a$). **B,** The venturi principle states that the pressure drop distal to a restriction can be closely restored to the prerestriction pressure if there is a dilatation of the passage immediately distal to the stenosis, with an angle of divergence not exceeding 15 degrees. Thus $P_c$ approximately equals $P_a$. The venturi is a widely used device to entrain a second gas to mix with the main-flow gas. The subambient pressure distal to the restriction draws in the second gas just past the restriction, and the increased outflow ($\dot{V}_c > \dot{V}_a$) is accommodated by the widened distal passage.

with the main-flow gas. Such entrainment takes place at the point of low pressure, the distal widening not only permitting pressure restoration but also providing ample space for the increased volume of the mixed gases. Reference will be made later to both the Bernoulli phenomenon and the venturi during discussions of equipment.

A distinction should be made here between the terms *flow* and *velocity*. Flow is a measure of the movement of a fluid *volume* per unit of time, and velocity is a measure of *linear* movement of a fluid per unit of time. For example, in two conducting tubes with different capacities, gases may move at the same velocity but at widely different flows. However, it should be evident that, in a given conducting system operating under a constant delivery pressure, changes in flow entering the system will elicit corresponding qualitative changes in gas velocities through the system. To this limited degree flow and velocity are directly related, but Fig. 3-19, *A*, shows us that the introduction of a restriction in the system necessitates an increase in postobstruction velocity to maintain a steady flow. We shall use these relationships shortly as we explore in more detail the mechanics of fluid flow.

Energy is the ability of a substance to perform work, and there are three kinds of energy in a moving fluid:

1. *Potential energy (PE)* is that energy due to the force of gravity acting on a volume of fluid elevated above its plane of horizontal flow. Its magnitude is dependent on the weight and height of the fluid, and it is best exemplified by a water tower reservoir. Potential energy can also be symbolized as *HW*, the product of height and weight.

2. *Pressure energy (P)* is the radial force exerted by a moving horizontal fluid and is demonstrated by measuring its lateral pressure while flowing through a pipe.

3. *Kinetic energy (KE)*, the energy imparted by the velocity of moving fluid, represents the amount of work performed by matter in motion against a resistive force.

For our purposes we do not need to consider units of measurement as we are interested only in the principles of energy relationships. Thus kinetic energy is expressed as *0.5 × density of the fluid × the square of the velocity of the fluid*, or *0.5 Dv$_2$*. The derivation of this can be found in standard textbooks of physics.

The Bernoulli theorem for a continuous fluid flow states that the sum of the potential, pressure, and kinetic energies at any given point in the stream will equal the sum of these energies at any other point.[18] However, in our area of interest, since we work with gas flows through tubing circuits under the force of a generated pressure, the factors of elevation and weights of gases are not applicable, and we can ignore potential energy. Thus we can set up an equation in reference to points *a* and *b* in Fig. 3-19, *A*, showing the relationships between pressure and kinetic energies:

$$P_a + 0.5\ Dv_a^2 = P_b + 0.5\ Dv_b^2$$

To make this equation more applicable to our needs in pulmonary physiology, we can alter it and rewrite it as a proportionality. If we assume we are dealing with a single gas, density will be a constant and can be dropped, giving the following proportional expression:

$$P_a - P_b \cong v_b^2 - v_a^2$$

Since the velocity at point *b* is greater than at point *a*, the pressure at *b* must be less than the pressure at *a*. This means that as gas flows through a stricture, its velocity *increases* and its pressure *decreases* and the magnitude of the pressure drop across the obstruction is proportional to the increase in the *square* of the velocity. Simply, the additional energy expended by the increased velocity reduces the amount of energy available to exert pressure. The implication of this effect is extremely important to the respiratory therapist. If therapeutic gas is applied to the airways of a patient with obstructive disease, the higher the flows delivered at a constant pressure the greater will be the velocities; and with increasing flows the difference between the squares of the preobstruction and postobstruction velocities will be widened. There will be an accompanying decrease in intraluminal pressure distal to the obstruction as the $P_a - P_b$ gradient enlarges.

Earlier it was noted that, given sufficient time, once airflow stops at end-inspiration, mouth, intraluminal, and alveolar pressures will equilibrate. The introduction of a turbulence-producing obstruction interferes with ventilation by hampering pressure equilization. Fig. 3-20 schematically compares laminar with turbulent flow, showing pressure relationships in smooth and obstructed conducting tubes, each of which terminates in an alveolus, *A*, which is inflated by the lateral pressure delivered to it. Fig. 3-20, *A*, depicts the low resistance and small pressure drop of laminar flow, $P_a - P_A$. Alveolar distending pressure is thus not much less than up-

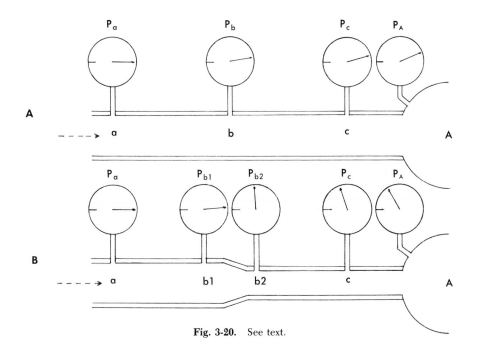

**Fig. 3-20.** See text.

stream pressure, and at end-inspiration rapid equilibration between $P_a$ and $P_A$ effects maximum alveolar inflation. Time is of relatively little importance. Fig. 3-20, *B*, shows that turbulent flow from an obstruction indicates high resistance and is accompanied by a large $P_a - P_A$ drop from the increased postobstruction gas velocity ($P_{b1} - P_{b2}$). Lateral alveolar distending pressure is considerably less than upstream pressure, and at end-inspiration, $P_a - P_A$ will still be large and the alveolus incompletely inflated. Here, time is very important, for, if upstream pressure can be held, $P_a$ and $P_A$ will gradually equilibrate to allow completion of alveolar filling. Perhaps the student can now see how the easily equalized pressure gradient from $P_a$ to $P_{b1}$ might prematurely stop downstream flow and leave the alveolus virtually uninflated.

There is yet another valuable clinical aspect to the Bernoulli phenomenon. Let us rewrite the above proportionality to include the density factor (eliminating the 0.5 as a constant):

$$P_a - P_b \cong D\ (v_b^2 = v_a^2)$$

Inspection shows that with a given increase in velocity the pressure drop across a restriction will be lessened if the gas density is reduced. Thus with obstructed airways, where the Bernoulli effect can be expected to exert a strong influence on the effectiveness of ventilation, distal pressure loss will be minimized with the use of low-density gases. This knowledge makes available to us a very valuable therapeutic tool, and we will see a practical use of the material just discussed when we consider the clinical use of helium.

*Tracheobronchial flow* is a descriptive term given to the mixture of laminar and turbulent flows found in the normal respiratory tract. Smooth gas flow through short segments of the tract is increasingly broken by the continuous branching of the airways, and even the relatively straight segments become progressively narrower with deeper penetration. Ventilation is thus the net sum of both laminar and turbulent flows, and effective alveolar pressure is related to the gas flow and tube radius in the laminar areas and the square of the gas velocity in the turbulent areas. The body's apparatus for moving air into and out of the lungs is designed to function against a normal balance of these resistances, but when they are increased by disease, the disability that results often requires the skilled services of respiratory therapy.

This is a good place to tie together the related factors of compliance, ventilatory frequency, flow, and airway resistance, which we have been describing individually. If his knowledge of these parameters is to have useful clinical meaning, the therapist must see the role played by each in reference to the others. Since the basic function of ventilation is the movement of air, the amount of air moved per unit of energy or pressure exerted will determine the efficiency of the system. This, we have already learned, is the description of compliance and is a measure of the elastic resistance of the lung-thorax system. However, we also know that the amount of air moved is dependent upon the state of the airways, the degree of their resistance to airflow. Thus, although the elastic resistance determines the pressure necessary to generate a given volume change, flow resistance determines the pressure needed for a given flow. From a practical point of view, then, the overall functional or *measured* lung-thorax compliance is really the net sum of the *actual* compliance of the system and the airway resistance. We can say that the general quality of airflow throughout the lungs is dependent upon the *uniformity of distribution* of both the elastic properties (actual compliance) in all areas of the lung and the flow-resistive properties (airway resistance) among all the airways. More specifically, it has been determined that, when flows are low, pulmonary air distribution is dependent upon lung elasticity and, when flows are high, upon airway resistance.[19]

Of clinical importance is the observation that in normal healthy subjects measured compliance does not vary as much with increased breathing rates as in patients with chronic bronchopulmonary disease, in whom measured compliance progressively drops as frequency increases. Thus the patient with obstructive disease needs increasing effort to move a given volume of air as he breathes at higher rates. Although his *actual alveolar compliance may be normal* (a possibility, even in diseased states), his measured compliance, or the volume of air he moves per unit of pressure, is depressed. Fig. 3-21 shows the reason for this. For a given volume of air per breath (tidal volume), as the frequency of breathing increases so does the flow, since the volume must be moved faster with each ventilatory excursion. At low frequencies with low

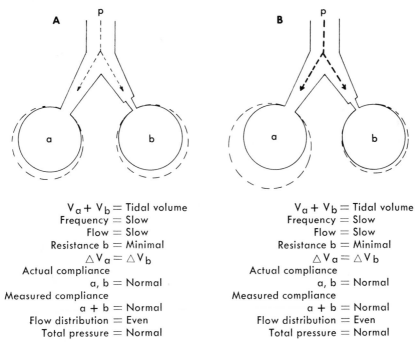

$$V_a + V_b = \text{Tidal volume}$$
Frequency = Slow
Flow = Slow
Resistance b = Minimal
$$\triangle V_a = \triangle V_b$$
Actual compliance
$$a, b = \text{Normal}$$
Measured compliance
$$a + b = \text{Normal}$$
Flow distribution = Even
Total pressure = Normal

$$V_a + V_b = \text{Tidal volume}$$
Frequency = Slow
Flow = Slow
Resistance b = Minimal
$$\triangle V_a = \triangle V_b$$
Actual compliance
$$a, b = \text{Normal}$$
Measured compliance
$$a + b = \text{Normal}$$
Flow distribution = Even
Total pressure = Normal

**Fig. 3-21.** The effect of airway resistance on measured total compliance is shown in sketches where one of each pair of alveoli, with normal actual compliance, is obstructed. The solid-line alveoli are at the resting level, the broken-line at end-tidal inspiration. *P* designates ventilatory pressure. In **A,** with a slow frequency, the obstruction has little effect on total ventilation, for the volume changes in the alveoli are equal. In **B,** the increased flow reduces the ventilation of alveolus *b*, while *a* compensates by hyperinflating. The increased ventilatory pressure, which attempts to overcome the resistance, lowers the measured, apparent, total compliance.

flows, the effect of resistance is minimal, and air is equally distributed between two alveoli because the actual compliance of the two pulmonary units determines the distribution of the air. With an increase in breathing frequency, as flow increases, the accompanying flow resistance of the obstruction causes a wide discrepancy in the distribution of flow to the alveoli while increasing the total pressure needed to move the air. Thus, for the overall functional compliance to remain constant in the presence of variable rates of breathing, the distribution of flow must remain constant. This requires that the elastic properties and the flow-resistive properties of all the pathways of the lung be uniformly distributed, a condition apparently found only in normal lungs. This view of *compliance* gives a more realistic picture of the relation between volumes and pressures than does the classic definition, described earlier.

## EXHALATION MECHANICS

Because of its clinical importance, the mechanics of exhalation deserves special consideration. It will be emphasized later that disturbances in exhalation produce some of the most frequent and severe examples of pulmonary disability. Whereas inhalation is a function of the active contraction of the several muscle groups described earlier, quiet exhalation is the result of *passive recoil* of elastic tissue of the lung, aided by the force of surface tension. At end-inspiration, ventilatory muscles "let go," allowing the lung-thorax to return to the resting level. Under conditions of stress, or in response to airflow obstruction, exhalation may be active through abdominal muscle action, forcing the diaphragm upward for more rapid emptying of the lung. Of critical importance in determining the passivity or activity of exhalation is the element of *time*. If the body's gas exchange needs, for a given level of physical exertion, can be satisfied by an effortless passive exhalation before the succeeding inhalation is triggered, supplementary muscular activity will not be needed; but if there is an increased gas exchange need, or if disease of the respiratory tract is impeding gas flow or uptake, or if there has been loss of lung-thorax elasticity, the body may require additional expiratory effort to move enough air from the lungs in *time* to satisfy the need. This effortful exhalation may be so energy consuming as to produce marked disability.

It should be evident that airway resistance to exhalation and loss of elasticity are important factors in determining ventilatory patterns. During quiet breathing, airway resistance to inhalation and exhalation in healthy subjects is about the same, even though the negative intrathoracic pressure of inhalation dilates and elongates the bronchioles and the rising pressure of exhalation narrows and shortens them. Forced exhalation, on the other hand, does increase resistance, and if exhalation is forced through normally patent airways and against negligible resistance, as in unobstructed hyperventilation, the high velocity of exhaled air creates its own resistance due to turbulence, but the expiratory muscular effort responsible is adequate to maintain smooth airflow. However, many pulmonary diseases damage and weaken the walls of the bronchioles. In such circumstances, should airway obstruction or loss of elasticity necessitate a strong expiratory effort to overcome resistance, the excessive positive pressures generated in the thorax may collapse the weakened bronchioles before the alveoli they drain are emptied. This condition of *air trapping* is a common com-

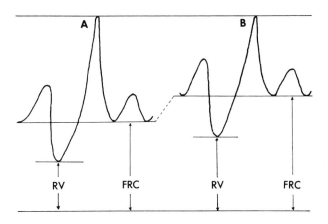

**Fig. 3-22.** Sketch **A** shows the resting level before, and **B** after, the effect of long-standing airway resistance and/or loss of lung elasticity, as the expansile thoracic springs dominate the pulmonary. Both functional residual capacity and residual volume enlarge. As disease progresses, loss of pulmonary flexibility decreases the expiratory reserve volume, further enlarging the residual volume, and continuing distention may depress the diaphragm to expand the total lung capacity.

plication of chronic bronchopulmonary disease, often posing a management problem for the respiratory therapist, and will be discussed more fully later.

With prolonged airway resistance or loss of elasticity, structural changes may occur in the chest. A major consequence of these disturbances is the gradual elevation of the resting level of the chest, as air trapping and/or inadequate recoil force prevent the lung-thorax from returning to its original, normal end-expiratory position. As shown in Fig. 3-22, this produces an increase in both the functional residual capacity and the residual volume. If uncorrected over a sufficient period of time, there is a progressive increase in the size of the thorax, especially in its anteroposterior diameter, the deformity descriptively called a "barrel chest." This is a remarkable phenomenon, since it most frequently occurs after the middle years, when the skeleton is well fixed, but it attests to the force exerted by the distended lung, coupled with the traction of accessory ventilatory muscles, to be described later. Because of the elevated resting level, the affected subject gives the appearance of holding his chest in the inspiratory position, a condition frequently seen in pulmonary emphysema.

## SUMMARY

The importance of the material covered in this chapter justifies a brief summary to emphasize a few clinical points of interest to the respiratory therapist. In good health the respiratory system is able to assure the body of a maximally effective ventilation, with a minimum of effort for any given level of need. Indeed, except under conditions of physical stress, we are generally unaware of the easy rhythmicity of our own breathing until it becomes impaired. Although we have not yet considered details of internal physiologic derangement of blood gas exchange that can upset the normal pattern of breathing, we should be impressed with the multitude of physical factors that influence ventilation and wonder at the ease with which it is accomplished.

The effective respiratory therapist must be observant. He must be able to judge, at least grossly, the general efficiency of his patient's ventilation on the basis of clinical observation. This means that he must have a clear mental picture of a *normal* breathing pattern for a given individual. He will note, for example, the rate and depth of tidal air exchange and attempt to determine whether the patient is hypoventilating or hyperventilating. He will evaluate the patient's work of breathing by looking for evidence of the use of accessory muscles of ventilation, the resting end-expiratory chest level, signs of inspiratory epigastric retraction or retraction of the costal margins, and evidence of expiratory abdominal contraction. He will observe the time relations between inspiration and expiration to see whether the normal inspiration-longer-than-expiration pattern is reversed. Such information will aid in carrying out, most efficiently and comfortably, his assigned treatment. Many times, of course, effortful breathing is obvious and the great effort to breathe is apparent at once. Such a patient can be described as short of breath at rest or at any specified level of activity. The therapist will frequently hear the term *dyspnea* used and he should understand its real meaning. Dyspnea is a symptom, a subjective feeling experienced only by the patient, not objectively observed by someone else. If a patient states that he is having difficulty breathing, then he is dyspneic. It means that he is uncomfortably aware of the need to work to breathe, and the therapist will be surprised at the number of patients who are obviously breathing with effort but who do not complain of it.

Although there are many pathologic aberrations in ventilatory patterns, there is one type with which the therapist should be familiar because of its frequency. This is referred to as *periodic breathing,* and while there are variations of it, the most common is known as *Cheyne-Stokes respiration.* It is characterized by alternating periods of hyperventilation and apnea. Tidal volume excursions get progressively deeper with each breath, reach a maximum, gradually get smaller in amplitude, and then cease completely. Each period of ventilation and apnea can last up to 20 seconds.[20] The "waxing and waning" pattern is characteristic and makes this disorder easy to recognize, even when the apnea may not be complete. Cardiovascular rather than respiratory factors are usually responsible for Cheyne-Stokes breathing, which is basically the result of cerebral oxygen want due to a reduced circulatory output of the left ventricle associated with obstructive cerebrovascular disease that reduces blood flow to the brain. Despite the apneic intervals, average blood carbon dioxide levels are usually low because of the hyperventilation. We are not concerned with the treatment of this condition but the therapist should be on the watch for it and call it to the attention of attending medical or nursing personnel whenever he notes it.

A less commonly encountered periodic pattern is *Biot's respiration.* This is somewhat similar to Cheyne-Stokes, except that the hyperventilatory phases are abrupt in onset and termination, without the crescendo-decrescendo character of Cheyne-Stokes. The respiratory efforts may vary in intensity, and the intervening apneic periods may be unequal and irregular. Biot's breathing is usually the result of severe brain damage, and although the exact mechanism is not known, many feel that there may be a reduced inhibitory action of the higher brain centers on the inspiratory function of the respiratory center, allowing periodic breakthrough of excessive inspiratory efforts.[21]

Chapter 4

# BLOOD GASES AND ACID-BASE BALANCE

The natural mechanisms of ventilation in good health and the techniques of respiratory therapy in the treatment of disease are designed to provide the circulating blood with sufficient oxygen for general cellular needs and to remove excess carbon dioxide. Failure to satisfy these two requirements subjects the blood to a reduced oxygen content *(hypoxemia)*, deprives tissue cells of oxygen *(hypoxia)*, and allows abnormal amounts of carbon dioxide to accumulate in the blood *(hypercapnia)*. Excessive ventilation or therapy, on the other hand, can overload the body with oxygen *(hyperoxemia, hyperoxia)* and reduce blood carbon dioxide to abnormally low levels *(hypocapnia)*. The genesis, clinical significance, and treatment of these pathologic states will be detailed later, but to prepare ourselves, in this chapter we will review the principles governing the actual movement of respiratory gases into and out of the circulation, the transportation systems that carry the gases between lung and body, and the intricate neurochemical mechanism that regulates spontaneous breathing. However, the respiratory gases, in addition to their participation in cellular metabolic needs, strongly influence the stability of the acid-base balance of the body, and we must include this aspect of physiology as an integral part of the overall study of blood gases. We will start with a discussion of the physical dynamics of alveolar blood diffusion and conclude with the physiologic and clinical aspects of acid-base balance.

## MECHANICS OF DIFFUSION

Our study of the physiology of the respiratory tract has now brought us to that critically vital structure, the perfused alveolus. So far we have been concerned with factors responsible for the mass movement of air from the atmosphere into the conducting airways. With air in the alveoli, we will now consider the mechanisms by which oxygen is extracted and made available to the body in exchange for carbon dioxide. For this we will have to think microscopically, for we will be dealing with gases at the molecular level and with the physical and chemical reactions in which they take part in their travels to and from body cells. We will first review the manner in which the respiratory gases overcome the boundary between the "inside" and the "outside" of the body, the alveolar wall, by the process of diffusion.

Diffusion is the movement of gas molecules from an area of relatively high partial pressure of the gas to one of low partial pressure. As all motion requires some driving force, so diffusion depends upon a pressure gradient. In our realm of interest, the

**117**

two gases with which we will be concerned, oxygen and carbon dioxide, not only must diffuse from one anatomic area to another but must also move through formidable obstructions—the alveolar wall–pulmonary capillary barrier (sometimes called the alveolar-capillary [A-C] membrane) and the body cell wall–systemic capillary barrier.[22] Thus, for gases to pass between the alveoli and the pulmonary capillary blood, there must exist a pressure gradient for each gas across this barrier, and the production and magnitude of these gradients will be of great concern to us from here on. Fig. 4-1 schematically illustrates the nature and structure of the A-C barrier, and if we keep in mind the minuscule size of a molecule of gas, we must be impressed with the task facing it in making the obstacle-ridden trip between alveolus and blood, and blood and tissue cell.

Since the A-C membrane is essentially a fluid barrier, the ability of gases to diffuse through it depends on two physical laws governing the passage of gas through liquid:

1. *Henry's law* states that the weight of a gas dissolving in a liquid at a given temperature is proportional to the partial pressure of the gas. The amount of gas that can be dissolved by 1 ml of a given liquid at standard pressure and specified temperature is called its *solubility coefficient* and varies *inversely* with the temperature. The solubility coefficient of oxygen in plasma, at 37° C and 760 mm Hg pressure, is 0.023 ml, and for carbon dioxide is 0.510 ml.

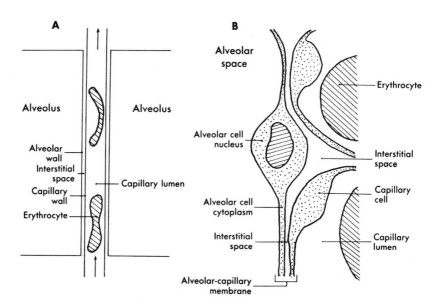

**Fig. 4-1.** Sketch **A** diagrams the relationship between the components of the alveolar-capillary (A-C) membrane, and **B** is a magnification sketch of a section through the structure. The *alveolar wall* is a cytoplasmic extension of the alveolar epithelial cells; it is separated from the adjacent capillary epithelial cells by a space, which may be real or potential, called the *interstitial* or intermembranous space. This space may contain tissue fibrils, and the accumulation of fluid here is of great clinical importance. The thickness of the A-C membrane varies from $0.4\mu$ to $2.0\mu$, depending upon the contents of the space. (Modified from Divertie, M. D., and Brown, A. L., Jr.: J.A.M.A. **187**:938, 1964.)

2. *Graham's law* states that the rate of diffusion (D) of a gas through liquid is directly proportional to its solubility coefficient and inversely proportional to the square root of its density (or gram-molecular weight). The number of milliliters of a gas that will diffuse a distance of 0.001 mm $(1\,\mu)$, over a square centimeter surface per minute, at 1 atm of pressure, is the *diffusion coefficient* of the gas.

Combining the above two properties, we can say that the relative rates of diffusion of two gases are directly proportional to the ratio of their solubilities and inversely proportional to the ratio of the square roots of their densities or gram-molecular weights. To illustrate this, let us compare the relative diffusibility of carbon dioxide with oxygen or, to state it another way, determine how much more or less diffusible is carbon dioxide than oxygen:

$$\text{Diffusibility of } CO_2 \cong \frac{\text{Sol coef } CO_2 \times \sqrt{\text{gmw } O_2}}{\text{Sol coef } O_2 \times \sqrt{\text{gmw } CO_2}}$$

$$\cong \frac{0.510 \times \sqrt{32}}{0.023 \times \sqrt{44}}$$

$$\cong \frac{0.510 \times 5.657}{0.023 \times 6.663}$$

$$\cong \frac{19}{1}$$

In other words, carbon dioxide is nineteen times as diffusible as oxygen.

*Exercise 4-1.* Given the following data, what is the diffusibility of gas B compared with gas A?

|          | Gas A | Gas B |
|----------|-------|-------|
| Sol coef | 0.25  | 0.65  |
| gmw      | 30    | 50    |

In cardiopulmonary physiology, knowledge of the diffusing capacity of the lung is sometimes helpful in evaluating pathologic conditions. Discussion of the laboratory techniques for measuring this function is not relevant here, but with the general concepts of diffusion just discussed in mind, we can relate its use to pulmonary evaluation. The expression *diffusion capacity of the lung* $(D_L)$ is defined as the number of milliliters of a specific gas that diffuse from the lung across the A-C membrane into the bloodstream each minute, for each mm Hg difference in the pressure gradient across the membrane. The two most common gases used to measure this function are low concentration carbon *monoxide* (CO) and oxygen, and in reporting values obtained we must identify the gas used. Thus average normal values are $D_{L_{CO}} = 17$ ml/min/mm Hg and $D_{L_{O_2}} = 20$ ml/min/mm Hg.[17]

Disease of the lung, if it modifies diffusion at all, always reduces diffusion. This implies that some abnormality has made it difficult for gas molecules to cross the A-C membrane in a reasonable period of time, in response to a normal pressure gradient. The clinical implications of this fact will be discussed further in Chapter 6.

## DIFFUSION GRADIENTS

The pressure gradient across the A-C membrane, so essential for gas diffusion, is dependent upon the concentrations of the gases in the inspired air and alveoli, as well as in the blood, and we will consider some of the physiologic normals. Since there is a continuous interchange in the alveoli of oxygen and carbon dioxide, each diluting the other, the alveolar concentrations of these gases are considerably different from their atmospheric concentrations. Table 4-1 presents some average normal values for *dry* inspired, alveolar, and exhaled air.

Correcting for the saturated state of these gases in the alveoli, we note that their alveolar partial pressures ($P_A$) at 1 atm are about:

| $O_2$ | $CO_2$ | $N_2$ | $H_2O$ |
|---|---|---|---|
| 100 mm Hg | 40 mm Hg | 573 mm Hg | 47 mm Hg |

At the circulatory end of the gradient, the respiratory gases in the blood also exert their own partial pressures. Although we have not yet discussed the transportation and utilization of the gases, we know that venous blood returning to the lung has less oxygen and more carbon dioxide than does arterial blood. Therefore the partial pressures will differ between the types of blood. The average normal venous ($P_V$) and arterial ($P_a$) partial pressures are shown in Table 4-2. If reference is made to oxygen or carbon dioxide tension in blood generally, without regard for its arterial or venous character, gas tensions may be symbolized as $P_{O_2}$ or $P_{CO_2}$.

An explanation is in order for the 90 to 100 mm Hg range of arterial oxygen tension listed in Table 4-2. The average $P_{a_{O_2}}$ of a large number of normal subjects would probably fall at about *95 mm Hg*, in a range that would extend from 90 mm Hg to perhaps 103 mm Hg. If the lung were a "perfect" organ, every alveolus would have exactly the same $P_{O_2}$ and the arterial blood leaving each alveolus would, through the process of diffusion to be described below, have exactly the same $P_{O_2}$ as each alveolus, about 100 mm Hg. We will see later, however, that the lung is not perfect and normally there are slight discrepancies between the ratios of ventilation to perfusion among the many A-C units. As a result, a sample of mixed arterial blood (blood from all areas of the lung returning to the heart for distribution through the systemic circulation) often has an oxygen tension less than that of an air sample taken from the lungs as a whole. In this text, for the sake of uniformity, mixed arterial blood will be assumed to have an oxygen tension of 95 mm Hg, the 5 mm Hg difference between it and

**Table 4-1.** *Composition of dry inspired, alveolar, and exhaled air*

|  | %$O_2$ | %$CO_2$ | %$N_2$, etc.[23] |
|---|---|---|---|
| Inspired air | 20.95 | 0.03 | 79.02 |
| Alveolar air | 14.0 | 5.6 | 80.4 |
| Exhaled air | 16.3 | 4.5 | 79.2 |

**Table 4-2.** *Gas partial pressures in venous and arterial blood*

| $P_{v_{O_2}}$ | 40 mm Hg | $P_{a_{O_2}}$ | 90-100 mm Hg |
|---|---|---|---|
| $P_{v_{CO_2}}$ | 46 mm Hg | $P_{a_{CO_2}}$ | 40 mm Hg |

alveolar oxygen tension constituting a normal *alveolar-arterial oxygen tension gradient*. This term will be used again later, with both normal and abnormal connotations. However, when describing physiologic events at the level of a single alveolus and its capillary, we will assume in the interest of simplicity that the A-C unit is "perfect" unless otherwise specified and that the local capillary-arterial oxygen tension is 100 mm Hg.

It should be noted that blood values for nitrogen partial pressure were not included. This by no means indicates that such a pressure does not exist. However, as far as the physiology of respiration is concerned, nitrogen is an *inert* gas in that it takes no part in metabolic gas exchange. It can be considered as a filler, taking up whatever space is not used by the two respiratory gases. Nitrogen diffuses readily between alveoli and blood, and the partial pressure it exerts is the difference between (1) the sum of the respiratory gas pressures and the atmospheric pressure and (2) the water vapor pressure. Nitrogen is of medical importance under certain circumstances and will be discussed further when indicated.

We can now correlate the above data on partial pressures and show how they make up gradients to promote a continuous and relatively smooth diffusion of respiratory gases. Consider the alveolus as a small pump that is constantly drawing in oxygen (air) and expelling carbon dioxide, thus maintaining alveolar partial pressures at *average* levels as described above. At any given moment the pressures in the alveolus will vary according to the time of the ventilatory cycle (or cycling of the alveolar pump), but samples of alveolar air over many cycles determine these average partial pressures. Two pressure gradient systems are established, one between alveolar oxygen (100 mm Hg) and venous oxygen (40 mm Hg) and a smaller one between venous carbon dioxide (46 mm Hg) and alveolar carbon dioxide (40 mm Hg). Oxygen, with its partial pressure maintained through the alveolar pump, diffuses from the alveolus into the pulmonary blood, *equilibrating* the $P_{O_2}$ of the blood with that of the alveolus. As the blood flows past the alveolus, it thus takes up oxygen and leaves the capillary as *arterialized* blood, with a $P_{O_2}$ in equilibrium with the alveolar oxygen, around 100 mm Hg. Simultaneously, carbon dioxide flows from the pulmonary capillary with its $P_{CO_2}$ of 46 mm Hg into the alveolus with its average $P_{CO_2}$ of 40 mm Hg. Again, the alveolar pump, by the regulated exhalation of carbon dioxide, maintains the gradient until the capillary blood has equilibrated with the alveolus, and the arterialized blood leaves the capillary with a $P_{CO_2}$ of 40 mm Hg. Fig. 4-2 illustrates the "perfect" diffusion gradients across the A-C membrane and the manner in which venous blood becomes arterialized.

We should note that the element of time is a critical factor in the diffusion of oxygen, although it is not directly related to the ability of the A-C membrane to exchange the gas. For blood to leave the pulmonary capillary adequately oxygenated, not only is the integrity of the membrane important but the blood must spend sufficient time in contact with the membrane to permit maximum diffusion. In the normal subject at rest, it takes about 0.75 second for a given point in the bloodstream to traverse the pulmonary capillary, and with the increased velocity of heavy exercise, about 0.34 second.[24] Most oxygen diffusion occurs at the beginning of the capillary; thus it would require a very severe diffusion defect to be solely responsible for inadequate oxygenation. However, since such pathologic conditions as fever, acute blood loss, and cer-

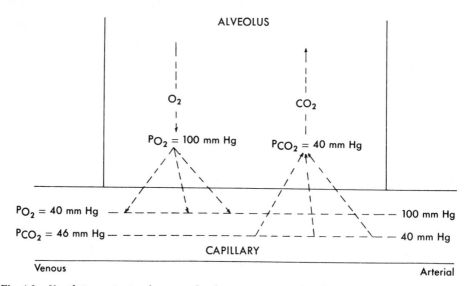

**Fig. 4-2.** Ventilation maintains the mean alveolar gas tensions as noted in the sketch. As blood enters the venous end of the pulmonary capillary, it loses its $CO_2$ and takes up $O_2$, until these two gases are in equilibrium with the mean alveolar tensions, and it leaves the capillary as arterial blood.

tain cardiac irregularities, to mention a few, can increase the cardiac output and blood velocity, it is reasonable to suppose that, when associated with sufficient pulmonary disease, the rapid flow of blood through the pulmonary capillaries might be a significant contributing factor to incomplete oxygenation.

Our discussion of gradients so far has centered about the A-C membrane, but for a clear picture of diffusion we must include the equally important gradients at the tissue cellular level, for it is to service the cells that the ventilation-transportation system exists. The respiratory gas gradients at the cell can be visualized as the reverse of those in the lung. As the metabolism of the cell depletes its store of oxygen, the intracellular $P_{O_2}$ drops below that of the blood entering the arterial end of the systemic capillary, and oxygen diffuses into the cell. At the same time the carbon dioxide diffuses from its higher pressure level in the cell into the capillary blood, and the blood becomes venous, returning to the lung to repeat its circuit. In a sense we are dealing with two sets of gradients (alveolar-blood and blood-cell, for both $O_2$ and $CO_2$) that provide gas transportation between the extremes of the two wider gradients of alveolus-cell for O and cell-alveolus for $CO_2$.

## OXYGEN TRANSPORTATION

The mechanism by which oxygen is carried between the alveolus and the body cell will be discussed first, to be followed by a description of the transportation of carbon dioxide; but it must be clearly understood that these two processes occur simultaneously, and it is only for convenience and clarity that we are separating them. Both gases are carried in the blood by virtue of their abilities to dissolve in blood or to combine with some of the elements of blood. An understanding of basic principles of gas transportation is essential for the safe and intelligent treatment of cardiopulmonary defects. Oxygen is carried in the blood in two so-called "compartments." One is the blood plasma, in which oxygen is dissolved in very small but important amounts, and the other is the hemoglobin of the erythrocyte, which carries the bulk of the load.

## Dissolved oxygen

As oxygen molecules diffuse into the blood, some go directly into solution in the plasma, and when this compartment is filled, the rest continue into the erythrocytes. The amount of oxygen that dissolves depends on the solubility coefficient of oxygen in plasma at body temperature. Thus for every 760 mm Hg pressure 0.023 ml of oxygen dissolves in each milliliter of plasma. In pulmonary physiology it is customary to refer to dissolved blood gases in terms of *volume percent* (vol%), which means so many *milliliters of gas per 100 ml of plasma.* Ml/dl could also be used, but by custom, in this circumstance, vol% is more common. Therefore for every 760 mm Hg pressure there are 2.3 vol% of dissolved oxygen, and this can be reduced to the basic factor of 0.003 vol% for *each* millimeter of mercury $P_{O_2}$. Calculation of the amount of oxygen that dissolves in plasma at any $P_{O_2}$ is simply: *Vol% = $P_{O_2}$ × 0.003.* In average normal arterial blood, with its $P_{a_{O_2}}$ of 95 to 100 mm Hg, the dissolved oxygen equals 0.3 ml of oxygen for each 100 ml of plasma. However, the $P_{a_{O_2}}$ of a subject breathing pure oxygen theoretically could reach 673 mm Hg, with dissolved oxygen of 2.02 vol%. The value of 673 is reached as follows: Recalling that physiologic gases are calculated in the dry state and assuming complete alveolar-arterial equilibrium with no $P_{O_2}$ gradient, we can calculate that the alveolar gases of a subject breathing pure oxygen at 1 atm have a pressure of 760 − 47 = 713 mm Hg (atmospheric pressure − water vapor pressure). After a subject has breathed 100% oxygen for several minutes, nitrogen that was in the alveoli during air breathing is completely washed out, leaving only oxygen and carbon dioxide. With a carbon dioxide tension of 40 mm Hg, alveolar (and presumably arterial) oxygen tension equals 713 − 40, or 673 mm Hg. A method of estimating $P_{A_{O_2}}$ at any concentration of inhaled oxygen employs the *alveolar air equation,* which will not be considered at this time (Appendix 12). Fig. 4-3 illustrates, by graph, the linear relationship between partial pressure of oxygen and volume percent of oxygen dissolved in the plasma.

## Combined oxygen

Most of the oxygen in the body is carried physically bound to or combined with the *hemoglobin* (Hb) of the erythrocytes. Hemoglobin is the "red stuff" of the blood, giving to blood its characteristic colors, and except in abnormal conditions, it is always confined to the erythrocyte. Should disease or disturbed physiology produce rupture of the red cells, the spillage of hemoglobin into the plasma is referred to as *hemolysis* of the cell with subsequent *hemoglobinemia.* Hemoglobin is a protein, *globin,* combined with an iron-containing compound called *heme.* It is a large and heavy molecule with a *physical* molecular weight of 66,700, but in its respiratory function its *physiologic* molecular weight is considered to be only 16,700. There are many different kinds of hemoglobin, designated by letters, A, C, E, F, G, H, I, J, K, S. Some of these types are variants of the normal; others are clinically pathologic. The differences in

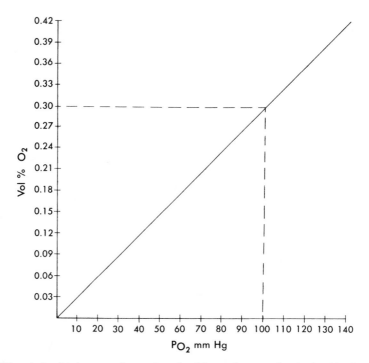

**Fig. 4-3.** The relationship between the number of milliliters of oxygen dissolved in blood and its consequent partial pressure is linear. Each 0.003 ml of $O_2$ dissolved in 100 ml of blood (vol% of $O_2$) exerts a pressure of 1 mm Hg. The dashed line emphasizes the fact that arterial blood, with an average $P_{O_2}$ of 100 mm Hg, has 0.3 ml of $O_2$ dissolved in each 100 ml.

the hemoglobin types lie in the structure of the globin portion, which is made up of many amino acids derived from diet.

We will soon see that the transportation of oxygen and of carbon dioxide in the erythrocyte are mutually dependent upon one another, since they alternate in using hemoglobin as a carrier; but first we will consider oxygen alone and then relate the two systems. Venous blood leaving the body cells still contains some oxygen, enough to maintain a partial pressure of about 40 mm Hg, but because of its depleted oxygen supply, most of its hemoglobin is called *reduced hemoglobin*. This is often symbolized simply as *Hb* or, since it has acquired a hydrogen ion in its participation in the transport of carbon dioxide from the cells (to be described and illustrated shortly), more properly as *HHb*. In the pulmonary capillaries, immediately upon release of carbon dioxide, the HHb converts to the potassium salt, *KHb*. In this form hemoglobin combines with oxygen molecules diffusing into the erythrocytes, becoming *oxyhemoglobin*, $Hb_{O_2}$, or better, $KHb_{O_2}$. One gram-molecular weight of oxygen, 32 g, can combine with 16,700 g of hemoglobin, and it is this factor that determines the physiologic molecular weight of hemoglobin as noted above. Because

$$\frac{1 \text{ mole } O_2}{16,700 \text{ g Hb}} = \frac{22,400 \text{ ml } O_2}{16,700 \text{ g Hb}} = \frac{1.34 \text{ ml } O_2}{\text{g Hb}}$$

each gram of hemoglobin is able to take up and carry 1.34 ml of oxygen. If we assume a normal hemoglobin concentration of 15 g/dl blood, the combined oxygen *capacity* is $1.34 \times 15 = 20.1$ ml $O_2$/dl blood, or *20.1 vol %*, and is directly related to the amount and quality of available hemoglobin.

However, the quantity of oxygen actually carried, or the content, is dependent upon the hemoglobin *saturation*. This refers to the amount of oxygen combined with hemoglobin in proportion to the amount of oxygen the hemoglobin is capable of carrying if it has its full load, and it is expressed as a percentage from the ratio content/capacity. Although the capacity can be calculated as above, if the presence of abnormal or inactive hemoglobin is suspected, in the laboratory the oxygen content can be chemically analyzed in volume percent; then by exposing the sample to air to allow it to combine maximally with oxygen, we can determine its capacity. If the content is one half the capacity, the saturation is reported as 50%. Because the lung is not a "perfect" organ, as described above, in the normal subject breathing room air at 1 atm pressure, the average saturation of mixed arterial blood ($S_{\bar{a}_{O_2}}$) is about 97%, and the average saturation of mixed venous blood entering the lung through the pulmonary circulation ($S_{\bar{v}_{O_2}}$) is about 70% to 75%. *Unsaturation* is the converse of saturation and refers to the degree to which blood is not saturated. Thus normal arterial blood may be considered to be 3% unsaturated, and venous blood, 30% unsaturated. Since saturation equals content/capacity, then content equals capacity times saturation, and the amount of oxygen combined with hemoglobin in average normal arterial blood with 15 g/dl hemoglobin equals:

$$1.34 \times 15 \times 0.97 = 19.5 \text{ vol\%}$$

It is worth our while to spend a moment here to clarify the mechanisms responsible for the normal 97% hemoglobin oxygen saturation of mixed arterial blood leaving the lungs. When there is no impediment to the diffusion of a normal amount of oxygen under normal pressure across the alveolar-capillary membrane, failure of mixed arterial blood to show 100% saturation of its available hemoglobin is the result of venous blood mixing with it. This combination is called a *venous admixture*, and it may be the result of a physical or anatomical shunt or a *ventilation/perfusion imbalance*.

**Shunt.** A condition whereby venous blood physically bypasses the lung without perfusing ventilated alveoli is termed a *right-* (venous blood) *to-left* (arterial blood) *shunt*. The mixed venous-arterial blood has a lower oxygen content and saturation than does pure arterial blood. There are two normal anatomical shunts that contribute to the 3% arterial unsaturation, and they are referred to as physiological because they are not due to pathology.[25]

*Thebesian venous drainage.* Thebesian veins are very small vessels that drain the myocardium and empty through minute openings into both atria. Those which communicate with the left atrium mix venous blood with arterial and may provide a major part of the normal arterial unsaturation.

*Bronchial venous drainage.* The airways, like all other body tissues, are perfused by the systemic circulation through the bronchial arteries and veins. Bronchial venous drainage, however, is quite unorthodox, and most of it enters the pulmonary veins (arterialized blood) directly, with only a few identifiable bronchial veins joining azygous and intercostal venous systems. Here, then, is another source of venous admixture to keep arterial oxygen saturation below 100%.

**Ventilation/perfusion imbalance.** Positional underventilation in proportion to perfusion of some alveoli may find venous blood perfusing incompletely ventilated lung tissue. Thus partially unsaturated blood mixes with fully saturated blood from other areas, creating a venous admixture. Such a phenomenon is likely to be found in dependent lung segments, especially during periods of relatively shallow breathing.

Pathological shunts and ventilation/perfusion ratios will be considered in Chapter 6.

Let us now consider those factors that are responsible for determining the degree of arterial oxygen saturation—*partial pressure of arterial oxygen, hydrogen ion concentration of the blood (pH), body temperature,* and *organic phosphates.* One of the most important fundamentals of pulmonary physiology is the relationship between oxygen saturation and these factors, graphically illustrated in the *oxygen dissociation curves,* which indicate the physiologic conditions under which oxygen combines with or dissociates from its hemoglobin carrier. When all the elements of ventilation, pulmonary air distribution, ventilation/perfusion ratio, and alveolar diffusion are able to achieve a $P_{O_2}$ of 100 mm Hg in arterial blood with a normal pH of 7.40 at body temperature, the arterial oxygen saturation will be approximately 97%.

**Partial pressure of oxygen.** Fig. 4-4 is the dissociation curve of blood at 37° C, showing the important relationship between $P_{O_2}$ and $S_{O_2}$ at three pH values. For the moment we will concern ourselves only with the middle curve. Note that the dissociation curve is not linear like that of the dissolved oxygen graph but is doubly curved. The upper end of the curve slopes gently downward to the left for a distance and then becomes steep in its middle segment, a characteristic of great physiologic importance. Note that the line at $P_{O_2}$ of 100 mm Hg meets the normal pH 7.40 curve at a point corresponding to a $S_{O_2}$ of 97%. Again note that even if some abnormality reduced the $P_{O_2}$ to 65 mm Hg, arterial blood would still be 90% saturated, but if the curve were linear, the $S_{O_2}$ would be only about 64%. The relatively flat upper part of the curve prevents wide fluctuations in saturation (and thus in content) in the presence of oxygen tension drop due to disease or environmental abnormalities, but below $P_{O_2}$ of 50 mm Hg, the drop in saturation becomes precipitous.

When arterial blood perfuses body tissues and equilibrates with the oxygen-poor cells, its $P_{O_2}$ drops to the venous level of about 40 mm Hg and its saturation to approximately 73%, but on its return to the lung, where it equilibrates with the alveolar $P_{A_{O_2}}$ of about 100 mm Hg, it again becomes 97% saturated. This portion of the curve, between $P_{O_2}$ of 100 mm Hg and 40 mm Hg, represents the loading and unloading of oxygen in the lung and at the body cell. If we stipulate a hemoglobin content of 15 g/dl, assume complete $O_2$ equilibration between blood and both lung and tissue cell, and assume that the pH remains at 7.40 (actually there is a slight shift of about 0.03 pH unit as blood varies between venous and arterial), we can calculate the total

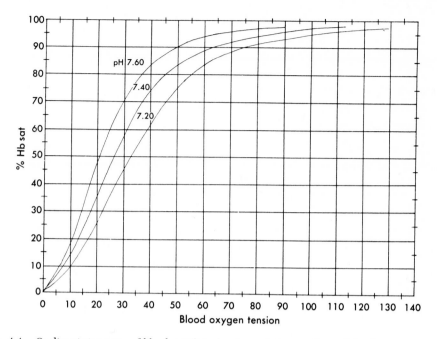

**Fig. 4-4.** $O_2$ dissociation curve of blood at 37° C, showing variations at three pH levels. For a given $O_2$ tension, the higher the blood pH, the more the hemoglobin holds onto its $O_2$, maintaining a higher saturation.

**Table 4-3.** *Oxygen content of arterial and venous blood*

|  | Vol % arterial $O_2$ | Vol % venous $O_2$ |
|---|---|---|
| Combined $O_2$ (1.34 × 15 × Sat) | 19.5 | 14.7 |
| Dissolved $O_2$ ($P_{O_2}$ × 0.003) | 0.3 | 0.1 |
| Total $O_2$ content | 19.8 | 14.8 |

volumes percent of oxygen (combined plus dissolved) in both arterial and venous blood, as in Table 4-3.

This arterial-venous (a-v) difference of 5 vol% represents the amount of oxygen given up to tissue cells and is referred to as the *average oxygen uptake*. Obviously, the uptake of all body cells at one time is not the same, but the blood reflects the mean of the body as a whole. It should be apparent that when physiologic abnormalities cause a low $P_{a_{O_2}}$ breathing room air, the resulting drop in arterial saturation can often be corrected by so elevating the alveolar $P_{O_2}$ with high oxygen concentrations that the $P_{a_{O_2}}$ will rise toward the upper end of the dissociation curve. Because of the continuing flattening of the upper curve, increasing $P_{a_{O_2}}$ values produce reducing increments of increase in saturation of hemoglobin, and 100% saturation is finally reached at $P_{a_{O_2}}$ of about 340 mm Hg.

***Hydrogen ion concentration of the blood (pH).*** The mechanism and clinical significance of blood pH changes will be discussed later, but it should be explained here that the path and shape of the oxygen dissociation curve depends on pH as well as on blood oxygen tension and saturation. An increase in $[H^+]$ (drop in pH) moves the curve to the right, and a decrease (rise in pH) moves it to the left, an immediate effect of the direct action of hydrogen ions on the hemoglobin molecule. This is known as the *Bohr effect*, and it demonstrates that hydrogen ions decrease the ability of hemoglobin to hold onto oxygen. Thus, as blood pH drops (increase in $[H^+]$), oxygen is released to the cells and saturation at a given $P_{O_2}$ is lowered. Conversely, with a rising pH (decrease in $[H^+]$ the affinity of Hb for $O_2$ is increased, saturation remains high, and oxygen is less available to the cells.

Even within the narrow range in which blood alternates between arterial and venous, the Bohr effect has physiologic importance. It was noted above that blood pH varies about 0.03 pH unit between venous and arterial, and this is illustrated in Fig. 4-5, which shows a segment of the normal dissociation curve. As blood becomes venous, $(V)$, its increased $CO_2$ content raises $[H^+]$ and lowers pH by a mechanism to be described in the next section. As a result, the $O_2$ curve moves slightly to the right, and at a given $P_{O_2}$ shows a lower $S_{O_2}$ than does the pH 7.40 curve, indicating release to the tissues of a greater volume of oxygen. In the lung, arterialized blood, $(A)$, loses $CO_2$, its pH rises, and it has an increased affinity for oxygen. The Bohr effect thus facilitates pulmonary uptake and tissue delivery of oxygen.

Fig. 4-5 illustrates variation in the shape and position of the oxygen dissociation curve with wide ranges of pH. Given a $P_{a_{O_2}}$ of 50 mm Hg, there is a difference of 15% saturation between pH 7.20 and 7.60. Variations in blood pH alone, with no change in oxygenation, can modify the oxygen content/capacity ratio of hemoglobin; or, to put it another way, the affinity of hemoglobin for oxygen is dependent on the pH of the blood. For example, in acidosis, the curve shows us that severe unsaturation of hemoglobin with oxygen may exist even with a near normal $P_{O_2}$. A clinically important observation can be made from the effects of the pH shifts of the dissociation curve. For a given $P_{O_2}$, because the blood is able to maintain a higher oxygen saturation

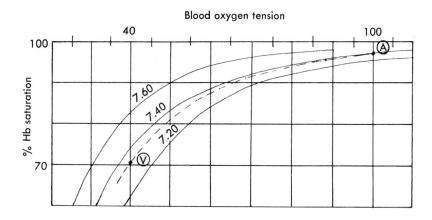

**Fig. 4-5.** Bohr effect. The dashed line indicates the physiologic shift in $O_2$ dissociation curve as changing blood $CO_2$ content alters blood pH between arterial, $(A)$, and venous, $(V)$, points.

in a state of alkalosis than in acidosis, alkalosis might seem to be a distinct advantage to the body economy and suggest the desirability of that state as a preventative of hypoxemia. However, let us compare the performances of both the pH 7.60 and pH 7.20 dissociation curves in a hypothetical situation. We will again assume a hemoglobin concentration of 15 g/dl and complete oxygen equilibration at $P_{O_2}$ of 100 mm Hg and 40 mm Hg, for arterial and venous blood, respectively. From the dissociation curves, we read oxygen saturations of 98% for arterial blood and 84% for venous blood at pH of 7.60 and corresponding saturations of 94% and 62% at pH of 7.20. We can now compute the a-v oxygen difference between the alveoli and tissue cells for each abnormal pH value, comparing them with the normal, as outlined in Table 4-4.

There is less than 1 vol% of oxygen difference between alkalotic and acidotic arterial blood, but after tissue perfusion the a-v oxygen difference of acidotic blood is more than double that for alkalotic. The important inference here is that alkalotic blood does not dissociate readily but rather holds onto its oxygen, making the oxygen less available to body cells than does normal or acidotic blood. This does not mean that acidosis is beneficial just because it releases oxygen more freely, for we will see that the acidotic state is generally a very unwholesome condition for the entire body physiology. Close inspection of the dissociation curves shows that if the arterial blood has a very low oxygen tension (40 to 50 mm Hg), the oxygen uptake difference between alkalotic and acidotic blood, at venous levels of 10 to 20 mm Hg $P_{O_2}$, is much less than at normal arterial values, but acidotic blood still releases more oxygen. The therapist will soon learn that the objective of treatment is to restore physiology as close to normal as possible.

Shifting positions of the oxygen dissociation curve are sometimes referred to as changes in the $P_{50}$. This is the partial pressure of blood oxygen that half saturates hemoglobin, providing about 10 vol% of oxygen bound to hemoglobin. As shown in Fig. 4-4, the $P_{50}$ of the normal middle curve is *26.5 mm Hg*. In contrast, the $P_{50}$ of blood with a pH of 7.60 is about 20.5 mm Hg and with a pH of 7.20, about 32 mm Hg. A dissociation curve that shifts to the left is said to have a low $P_{50}$ and to the right, a high $P_{50}$. A low value tells us that something has happened to increase the affinity of hemoglobin for oxygen. The hemoglobin holds the oxygen more firmly than normal, and less pressure is needed to bind the two. It is harder for oxygen to dissociate from hemoglobin, thus its availability to tissues is reduced. A high $P_{50}$ tells us that something has weakened hemoglobin's intrinsic ability to hold on to oxygen and that a higher gas pressure is needed for binding. Oxygen escapes hemoglobin easier and is more readily available to tissues. We can say therefore that a high pH, or a low $[H^+]$,

**Table 4-4.** *Arterial-venous (a-v) oxygen difference at three pH levels*

|  | *Total vol% arterial $O_2$* | *Total vol% venous $O_2$* | *a-v vol% $O_2$* |
|---|---|---|---|
| pH 7.60 | 20.0 | 17.0 | 3.0 |
| pH 7.40 | 19.8 | 14.8 | 5.0 |
| pH 7.20 | 19.2 | 12.6 | 6.6 |

produces a low $P_{50}$ oxygen dissociation curve (leftward shift), and a low pH, or high [$H^+$], produces a high $P_{50}$ curve (rightward shift).

**Body temperature.** Fig. 4-6 illustrates the influence of body temperature on oxygen saturation and dissociation. It is customary to measure oxygen tension at a temperature of 37° C, then by the use of tabulated factors or nomograms, correct tension and saturation to the patient's actual temperature. Many combinations of pH and temperature can produce a host of possible curves. The therapeutic use of low body temperature (hypothermia) employs the principle of reduced oxygen need and utilization under conditions of cooling. This effect is evident in the lower a-v oxygen differences shown on the low temperature dissociation curve. (Compare with pH effect described above.)

**Organic phosphates.** In the area of general metabolism, organic phosphate compounds play vital roles in many cellular biochemical reactions and are essential to the transfer of energy on which cellular function depends. Within the past few years, attention has been directed to the involvement of phosphates in respiration, a phenomenon long known but little appreciated. The two most significant organic phosphates in this reference are *2,3-diphosphoglycerate (DPG)* and *adenosine triphosphate (ATP)*, but in the interest of brevity and because of its relatively greater importance, we will describe DPG as the prototype.[26-31]

DPG is found *in the erythrocyte,* where it is formed as one of the chief end products of glucose metabolism, and it is bound to unsaturated hemoglobin. Like hydrogen

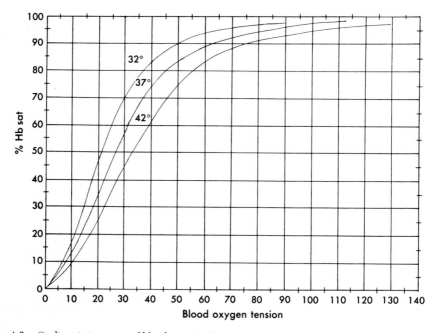

**Fig. 4-6.**   $O_2$ dissociation curve of blood at a pH of 7.40, showing variations at three temperatures. For a given $O_2$ tension, the lower the temperature, the more the hemoglobin holds onto its $O_2$, maintaining a higher saturation.

ions, *DPG decreases the affinity of hemoglobin for oxygen*, high levels expediting oxygen release and low levels its retention by hemoglobin. By chemical measurement, its normal concentration is 4.0 to 5.25 mM/$\ell$ of erythrocytes.

It should be apparent that DPG shifts the oxygen dissociation curve to the right (high $P_{50}$) to promote oxygen unloading at the tissues. Three factors modify the action of DPG, with results that are of clinical interest to us.

*Hypoxia.* DPG concentration increases with hypoxia of any cause, shifting the dissociation curve to the right to make up for the hypoxia by increasing the availability of oxygen to the tissues.

*Anemia.* As hemoglobin concentration drops, DPG increases about 0.23 mM for each gram per deciliter loss of hemoglobin. This response may compensate for up to half the oxygen deficit due to the anemia and may account for the lack of hypoxic symptoms, so frequent even in severe anemia.

*Blood pH.* DPG concentration varies directly, about 5%, with each 0.01 pH unit change. Thus a shift of the dissociation curve due to the Bohr effect is countered, to some degree, by a reverse shift from DPG action.

## CARBON DIOXIDE TRANSPORTATION

As oxygen diffuses from the blood into the body cells, carbon dioxide moves from cells to blood and is transported to the lung for excretion, but we must remember that all of the carbon dioxide carried in venous blood to the lung is not removed, enough remaining to exert a partial pressure of 40 mm Hg in the arterial blood. The mechanics of $CO_2$ transportation is more complicated than that of oxygen, but it must be understood clearly, for the amount of $CO_2$ in transit is one of the major determinants of the acid-base balance of the body. Fifty to 60 vol% of carbon dioxide are carried in three plasma and three erythrocyte compartments: *in plasma*—bound to protein, as bicarbonate, and in physical solution; *in erythrocytes*—dissolved in erythrocyte water, combined with hemoglobin, and as carbonic acid.

Fig. 4-7 is a schematic diagram of both $CO_2$ and $O_2$ transport in the blood, and their exchange at both body cell and the lung. The horizontal rectangle represents an erythrocyte suspended in plasma. The left side of the diagram shows the alveolar-capillary barrier and gas exchange in the lung, and the right side, the diffusion of gases across the cellular membrane. Solid arrows indicate the direction of gas movement, the molecules or ions that react with one another, and the products of their reactions. Dashed-line arrows identify the dissociation of compounds into molecules or ions. Circled numbers on the right index horizontal reactions for reference in the following discussion. Because our primary interest in these pages is with $CO_2$, we will only note in passing the basic elements of oxygen transport, shown at the top of the diagram. Oxygen diffuses from alveolus into plasma, on the left, and some goes directly into solution. This is only a small volume, and when the perfusing blood is quickly saturated, the remaining $O_2$ enters the erythrocyte, where it reacts with reduced potassium hemoglobin made available by the dissociation of potassium bicarbonate of the $CO_2$ system. When the erythrocyte reaches a systemic capillary (right half of Fig. 4-7), the oxyhemoglobin separates into reduced KHb and $O_2$. The latter

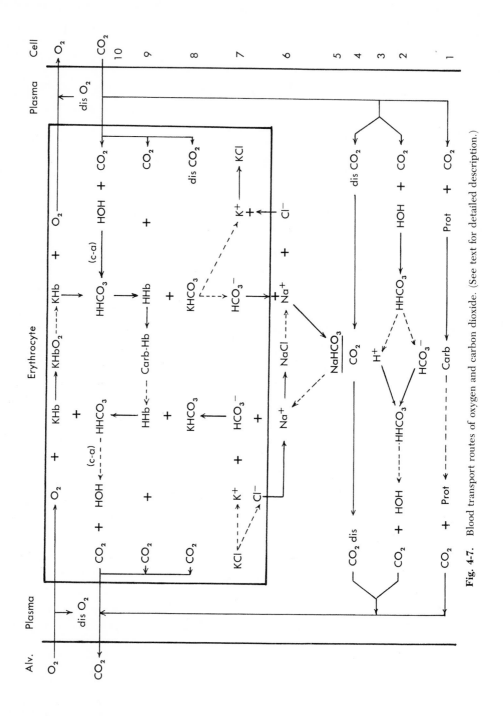

**Fig. 4-7.** Blood transport routes of oxygen and carbon dioxide. (See text for detailed description.)

diffuses out of the erythrocyte, into plasma solution and thence into the cell, leaving a smaller amount dissolved in the plasma after cellular perfusion than after alveolar. The reduced hemoglobin is now ready to participate in $CO_2$ carriage.

### Plasma transport of carbon dioxide

*Bound to protein.* As $CO_2$ leaves the cell, ⑩, a very small amount of it combines with plasma protein to form a complex called a *carbamino compound* ①. This fraction of the $CO_2$ in the blood is relatively insignificant, comprising only 1.12 vol% of the total.

More of the $CO_2$ goes into physical solution in the plasma, ③, but once dissolved, follows two different pathways.

*Bound as bicarbonate.* In solution one fraction of the $CO_2$ reacts with plasma water, ②. By hydrolysis the $CO_2$ and water form carbonic acid which at once is ionized into H and $HCO_3$ ions. These hydrogen ions are an important and significant portion of the total circulating hydrogen ion concentration that governs our acid-base balance. The bicarbonate ion becomes part of what is referred to as the *alkaline reserve* of the body, also important in acid-base regulation.

*Dissolved in plasma.* The other fraction of dissolved $CO_2$ remains in physical solution, unchanged, ④. This dissolved volume of $CO_2$ is about 1000 times as great as that which hydrolyzes into carbonic acid, a proportion that remains remarkably constant. This ratio is exceedingly useful to us. While we would like to be able to measure the concentration of the hydrogen ions from carbonic acid ionization, this is not technically feasible for clinical use. We can measure the amount of dissolved $CO_2$ very easily, however, and because of the ratio of $CO_2$ to $H^+$, can deduce concentrations of the latter.

### Erythrocyte transport of carbon dioxide

*Dissolved in erythrocyte.* Another insignificant portion of $CO_2$, after it has diffused through the erythrocyte membrane, goes into physical solution in the erythrocyte water and is noted here only for completeness ⑧.

*Combined with hemoglobin.* A larger fraction of the gas combines with the *reduced acid* hemoglobin (HHb), made available by the release of oxygen to the tissues and, because hemoglobin is a protein, forms carbamino-hemoglobin ⑨, somewhat similar to its combination with plasma protein. This is a very rapid reaction, and since the combining power of reduced hemoglobin with carbon dioxide is greater than that of oxyhemoglobin, the gas is readily picked up at the cell and discharged at the lung. The carbamino-Hb constitutes from 8% to 10% of the total $CO_2$ transported but 20% to 25% of the $CO_2$ released in the lung.

*As carbonic acid.* The major portion of the transported $CO_2$ is hydrated in the red cell to $H_2CO_3$, a normally slow process that is speeded up by an enzyme catalyst called *carbonic anhydrase* (c-a). The following sequence of steps then takes place: The carbonic acid immediately ionizes, as it does in the plasma. The reduced KHb, available after the release of $O_2$, reacts with the newly formed $HHCO_3$ (shown vertically on the diagram) to produce reduced hemoglobin (HHb), referred to above, and potassium bicarbonate ($KHCO_3$), (9) and (8). As soon as the $KHCO_3$ is formed, it ionizes and the $HCO_3^-$ *diffuses out of the erythrocyte* into the plasma, as part of an interesting maneuver known as the "chloride shift," or the Hamburger phenomenon. To maintain ionic equilibrium, if one ion leaves the red cell, another must enter to replace it. Large amounts of NaCl are present in plasma, and as the bicarbonate ions leave the red cell, chloride ions enter in exchange, (6). The sodium of the plasma NaCl then combines with the bicarbonate from the red cell to form $NaHCO_3$, (5), and the released potassium in the erythrocyte combines with the shifted chloride from the plasma to produce KCl, (7).

The student should need no further guidance in interpreting the remainder of Fig. 4-7, showing reversal of the reactions just described, as blood reaches the lung and $CO_2$ is moved from blood to alveolus in exchange for oxygen from alveolus to blood. Later in the text we will have much to say about another ratio shown in the diagram, that between $NaHCO_3$ and dissolved $CO_2$ at lines (4) and (5). Our clinical understanding and evaluation of acid-base balance is built on this approximately 20:1 relationship.

Just as there is a relationship between blood $P_{O_2}$ and oxygen saturation of hemoglobin, expressed by the oxygen dissociation curves, so there is a relationship between blood $P_{CO_2}$ and whole blood content of $CO_2$, calculated in volumes percent. This too can be graphically demonstrated in so-called $CO_2$ *dissociation curves,* as shown in Fig. 4-8. The first point to note is the influence of oxygen saturation on the $P_{CO_2}$-$CO_2$ content ratio. We know that $CO_2$ levels modify the oxygen dissociation curve (Bohr effect), and we now see that $S_{O_2}$ determines the course of carbon dioxide dissociation. This is called the *Haldane effect.* Fig. 4-8, *A*, shows the curves of $CO_2$ dissociation for three levels of blood $O_2$ saturation, two of which are physiologic values, and the third an extreme for contrast. These might be called "laboratory curves," since they are experimentally determined by subjecting samples of whole blood to various oxygen saturations and measuring the $CO_2$ content of each at different $CO_2$ tension exposures.

The purpose of the curves is to show how $CO_2$ dissociates from, or leaves, the blood as its partial pressure drops or, contrarily, the increasing amounts of $CO_2$ accumulating in the blood as tension rises. The graphs indicate how this relationship depends on oxygen saturation. Fig. 4-8, *B*, shows selected segments of the curves to include the physiologic range of $P_{CO_2}$, from the arterial point (A), with a $P_{CO_2}$ of 40 mm Hg, $S_{O_2}$ of 97.5%, and $CO_2$ content of 48 vol%, to the venous point (V), with a $P_{CO_2}$ of 46 mm Hg, $S_{O_2}$ of 70%, and $CO_2$ content of 53 vol%. Since oxygen saturation changes from arterial to venous blood, the true physiologic $CO_2$ dissociation curve must lie somewhere between the two "laboratory curves" for arterial and venous saturation, and such a curve is shown as a dashed line in Fig. 4-8, *B*. The student can see that at (A), with its high $S_{O_2}$, the $CO_2$ capacity for a $P_{CO_2}$ of 40 mm Hg is low, thus encouraging the excretion of the gas in the lung. At (V), with its lower $S_{O_2}$, the capacity of the blood to hold $CO_2$ at a given partial pressure increases, facilitating the removal of the gas from tissue cells. The student should also note that it is at this venous point, (V), that the dissociation of oxyhemoglobin takes place, indicated in the

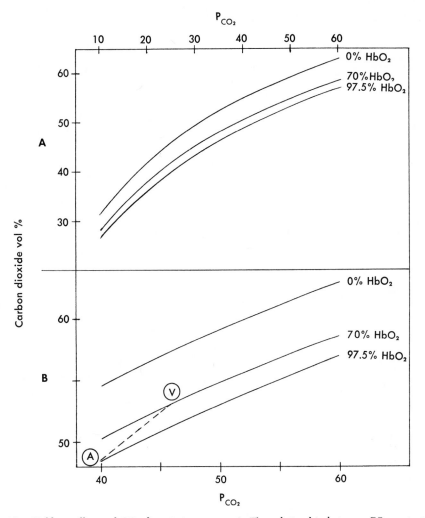

**Fig. 4-8.** Haldane effect and $CO_2$ dissociation curves. **A,** The relationship between $CO_2$ content and tension at three levels of Hb saturation. **B,** Close-up of the curves between $P_{CO_2}$ of 40 mm Hg and 60 mm Hg (see text for details). (Modified from Comroe, J. H., Jr., et al.: The lung, Chicago, 1962, Year Book Medical Publishers, Inc.)

RBC rectangle of Fig. 4-7, whereby oxygen is released, and reduced KHB is made available to react with $H_2CO_3$.

In summarizing respiratory gas transportation, let us remember that the many processes described do not take place in intermittent stages but occur rapidly, simultaneously, and continuously. The close correlation and interdependence between oxygen and carbon dioxide transportation is evidenced by the Bohr and Haldane effects. Also, although Fig. 4-7 is limited to only half of the $CO_2$ circuit, in the interest of economy, it can also serve to illustrate reactions that occur when blood reaches the lung, by visualizing the same processes with the directions of the arrows turned about.

**Table 4-5.** *Carbon dioxide content of arterial and venous blood*

| | Arterial | | Venous | |
|---|---|---|---|---|
| | *Vol %* | *mM/ℓ* | *Vol %* | *mM/ℓ* |
| Combined $CO_2$ | 53.5 | 24.0 | 60.4 | 27.1 |
| Dissolved $CO_2$ | 2.7 | 1.2 | 3.1 | 1.4 |
| Total $CO_2$ | 56.2 | 25.2 | 63.5 | 28.5 |
| $P_{CO_2}$ | 40 mm Hg | | 46 mm Hg | |

Most of the $CO_2$ is carried in the plasma but must pass through the erythrocyte as $HCO_3^-$ by the chloride shift mechanism. Of critical importance is the relationship between the $CO_2$ that is carried as the compound sodium bicarbonate and that which is in physical solution in the plasma. The former is referred to as the *bound* $CO_2$, and the latter as the *dissolved*. Under normal conditions the ratio of the bound to the dissolved $CO_2$ is remarkably constant at 20:1. It will be seen in the next few pages that such a ratio is essential to maintain normal acid-base balance of the blood. It was noted earlier that the amount of physically dissolved $CO_2$ is directly proportional to the amount of $CO_2$ that is hydrolyzed in the plasma to carbonic acid; thus the dissolved $CO_2$ represents the amount of this acid present in plasma. The 20:1 proportion of combined to dissolved $CO_2$ is therefore a ratio between an *acid salt* and a *weak acid*, an important concept of buffering to be discussed with acid-base balance.

Because the carriage of $CO_2$ involves chemical reactions, the chemical quantitative expression of *millimoles per liter* (mM/ℓ) is more frequently used than volumes percent (vol%) to indicate amounts of the gas in the blood. The calibration is 1 gmw $\times$ $10^{-3}$ of $CO_2$ per liter of plasma. The actual measurement of blood $CO_2$ in the laboratory is done as volumes percent but is converted to millimoles per liter according to the following principle (as noted on p. 6, the molar volume of $CO_2$ to be used here is 22.3 liters)[31a]:

(1) Vol% = ml $CO_2$/100 ml plasma
(2) 1 mM $CO_2$ = 1 gmw $CO_2$/1000 = 22,300 ml/1000 = 22.3 ml
(3) 1 mM $CO_2$/ℓ = 22.3 ml $CO_2$/1000 ml plasma = 2.23 ml $CO_2$/100 ml plasma
(4) Therefore, *mM $CO_2$/ℓ = vol% ÷ 2.23*

Average values for $CO_2$ content of venous and arterial blood are listed in Table 4-5.

## ACID-BASE BALANCE

For optimum function of the body cells, the chemical reactions of their environment (body fluids and blood) must remain within a specific narrow range. Deviations of a body pH above and below the normal range interfere with cellular metabolism and at extreme levels cause death of the cells. Survival is unlikely when pH drops below 7.0 and probably when it exceeds 7.80. The net result of all the interreactions of substances in the body should produce a hydrogen ion concentration [$H^+$] to maintain a blood pH of 7.35 to 7.45 with an average normal of *7.40 for arterial blood*, just slightly alkaline. The pH is influenced by food, drink, and disease, but the body has a great capacity for maintaining a normal reaction in the face of factors that would change it. Maintaining a normal acid-base balance is one of the body's more important functions and one in which respiration plays a major role. Should the blood pH fall below the normal range, becoming *less* alkaline, a state of *acidemia* is said to exist; should it rise above the range, becoming more alkaline, *alkalemia* exists. This terminology is in keeping with the recommendations of a select committee representing the American College of Chest Physicians, and the American Thoracic Society.[32] They define acidemia as a state of the blood with a pH less than normal, and alkalemia as a state with a pH greater than normal. Other acid-base terms will be defined later, but at this point we will describe physiologic buffers and their importance to acid-base chemistry.

### Buffers and the Henderson-Hasselbalch equation

A "buffer system" is a combination of a *weak acid* and a *salt* of that acid, and when introduced into a chemical reaction, it limits or buffers large changes in hydrogen ion concentration to prevent wide swings in pH. Although the industrial use of buffers is extensive, we are interested only in a few biologic systems, among which the following are worth identifying:

(1) *In plasma*
Carbonic acid/sodium bicarbonate $\quad\quad$ $H_2CO_3/NaHCO_3$
Sodium *acid* phosphate/sodium
$\quad$ *alkaline* phosphate $\quad\quad\quad\quad\quad$ $NaH_2PO_4/NaHPO_4$
Acid proteinate/sodium proteinate $\quad$ HProt/NaProt
(2) *In erythrocytes*
Acid hemoglobin/potassium hemoglobin $\quad$ HHb/KHb
Potassium *acid* phosphate/potassium
$\quad$ *alkaline* phosphate $\quad\quad\quad\quad\quad$ $KH_2PO_4/K_2HPO_4$

The $H_2CO_3/NaHCO_3$ is by far the most important of all the buffers and will be used exclusively in the following to describe the detailed function of a buffer.

If a *strong* acid is added to a buffer pair, the chemical reaction will yield a *weak* acid and a neutral salt, and a *strong* alkali will yield a *weakly* alkaline salt and water. Thus, if HCl is added to the carbonic acid/sodium bicarbonate mixture, the strong acid will react with the bicarbonate of the buffer:

$$HCl + \frac{HHCO_3}{NaHCO_3} \longrightarrow HHCO_3 + NaCl$$

This converts the strong acidity of HCl to the relatively weak acidity of $H_2CO_3$, and the increase in $[H^+]$ is slight. Similarly, if NaOH is added to the same buffer, it will react with the $H_2CO_3$ of the mixture:

$$NaOH + \frac{HHCO_3}{NaHCO_3} \longrightarrow NaHCO_3 + HOH$$

The strong alkalinity of NaOH is "buffered" into the relatively weak alkalinity of $NaHCO_3$. It is evident that eventually the buffer will be used up, but in the meantime the $[H^+]$ of the reaction, and thus the pH, will change gradually rather than abruptly.

In a buffer pair the weak acid is slightly ionized, whereas its accompanying salt is almost completely ionized, and the $[H^+]$ of the buffer system is proportional to the ratio between the concentration (in moles per liter) of the free acid and the acid "bound" by base as the salt. The $[H^+]$ and pH of any buffer pair can be calculated if the concentration composition of the mixture and the equilibrium (ionization) constant of the weak electrolyte (the acid) are known. Using the simple expression for the ionization of a weak acid, we will demonstrate how it can be modified to determine the reaction of the buffer. The dissociation of carbonic acid (written as $HHCO_3$) is:

$$HHCO_3 \rightleftharpoons H^+ + HCO_3^- \quad \text{(very slight ionization)}$$

thus

$$\frac{[H^+][HCO_3^-]}{[HHCO_3]} = K_{ac}$$

and

$$[H^+] = K_{ac} \frac{[HHCO_3]}{[HCO_3^-]}$$

In this buffer mixture, since most of the acid is un-ionized ($[H^+]$ is very minute), the molar concentration of un-ionized acid in the numerator of the preceding ratio for all practical purposes is the same as the known acid concentration that was used to prepare the buffer. On the other hand, because the salt $NaHCO_3$ is almost completely ionized:

$$NaHCO_3 \rightleftharpoons Na^+ + HCO_3^- \quad \text{(complete ionization)}$$

the value of $HCO_3^-$ in the above denominator is approximately the same as the total molar concentration of the salt used in the buffer. Thus, the above ionization equation for a weak acid can be rephrased to express the ionization of a buffer system, of which it is a part, by substituting molar concentration of the buffer *salt* in place of the bicarbonate ion:

$$\text{Molar concentration } H^+ = K_{acid} \times \frac{\text{Molar concentration } HHCO_3}{\text{Molar concentration } NaHCO_3}$$

From the foregoing is derived the *Henderson-Hasselbalch equation*, which is a cornerstone of the clinical application of the principles of acid-base balance. Since pH is the negative log of the hydrogen ion concentration used as a positive number, the buffer ionization equation can be rewritten to allow calculation of the pH:

$$H^+ = K_{ac} \times \frac{M/\ell \text{ acid}}{M/\ell \text{ salt}}$$

$$\log H^+ = \log \left[ K_{ac} \times \frac{M/\ell \text{ acid}}{M/\ell \text{ salt}} \right]$$

$$\log H^+ = \log K_{ac} + \log \left[ \frac{M/\ell \text{ acid}}{M/\ell \text{ salt}} \right]$$

$$pH = -\log K_{ac} - \log \left[ \frac{M/\ell \text{ acid}}{M/\ell \text{ salt}} \right]$$

$$pH = pK + \log \left[ \frac{M/\ell \text{ salt}}{M/\ell \text{ acid}} \right]$$

$$pH = pK_{ac} + \log \left[ \frac{M/\ell \text{ } NaHCO_3}{M/\ell \text{ } H_2CO_3} \right]$$

Note the use of the term *pK*. Similarly to pH, pK means the *negative log of the equilibrium constant of the acid component of the buffer system*, used as a positive number. Because laboratory techniques make it easier to determine the amount of *dissolved* $CO_2$ in the blood than the $H_2CO_3$ content and because the dissolved $CO_2$ is directly proportional to the blood $H_2CO_3$, the concentration of dissolved $CO_2$ is used in the equation in place of the *acid*, with a compensatory change in the ionization constant. Under physiologic conditions the carbonic acid ionization K has a value of $7.85 \times 10^{-7}$, which is easily converted by calculation into a pK of *6.1*. Also, the importance of the numerator of the equation, usually referred to as "base" rather than salt, lies in the $HCO_3$ ion, since it represents and includes "bound" acid. Finally, because of the small quantities involved, it is more convenient to calibrate concentrations as millimoles per liter than moles per liter. The Henderson-Hasselbalch equation, as it applies to the $H_2CO_3/NaHCO_3$ buffer system for determination of blood pH, can be summarized as follows:

$$\text{(1)} \quad pH = 6.1 + \log \left[ \frac{\text{mM}/\ell \text{ of bicarbonate}}{\text{mM}/\ell \text{ of dissolved } CO_2} \right]$$

$$\text{(2)} \quad pH = 6.1 + \log \left[ \frac{[HCO_3^-]}{[\text{dissolved } CO_2]} \right]$$

## Application of the H-H equation

Since carbon dioxide, both dissolved in solution and combined as bicarbonate, is intimately involved in acid-base balance, it is easy to see why ventilation is so important in regulating this balance and why a clear understanding of this relationship is necessary for those treating respiratory diseases. We will discuss in some detail those factors involved in the acid-base equation and learn to use the equation for better understanding of acid-base physiology. For our purposes the term *acid-base balance* refers to the ratio between carbonic acid and its salt, the base sodium bicarbonate. In evaluating this balance, we can measure in the laboratory certain blood values, which we then apply to the equation for whatever information is desired. So first we must be acquainted with some of the terms used. *Total $CO_2$ content* means all the $CO_2$ that can be chemically extracted and measured from a blood sample. This includes the *sum* of the combined $CO_2$ (as bicarbonate) and the dissolved $CO_2$; and it is measured as volumes percent and converted to millimoles per liter as described earlier. The *dissolved $CO_2$* is that fraction of the blood gas which is in solution in the blood plasma. The *combined $CO_2$*, also called *bound $CO_2$*, *base*, and *bicarbonate*, refers to that portion of the total $CO_2$ which is contained in the blood bicarbonate. This can be measured directly by chemical analysis (not clinically applicable), computed as the difference between the total and the dissolved $CO_2$, or calculated from the H-H equation.

Laboratory technology makes it easy and quick to measure directly the partial pressure of $CO_2$ in a blood sample. The $P_{CO_2}$ can be converted to millimoles per liter very simply by a factor, the derivation of which is outlined below:

(1) 1 mole $CO_2$ = 22,300 ml at 760 mm Hg pressure
(2) 1 mM $CO_2$ = 22.3 ml
(3) Sol coef $CO_2$ at 760 mm Hg = 0.51 ml $CO_2$/ml plasma

(4) Thus the ml $CO_2$/ml plasma at any $P_{CO_2} = \dfrac{P_{CO_2} \times 0.51}{760}$

(5) The ml $CO_2/\ell$ plasma $= \dfrac{P_{CO_2} \times 0.51 \times 1000}{760}$

(6) The mM $CO_2/\ell$ plasma $= \dfrac{P_{CO_2} \times 0.51 \times 1000}{760 \times 22.3}$

$$= P_{CO_2} \times 0.03014$$

The normal arterial $P_{CO_2}$ value of 40 mm Hg, multiplied by the factor 0.03 gives a concentration of dissolved $CO_2$ of *1.2 mM/$\ell$*.

Let us assume that an arterial blood sample yields a total $CO_2$ content of 56.2 vol%, which converts to a concentration of 25.2 mM/$\ell$, and the $P_{CO_2}$ is 40 mm Hg, or 1.2 mM/$\ell$. The bicarbonate value is the *difference* between these, or 24 mM/$\ell$. The H-H equation can now be used to determine the arterial pH:

$$pH = 6.1 + \log\left[\frac{24}{1.2}\right]$$
$$= 6.1 + \log 20$$
$$= 6.1 + 1.301$$
$$= 7.40$$

A critical point to learn here is that the blood pH depends on the *ratio* of the bicarbonate to dissolved $CO_2$ rather than on the absolute value of each. As long as the ratio is 20:1, the pH will always be 7.40. The values could be 12:0.6 or 48:2.4 or any other combination to yield 20. Reference was made to this in the discussion of $CO_2$ transportation, and the student should now be beginning to understand the true meaning of "acid-base balance."

The total $CO_2$ blood content plays no role in contemporary blood gas or acid-base evaluation. Before the days of current instrumentation, volumetric measurement of the milliliters of $CO_2$ per 100 milliliters of blood was the only readily available clinical technique, and although it indicated some abnormalities, it was far from adequate. The importance of evaluating $HCO_3$ and dissolved $CO_2$ individually will be emphasized a little later, and since total $CO_2$ includes both of these fractions, variations in it do not differentiate between them. For example, because the $HCO_3/CO_2$ ratio has such a relatively high numerator, an increase in $HCO_3$ of 50% gives a total $CO_2$ of 37.2 mM/$\ell$, or 82.9 vol%, noticeably greater than the normals of 25.2 mM/$\ell$, or 56.2 vol%. Yet an equally significant 50% increase in dissolved $CO_2$ is reflected in a small total $CO_2$ change to 25.8 mM/$\ell$, or 57.5 vol%. Despite its clinical uselessness, total $CO_2$ will be included in exercises later to enhance the student's understanding of the relationships of all the factors involved in acid-base balance and to show him how this volumetric procedure may be used as a backup in the laboratory should equipment failure prevent direct measurement of one of the H-H equation variables.

Of the three variables in the H-H equation, any one obviously can be calculated if the other two are known. In actual cardiopulmonary practice, compact equipment now available makes it convenient to measure pH, $P_{CO_2}$, and $P_{O_2}$ on the same blood sample, a procedure much easier than the chemical analyses of total $CO_2$ and $HCO_3$. Nomograms and charts are also available to show the relation among the various factors. However, to understand fully these relationships the student should know how to use the H-H equation to solve for an unknown, given two known data . For practice in performing such exercises, the following equations are listed for reference. Some merely represent differences between calculated values, and others are algebraic rearrangements of the H-H equation, one example of which is detailed in Appendix 10.

(1) $mM/\ell = vol\% \div 2.23$

(2) Dissolved $CO_2$ in $mM/\ell = P_{CO_2} \times 0.03$

(3) $P_{CO_2} = \dfrac{\text{Total } CO_2 \text{ in } mM/\ell}{0.03 \times [1 + \text{antilog } (pH - 6.1)]}$

(4) Total $CO_2$ in $mM/\ell = HCO_3$ in $mM/\ell$ + dissolved $CO_2$ in $mM/\ell$
$\qquad\qquad\qquad = P_{CO_2} \times 0.03 \times [1 + \text{antilog } (pH - 6.1)]$

(5) $HCO_3$ in $mM/\ell = $ Total $CO_2$ in $mM/\ell$ − dissolved $CO_2$ in $mM/\ell$
$\qquad\qquad\qquad = P_{CO_2} \times 0.03 \times [\text{antilog } (pH - 6.1)]$

Following are examples of acid-base calculations:

1. *Given:* Arterial $P_{CO_2} = 52$ mm Hg, and total arterial $CO_2$ content = 62 vol%
   *Calculate:* Arterial pH

*Solution:*
Dissolved $CO_2 = 0.03 \times 52 = 1.56$ $mM/\ell$
Total $CO_2 = 62 \div 2.23 = 27.8$ $mM/\ell$
$HCO_3 = 27.8 - 1.56 = 26.24$ $mM/\ell$

$pH = 6.1 + \log \left[ \dfrac{26.24}{1.56} \right] = 6.1 + 1.225$

$pH = 7.33$

2. *Given:* Arterial pH = 7.24, and arterial $P_{CO_2} = 56$ mm Hg
   *Calculate:* Dissolved $CO_2$, total $CO_2$, $HCO_3$

*Solution:*
Dissolved $CO_2 = 0.03 \times 56$ $\qquad\qquad\qquad = 1.68$ $mM/\ell$
Total $CO_2 = 1.68 \times [1 + \text{antilog } (7.24\text{-}6.1)]$
$\qquad\qquad = 1.68 \times [1 + \text{antilog } (1.14)]$
$\qquad\qquad = 1.68 \times 14.8$ $\qquad\qquad\qquad = 24.9$ $mM/\ell$
$HCO_3 = 24.9 - 1.68$ $\qquad\qquad\qquad\qquad = 23.2$ $mM/\ell$

3. *Given:* Arterial pH = 7.58, and total arterial $CO_2$ content = 19.2
   *Calculate:* $P_{CO_2}$

*Solution:*
$P_{CO_2} = \dfrac{19.2}{0.03 \times [1 + \text{antilog } (7.58\text{-}6.1)]}$

$= \dfrac{19.2}{0.03 \times [1 + \text{antilog } (1.48)]}$

$= \dfrac{19.2}{0.03 \times 31.2}$

$= 20.3$ mm Hg

The answers to such calculations can be checked by fitting them into the H-H equation to see whether the equation balances.

### Exercise 4-2

| Given | | Calculate |
|---|---|---|
| (a) $P_{CO_2} = 32$ mm Hg | Total $CO_2 = 55$ vol% | pH |
| (b) $P_{CO_2} = 56$ mm Hg | Total $CO_2 = 66$ vol% | pH |
| (c) $P_{CO_2} = 72$ mm Hg | Total $CO_2 = 30$ vol% | pH |

(d) Total $CO_2$ = 55 vol%    pH = 7.26    $P_{CO_2}$
(e) Total $CO_2$ = 44 vol%    pH = 7.55    $P_{CO_2}$
(f) Total $CO_2$ = 30 vol%    pH = 7.35    $P_{CO_2}$
(g) $P_{CO_2}$ = 55 mm Hg    pH = 7.41    Total $CO_2$; $HCO_3$
(h) $P_{CO_2}$ = 38 mm Hg    pH = 7.52    Total $CO_2$; $HCO_3$
(i) $P_{CO_2}$ = 26 mm Hg    pH = 7.30    Total $CO_2$; $HCO_3$

## CONTROL OF VENTILATION

Although the general principles of ventilation were covered in Chapter 3, a discussion of the factors regulating it was delayed so that it could be included at this point. Because ventilation is as deeply involved with the body's acid-base homeostasis as it is with the mechanics of air movement, it was felt that the student should first be exposed to the fundamentals of blood gas transport and acid-base balance. Also, it was believed that this sequence would make for a smooth transition into the discussion of clinical acid-base problems with which this chapter closes.

Until fairly recently, the central control of ventilation was believed to rest in a single *respiratory center* located in the medulla of the brain. It was further believed that, as arterial blood perfused the highly specialized cells of the center, the partial pressure of its contained carbon dioxide was sensed by the cells, and if the $P_{CO_2}$ was higher than normal, impulses from the center stimulated the ventilatory muscles to blow off excess carbon dioxide; if the pressure was low, ventilation was depressed to allow the gas to be retained. Similarly, oxygen lack and excess supposedly increased and decreased breathing, respectively. Contemporary studies of the mechanics of the ventilatory system, however, have made it clear that its control is exceedingly complex, and our knowledge of it is incomplete and often speculative. The problem of trying to present a clear picture of this vital process is further complicated by conflicting and contradictory data and opinions. We will briefly discuss those factors that seem to be most generally accepted as the prime determinants of ventilation and consider one possible pattern of their interrelationships. The neural and chemical structures that control ventilation are divided into the two categories of *peripheral* and *central*, depending upon their location outside or within the brain; Fig. 4-9 schematically outlines their various roles.

Instead of one cerebral respiratory center, there are at least three, one in the medulla and two in the pons. In addition, there is a less well-located area in the medulla containing *chemoreceptors*, which will be described below. Similar chemoreceptors are found among the peripheral stimulators, along with reflexes from the lung and a variety of other organs and tissues.[33] We will discuss the relationships among these factors without necessarily confining ourselves to a sequence depending on their central or peripheral locations.

The *medullary center* can be considered to have two major functions. First, it acts as a coordinator for stimuli reaching it from all other areas involved in ventilatory control. These stimuli carry information concerning the somatic gas exchange needs and the data from sensory, chemical, and other factors that can modify breathing. It is the medullary center's task to match these needs and influences and to determine the ventilatory pattern most useful to the body as a whole, on a breath-to-breath basis.

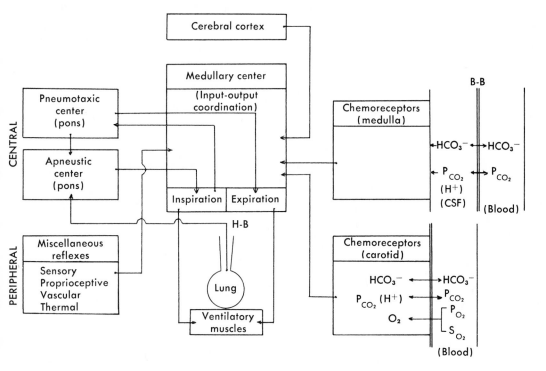

**Fig. 4-9.** Ventilatory control. Diagram of relationships between central and peripheral factors regulating breathing. (See text for details.)

Second, the medullary center sends its nerve impulses to the muscles of ventilation through two subcenters that individually control the inspiratory and expiratory phases of breathing. Thus, instead of acting as the sole regulator of ventilation, responding directly to carbon dioxide and oxygen levels as once believed, the medullary center is more of a final determinant of breathing patterns, responding to autonomic stimuli as well as to the voluntary stimuli of the higher centers of the cerebral cortex, which can override them all.

*Chemoreceptors* are groups of specialized nerve cells that can differentiate between concentrations of hydrogen ions and oxygen in the fluid perfusing them. There are two sets of chemoreceptors, one diffusely distributed in the medulla of the brain, known as *medullary* or *central chemoreceptors*, and the other located in the bifurcations of both carotid arteries, called *peripheral chemoreceptors*, or *carotid bodies*. Similar structures are located in the arch of the aorta, the *aortic bodies*, but since these are more concerned with cardiovascular than with ventilatory control, we will use the carotid bodies as representative of peripheral receptors for our discussion.[34, 35] As indicated by the sketch in Fig. 4-9, both central and peripheral chemoreceptors send impulses to the medullary center, and while there are similarities in their functions, there are also significant differences. We will consider first the effect of hydrogen ions on chemoreceptors, then the effect of oxygen.

Circulating hydrogen ions come from two sources: (1) dissolved $CO_2$ that hydrolyzes into $H_2CO_3$ and that in turn dissociates into H and HCO ions; and (2) ionization of other acids in the blood, both normal and abnormal. We know that the hydrogen ion concentration is directly proportional to the ratio of the concentrations of dissolved $CO_2$, reflected as $P_{CO_2}$, and the bicarbonate ion: thus $[H^+] \cong P_{CO_2}/HCO_3^-$. The membrane of the peripheral chemoreceptor cell is only slightly permeable to ions such as H and $HCO_3$ so that they move slowly across this barrier, but it readily allows passage of the un-ionized dissolved $CO_2$. Therefore, should the blood carbon dioxide level rise because of increased metabolic production or because of inhalation of the gas, its rapid diffusion quickly raises carotid receptor intracellular carbon dioxide, increases the $CO_2/HCO_3^-$ ratio, and elevates the hydrogen ion concentration. This increase in cellular hydrogen ion concentration triggers nerve impulses from the chemoreceptor to the medullary center, indicating the need to step up ventilation to blow off excess $CO_2$. Conversely, an excessive removal of blood carbon dioxide, as by a period of voluntary hyperventilation, leaves a relative surplus of intracellular bicarbonate ion over carbon dioxide, and when overbreathing ceases, the lowered hydrogen ion concentration causes an interval of apnea as the medullary center is instructed to reduce breathing and allow a buildup of blood carbon dioxide to normal. These responses to $CO_2$ tension changes, mediated through the carotid bodies and the medullary center, are of course dependent on a reactive and functional ventilatory system. Hypercapnia or hypocapnia due to pulmonary abnormalities, which manifest as hypoventilation or hyperventilation, may cause hydrogen ion changes as described, but because of pulmonary disease there will be no ventilatory system responses. Further, the influence of the central chemoreceptors, to be described below, on chronic states of carbon dioxide changes, or in conditions of primary ventilation defects, is probably more important than is that of the peripheral sensors.

In contrast, peripheral chemoreceptor reaction to changes in blood hydrogen ions due to fluctuations in bicarbonate ion levels is slow because of the poor diffusibility of the ion across the cell membrane. Metabolic (nonrespiratory) disturbances such as increases in fixed or abnormal acids circulating in the blood can deplete the available bicarbonate ions and, by thus increasing the blood $P_{CO_2}/HCO_3^-$ ratio, raise its $[H^+]$. This sets up a bicarbonate concentration gradient from chemoreceptor to blood, and although diffusion of the ion is slow, bicarbonate eventually leaves the cell, increasing the intracellular $P_{CO_2}/HCO_3^-$ ratio, elevating $[H^+]$, and stimulating hyperventilation. The increased breathing in turn depletes blood carbon dioxide, lowers the $P_{CO_2}/HCO_3^-$ ratio, and tends to return the blood hydrogen ion concentration toward normal. On the other hand, metabolic increases in blood bicarbonate, as by ingestion or infusion of the ion, or relative increases, as from renal or emetic loss of fixed normal acids, can reverse the bicarbonate ion gradient and eventually lower the hydrogen ion concentration within the receptor cells. Reduced ventilation then retains carbon dioxide in the blood to balance the elevated bicarbonate and normalize the $[H^+]$.

There is an interesting difference between the operation of the central chemoreceptors and the carotid bodies, although the principles described for the latter generally apply to the former.[36] Where the peripheral chemical sensors are perfused directly by the blood, the medullary cells are separated from the blood by circulating *cerebrospinal fluid (CSF)*, and between these two systems there is a semipermeable membrane referred to as the *blood-brain barrier (B-B* in Fig. 4-9). Anatomically, this is found at surfaces where perfusing capillaries are in contact with the CSF in the arachnoid space of the brain. The barrier is nearly, if not completely, impermeable to many ions, including H and $HCO_3$, but is rapidly permeable to undissociated dissolved $CO_2$. Also, it should be noted that the CSF is not simply a filtrate of blood plasma, since it may contain concentrations of ions not in equilibrium with the blood. Exchange across the blood-brain barrier, in addition to the pressure gradient diffusion of readily diffusible substances like $CO_2$, also involves a physicochemical process known as *active transport* for substances to which the barrier is impermeable by diffusion. Active transport is a phenomenon found in other body systems and is too complex to describe here, but basically it uses cellular energy to move substances through biologic membranes in the face of opposing concentration gradients across such barriers. Thus bicarbonate can cross the blood-brain barrier by the active transport mechanism without dependence upon a pressure difference across the membrane. While this process is not as fast as the rapid movement of diffusible carbon dioxide, it gives the central receptors considerable versatility in adjusting to blood chemical needs more quickly than would reliance on the slow diffusion of the ion.

The role of the medullary chemoreceptors in regulating ventilation to acute carbon dioxide changes (other than those due to mechanical ventilatory disorders) is the same as that described for the carotid mechanism, and the two systems function in concert. Variations in blood carbon dioxide are quickly answered by the responses of CSF hydrogen ion concentrations, since carbon dioxide easily crosses the blood-brain barrier. Because hydrogen ions, like bicarbonate, diffuse poorly across cell membranes, it is probable that the central chemical sensors are activated by the hydrogen ions bathing their surfaces, rather than by ions generated within them. At any rate a high concentration of hydrogen ions in the CSF causes the central chemoreceptors to stimulate the medullary center into increased ventilation, and a low concentration retards it. Like its peripheral counterpart, the central chemoreceptor cannot correct a malfunctioning ventilatory system.

An example of the combined action of both sets of chemoreceptors in response to metabolic acidosis will best illustrate how the function of the central receptors differs from the peripheral receptors. Let us imagine the incursion of a disease-generated acid into the blood, and consider in an artificial stepwise sequence some of the subsequent events. First, the excessive number of hydrogen ions depletes much of the circulating bicarbonate buffer, creating gradients for bicarbonate from CSF and carotid body cells to the blood. As bicarbonate leaves the cells and CSF, cellular and CSF $P_{CO_2}/HCO_3^-$ ratios and $[H^+]$ are raised, and the medullary center is signalled to stimulate hyperventilation. The increased breathing, however, gradually eliminates some of the blood carbon dioxide, initiating diffusion of the gas from carotid cells and CSF, dropping their hydrogen ion concentrations and retarding the hyperventilation. The active transport mechanism of the blood-brain barrier now becomes active, moving more bicarbonate out of the CSF to raise the hydrogen ion concentration and reestablish hyperventilation. Metabolic alkalosis can provoke a mirror image response of this sequence, with reactions moving in opposite directions. We can generalize by stating that, in the face of metabolic hydrogen ion changes in the blood, both central and peripheral chemoreceptors work together to effect rapid ventilatory correction, but the central sensors, through the energy of the blood-brain barrier active transport, better stabilize responses for prolonged action.

The effect of oxygen on ventilation is mediated almost entirely through the peripheral carotid bodies, another difference between the two sets of chemical sensors.[37] The carotid bodies are sensitive to both blood oxygen tension and content, a reduction in either stimulating the medullary center to increase ventilation, and a combination of subnormal tension and amount of gas having an additive effect on the amplitude of breathing. Conversely, high oxygen tensions can reduce ventilation, which will be mentioned later in the discussion of oxygen therapy. Finally, the maximum stimulation to breathing results from a combination of hypoxemia and hypercapnia acting together on the chemoreceptors.

The reaction of the peripheral chemoreceptors to hypoxemia is modified by the effect of hydrogen ion concentration on the receptors, in a paradoxical manner. Responding to a drop in oxygen tension, the carotid bodies stimulate the medullary center to increase ventilation. However, the resulting hyperventilation reduces blood carbon dioxide, setting up a diffusion gradient that moves carbon dioxide from both peripheral and medullary chemoreceptors, lowering their hydrogen ion concentrations and retarding ventilation despite the hypoxemic stimulus. Given sufficient time, the active transport will move bicarbonate ions out of the CSF, elevating the hydrogen ion concentration and improving ventilation. This phenomenon is responsible for a sequence sometimes seen in prolonged oxygen deficit, in which initial hyperventilation is followed by depressed breathing and finally by the return of hyperventilation.

Another relationship between the simultaneous effects on ventilation of oxygen and hydrogen ions is illustrated by the state of chronic hypoventilation. If hypercapnia, with its elevated blood and chemoreceptor hydrogen ion concentration, is of long standing, the active transport of the blood-brain barrier will have time to move bicarbonate ions into the CSF and restore the latter's hydrogen ion concentration to normal. This removes the usual stimulating effect on breathing of a high carbon dioxide level and leaves ventilatory drive almost entirely to the low blood level of oxygen, which is also a product of hypoventilation. Sustained spontaneous ventilation is thus dependent upon a degree of hypoxia, the therapeutic correction of which may lead to the cessation of breathing.

The *apneustic center* is located in the lower portion of the pons and is referred to as a pontine center. Apneusis is a condition in which ventilation stops in the inspiratory position. In such instances the resting level is end-inspiratory rather than end-expiratory, although the apneustic level is at the end of *full* inspiration. The apneustic center, if unrestrained, promotes deep and prolonged inspiration, but normally it is controlled by the *pneumotaxic center* and *inflation reflexes (Hering-Breuer)* from the lung, to be described below. Disease of the pons leading to abnormal stimulation of the apneustic center can produce apneustic breathing, a gasping type of ventilation with maximal inspiration.

The *pneumotaxic center* is also in the pons, located slightly higher than the apneustic. As noted above, it controls the effect of the apneustic center and encourages a rhythmic ventilation. It has been suggested that the pneumotaxic center receives impulses from the medullary inspiratory subcenter and in turn sends impulses to the medullary expiratory subcenter, thus limiting the extent of inhalation.

An *inflation reflex*, commonly called the Hering-Breuer reflex (*H-B* in Fig. 4-9), carries impulses from the lung to the brain through the vagus nerve. Sensory receptors in the lung or bronchioles respond to the stretch of the distending lung and relay inhibitory impulses to the central control through the apneustic center, inhibiting the latter's function and limiting further inflation. By restricting unnecessary inhalation, the inflation reflex assists the respiratory system in moving a volume of air adequate to supply the alveoli, with a minimum of energy expenditure.

There are several *miscellaneous reflexes*, widely scattered sensing devices that contribute to the total data on which the medullary center depends. Included are reflexes that respond to pain, temperature, tissue pressure and stretch, and circulatory dynamics. In the interests of economy of time and space, these will not be detailed here, but the student is encouraged to study them on his own so he will have the broadest possible view of this important feedback system.

In summary we can say that the *medullary center* receives nerve impulses from a wide variety of sources throughout the body, analyzes them, determines the necessary level of breathing, and through inspiratory and expiratory subcenters stimulates the ventilatory muscles into appropriate action. In the background, as it were, the pontine *apneustic center*, with its inherent ability to produce a full and sustained inhalation, acts as a sort of guarantee against failure of the lung to expand. The *pneumotaxic center*, also in the pons, keeps the apneustic center in check, and in addition correlates inspiratory and expiratory impulses from the medullary center and helps to maintain a rhythmic ventilation. The *Hering-Breuer stretch reflex*, originating in bronchiolar or alveolar walls, modifies the apneustic center's action by limiting inhalation and helps the medullary center establish a smooth and easy combination of tidal volume and rate. A large number of miscellaneous stimuli bring sensory, pressure, thermal, circulatory, and probably other information to the medullary center for the latter's consideration of ventilatory needs. The greatest influences, however, come from blood and cerebrospinal fluid hydrogen ion concentration and oxygen content stimulation of medullary and carotid chemoreceptors. These help correlate ventilation with acid-base balance as well as with gas exchange needs. Finally, the entire autonomic ventilatory control complex is subject to voluntary override by the higher areas of the cerebral cortex. Such a summary is oversimplified, and because of knowledge gaps, may be inaccurate in some details, but it does present a practical picture of at least the major factors responsible for control of ventilation.

## CLINICAL ACID-BASE STATES

When we consider the acid-base balance from a clinical, or patient-oriented, point of view rather than seeing it only as a chemical reaction in blood, we speak of *acidosis* and *alkalosis*. The suffix *-osis* is "a word termination denoting a process, especially a disease or morbid process, and sometimes conveying the meaning of abnormal increase."[38] Thus acidosis is a pathological state that can, but does not necessarily, produce acidemia, and alkalosis a state that may include alkalemia. Acidosis is characterized by *hypercarbia* (hypercapnia; elevated arterial $CO_2$ tension) when it is due to respiratory disease, and *hypobasemia* (lowered arterial $HCO_3$ concentration) when it is due to metabolic or nonrespiratory causes. Alkalosis is characterized by *hypocarbia* (hypocapnia; lowered arterial $CO_2$ tension) when it is due to respiratory disease, and *hyperbasemia* (elevated arterial $HCO_3$ concentration) when it is due to metabolic or nonrespiratory causes.[32] In the pages immediately following, we will differentiate in some detail between acidosis and alkalosis, and in each of these categories, between respiratory and metabolic. We will introduce the very important concept of *compensation.*

Perhaps the student is still not clear about proper uses of the "emias" and the "oses" in acid-base communication. This is understandable, and in many instances analyzing the subtleties of definitions may be more time consuming than it is worth. From habit, if nothing else, when talking generally about clinical states and problems we will use the "oses" and reserve the "emias" for specific references to blood pH levels.

**Table 4-6.** *Table of acid-base states*

| *Normal balance* | $\dfrac{24\ mM/\ell}{1.2\ mM/\ell}$ *(40 mm Hg)* | *Ratio* $\dfrac{20}{1}$ | *mM/$\ell$ H$^+$* 40 | *pH* 7.40 |
|---|---|---|---|---|
| Respiratory acidosis | $\dfrac{24\ \text{mM}/\ell}{2.4\ \text{mM}/\ell}$ (80 mm Hg) | $\dfrac{10}{1}$ | 80 | 7.10 |
| Respiratory acidosis (compensated) | $\dfrac{48\ \text{mM}/\ell}{2.4\ \text{mM}/\ell}$ (80 mm Hg) | $\dfrac{20}{1}$ | 40 | 7.40 |
| Respiratory alkalosis | $\dfrac{24\ \text{mM}/\ell}{0.6\ \text{mM}/\ell}$ (20 mm Hg) | $\dfrac{40}{1}$ | 20 | 7.70 |
| Respiratory alkalosis (compensated) | $\dfrac{12\ \text{mM}/\ell}{0.6\ \text{mM}/\ell}$ (20 mm Hg) | $\dfrac{20}{1}$ | 40 | 7.40 |
| Metabolic acidosis | $\dfrac{12\ \text{mM}/\ell}{1.2\ \text{mM}/\ell}$ (40 mm Hg) | $\dfrac{10}{1}$ | 80 | 7.10 |
| Metabolic acidosis (compensated) | $\dfrac{12\ \text{mM}/\ell}{0.6\ \text{mM}/\ell}$ (20 mm Hg) | $\dfrac{20}{1}$ | 40 | 7.40 |
| Metabolic alkalosis | $\dfrac{48\ \text{mM}/\ell}{1.2\ \text{mM}/\ell}$ (40 mm Hg) | $\dfrac{40}{1}$ | 20 | 7.70 |
| Metabolic alkalosis (compensated) | $\dfrac{48\ \text{mM}/\ell}{2.4\ \text{mM}/\ell}$ (80 mm Hg) | $\dfrac{20}{1}$ | 40 | 7.40 |

Let us now consider the nine fundamental acid-base conditions and their chemical characteristics, as listed in Table 4-6.

When several factors work together to maintain a physiologic balance and one of the factors behaves abnormally to threaten the equilibrium, the other factors readjust their levels of function in an attempt to make up for the deficiency and maintain stability of the system. This is called *physiologic compensation.* Thus each of the four types of acid-base upsets can exist as uncompensated or compensated. The differentiation is not as clear-cut as indicated in the table, which is exaggerated for emphasis. In fact, compensation actually starts as soon as the balance is upset, and although we have shown the disturbances in equilibrium and their compensation as isolated stages purely for demonstration purposes, it should be appreciated that these processes occur simultaneously. Finally, compensation is often incomplete, becoming less effective as the imbalance increases until it eventually breaks down. For the severe levels of decompensation shown, full physiologic compensation would be impossible, and all degrees of partial compensation could be found in a real clinical situation.

The following general rule will help to keep acid-base disturbances in a reasonable mental order: *respiratory* disorders upset the *denominator* of the acid-base ratio because ventilation regulates the blood $CO_2$, and compensation attempts to adjust the numerator to restore a 20:1 ratio; *metabolic* disorders upset the *numerator* of the ratio as bicarbonate is either increased or decreased, and compensation attempts to adjust the denominator. The dissolved $CO_2$ can be changed, either primarily or as a secondary compensation, only by modifying the ventilatory pattern with hypoventilation or hyperventilation. The $HCO_3$ compensates by an increase in production or by varying the amounts excreted in the urine.

## Respiratory acidosis

Respiratory acidosis is *always* the result of *alveolar hypoventilation* with its retention of $CO_2$ in the arterial blood. The hypoventilation may be due to (1) chronic cardiopulmonary disease with failure of the ventilatory control system, (2) neuromuscular or skeletal disease with inadequate ventilatory muscular action, or (3) the action of drugs such as narcotics and sedatives, which depress respiratory center action. Regardless of cause, there is an increase in the partial pressure of arterial $CO_2$ and, depending upon the state of compensation, a drop in arterial pH.

Compensation begins as soon as the $CO_2$ starts to accumulate and is a major function of the kidney. The body attempts to increase the amount of bicarbonate, keeping pace with the rising dissolved carbon dioxide, to maintain the necessary 20:1 ratio for a pH of 7.40. Reference to Fig. 4-7 will recall the mechanism of the chloride shift, whereby, as the amount of $CO_2$ increases in the blood, chloride moves out of the plasma into the erythrocyte in exchange for bicarbonate. As a result, during the compensation for respiratory acidosis, the level of plasma chloride drops and the bicarbonate increases. It is here that the action of the kidney is of extreme importance, for the kidney uses two mechanisms to regulate the essential electrolyte levels. First, it selectively rejects the excretion of the bicarbonate ion in the urine, conserving it in the plasma for its use as a blood buffer. At the same time it also reduces the excretion of sodium, retaining it to combine with the increased amounts of bicarbonate. The additional amounts of sodium bicarbonate thus made available to counter the increasing retained carbon dioxide are referred to as the *alkaline reserve*. Second, in place of sodium the kidney removes from the blood increasing amounts of hydrogen ion, as HCl and $NH_4Cl$. This serves the dual purpose of maintaining electrolyte balance, by substituting one positive ion for another in the urine; but most important, for the health of the body, it reduces the overall acidity of the blood. In a sense the perceptive kidney, recognizing that retained carbon dioxide represents increasing amounts of carbonic acid, removes as many hydrogen ions as it can from the blood to "compensate" for the respiratory-induced acidity. If the onset of respiratory acidosis is rapid and acute, renal compensation may not be able to keep up with the rising carbon dioxide on a minute-by-minute basis, and the compensatory exchange of hydrogen for bicarbonate may not reach its maximum efficiency for 3 or 4 days. In slowly developing acidosis, as is often seen with chronic pulmonary disease when repeated infections and the progressive lung destruction span months or years, the compensatory process may adjust proportionately to the acidosis. In such instances pH levels may be maintained stable, within the normal range, not less than 7.35. It should be emphasized that, because kidney action can prevent a serious drop in pH, this does not mean that acidosis is absent. Examination of arterial blood would reveal an elevated $P_{CO_2}$, and this is conclusive evidence of respiratory acidosis in a patient with ventilatory failure, but an acidosis compensated by renal action. As should be anticipated, there is a limit to which the body can compensate an acid-base upset, beyond which there is a "break" in compensation. This point varies considerably among patients, and in uncomplicated chronic respiratory disease the kidney can often maintain a normal arterial pH in the face of a high $P_{CO_2}$. One study concluded that renal compensation was rarely complete for a $CO_2$ tension greater than 70 mm Hg,[39] while another cites compensation for, and good tolerance of, tensions up to 90 mm Hg.[40] The therapist will see many patients with varying degrees of hypercarbia and accompanying acidemia, and frequently they will have associated conditions that influence acid-base balance, especially metabolic disorders and cardiac failure.

In pulmonary emphysema, for example, slowly progressive alveolar hypoventilation can produce a chronic hypercarbia that may be countered by a migration of $HCO_3$ ions into the CSF, maintaining there a normal $[H^+]$ bathing the medullary chemoreceptors. This same hypoventilation also fails to supply the alveoli with adequate oxygen so that hypercarbia is accompanied by hypoxemia and cellular hypoxia. Under such a circumstance the most active stimulus to ventilation is the low arterial $P_{O_2}$, mediated through the carotid bodies and referred to as the *hypoxic drive*. This is not an efficient mechanism, for it requires a steady state of hypoxia to perpetuate a tidal air exchange. Should the hypoxia manage to effect enough ventilation to improve oxygen uptake, a simultaneous drop in blood $CO_2$ would draw $CO_2$ from the CSF, leaving there an excess of $HCO_3^-$, which in turn would stop the drive. This paradoxical antagonism between these two important components of the respiratory control system, which places the patient in great jeopardy, may be one of the most important physiologic casualties of chronic respiratory failure. It is important to note that hypoxia must be present for the chemoreceptor drive to function and that this function ceases when hypoxia is corrected. Here is a circumstance in which **indiscriminate use of oxygen can be fatal.** In ventilatory failure, respiratory exchange is inadequate for prolonged survival, but *some* ventilation is better than *none*, even though it maintains a state of hypercarbia and hypoxia. Should the patient be given oxygen to relieve his hypoxia, the chemoreceptors will cease to function, and *breathing will stop.* In this state of apnea, acidemia and cellular acidosis will rapidly increase to a fatal level and the patient will expire, often with a paradoxically healthy-appearing pink complexion. This is a very real risk in the treatment of patients in failure and must be guarded against by all those involved in the patient's management. Safe and effective techniques will be discussed elsewhere.

The patient in respiratory acidosis will manifest hypoventilation in one of two ways. His tidal volume will be small, sometimes with barely perceptible chest and epigastric motion, or he will be tachypneic, with rapid shallow movements that accomplish little more than ventilation of the dead space. Laboratory examinations will show a low pH, an elevated $P_{CO_2}$ and $HCO_3$, a low serum Cl, and an acid urine. If acid-base compensation is poor, the patient's mental state will be obtunded or he may be in a coma, and almost always the ventilation is enough impaired that hypoxia produces visible cyanosis. Although much of the management is directed toward the underlying disease, the most critical treatment is the correction of hypoventilation, usually best accomplished by assisting the patient with mechanical ventilators or controlling his breathing completely. *While being adequately ventilated,* the patient can be given oxygen as needed to correct his hypoxia, blood gas and pH determinations being used frequently to monitor the effectiveness of therapy. Other details of management will be considered later.

### Respiratory alkalosis

Alveolar hyperventilation removes $CO_2$ from the blood, dropping the $P_{CO_2}$ to low levels and elevating the pH. The respiratory center can be stimulated to excessive activity by brain injury or a tumor's increasing pressure on the center, by excessive salicylate ingestion, by fever, by inflammation of the brain, or by emotional stimuli. Of immediate concern to the respiratory therapist, however, is the hyperventilation that *he* can induce by the use of mechanical ventilators. Artificial ventilation of a patient with a normal respiratory tract can easily be overdone and the patient hyperventilated into respiratory alkalosis. The therapist must watch carefully to prevent this development.

Compensation is accomplished by an increased renal excretion of bicarbonate, retention of chloride, and reduction in both the formation of ammonia and excretion of acid salts. This lowers the blood bicarbonate level, bringing the acid-base ratio back toward 20:1 and reducing the pH.

Alkalosis is as hazardous to the patient as is acidosis. He is seen to be breathing deeply, and his blood shows an elevated pH, a depressed $P_{CO_2}$, and depending upon the degree of compensation, low bicarbonate and total $CO_2$ levels. Serum chloride may be slightly elevated, and the urine alkaline. The patient may complain of *paresthesias* of the extremities, a sensation of "pins and needles" or of the extremities "being asleep." Reflexes are hyperactive, true tetanic contractions may occur, and somnolence increasing to coma may develop. One of the major complications of alkalosis is its impairment of cerebral circulation, as a rapid decrease in $P_{CO_2}$ produces a contraction of cerebral arterioles, with a reduction in blood flow to the brain. This can be severe enough to cause speech difficulty and muscular paralysis, which may be permanent. Hypocarbia also predisposes the patient to serious disturbance in cardiac rhythm (arrhythmia), which may lead to arrest. Treatment is usually directed toward the underlying cause, but symptomatic relief can often be obtained by the use of sedation to suppress the respiratory center and by the inhalation of carbon dioxide to build up the blood $P_{CO_2}$.

### Metabolic acidosis

In metabolic disorders, acid-base balance is dependent upon the electrolytic balance in the body, or the relation between the positively charged ions (cations) and the negatively charged ions (anions).[41,42] The former consist of Na, Cl, K, Mg; the latter, $HCO_3$, protein (serum protein and hemoglobin), $HPO_4$, Cl, $SO_4$, and organic acids. The $HCO_3$, protein, and $HPO_4$ ions we already know comprise the buffer systems of the body and are appropriately named *buffer anions*. The remaining anions are designated as *fixed anions*. The cations are combined with a variety of anions, and those that are in combination with the buffer anions (mostly sodium as $NaHCO_3$, but small amounts of the other cations as well) are termed *buffer cations*, and sometimes *buffer base* or *total body buffer*. The remaining cations, combined with other than buffer anions, may be considered as *fixed cations*. The sum of the anions must equal the sum of the cations, and they are measured in $mEq/\ell$ or $mM/\ell$, depending upon the ion.

The total ionic content of plasma in concentration per liter is depicted schematically in Fig. 4-10. Here, two columns contain the cations and anions, and their average normal values are indicated. Carbonic acid dissociates so little that it is indicated in both columns as $mM/\ell$ of $CO_2$. The buffer anions are clearly delineated from the fixed anions; the buffer cations are not different cations from the fixed cations but rather are portions of the latter that are combined with buffer anions. It can be seen, for example, that if chloride should decrease in amount, the buffer anions would increase to keep the total unchanged. Also, it is easy to visualize a loss of sodium, with an accompanying loss of bicarbonate, and chloride expanding to replace the bicarbonate. Thus the interchanges between the electrolytes due to metabolic reactions modify the buffer anions and through changes, especially in the $HCO_3$, regulate pH. Although the metabolic relation to acid-base balance is not of primary concern to the respiratory therapist, a general understanding of the basic principles should be of interest to him, since many of his patients will have systemic diseases associated with the respiratory.

Any systemic disease that causes a depletion of the fixed cations (or buffer base), or an increase in the fixed anions, can produce metabolic acidosis. The production of abnormal acids in the blood, or the retention of acids through failure of the kidney

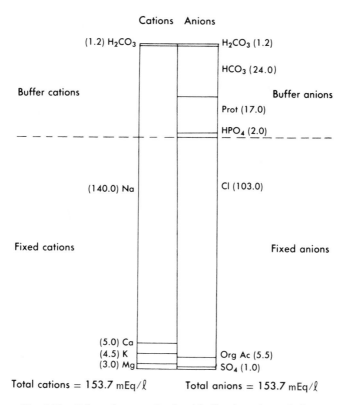

Cations    Anions

(1.2) H₂CO₃ ——— H₂CO₃ (1.2)

HCO₃ (24.0)

Buffer cations                    Buffer anions

Prot (17.0)

HPO₄ (2.0)

(140.0) Na                  Cl (103.0)

Fixed cations                    Fixed anions

(5.0) Ca
(4.5) K                    Org Ac (5.5)
(3.0) Mg                   SO₄ (1.0)

Total cations = 153.7 mEq/ℓ        Total anions = 153.7 mEq/ℓ

**Fig. 4-10.**   Balance between fixed and buffer electrolytes of plasma.

to excrete them, will replace buffer anions. This may be viewed as the depletion of the buffer ions while neutralizing the acids. Again, in the plasma $HCO_3$ is the major anion involved, since the most prevalent protein, Hb, is found only in the erythrocyte and phosphate is present in only small amounts. Keeping in mind the H-H equation, we can conveniently visualize an abnormal buildup of acids in the body (especially organic) with which the plasma $HCO_3$ reacts to neutralize the acidity. This effort depletes the available $HCO_3$, lowering the numerator of the H-H equation and reducing blood pH. Retention of chloride, incident to an excessive intake of this ion, will replace some of the bicarbonate in the anion column, lowering the blood pH. Surprisingly, and somewhat paradoxically, loss of potassium, which might be expected to produce acidosis, raises the pH. This is the result of a complex chain of electrolytic exchanges by which there is, in the presence of potassium loss, a disproportionately larger renal loss of chloride so that the net result is an increase in bicarbonate.

Compensation for metabolic acidosis is by an increase in the respiratory removal of $CO_2$ proportionately to the bicarbonate through the mechanism of hyperventilation. It should be noted in Table 4-6 that, from the blood findings alone, it is not possible to distinguish between *compensated* respiratory alkalosis and *compensated* metabolic acidosis. In this case the clinical picture of the patient's condition will be the deciding factor. The treatment of metabolic acidosis is obviously that of the underlying disease, since the respiratory abnormality is a compensatory act and not a re-flection of respiratory disease.

### Metabolic alkalosis

It is apparent that metabolic alkalosis is the product of any systemic disease that causes an excess of buffer through a relative increase of fixed cations over fixed anions. This can be the result of the loss of chloride of gastric HCl in protracted vomiting, the retention of large amounts of sodium by the ingestion of alkalis (the sodium thus combining with additional bicarbonate), the disproportionate loss of chloride over sodium common with use of diuretics, or the effect of potassium loss just mentioned. (This is often found in potassium loss that occurs with intubation and drainage of the bowel, long-term use of corticosteroids, or a reduced potassium intake.) Compensation is attempted by a conservation of $H_2CO_3$ through hypoventilation to raise the acid denominator of the H-H equation and to restore a 20:1 ratio. Again note that *compensated* metabolic alkalosis is indistinguishable chemically from *compensated*

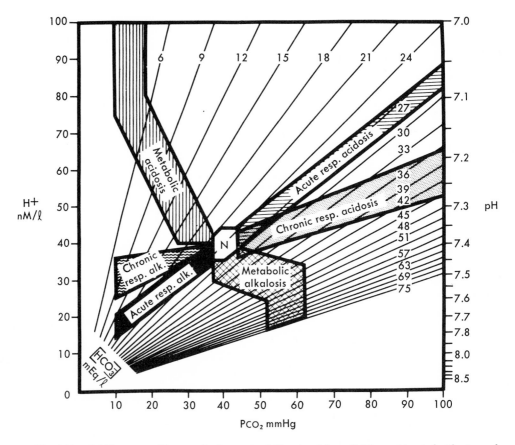

**Fig. 4-11.** Acid-base map. (See text for description.) (Reprinted from Goldberg, M., et al.: The Journal of the American Medical Association, Jan. 15, 1973, Vol. 223. Copyright 1973, American Medical Association.)

respiratory acidosis, which emphasizes the fact that diagnostic reliance cannot be placed completely on the laboratory.

### Mixed acid-base states

By now it may be obvious to the student that combinations of disorders may occur in the same patient.[43, 44] Any of the four respiratory states may coexist with any of the four metabolic states, and patients with simultaneous respiratory and metabolic diseases often present complicated pictures. Referred to earlier, and emphasized again, is the patient with respiratory acidosis who swings rapidly into respiratory alkalosis because of too vigorous therapy and thus demonstrates not simultaneous but alternating acid-base disorders. It is theoretically possible for a respiratory imbalance in one direction to be offset by a metabolic imbalance in the other, with a resulting normal pH. Differentiation between these possibilities is a medical problem requiring the finest diagnostic acumen and intelligent use of the laboratory, and the difficulties encountered should be appreciated by the respiratory therapist.

When acid-base status is very labile, responding to both metabolic and respiratory stimuli, it is sometimes helpful to monitor the blood gas changes with a so-called *acid-base map*. There are many formats available, one example of which is illustrated in Fig. 4-11. The areas of acid-base abnormalities surrounding a central normal axis were plotted as 95% confidence bands or limits, based on the clinical and statistical analysis of a large number of patients with a wide variety of acid-base imbalances. Such a confidence limit simply means that in all probability, of 100 patients whose arterial blood gas data projection lines intersect in a given designated area, 95 have that disorder. Intersects outside the mapped areas indicate mixed acid-base problems.

It is strongly emphasized that such a device gives no information not available in a simple flow chart, is no substitute for a solid understanding of acid-base physiology, and does not provide an automatic, foolproof diagnosis. It does, however, give a visual running account of sequential relationships between blood gas values and the probable clinical states they represent. It remains for each student to decide whether or not a learning tool such as this is best for him.

# Chapter 5

# CARDIOVASCULAR SYSTEM

In view of the great volume of texts written on the structure, function, and pathology of the heart, it is unnecessary for us to undertake a comprehensive review of cardiology. However, because the functions of the heart and lungs are so interrelated, it is felt that a brief explanation of some selected features of the cardiovascular system is pertinent, with emphasis on those aspects relating most directly to principles and practice of respiratory therapy. From references already made, it should be apparent to the therapist that he will frequently be called upon to treat patients with both pulmonary and cardiac diseases, and in his approach to his work he should always be aware of *cardiopulmonary* function. With this as a start, it is hoped that he will be encouraged to pursue the topic further as his interest and experience develop.

## CARDIAC CYCLE

In the performance of its function as a pump, the heart works through a ceaseless series of cycles, from the prenatal period to the moment of death. Each cardiac cycle is composed of a contraction of the myocardial fibers, followed by a period of rest. Contraction of the involuntary muscle is achieved by a forceful shortening of each fiber so that, as the total muscle mass contracts, it builds up a pressure in the cavities it encloses, reduces their volumes, and expresses their contents into the cardiac outflow tracts. Nerve impulses from the higher centers of the central nervous system are carried to the heart by the vagus nerve, which contains parasympathetic fibers, and by sympathetic nerves arising from the upper thoracic segments of the spinal cord. The former inhibit heart action, the latter stimulate it, and the net sum of the constant barrage of impulses through these channels determines the final controlling influence.

Within the heart itself, a highly specialized system of conducting tissue is responsible for the precisely timed distribution of impulses to all parts of the myocardium. Under suitable conditions the intact heart removed from all nerve connections can continue to beat for a period of time, which fact demonstrates that, despite its control over cardiac contraction, the central nervous innervation is not essential for heart action. There must be, therefore, an automatic stimulus in the heart capable of maintaining contraction but, in the intact subject, greatly influenced by the central nervous system. This is labeled the *conduction system* of the heart. Fig. 5-1 schematically illustrates the major portions of this system: the sinoatrial node (sinus node), the

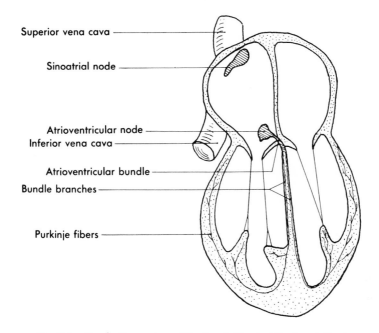

Superior vena cava

Sinoatrial node

Atrioventricular node
Inferior vena cava

Atrioventricular bundle
Bundle branches

Purkinje fibers

**Fig. 5-1.** Conduction system of the heart. (See text for description.)

atrioventricular node (A-V node), the atrioventricular bundle (bundle of His), and the bundle branches and Purkinje fibers. The histology of the conduction system is that of highly specialized muscle fibers rather than nerve fibers but capable of conducting muscle-stimulating impulses.

*Sinoatrial node (sinus node).* The sinoatrial node is called the *pacemaker* of the heart and is a small nodule of conducting tissue, about ¾ inch long, located in the muscle of the right atrium just in front of the opening of the superior vena cava. The sinus node initiates electrical impulses (to be described later), which radiate from it in the fashion of circular ripples from a stone dropped into water. Traveling at a rate of 1000 mm/sec, these impulses are discharged at variable rates, from 50 to 90 per minute but average about 70 per minute at rest. They excite the atrial myocardium to contract, both atria functioning simultaneously. The discharge rate of the sinus node is modified by nervous control, increased by the sympathetic nerves, and inhibited by the parasympathetic through vagal innervation. Cardiac rate can be increased by excessive stimulation of sympathetic nerves or by drugs simulating sympathetic action, and the heart can be slowed or stopped by parasympathetic action, especially through the action of certain reflexes carried by the vagus nerve. Both effects are of considerable clinical importance.

*Atrioventricular (A-V) node.* Similar in structure to the sinus node, the A-V node is located in the right atrium on the lower part of the interatrial septum just above the septal leaf of the tricuspid valve. It functions as a pickup and relay station for sinus impulses. With no structural connection to the sinus node, the A-V node is stimulated by the radiating sinus impulses, and it relays these onward into the ventricles. Should the sinus node fail to function because of disease, the A-V node then assumes the duties of pacemaker, but it is less effective than the sinus node.

*Atrioventricular bundle (bundle of His).* A well-defined bundle of muscular tissue originates at the A-V node and runs horizontally forward over the septal tricuspid valve leaf to the upper part of the interventricular septum. The sinus impulse received by the A-V node is transmitted through the bundle and is thus carried to the myocardium of the ventricular chambers. This is the only conduction link between atria and ventricles, and when it is damaged or destroyed by disease, a condition of *block* is said to exist, a cardiac condition commonly encountered in clinical medicine.

*Bundle branches and Purkinje fibers.* On the upper part of the interventricular septum, the A-V bundle terminates by dividing into two *bundle branches*, the right and left, each going to its respective ventricle. The bundles pass down the septum, beneath the endocardium, giving off branches to the papillary muscles, and then continue into the ventricles, where they divide into innumerable fine filaments and form a network (Purkinje fibers) interlacing the depths of the ventricular muscle. The impulse, originating in the sinus node, is carried at a rate of some 5000 mm/sec to every portion of the ventricles, in effect stimulating all myocardial fibers simultaneously, for uniform contraction of both ventricles.

The sequence of the cardiac cycle is contraction of both atria, driving blood into the ventricles, followed by contraction of both ventricles, which expels the blood into the cardiac outflow tracts. These phases of muscular contraction are respectively called atrial and ventricular *systole.* After systole both sets of chambers enter a period of rest and muscular relaxation called *diastole.* Because systole and diastole of the two sets of chambers are not of uniform duration, there is some overlapping, schematically illustrated in Fig. 5-2, which shows the start of a cardiac cycle with ventricular systole, as a matter of convenience. Note that the atria spend most of their time in diastole, during which time blood flows into these chambers from the venae cavae and pulmonary veins and, with the tricuspid and mitral valves closed, the atria distend with blood. After about 0.3 second of atrial diastole, a point corresponding to the end of ventricular systole, the atrioventricular valves open and atrial blood flows into the ventricles. Then, at 0.7 second, atrial systole occurs for a brief 0.1 second, forcibly ejecting the last of the atrial blood into the ventricles. During atrial diastole, ventricular systole takes place, for about 0.3 second; then as the A-V valves open, the semilunar valves close and the ventricles enter their diastolic phase. For approximately 0.4 second, atrial and ventricular diastoles coincide and the entire heart is quiet, as blood is flowing by gravity from atria into ventricles. It is important to note that myocardium has a peculiar quality that assures the heart of maximum contractile effort. Once systolic contraction begins, the fibers are *refractory,* or resistant to further stimulation, until they have had time to recover and regain their energy. This means that repeated stimuli cannot maintain them in a state of continued contraction, which would eventually lead to serious fatigue. The refractory period of the myocardium is maintained through systole and for an additional period of time approximately equal to the duration of systole, when it once again is responsive to stimuli.

The heartbeat, as palpated through the chest wall and at the peripheral arterial

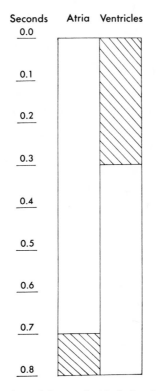

Seconds   Atria  Ventricles

**Fig. 5-2.** The duration and relationships of the systolic (shaded) and diastolic (clear) components of the cardiac cycle are shown for a rate of 75 beats per minute.

pulses, reflects the force of ventricular systole only, since the contraction of the atria is not sufficiently strong to be transmitted. The pause between beats consists of ventricular diastole, the last part of atrial diastole, and the unnoticed atrial systole. It is apparent that as the heart rate varies, the duration of the cycle segments will vary inversely. Thus rapid rates (tachycardia) often associated with disease not only reduce the rest periods of the myocardium but also, by shortening filling time, can reduce the cardiac output per beat (stroke volume).

## ELECTROPHYSIOLOGY OF THE HEART

As with other muscles, contraction of myocardial fibers is an electrical phenomenon consisting of the buildup and discharge of a minute electrical current. A strip of muscle fiber may be visualized as covered with positive and negative charges, these charges being equally distributed throughout the strip so that in the resting state the net electrical charge is neutral. With an electrical potential present, the muscle strip is polarized and is neither predominately positive nor negative. Should a portion of a muscle strip become excited or activated, or suffer injury, the area so affected becomes electronegative in relation to the rest of the muscle, as the zinc electrode of a battery is electronegative to the copper electrode. With this disruption in the even distribution of the electric charges, zones of opposite polarity are formed and a current flows from the positive to the negative zone. The muscle strip undergoes a process of *depolarization,* whereby all of the charges are used up in the current flow, until the strip is completely depolarized, or without electric potential. Functionally, this is the stage of muscle contraction, or cardiac systole. During diastole the muscle strip undergoes *repolarization,* with reestablishment of the original polarity. This process proceeds in the reverse direction from depolarization, starting with the end of the strip most recently depolarized, and since it involves zones of opposite polarity, a current is also produced during repolarization. Fig. 5-3 schematically demonstrates those two important phenomena. The rectangles represent muscle strips; those fully shaded at the top of the left column and the bottom of the right column

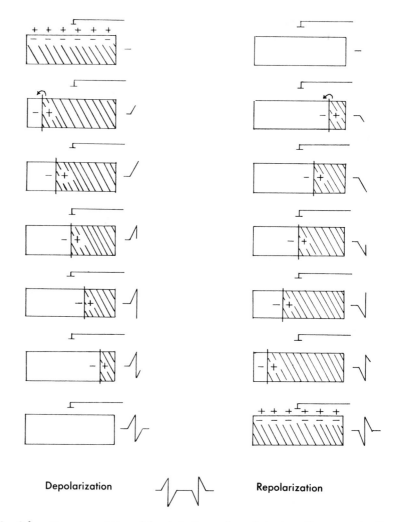

Depolarization        Repolarization

**Fig. 5-3.** Schematic representation of depolarization and repolarization of heart muscle. (See text for description.) (Modified from Barker, J. M.: The unipolar electrocardiogram, New York, 1952, Appleton-Century-Crofts.)

are in the resting, polarized state, with equal numbers of positive and negative charges. Over the center of each strip is an electrode to pick up current flow and lead it to a recording device that will translate the flow into a curve. The recorder is so designed that when the electrode is opposite positively charged tissue, an upright curve is written, and when opposite negative, a downslope. Representative curves are illustrated adjacent to each rectangle.

Because the polarized strip in the left column has a net neutral charge evenly distributed about it, no current flows and the electrode records a straight, or *iso-electric* line. After a suitable stimulus, depolarization begins as a zone of negativity at the left end of the strip, and this depolarized area is delineated in the illustrations from the remainder of the still polarized muscle by a vertical boundary line. The opposite side of the boundary is positively charged, and the direction of current flow is depicted by arrows. As depolarization progresses, the electrode is faced with the approaching positive charge and records an upstroke. When the boundary is directly beneath the electrode, because it is neither positive nor negative, the curve drops to the isoelectric line. Almost at once, strong negative charges are recorded, the curve drops sharply below the baseline, and as the negativity moves gradually away from the electrode, its influence wanes, the curve returning up to the baseline. At this point the strip is completely depolarized and charges are absent. The right column

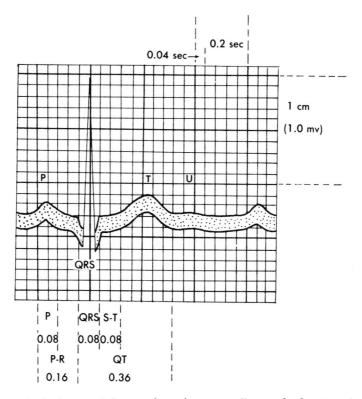

**Fig. 5-4.** Sketch of a normal electrocardiographic pattern. (See text for description.)

shows the repolarization proceeding in the opposite direction, recording curves that are the reverse of those of depolarization.

The above principles are widely used in diagnostic electrocardiography and in monitoring devices for the continued observation of cardiac action in acutely ill patients. The electrical characteristics of the intact heart are more complex than those of the isolated muscle strip, and the currents recorded by the electrodes are the net sums of many currents in the areas being explored. It is not intended to present a course in electrocardiographic interpretation, but only to describe the basic major features of this important diagnostic tool.[45] Fig. 5-4 represents a typical "average" electrocardiographic segment, showing the characteristic curves recorded from a normal heart. The electrocardiographic machine amplifies the small electric currents brought to it by the electrode leads and passes them through a *galvanometer*, in which is located a pivoted writing arm called a *stylus.* Depending on the polarity of the current passing through the galvanometer, the stylus is attracted to one or the other pole of the galvanometer magnet. By convention, positive deflections move the stylus upward, and negative deflections downward. The movements are recorded on specially calibrated graph paper, which moves at a fixed speed, and the curves thus written can be measured in terms of voltage (vertical amplitude) and time (horizontal distance). Many different leads are used to give various electric "views" of the heart. For monitoring purposes one lead is employed and the current projected through a cathode tube onto a fluorescent screen, where the record of each heartbeat can be seen as it is formed. Such an instrument is called an *oscilloscope.*

Although the contour of each lead differs from the others, the major components of an electrocardiographic tracing are illustrated in Fig. 5-4. The bold vertical lines represent time intervals of 0.2 second, subdivided into increments of 0.04 second. Bold horizontal lines are 1 cm apart, measuring an amplitude of 1.0 millivolt (mv), and each interval between represents 0.1 mv. Some normal values of amplitude and duration are indicated in the illustration. The P wave records the electrical activity of atrial systole, whereas the QRS complex represents ventricular depolarization. The P-R interval (actually, the P-QRS interval) is the length of time taken by the atrial impulse to reach the ventricles. The QT time is referred to as electrical ventricular systole (not mechanical systole). Diastole extends from the end of T to the next P and often contains a small U wave, the significance of which is not well understood. The S-T interval is the pause between ventricular depolarization and repolarization and represents a period of *absolute* ventricular refractoriness, during which the ventricles cannot be stimulated, since they have not yet become polarized. Ventricular repolarization records the T wave, during which time the ventricles are only relatively refractory, since they can respond to stimuli in proportion to the degree that repolarization has been completed. After the T, of course, ventricular myocardium is fully responsive.

## SYSTEMIC BLOOD FLOW

With each ventricular systole approximately 60 to 70 ml of blood leave each ventricle so that the stroke volume of the heart is 120 to 140 ml. Obviously, the minute volume, or cardiac output, will depend on the stroke volume and the cardiac rate, a situation analogous to the relation between the ventilatory tidal volume, rate, and minute volume. The speed and power with which systemic arterial blood will disseminate to all parts of the body depend on a balance between two forces—that of left ventricular contraction and that of the resistance of the arterial tree. The latter is referred to as the *peripheral vascular resistance,* an important factor in determining systemic blood flow. Peripheral vascular resistance may be defined as the resistive force against which the left ventricle has to pump, it is produced by the "tone" of the arterial tree. It should be recalled that arteries contain both elastic and muscle fibers in their structure and the arterial system as a whole is a continuously branching and narrowing arborization of channels. The elastic recoil of the larger arteries provides the initial resistance to the bolus of blood expelled from the left ventricle, whereas the tone of the muscle fibers of the smaller vessels maintains resistance distally. The apposition of the forces of ventricular contraction and peripheral resistance makes for a relatively smooth flow of blood with a minimal surge effect, which would result if a strong jet of blood were propelled into a rigid conducting system. If the system were flaccid, the ejection force would be dissipated before the stream reached the distal vessels, and again the flow would be uneven. Under the impact of the left ventricular blood, the proximal aorta stretches across its diameter to accommodate the blood volume; then as the aortic valve closes, the elastic aorta recoils. The recoil force is exerted against the column of blood in the arterial system and, since the valve does not yield, forces the blood distally. A wave of expansion and contraction, gradually diminishing, thus carries the blood through the major arteries, with no significant loss of velocity. The smaller arteries and arterioles maintain resistance and also determine the quantity of distal blood flow by appropriate contraction and relaxation of their muscle fibers. The function of these fibers, which is under reflex nervous control, assures adequate blood supply to those areas of the body in greatest need.

Each left ventricular contraction must be of sufficient force to impel the systemic column of blood in a continuous circuit, carrying the venous blood back to the right heart, much of the way against gravity. This force is called the left ventricular systolic pressure. Direct measurement of this pressure can be made only by the technique of threading a catheter into the chamber, attaching the proximal end to a pressure recording device. However, an excellent approximation of this ejection force can be reached by measuring the pulsatile force transmitted to the column of blood in the brachial artery. This is the measurement of the familiar *blood pressure.* An inflatable cuff is secured about the upper arm and is connected by a rubber tube to a mercury manometer. By means of a hand bulb, the cuff is inflated until the brachial arterial flow is occluded, the inflating pressure being transmitted to the manometer. The cuff pressure is gradually released until blood just starts to flow again in the artery, and at this precise moment the manometer pressure is noted. At this point the force of left ventricular contraction is enough to overcome (or is equal to) the pressure in the cuff as recorded by the manometer. It is reported as so many millimeters of mercury. In practice, the escape of blood past the occlusion of the cuff is determined by listening with a stethoscope over the artery in the antecubital fossa, at which time a characteristic sound is heard. this is the *systolic* blood pressure, with a wide range of normal from about *90 to 150 mm Hg* and an average in the adult of approximately *120 mm Hg*. After noting the systolic pressure, if the examiner continues to listen while still releasing cuff pressure slowly, he will hear a rather abrupt and definite muffling of the arterial sound and finally a disappearance of the sound. The muffling is generally considered to coincide with the elastic recoil of the artery on the blood column and with the closure of the aortic valve. The pressure noted at this time is called the *diastolic* blood pressure and has a normal range of *70 to 90 mm Hg* with an average of 80 mm Hg. Some consider the true diastolic point to be the pressure at the disappearance of the sound. A blood pressure reading should properly include three components, one systolic and two possible diastolic pressures, as for example, 120/80/68. The third figure is rarely used in common practice, however, and only the systolic and first diastolic pressures are recorded, as 120/80.

The physiologic significance of blood pressure values can be summarized in a simplified manner as follows:

*Elevated systolic pressure* implies an increase in the resistance of the arterial tree, such as occurs with pathologic thickening of arterial or arteriolar walls, and/or reduction in their elasticity.

*Reduced systolic pressure* indicates a drop in conducting system resistance, as may result from peripheral vascular collapse, a state of shock, or weakness of the left ventricular myocardium.

*Elevated diastolic pressure* is consistent with an increase in peripheral resistance, often accompanying systolic pressure increase, but it usually implies more advanced resistance than does a systolic increase alone.

*Reduced diastolic pressure* is found with a loss of resistance or myocardial weakness, as described above, but also occurs with an incompetent aortic valve, which allows retrograde flow of blood back into the left ventricle during diastolic recoil.

Although much of the systolic thrust of the left ventricle has been dissipated by the time capillary blood has perfused tissue cells, the return venous circulation is under a significant head of pressure. Venous return is dependent on the impetus of the arterial flow, aided by the "milking" effect exerted on the veins by surrounding muscles (especially of the lower extremity), the tone of the abdominal musculature, and the negative inspiratory intrathoracic pressure. Thus venous return from the lower limbs is more effective when leg muscles are active than when at rest, a matter of some practical importance, whereas return flow from the head and neck is dependent upon gravity and the intrathoracic negative pressure. The effect of intrathoracic pressure on venous return to the heart is of considerable importance to the respiratory therapist, as it relates directly to his work. Spontaneous natural breathing is characterized by a relatively long inhalation followed by a short exhalation, so that the time interval of falling intrathoracic pressure is greater than the time of rising pressure; and we know that except under conditions of forced exhalation, thoracic pressure never exceeds ambient.

The thorax thus acts like a large suction pump, aiding the venous blood in its return to the heart, and by virtue of the ventilatory pattern, maximum return occurs during inhalation. It can be properly inferred, then, that any condition which raises the mean intrathoracic pressure will impede the venous return; and it readily follows that if the volume of blood returning to the heart is reduced, the cardiac output will drop. We can easily demonstrate the effect on venous flow of increased intrathoracic pressure by holding the breath, straining, and then observing the color changes in the face from stasis of blood in the veins. Under some conditions we can note marked distention of the superficial veins of the neck. If such a buildup of thoracic pressure is significant and prolonged, venous blood unable to return to the heart will pool in venous reservoirs of the liver and abdominal circulation.

It is pertinent to observe here that one of the major tools of respiratory therapy, the positive-pressure ventilator, is a potential prime offender in this regard, a matter that will be discussed in detail later. Because the venous pressure varies greatly in different parts of the body and with position of the body, its measurement is made under standard conditions. A vein in the antecubital fossa is chosen as the site, and the patient is placed in a flat supine position with the arm supported so that the antecubital fossa is at the same level as the right atrium of the heart. A needle is inserted into the vein and is attached to a special manometer so that the pressure of the column of blood in the vein is balanced against a column of *saline* in the manometer. The normal range of venous pressure is very wide, from 50 to 110 mm of *water*.

Venous pressure measurements have been used for many years to evaluate the retarding effects on venous return of weakness of the right ventricle. In some circumstances elevated venous pressure is readily apparent by visible distention of cervical veins, an important clinical sign. Because peripheral venous pressure (in an extremity) is difficult to measure uniformly, is subject to so many influences, and has such a wide normal range, it has generally been replaced by measurement of the central venous pressure, which will be described later in a discussion of acute circulatory failure.

## PULMONARY BLOOD FLOW

The pulmonary circulation, when compared with the systemic circulation, is a low-pressure system. The total circuit distance from right ventricle to left atrium is short, and the pulmonary capillary bed is extensive so that relatively low pressures suffice for blood flow. As an average, the pulmonary artery pressure is about 25/8 mm Hg. It should be apparent that recording pulmonary pressure is not as simple as measuring the systemic pressure and can only be accomplished by means of intracardiac catheterization. By this technique it is possible to measure pressures in the right atrium, the right ventricle, and for a considerable distance into the pulmonary arteries. Such serial readings make it possible to differentiate between lesions, for example, stenotic heart valves, which lead to increased pressures within the heart in the presence of a normal pulmonary system, and an actual increase in the peripheral resistance of the pulmonary arterial tree. Many of the diseases with which the respiratory therapist will have contact produce thickening and/or narrowing of the pulmonary vessels, the resulting increased resistance requiring added ejection force of the right ventricle. Also, destruction of a sufficient portion of the pulmonary capillary bed by disease of the lung, even in the presence of normal remaining vessels, may produce resistance to right heart output, since the same output is forced through a smaller cross-sectional capillary bed. Whenever resistance to pulmonary flow is present, the right ventricle is put under strain and, if persistent, will lead to weakening of the right ventricle. If this is due to pulmonary disease, the effect on the heart is called *cor pulmonale*, or "pulmonary heart," to be described shortly.

Despite the vital importance of the pulmonary arterial blood supply, we cannot overlook the systemic component of the total pulmonary blood flow.[46] The student is encouraged to review the anatomic relationships of the bronchial arteries and note that, whereas the pulmonary arteries give off no visceral branches before the level of the alveoli, the bronchial vessels supply the entire length of the bronchial tree to the bronchioles with oxygenated blood. The returning bronchial venous blood follows an interesting variety of routes, which have some clinical significance. The accompanying bronchial veins are imperfect and irregular and can probably accommodate no more than one third of the bronchial venous blood as they empty into the azygos vein. From the distal portions of the airways, bronchial venous blood drains into the *pulmonary veins* (arterialized blood) and thus contributes to the normal small degree of unsaturation of the systemic arterial blood. At the capillary level there are microscopic communications between bronchial and pulmonary capillaries. Here there is a mixture of arterialized systemic blood (bronchial capillaries) with venous blood (pulmonary capillaries). This relationship is unimportant under normal circumstances, but in certain disease states in which there is interruption of pulmonary arterial flow, these communications may become grossly enlarged and provide a significant volume of blood perfusing alveoli, even though it is arterial. This so-called *bronchial collateral flow* can reach tremendous proportions in destructive pulmonary diseases, best exemplified by bronchiectasis.

At this point the essentials of *acute pulmonary edema* will be described because, although not necessarily the product of intrinsic lung or heart disease, edema of the lung involves a serious disruption of the pulmonary circulation and marked interference with pulmonary gas exchange. It can provoke an acute, life-threatening clinical situation frequently encountered not only in the hospital emergency room but also on inpatient divisions, and the respiratory therapist plays an important role in its treatment. Theoretically, edema of the lung can be of three types: intracellular, interstitial, and alveolar, but our present interest will be centered about the alveolar edema.[47]

Acute pulmonary edema is a condition in which there is a rapid movement of some or all of the blood components across the pulmonary capillary wall into the minute pericapillary space, from which they flow into the alveoli, alveolar ducts, and bronchial tree. Among the many factors that determine the degree of edema are (1) the net osmotic pressure across the capillary wall, between the blood and interstitial lung fluid, (2) the permeability (ease of penetration) of both capillary and alveolar walls, and (3) the capacity of the pulmonary lymphatic drainage, or the ease with which the lymphatics can remove excess interstitial fluid. An upset of the physiologic balance among these factors, whatever the cause, can produce an outpouring of fluid (transudation) into the lungs in a matter of minutes. Despite the frequency with which acute pulmonary edema occurs, little is known about the exact mechanism responsible for it. Presumably a precipitating underlying disease stimulates some autonomic nervous system reflexes that enhance alveolar-capillary permeability. Afferent autonomic nerve endings are found in many organs (heart, vessels, lungs, hollow viscera of the abdomen) that communicate through brain centers with efferent nerves supplying peripheral and pulmonary blood vessels. Abnormal reflexes can be initiated that upset the usual balanced vasomotor tone responsible for smoothly related pulmonary flow and hydrostatic pressure.[48]

Acute pulmonary edema is more a clinical syndrome than a disease entity and accompanies a variety of specific diseases. Among the latter, in which acute edema may play a significant role, are cardiovascular disease, especially coronary heart disease, heart failure, valvular disease, lung diseases, severe infections, brain injury, metabolic disorders, extensive surface burns, and severe body trauma. The acute edema itself may be responsible for the loss of a great enough volume of circulating fluid to precipitate a serious state of shock (acute circulatory failure, see below), but the outstanding signs and symptoms are the result of the extensive obstruction of airways and alveoli, with resulting hypoxemia and impaired ventilation. Often the onset of acute pulmonary edema may be preceded by a sense of anxiety and then openly manifest itself by sudden dyspnea. The fluid permeating the respiratory tract is churned into a froth by the rapidly moving tidal air exchange, is often pink or frankly blood tinged, and may be of such quantity as to bubble from the mouth under the stress of the patient's strenuous breathing. The neck veins may be markedly distended, and frequently the blood pressure is elevated, unless shock is present. Air passing through the edema fluid produces bubbling sounds known as *rales*, which often can be heard by the unaided ear as well as by the stethoscope, and not rarely the wheezing sounds of air moving through narrow passages are also present. The patient labors hard to breathe and is usually severely cyanotic from his severe obstructive hypoxemia. The treatment of acute pulmonary edema will be discussed later, but the student can certainly perceive that therapy will be of a dual nature—that of the underlying disease and of the edema itself.

## CORONARY BLOOD FLOW

Although we are not concerned with specific diseases at this point, because of the great prevalence of coronary heart disease—especially in the age group comprising the bulk of patients receiving respiratory therapy—a few observations should be made of this important segment of the cardiovascular system. If the student reviews the anatomy of the heart, he will recall that the myocardium receives its blood supply through the coronary arteries and that these vessels are the first branches of the aorta, thus assuring that perfusion of the myocardial cells will be supported by the maximum delivery pressure of the left ventricle. Not only is the contractility of the heart muscle dependent upon an adequate blood flow but the conducting system of the heart is very sensitive to circulatory interference. Because the work demand of the heart is so variable and the organ's response to demand must be prompt, the circulatory system of the heart must be flexible and able to adjust blood flow from moment to moment. As long as the coronary vessels are normal in structure, this presents no problem; but when diseased, they subject the function of the entire body to a serious hazard.

From the middle years on, the incidence of impaired coronary circulation increases, yet despite the prevalence of coronary artery disease, relatively little is known about its specific causes. It is believed that the vessels may respond to unknown stimuli, neurogenic or humoral, by a spastic contraction of their muscle fibers. Such episodes reduce the blood flow to the myocardium, often with drastic but usually transient effects, most frequently manifested by acute chest pain. A recurring condition, it is clinically referred to as *angina pectoris* (literally, "pain in the chest"). The coronary vessels are also subject to the same sclerosis, or hardening process, that so often affects the general arterial tree. Attributed to such factors as the degeneration of aging, toxic effects of nicotine directly or indirectly, cholesterol ingestion, neurogenic stimuli, and many others, thickening of the coronary arterial walls effectively and permanently reduces their caliber and elasticity. Such vessels are unable to respond to myocardial need for a rapid increase in cellular perfusion and seriously handicap the cardiac function. Further, the arteries, whether already damaged or not, are subject to the formation of thromboses (blood clots) from causes that again are not clear, with acute or gradual occlusion of their lumens. The respiratory therapist will have frequent occasion to see patients suffering from acute coronary occlusion, many of whom are ill enough to require the services of specialized care units in the hospital.

Interference with myocardial perfusion damages the muscle cells, and when such damage is severe enough to be permanent, the affected myocardium is replaced with fibrosis. Over a period of time the accumulation of fibrosis can reach a point at which there is not enough normal-functioning myocardium for adequate cardiac function, and heart failure develops. Also, should myocardial circulatory insufficiency involve a segment of the conducting system of the heart, rate and rhythm disturbances will be an important part of the clinical picture. The term *infarction* is given to a localized area of the heart where myocardial cells have been replaced by scarring, and *diffuse myocardial fibrosis* to a more generalized distribution of fibrous replacement.

It should be emphasized that the myocardium is very susceptible to hypoxia, and the coronary vessels, to a sudden drop in arterial carbon dioxide tension. These facts must be kept in mind by the respiratory therapist, and although he may be treating a patient primarily for a respiratory ailment, he should acquaint himself with the general state of the patient's myocardial health.

## CARDIOVASCULAR FAILURE

The respiratory therapist will have constant contact with patients in heart failure, and he must be aware of the basic physiologic defects involved. A heart is considered to be in failure when it can no longer fulfill its function of ensuring adequate cellular perfusion to all parts of the body without assistance. Such a state is called *cardiac decompensation*. With its underlying disease still present but its function restored by supportive therapy (i.e., digitalis, bed rest, etc.), the heart is said to be in a state of *compensation*, full or partial. A heart may decompensate because of an increase in the work load imposed on it (increased resistance in the circulation, defective function of the cardiac valves), a decrease in the ventricular contractile power (myocardial damage from fibrosis, infection, toxins), or a combination of both. There are a host of classifications of cardiac and vascular functional derangements, based on physiologic and clinical criteria, but it would be inappropriate to attempt to summarize briefly, with any degree of clarity in these few pages, that which is not done with much uniformity in large texts. Because our purpose is to provide the respiratory therapist with a basic orientation to those forms of disease relative to his work, we will describe but two types of cardiovascular incompetence that are of great importance to him: *congestive heart failure* and *acute circulatory failure*.

## Congestive heart failure

The term *congestive* implies an overcrowding and refers to a packing of vessels with blood as a result of a backup of circulation. In this type of failure, since the forward flow of blood is reduced, the blood backlogs in the return vessels, which become distended, and there is pooling in venous and capillary reservoirs. Velocity is reduced, and there is interference with cellular gas exchange. There are two types of congestive failure, which need differentiation, *left ventricular congestive failure* and *right ventricular congestive failure*.

*Left ventricular failure.* Strong though it is, the left ventricle can fail if it is opposed by increasing resistance in the systemic circulation or if the myocardium is weakened by disease. Blood returning to the left heart from the lung cannot be ejected rapidly enough, and it backs up in the pulmonary circulation. Vessels in the lung, especially the arterioles, capillaries, and veins, become "passively" congested. Often pressure in these channels increases to the point that blood water is forced from them into the pulmonary pericapillary and interstitial spaces and the alveoli. Although this state justifies the title of pulmonary edema, there are some important differential points that separate it clinically from the acute pulmonary edema discussed above. The edema produced by left ventricular failure is of a passive nature, due to the increased hydrostatic pressure of blood stasis in the pulmonary circulation. This is entirely different from the "active" acute edema, which is the result of dynamic changes in the A-C membrane and its environment, mediated through nerve reflexes in response to disease that may be remote from the lung. In addition to etiologic and physiologic differences, the functional impairments of these two types of edema vary. However, it should be emphasized that a patient with passive pulmonary congestion and edema may also be subject to a superimposed acute edema, a not infrequent occurrence. We have already noted that acute pulmonary edema generally has an abrupt onset, runs a stormy course, and is of relatively short duration. Passive edema, on the other hand, is always due to heart disease and is chronic in nature. The extravasation of fluid into the lung is of much smaller volume than that of acute edema, and its clinical and physiologic effects upon ventilation are of different quality.

Whereas the functional impairment in respiration of acute pulmonary edema is generally obstructive in nature, that of passive congestion and edema is less easily categorized. The congested pulmonary vessels and edema fluid are space occupying and encroach on alveolar air space, with reduction especially noted in the vital capacity. With engorgement of the vessels and perivascular and interstitial fluid increased, the lung becomes less flexible, and loss of pulmonary compliance is an important sequela to left heart failure. The congested vessels also offer increased resistance to the work of the right ventricle, putting it under strain. Of great significance is the combined effect of pulmonary congestion and edema to disrupt normal ventilation-perfusion relationships, interfere with alveolar gas exchange, and produce hypoxia. It is reasonable to suppose that if sufficient edema fluid should accumulate in alveoli and perhaps terminal bronchioles, it would obstruct airflow to the alveoli. In this respect, chronic passive edema may simulate, but to a lesser degree, the effect of acute edema. However, much of the edema of passive congestion may be interstitial, exerting its influence by increasing the thickness of the A-C membrane, creating a "diffusion defect" for oxygen rather than an obstruction to ventilation. It is very probable that both obstruction and diffusion interference play simultaneous or reciprocating roles, depending upon the exact dynamics of the congestion at any given time. Because the quantity of pulmonary blood flow can be variable in left heart failure, depending on the degree of compensation or decompensation, its relation to ventilation will also be an important determinant in effective gas exchange. Thus obstruction, diffusion defect, and disturbed ventilation-perfusion relationships may all be important effects of chronic passive edema. These conditions will be described more generally, individually, in the next chapter. Finally, the hydrostatic pressure in the congested lung vessels and in the lymphatics of the thorax may reach such heights that fluid will escape into the pleural space, producing a hydrothorax (literally, "water in the chest"). Up to several liters may accumulate here, and because of the obvious effect of lung compression by the fluid, we see that restriction of lung expansion is also a potential risk of left heart failure.

**Right ventricular failure.** The most frequent cause of failure of the right ventricle is preexisting failure of the left ventricle, and we have already noted that increased back pressure in the pulmonary circulation can produce a pulmonary hypertension, the resistance of which can strain the capacity of the right ventricle beyond its normal compensation. In addition, other intrinsic cardiac diseases, valvular and congenital, can overburden the right heart, but we are interested in a specific type of right failure—that due to pulmonary disease. *Cor pulmonale* implies compromise of the right ventricle, by the effects of intrapulmonary pathology, and is characterized by right ventricular enlargement (hypertrophy, a thickening of the myocardial wall; or dilatation, an enlargement of the chamber due to stretching of the myocardial fibers; or both) associated with pulmonary disease known to interfere with right ventricular function.[49] The disease so affecting the right heart usually produces an elevated pressure in the pulmonary circulation, but pulmonary hypertension itself does not constitute cor pulmonale.

Cor pulmonale is most commonly seen, and has been best documented, in the disease complex of which we will learn more later, obstructive bronchitis–pulmonary emphysema. Studies of this condition, along with others characterized by ventilatory failure, indicate that the most important elements in the genesis of cor pulmonale are probably bronchiolar obstruction, alveolar hypoventilation, and hypoxia.[50] The exact interrelation of these factors is not entirely clear, but it has been suggested that hypoxia may exert its influence directly on the myocardium. On the other hand, the effect of chronic hypoxia may be more indirect, perhaps initiating a rise in cardiac output and a subsequent elevation of pulmonary arterial pressure. Others place more emphasis on the prerequisite of chronic airway obstruction as a prime mover in the development of right heart strain but with hypoxia and hypercapnia as necessary factors.[51] Whatever the mechanism, the right ventricle is subjected to increasing resistance in providing pulmonary perfusion, and it responds by increasing its mass of myocardial tissue for greater contractile force (hypertrophy) or by elongating its myocardial fibers for greater contractile leverage, enlarging the ventricular cavity (dilatation); or the two may exist together. The right side of the heart becomes prominent by x-ray examination and shows certain electrocardiographic patterns suggesting enlargement.

When the right ventricle fails, it can no longer maintain an adequate output (although the early signs of impending failure may be an increased output) and stasis or congestion occurs in the systemic circulation that supplies it. There is pooling of blood in the veins of the lower extremities and in the venous and capillary beds of the abdominal viscera, especially in the liver. Again, with the weakened right ventricle unable to accommodate the returning venous blood, hydrostatic pressure in the veins promotes the escape of fluid into surrounding tissues, producing edema of the feet and legs, demonstrable swelling of the liver (hepatomegaly), and the outpouring of fluid into the abdominal cavity (ascites). With pure right failure there may be no signs of circulatory embarrassment of the lung, only evidence of its underlying disease. Distention of the superficial neck veins, especially in the supine position, may be a prominent feature of right heart failure, and there will be an expected elevation of peripheral venous pressure.

In summary, because the heart is a mated pair of pumps, each with its own circuit but with each circuit interacting with the other, it is easy to see that each pump is subject to individual failure. Because of the relationship of the two pumps, we can see how the right can fail without materially affecting the left but that failure of the left will eventually strain the right to the point of decompensation. The therapist will see many patients with diseases of the cardiovascular system who will have both left and right congestive heart failure and who will demonstrate to varying degrees any or all of the signs and symptoms characteristic of each.

## Acute circulatory failure

*Acute circulatory failure* is a term that embodies a large number of different diseases and conditions with a variety of etiologies, but they all have one thing in common—a serious drop in cardiac output due to either cardiac or noncardiac causes, with subsequent tissue hypoxia. In contrast to the reduction in cardiac output found in the congestive heart failures discussed above, that which characterizes acute circulatory failure occurs rapidly, allowing the body little time to adjust to the acute change. The student will encounter this condition frequently, will often be part of the therapeutic team involved in its management, and will soon get accustomed to hearing it referred to as "shock." The name *shock* is not a precise one, since it may have different connotations for different people, and although some have recommended its discontinuance, a name once established is difficult to change.[52] Shock involves many interacting physiologic phenomena of great complexity, and there is no unanimity on classification, either clinical or physiologic. Since we do not wish to get embroiled in controversial theories, but rather wish to develop a practical clinical appreciation of this significant condition, we will describe the cardinal features of shock as a composite of those characteristics most frequently accepted.[53-55]

We will avoid the complex classifications of shock that involve the many specific etiologies and describe it as an abnormal physiologic state with a disproportion between the circulating blood volume and the size of the vascular bed, which leads to circulatory failure (the inability to maintain an adequate minute volume of blood flow for tissue needs) and cellular hypoxia. The three important factors in its genesis are the *blood volume*, the *effectiveness of the cardiac pump*, and the *"tone" of the peripheral vasculature*. Should one or more of these fail, shock will develop if the remainder cannot compensate for the deficiency. With the major component of the shock syndrome a reduced cardiac output, we can rightfully expect there to be an accompanying drop in arterial blood pressure. It is these two factors that subject the body tissues to the risk of hypoxia, since adequate cellular gas exchange requires both a minimum blood volume and a perfusing pressure. In the presence of this threat, the body must protect its most hypoxia-sensitive vital organs, the brain and heart, from oxygen want.

Compensation consists of redistributing the arterial circulation to assure adequate cerebral and cardiac perfusion, even at the expense of other tissues, especially the abdominal organs and peripheral areas (skin). This is accomplished by widespread vasoconstriction to shift the available blood flow to the two vital structures and also to maintain suitable blood pressure through an increase in peripheral resistance. The blood pressure may continue to fall, a characteristic of shock, but cerebral and cardiac perfusion can remain ample for a long time. Should the shock state progress into what is termed *irreversible shock*, compensation will fail and vasoconstriction may give way to vasodilatation at the capillary and venular level, with the pooling of large volumes of blood in the capillary beds. This further reduces the circulating blood volume (hypovolemia) and initiates a vicious cycle that may continue to death.

There are some types of acute circulatory failure that initially show vasodilatation rather than vasoconstriction, and in these the underlying disease prevents the constrictor compensation just described. It is perhaps evident to the student that there can be a period of imminent or potential shock before the classical symptoms of hypotension warn of falling cardiac output. Patients suspected of having conditions predisposing to shock are carefully observed for its signs.

We can summarize in a brief outline the major causes of reduction in cardiac output.

1. *Reduction in blood volume*
    a. Loss of blood by hemorrhage
    b. Extravasation of blood or plasma from vessels into intercellular spaces, as a result of damage to capillaries and larger vessels by trauma and surgery
    c. Dehydration, with loss of fluid through skin, kidney, gastrointestinal tract
2. *Reduced venous return from capillary and venular pooling*
    a. Vasodilatation, due to loss of vasomotor stimuli from toxins (bacterial sepsis)
    b. Vasodilatation, due to loss of vasoconstrictor action, as from spinal anesthesia
3. *Failure of cardiac pump action*
    a. Cardiac filling defect, as from tamponade (compression of heart from pericardial fluid) and tachycardia (insufficient diastolic filling time due to rapid rate)
    b. Cardiac emptying defect, as from an obstructing intracardiac thrombus, large pulmonary embolus
    c. Impaired cardiac function, especially from myocardial infarct

From a practical point of view, the respiratory therapist will see patients go into shock mostly as the result of severe trauma (automobile or industrial accidents, gunshot wounds), extensive surgery (manipulation of viscera, loss of blood and plasma), massive acute blood loss, and overwhelming sepsis (blood invasion by bacteria). There are two special circumstances of shock that are of particular interest to the therapist. First is the circulatory failure that can follow a disturbance in intrathoracic pressure. Any disorder that can produce a significant elevation in intrapleural pressure, elevating the mean pressure from the negative to the positive range, by virtue of interfering with venous return through the thoracic vessels and by restricting diastolic filling of the heart, can generate shock. It cannot be emphasized too frequently or too strongly that this is an inherent risk in the use of positive pressure ventilating equipment. Second, a condition sometimes referred to as shock lung, but more properly called adult respiratory distress syndrome, is a serious pulmonary consequence of acute circulatory collapse. It will be dealt with in more detail in our consideration of ventilatory failure but is noted here to emphasize the need for respiratory therapists to learn as much about shock as they can.

The clinical picture of shock will be a familiar one to the therapist in a general hospital. The patient may be restless or apathetic and lethargic, but he will show marked physical weakness. His skin will be pale, cold, and moist or will show a grayish cyanosis. The superficial veins will be collapsed and difficult to find, a point of considerable therapeutic concern. The blood pressure will be low, at least less than 80 mm Hg, systolic, and in severe states may be so weak as to be unobtainable, and the peripheral pulse will be faint or "thready" and rapid. Urinary output falls off as kidney perfusion is seriously compromised. Body temperature is often below normal. It is beyond the scope of this text to detail the particulars of therapy, which frequently taxes the ingenuity of the medical attendants, but among all the necessary supportive measures it should be evident that the administration of oxygen is of prime importance. The alert therapist will observe the other techniques employed to maintain maximum tissue perfusion, including the "shock position," fluid and blood replacement, and cardiovascular stimulants.

Of high priority in the management of the acutely ill patient whose cardiovascular status is in doubt or who is in frank shock, is the measurement of *central venous pressure (CVP)*.[56,57] As the name implies, CVP is the pressure in the large veins within the body as opposed to the pressure in a single extremity earlier described as peripheral venous pressure. CVP is measured by a water manometer often attached at a proper height to the head of the patient's bed. The manometer is in line with a catheter introduced into antecubital, internal jugular, or subclavian, veins percutaneously (threaded through a needle inserted in a vein) or by cutdown (directly into a vein exposed by surgical incision of the skin). It is advanced until its tip is in the superior vena cava.

CVP reflects the sum of the action of the pumping heart, the circulating blood volume, and peripheral vascular tone. Its normal range is 8 to 12 cm of water. Venous flow is controlled by cardiac output, and a deficit in cardiac contractibility causes blood to backlog in venous reservoirs, elevating the CVP providing the blood volume remains stable. If the heart is normal, CVP will drop with a decrease in circulating volume, or when peripheral vasodilatation causes venous pooling and a reduced venous return. It is thus an aid in the differentiation between cardiac failure and shock and is a good guide to fluid replacement therapy.

In addition to pressure in the central venous system, the vena cava indwelling line allows serial sampling of blood for determination of *central venous oxygen saturation* ($CVS_{O_2}$). Blood in the vena cava is pooled blood, a mixture from all parts of the body, representative of average metabolic activity from the body as a whole. $CVS_{O_2}$ is a much more accurate reflection of general oxygen usage than is saturation from a peripheral vein and is useful in estimating cardiac output. As cardiac output falls, less blood per unit of time perfuses cells. With a slowing of blood flow, blood-cell contact time increases, and more oxygen than normal is extracted from the perfusate. Mixed venous blood sampled from the superior vena cava thus has a low oxygen saturation. This is a very useful tool to monitor the progress of myocardial infarction, since experimentation has demonstrated that a drop in $CVS_{O_2}$ below 55% indicates a beginning fall in cardiac output and probable early complicating cardiac failure.[58,59]

Increasing use is being made of another, but similar technique for cardiovascular evaluation and monitoring, which might be considered a third generation development from the relatively simple and crude peripheral venous pressure measurement. The *Swan-Ganz catheter* represents a sophisticated, electronically monitored complex version of the central venous catheter.[60,61] The basic Swan-Ganz catheter itself is double walled with one channel open at the distal end and the other terminating at an inflatable balloon just before the tip. Proximally, the catheter is attached to a heparinized saline flush reservoir by a flow control unit, and through special pressure tubing, to a pressure transducer. Output from the transducer is carried to a monitor capable of at least two tracer recordings, the cardiac beat and intravascular pressures.

The Swan-Ganz catheter is introduced into a peripheral vein by surgical cutdown under strict asepsis and is advanced into the right atrium or ventricle. Pressure wave forms on the oscilloscope monitor enable the operator to plot the position. Air is instilled in the balloon, and the catheter is literally floated through the pulmonic valve into a pulmonary artery with the blood flow, until it wedges and can go no farther. The balloon is deflated to avoid obstructing blood flow to the surrounding lung.

It is not as easy or as desirable to attempt to withdraw blood samples through a Swan-Ganz catheter as through a simple CVP line for fear of clotting the lumen. The prime value of this elaborate procedure is its ability to transmit the so-called *pulmonary capillary wedge pressure (PCW)*. With the tip of the catheter advanced until the caliber of the pulmonary artery branch stops it, if the balloon is momentarily inflated, the pressure recorded in this wedged position is the pressure across the pulmonary capillary from the pulmonary venous system. It has been shown to reflect two important cardiac forces: (1) the mean left atrial pressure (average of the systolic and diastolic pressures in the left atrium over each cardiac cycle), and (2) the left ventricular end-diastolic pressure (pressure in the blood-filled left ventricle just prior to its systolic contraction).[62] The PCW, when elevated, is the major signal of the development or presence of pulmonary congestion and edema, since it relates directly to the volume of blood in the pulmonary venous bed. Thus anything impeding the flow of blood out of the left ventricle will cause a back pressure (as long as the mitral valve is patent) through the left atrium and the pulmonary veins to the tip of the catheter wedged into a small vessel on the arterial side of the pulmonary capillary.

Studies comparing the effectiveness of CVP with PCW have shown that CVP does not accurately reflect pulmonary venous distending pressure in patients with myocardial infarction and does not correlate with x-ray evidence of left ventricular failure as well as does the PCW.[63] Which monitoring technique is used, if any, for a given patient is a clinical decision of the responsible attending physician.

In summary, we can say that pulmonary venous pressure measurements are employed to detect signs of left ventricular failure, especially in the early stages of myocardial infarction, and to determine the adequacy of circulating blood volume. In the latter circumstance CVP or PCW catheters are useful in the management of shock and in fluid replacement therapy of any acutely ill patient. The therapist will see some patients on mechanical ventilation monitored with CVP or PCW pressure measurement, especially those whose ventilatory failure is complicated by shock, cardiac disease, or fluid-electrolyte problems.

## CARDIAC ARRHYTHMIAS

The importance of the cardiac arrhythmias lies not so much in their relation to respiratory therapy directly as in the frequency with which they occur in the hospital population most apt to be serviced by respiratory therapy. In the performance of his duties, the respiratory therapist will see and hear much attention directed to this class of cardiac disorders, and especially in critical care units he will see visual evidence of them on oscilloscope monitor screens. As with the preceding examples of heart disease, we will outline the minimal features of arrhythmias most commonly encountered in hospital practice, ignoring the more bizarre, and leave it to the individual therapist to supplement this material with independent reading, according to his interest.

Although *dysrhythmia* (a malfunctioning rhythm) is probably more accurate, *arrhythmia* has become the standard expression for a cardiac rhythm that deviates from the usual and natural pattern, interrupting the automatic rhythmic heart action that was initiated before birth. Many of the rhythm disturbances can be diagnosed with certainty only by the electrocardiogram, others can be readily detected clinically, and the presence of yet others may be highly suspected. The presence of an abnormal heart rhythm is not necessarily a bad omen, since many of them are innocuous and occur in normal hearts; but others may indicate serious underlying pathology, and a few signify imminent death. A simple physiologic concept must be understood if one is to appreciate the great variety of abnormal rhythms to which the heart is subject. We have already established that the sinus node (sinoatrial node) is the normal focus for the start of cardiac contraction, but any site in the myocardium or the conducting system is capable of initiating excitation. It is as though an almost infinite number of trigger points are kept subdued by the normal action of the dominant sinus node but express themselves when some factor causes the latter to lose its tight control. We will briefly describe the following, all of which the therapist may expect to see in the general hospital: sinus arrhythmia, premature contractions, paroxysmal tachycardia, atrial flutter, atrial fibrillation, ventricular fibrillation, atrioventricular block, and sinus arrest.[64, 65]

### Sinus arrhythmia

The most frequent and least harmful of all the arrhythmias, sinus arrhythmia, is a normal variant in the young but can be found at almost any age. It is characterized by a change in cardiac rate synchronous with the respiratory cycle, as the heart rate increases during inspiration and decreases with expiration. It can be exaggerated by inspiratory breath holding and eliminated by exercise. The mechanism for its presence is an alteration in the strength of vagal (parasympathetic) influence on the normal pacemaker. Presumably, during inspiration the increased vagal impulses brought into play by the Hering-Breuer reflex quantitatively detract from the vagal impulses serving the sinus node. With lessened parasympathetic inhibition during this phase of respiration, the excitation rate of the node increases with a similar response by the ventricles. This condition has no pathologic implications, and no treatment is indicated.

### Premature contractions

Localized areas of the atria, atrioventricular (A-V) node, and ventricular myocardium may initiate an excitation impulse independently of the sinus node. Because they occur away from the normal focus of stimulation, they are referred to as *ectopic foci*. Premature contractions may be prognostically benign or serious, since they can occur in both normal and diseased hearts. They result from the irritation of some spot in the myocardium or conducting system by a variety of stimulants, among which the following are frequent offenders: excitement, anxiety, smoking, alcohol ingestion, fatigue, gastrointestinal disturbances, and procedures such as thoracic surgery, cardiac catheterization, and digitalis (a vital drug used in the treatment of heart failure but which can irritate the myocardium).

The premature contraction is a sort of "extra" beat and is so named because it is activated before a normal beat would be expected, inserting itself between two normal contractions. If the stimulus is great enough or there is more than one stimulus, there may be a short string of premature contractions. Also, in pathologic states different stimuli may generate impulses from more than one ectopic focus. There are three general types of premature contractions: atrial, nodal, and ventricular. In the first an ectopic atrial impulse follows the usual path, and the extra beat cannot be distinguished from a normal. A nodal premature contraction starts in the A-V node (not the sinus node) and also follows the usual path into the ventricles, but because it travels a shorter distance than a sinus impulse, characteristic time measurements on the electrocardiogram identify it. Since a ventricular premature contraction starts at the opposite end of the excitation chain, its path through the ventricular muscle is grossly abnormal, and the electrocardiographic configuration is often quite bizarre. Ventricular extra systoles may occur with regularity, alternating with normal sinus beats, producing a coupled rhythm referred to as *bigeminy.*

An interesting characteristic of premature contractions, which can sometimes be noted clinically and usually by the electrocardiograph, is the slighly longer than normal refractory period of myocardial fibers. Because the extra ectopic stimulus occurs out of phase, it interferes with the usual sequence of excitability and refractoriness and causes a lag before the next following contraction. This is called a *compensatory pause.* In an atrial premature contraction the ectopic impulse encompasses the sinus node, which must wait until it recovers before it can initiate its own normal beat. Thus the interval between the premature beat and the next normal one is longer than the interval between two normal beats. After ventricular extra contractions, and usually nodal ones as well, the ventricles are refractory to the next normal sinus impulse, leading to a longer pause that is designated as "fully compensated." In this instance the time interval between the normal beats preceding and following the ectopic is exactly twice the time interval between any two other normal beats.

The clinical significance of premature contractions generally depends on the patient's tolerance of them, their frequency, and the presence or absence of underlying disease. Symptoms may be absent, or the patient may complain of "palpitations" or a "thumping" in the chest. The patient is actually aware of the *absence* of heart action during the compensatory pause as well as the difference in contractile force between normal and some abnormal beats. Sometimes dizziness and a sense of fullness in the chest or neck are bothersome.

## Paroxysmal tachycardia

Chains or bursts of atrial, nodal, or ventricular premature contractions constitute paroxysmal tachycardia, which may last for prolonged periods of time. During an attack, the cardiac rate may range from 160 to 240 per minute. The rhythm is usually regular, is not affected by breathing or exercise, and may terminate abruptly. Atrial and nodal paroxysms can often be stopped by strong vagal stimuli, accomplished by exerting pressure on the eyeballs or carotid sinus, or by gagging. Ventricular ectopic foci will not respond to these maneuvers, since the ventricular myocardium is less influenced by vagal innervation than is the atrial.

From a clinical point of view, this abnormality may be functional (not due to organic disease) or due to cardiac disease. It often produces weakness and dizziness, and if prolonged, there will be a drop in cardiac output due to the sharp reduction in diastolic filling time from the rapid rate. A diseased heart may be thrown into congestive failure, and shock is a real threat. There is also the risk that paroxysmal tachycardia will progress to the very grave ventricular fibrillation, to be described below. Its presence is always an indication for careful observation, and drug therapy of the arrhythmia is a usual precaution.

### Atrial flutter

In atrial flutter, there is either a rapid circular movement of a stimulus or a repetitive single ectopic focus exciting the atria at rates of 200 to 350 per minute, with a clocklike regularity. It is named from the flutterlike contraction imparted to the atria. The refractoriness of the A-V node does not permit it to transmit usually more than 180 impulses per minute, so many of the atrial signals are blocked. The ratio of blocked to transmitted impulses may be constant in a given instance, such as 2:1, 3:1, 4:1, etc.

Flutter is usually due to disease, and even with a partial block the ventricular rate is still high enough to compromise cardiac filling and output. Because of the fixed atrioventricular ratio, the cardiac rate does not increase with exercise, even in those instances in which the block may permit a nearly normal rate. This interferes with the normal cardiac reserve and its response to exercise.

### Atrial fibrillation

Atrial fibrillation is the most common of the significant abnormal rhythm disturbances and is the usual end point of a preexisting flutter, although a flutter is not a prerequisite. Fibrillation always means cardiac pathology. The atria are subjected to a completely uncontrolled, randomly irregular barrage of impulses at rates of 350 to 500 per minute. The A-V node transmits as many of these as it can, and the result is a chaotic ventricular response of grossly irregular contractions of varying intensities. Some of the contractions are too weak to be palpated in the peripheral pulses, and this leads to a *pulse deficit,* a discrepancy between the cardiac rate as counted over the chest and the rate of arterial pulsations.

The therapist will see many patients with this defect, since its causes span the extremes of life. It is a common sequela to such childhood diseases as rheumatic fever and is often seen with degenerative cardiac diseases of later years. It is not incompatible with fairly normal activity, and many people carry it for years. However, the fibrillation (weak, shaky, ineffectual contraction) of the atria promotes poor atrial emptying, with the retention of blood in these chambers and the subsequent risk of intra-atrial thrombus formation, often a source of future emboli. For this reason attempts are usually made to convert such hearts to a normal rhythm. Atrial fibrillation is readily detected by physical examination, but its electrocardiographic picture is characteristic, with the absence of definitive P waves and their replacement by an irregularly wavy baseline.

## Ventricular fibrillation

So grave as to be imminently fatal if not quickly corrected, ventricular fibrillation consists of a rapid tremulous shaking of the ventricular myocardium completely incompatible with any useful cardiac output. Frequently preceded by persistent or recurring ventricular paroxysmal tachycardia, fibrillation can be caused by many conditions, among which are electric shock, anesthesia, mechanical irritation of the heart, severe hypoxia, myocardial infarction, and large doses of digitalis or epi-nephrine. The rapid drop in cardiac output produces an acute cerebral hypoxia, often manifested by convulsions, and death ensues within a few minutes. From a functional viewpoint, ventricular fibrillation may be considered a form of "cardiac arrest," for although there is some ventricular activity, it is of no value. This abnor-mality, like sinus arrest to be described below, constitutes a true emergency situation, with survival dependent upon the immediate application of the techniques of emer-gency resuscitation.

## Atrioventricular block

Disorders of the myocardium such as inflammations, infarction or arteriosclerotic ischemia, and digitalis toxicity can reduce or destroy the ability of the A-V node or the bundle of His to transmit the sinus impulse to the ventricles. If every impulse is conducted but with a prolonged time (prolonged P-R interval on the electro-cardiogram), the block is considered as *first degree.* If some impulses are conducted but others dropped, the block is *second degree.* If no atrial impulses are conducted to the ventricles, the block is *third degree,* or "complete." The last is the most im-portant, for with no sinus impulse the ventricles must develop their own pacemaker and are able to do so only at very slow rates of between 25 and 45 per minute. Under conditions of stress, or in the presence of other arrhythmias, the bradycardia may be inadequate for cerebral blood flow, and the heart may even stop for several seconds. Acute unconsciousness may occur without warning, the so-called *Stokes-Adams syn-cope* (fainting). Convulsions and death may accompany such episodes. The disability of complete heart block is obvious and the need for treatment urgent.

Some patients with bradycardia, heart block, or arrhythmias that interfere with cardiac function, respond to medical therapy, whereas others are realizing new leases on life with the use of electronic pacemakers, or pulse generators, permanently implanted in their bodies. Therapists will frequently serve patients with cardiac problems and should know at least the general nature of pacemakers. Fundamentally, an artificial pacemaker is a battery-operated device that emits an electrical charge, which is carried by a conducting catheter (electrode) into the right atrium or ven-tricle. Usually the catheter is firmly impacted against the right ventricular wall, and the generated signal stimulates the myocardium into contraction. The therapist may see temporary pacemakers placed in patients during acute episodes of block. For use limited to only a few days, the temporary pulse generator is kept outside the body, a small boxlike unit attached to or near the patient by pins, tape, or other means. The electrode catheter is often introduced into the heart through a jugular vein of the neck. Once cardiac stability is achieved, the temporary unit is removed and the patient continued on other therapy, or it is replaced by a permanent implanted instrument.

Permanent pacemakers are placed in a subcutaneous pocket usually just below either clavicle, and can be easily recognized by a prominent bulge with an overlying scar. The electrode follows one of the large veins into the heart. Occasionally, the pulse generator pocket may be on the upper abdominal wall with the electrode traveling subcutaneously to its attachment on the external surface of the heart, but these are less common than the intracardiac type. Some pulse generators need replacement for battery failure after 2 or more years, while others can be recharged regularly by the patient for longer battery life. Nuclear-powered generators are almost a certainty for the future.

Pacemakers can be programed a number of ways, and it is not relevant for us to go into more detail. Suffice it to say that some have preset rates at which they stimulate the heart, while others function on demand in case of failure of the natural spontaneous mechanism.

### Sinus arrest

Like ventricular fibrillation, sinus arrest is a second cause of sudden cardiac standstill. The basic defect is failure of the sinus node to initiate an impulse and may be considered a suppression of the node by overwhelming vagal impulses. An ectopic pacemaker may compensate, but often the entire stimulus production of the heart is adversely affected, and no contraction occurs. Death is obvious unless excitation can be resumed. Sinus arrest is likely to accompany the early stages of anesthesia or certain bodily manipulations that are able to set up a strong vagal reflex. These include instrumentation during such examination of body cavities as cystoscopy, bronchoscopy, or pharyngeal probing and occasionally traction on thoracic organs during surgery. Many hearts so affected are perfectly normal and need only a stimulus such as massage or a sharp blow to the sternum to set them back into rhythmic activity.

•   •   •

Of special interest to the respiratory therapist are three factors related to cardiac arrhythmias, summarized briefly here. Prolonged deep hypoxia can stimulate the production of ectopic foci of excitation and precipitate conduction block in a myocardium already partially ischemic. Physical manipulation of the body can trigger vagal reflexes that are able to arrest heart action by inhibiting the sinus node. Although such incidents are uncommon, presumably moving the head or neck of some patients or initating pharyngeal vagal stimuli by instrumentation are among maneuvers with this potential risk. Finally, high blood levels of carbon dioxide in themselves, or because of the accompanying reduced blood pH, can activate ectopic focal activity. It is also believed that a sudden reduction in a previously elevated carbon dioxide tension can stimulate ventricular arrhythmias.[66, 67] These points must be kept in mind in the treatment of patients in ventilatory failure.

## CONGENITAL HEART DISEASE

No attempt will be made to classify and describe this large and important group of cardiac abnormalities, for the number of texts and articles in the literature on the subject are so vast that the student can find material to any desired depth of sophistication for his own self-study. A few principles will be discussed that should make further pursuit of the subject more meaningful.

Congenitally deformed hearts are the victims of incomplete or erroneous prenatal development, occasionally the result of maternal disease, but most often are due to some unknown cause. The scope of defects ranges from the slight, compatible with normal life, to the severe, incompatible with more than a few minutes of survival. Most defects are detected during childhood or adolescence, and because many are increasingly benefited by surgery, every attempt is made to establish an accurate diagnosis and prognosis. The respiratory therapist, in a hospital actively engaged in cardiac surgery, will have occasion to see many patients with congenital heart disease, since many of them have associated respiratory problems, and postoperative care often uses respiratory therapy services.

The two broad classifications of congenital disease that concern us here are *acyanotic* (absence of cyanosis) and *cyanotic* congenital defects. The differentiation between the two depends on whether significant amounts of unsaturated blood mix with arterialized blood to produce cyanosis. Many congenital defects consist of communications between the two sides of the heart through septal defects, or openings in the interatrial and interventricular septa. These are called *intracardiac shunts*, since blood can pass from one side of the heart to the other without following the usual channels. Because the pressure in the left heart is greater than in the right, an uncomplicated septal defect will shunt blood from the left to the right. In other words, variable amounts of left heart blood, depending upon the size of the imperfection, will pass directly into the right heart, mixing arterialized blood with venous. This, of course, does not produce cyanosis. However, the increased load of blood perfusing the lung, some of which is coming back for a second round, increases the pressure in the pulmonary circulation. Physical exercise may further raise the pulmonary pressure temporarily to a level that exceeds the systemic pressure, reversing the pressure gradient across the septum and converting the shunt from a left-to-right to a right-to-left. During this interval, venous blood will mix with arterial and may produce cyanosis. Also, progressive pulmonary hypertension may strain the right ventricle to the point of failure, and an interatrial shunt may be reversed to cause cyanosis. If narrowing of the pulmonary valve or the pulmonary artery is part of the cardiac defect complex, cyanosis will be present from the early stages in the presence of associated septal openings because of initial pulmonary hypertension. There are conditions that permit cyanosis even in the absence of pulmonary hypertension, for example, septal defects so large that venous blood mixes with arterial even without a reverse gradient, or an aorta that arises from the right ventricle. Generally speaking, however, the presence or absence of cyanosis in septal cardiac defects depends upon the presence or absence of high pressure in the pulmonary circulation.

# Chapter 6

# CLINICAL CARDIOPULMONARY PATHOLOGY

The purpose of this chapter is to consider some of the disturbances in cardiopulmonary physiology with which the respiratory therapist can be expected to come into frequent contact. The topics to be discussed will not constitute specific disease entities but rather will consist of some of the major physiologic changes that underlie the common respiratory disorders. This might be a good point to mention a basic philosophy of respiratory therapy. Generally speaking, respiratory therapy is not directed toward the cure of disease in the sense of removing a specific etiology. A surgeon removes an inflamed appendix and cures the clinical condition of acute appendicitis; a physician administers an antibiotic and cures a disease by destroying the causative organism. In contrast, respiratory therapy is fundamentally supportive or symptomatic in nature. In the former instance, therapy helps to maintain respiratory and cardiac integrity until more etiologically specific treatment can be effective, and in the latter, it attempts to counter the effects of disease and to help restore maximum function. In a broad sense, then, and with some obvious exceptions, the technology of respiratory therapy is concerned not so much with what the disease under treatment is as with what the disease has done to cardiopulmonary physiology. Although it is important that an effective therapist have a practical working knowledge of relevant clinical diseases, it is far more important that he understands the malfunction of respiration brought about by these diseases.

With this in mind, we will discuss major features of five pathologic conditions, some or all of which are common to cardiopulmonary disease in general—hypoxia, airway obstruction, pulmonary distention, pulmonary restriction, and ventilation-perfusion imbalance. It will be evident below that hypoxia can be caused by many factors, including the other four pathologic states here listed. Thus, theoretically at least, because it is a consequence of so many abnormalities, perhaps hypoxia should not be discussed in parallel with the others. However, its importance as the greatest hazard of all oxygen-dependent creatures, and as the prime object of our therapy, gives hypoxia top priority and our attention first.

## HYPOXIA

*Hypoxia* is a general term that means an inadequate availability of oxygen for cell function, whereas *hypoxemia* refers to a diminution in the actual content of oxygen in blood and implies tissue hypoxia but does not indicate what tissue or to what degree.[68-70] Although there is an obvious difference in their meanings, the two are frequently used interchangeably, and as a matter of convenience, the shorter term, *hypoxia,* will be used in the following text. It will be assumed that the reader can make his own mental differentiation between them according to usage of the terms. It is even more important that the student clearly understand the difference between two quantitative expressions of blood oxygen content, *arterial oxygen saturation* and *arterial oxygen tension.*

Since a major step in the process of oxygen transport is the union of oxygen with hemoglobin, the degree to which hemoglobin is saturated with oxygen is a valuable indication of the efficiency of the hemoglobin carriage. The question frequently arises as to which is the better gauge of oxygenation—hemoglobin saturation with oxygen or blood oxygen tension. It should be emphasized that neither tells us what we would really like to know—the level of oxygen in tissue cells. Both tell us only of oxygen's availability in the circulating arterial blood or give us a rough idea of its utilization by the body if measured in mixed venous blood.

*Hemoglobin oxygen saturation* is an implied quantitative measure of volumes of oxygen per volumes of blood and might seem to be more relevant to our needs than oxygen tension. It is clinically important and useful information but in itself is incomplete without knowledge of the hemoglobin concentration, the grams of hemoglobin per 100 ml of blood. Two subjects, one with 15 g/dl and the other with 7.5 g/dl, may both be 96% saturated with oxygen, but obviously 96% of 15 g of hemoglobin per deciliter of blood represents more oxygen than does 96% of 7.5 g. The product of hemoglobin concentration, hemoglobin oxygen saturation, and the factor 1.34 allows a rapid estimation of the actual volume of oxygen in 100 ml of blood.

*Blood oxygen partial pressure* is widely used in determining hemoglobin oxygen saturation. Saturation can be measured directly by time-consuming chemical analysis, but it is much more conveniently estimated from the easily measured blood oxygen tension and an oxygen dissociation curve, properly adjusted for pH and temperature. At the upper end of the dissociation curves, saturation changes very slightly with changes in $P_{O_2}$. As a result, a drop in saturation of only 3% between two samples might seem no cause for alarm, but it can represent a tension drop of 20 mm Hg or more, certainly indicative of some abnormality. $P_{O_2}$ measurements avoid overlooking slight but significant oxygen content changes. Finally, because partial pressure is a kinetic parameter, it gives us some idea of the molecular force available to oxygen in its diffusion efforts across physiological barriers. A useful index of abnormal oxygen transport as a cause of hypoxemia is a comparison of oxygen tensions in alveolar gas and arterial blood, called the alveolar-arterial oxygen tension gradient. The clinical use of this measurement will be discussed later, but it obviously requires use of tension rather than saturation data.

It is apparent therefore that there is no single better way of metering blood oxygen content. Both saturation and tension values give the most complete picture so far available to us.

## Classification of hypoxia

There are many classifications of types of hypoxia, but the following includes the principal causative factors.

***Reduced alveolar oxygen.*** Reduced alveolar oxygen can result from either low ambient $P_{O_2}$ or hypoventilation.

*Low ambient $P_{O_2}$.* Breathing a mixture with a low concentration of oxygen at atmosphere, or normal oxygen at subatmosphere, provides an inadequate alveolar oxygen tension for normal diffusion into pulmonary blood. A common example of this problem is encountered during travel to high altitudes, where the unaccustomed visitor often suffers ill effects of hypoxia for several days, the so-called "mountain sickness," or hypobarism.

*Hypoventilation.* Always associated with hypercapnia, hypoventilation reduces the amount of air ventilating the alveoli so that there is not enough oxygen available for normal arterial saturation.

***Impaired alveolar-capillary diffusion.*** Faced with pathologic changes in any of the structures of the A-C membrane, such as fibrosis, granuloma, proliferation of connective tissue, or interstitial edema, fewer oxygen molecules will be able to penetrate the barrier even with normal alveolar gas tension, and the arterial tension will be considerably less than the alveolar. The student may see this condition referred to in the literature as *alveolar-capillary block*, but in current terminology it is more properly called a *diffusion defect*. A pure diffusion defect is relatively uncommon, and because it is often absent in some conditions in which the pathology would seem to make it probable, much is not known about its exact mechanism. The diagnosis of impared diffusion is basically a laboratory procedure, and further reference will be made to it during the discussion on ventilation-perfusion imbalance.

***Anatomic shunts.*** A shunt is a bypass, or a short circuit, and in a cardiopulmonary sense it consists of a direct communication between the arterial and venous circulations. The result of congenital defects, disease, or trauma, a shunt may consist of a local communication between a peripheral artery and a nearby vein, or a large defect in the septa separating the left and right chambers of the heart. The latter type is the most clinically important; it is common in congenital heart disease and is described in Chapter 5.

***Hemoglobin deficiency.*** Hemoglobin deficiency may be of two varieties, absolute or relative.

*Absolute.* Anemia, with a quantitative lack of circulating hemoglobin, can seriously impair the oxygen-carrying capacity of the blood, even in the presence of normal supply and adequate diffusion.

*Relative.* For adequate oxygenation not only must there be enough hemoglobin, but it must be capable of transporting oxygen because abnormal hemoglobin can produce clinically significant hypoxia. For example, carbon monoxide in a breathing mixture will combine with hemoglobin much faster than will the oxygen present, and it forms carboxyhemoglobin, which is incapable of carrying oxygen. It is this mechanism that makes carbon monoxide such a lethal agent. Another abnormal form of hemoglobin is methemoglobin, an oxidized (not oxygenated) form in which the iron is in the ferric instead of the normal ferrous state. The result of hereditary defects or the ingestion of certain drugs in toxic doses, methemoglobin, like carboxyhemoglobin, is unable to transport oxygen and is an important cause of hypoxia.

**Circulatory failure.** Should the systemic circulation lose its thrust, there will be reduced tissue cell perfusion with resulting hypoxia. This may also be of two types, generalized or local.

*Generalized.* In the presence of generalized circulatory failure, as in shock or with a failing heart, oxygen deprivation will be widespread.

*Local.* Venous or arterial obstruction can interfere with local circulation, causing tissue hypoxia of the affected area.

**Histotoxins.** Chemical substances that interfere with the enzyme systems of body cells responsible for oxygen utilization can produce lethal cellular hypoxia, in the presence of adequate oxygen supply. Cyanide poisoning is one of the best known clinical examples of this category.

**Ventilation/perfusion ratio imbalance.** Because of the clinical importance of this cause of hypoxia, its principles and the consequences of its disturbance will be discussed in considerable detail later in this chapter under its own heading.

## Acute hypoxia

Acute hypoxia is caused by a rapid reduction of available oxygen as from asphyxia, airway obstruction, blockage of alveoli by the fluid of edema or infectious exudate, abrupt cardiorespiratory failure, and acute hemorrhage. Some patients, depending on the cause, may exhibit hypoventilation and others, hyperventilation to the point of "air hunger," a seemingly insatiable attempt to breathe more and more air. In the latter, hyperpnea is usually present, and the increased ventilatory volume blows off excess carbon dioxide, dropping the blood level significantly and elevating blood pH. Arterial oxygen tensions and saturation are both low. If the degree of hypoxia is less than critical, the mental state it produces has been likened to that of alcoholic intoxication.[71] Headache is a frequent complaint, and there is often mental confusion. However, in the early stages of oxygen deprivation, mental stimulation may be strikingly evident, the subject reacting in a euphoric and sometimes hilarious manner. This is followed by a state of depression and drowsiness. Muscle weakness ensues, accompanied by lack of coordination, and as the hypoxia progresses, there is serious loss of discrimination and judgment.[72] With a more sudden hypoxia, there may be an acute abrupt loss of consciousness; this is not common except in those instances when the subject finds himself suddenly in an airless environment, such as a gas-filled compartment.

The most critical target organ of hypoxia is the central nervous system, and with a few exceptions, survival of acute hypoxia depends on its effect on the brain. One of the early responses of the brain is vasodilatation and an increased cerebral blood flow. However, because nerve tissue is so vulnerable to oxygen lack, a few minutes of severe hypoxia may produce irreversible damage to brain cells, and prolongation of lesser degrees can lead to death or permanent damage. Comas of days' or weeks' duration are not uncommon; and the half-living vegetative existence of the not-quite-dead brain may be the most tragic consequence of hypoxia.

Other organs are affected by hypoxia. Although the healthy heart can tolerate hypoxia to a considerable degree, one slightly compromised by disease may suffer seriously. This is especially evident in the patient with subclinical cardiac disorders (not quite to the symptom-producing stage), such as early or mild coronary artery narrowing or early heart failure. Functioning with a minimum reserve, such hearts, when perfused with hypoxic blood, will be adversely affected. Myocardial fibers, with a high oxygen demand, may weaken or die, or the cardiac rhythm may be seriously disturbed. Patients with known or suspected heart disease, especially those in the middle and older age groups, must be watched very closely, from the cardiac point of view; electrocardiographic changes are frequent indications of impending or actual myocardial hypoxia. Kidney cells also require constant and adequate oxygenation, and hypoxia can precipitate renal failure, interfering with the ability of the kidney to maintain normal electrolyte and water balance and to eliminate waste products efficiently. Finally, the carbon dioxide transport mechanism is less effective with hypoxia, since oxyhemoglobin is needed to displace carbon dioxide in the lung.

The depth of hypoxia that the body can tolerate and still survive is a matter of considerable interest. There are so many obvious modifying variables, such as the state of the circulation (especially the cerebral), the general body cellular health, the total metabolism, and the intensity of therapy, that there is no clear-cut lower limit of oxygenation. A guiding rule of thumb for some time has held that an arterial $P_{O_2}$ below 20 mm Hg is probably incompatible with life[73]; yet values as low as 9 mm Hg followed by recovery are known from my own experience. It is most likely that the modern therapy of respiratory failure has reduced the hypoxic threshold of viability. A more practical guide that the therapist may encounter is the so-called *rule of three,* which describes, as at least temporarily acceptable as minimal oxygenation, an arterial oxygen tension that is three times the value of the inspired oxygen concentration. It should be apparent that such a gimmick has no scientific basis, since it employs unlike terms of measurement. It is simply an expression of clinical observation that tells us the oxygen uptake and transport are probably holding their own if the $P_{a_{O_2}}$ follows the rule or are decompensating if it does not.

Special mention will be made of a common sign of hypoxia, *cyanosis,* present in both acute and chronic hypoxia although not invariably in either. Cyanosis is a blue or gray-blue color imparted to skin, mucous membranes, and nail beds in the presence of hypoxia. Evaluation of the degree of cyanosis, or even its presence, depends upon the perception of the examiner, modified by such factors as the ambient lighting, the color of the environment, and especially the skin color of the subject. In dark-skinned patients cyanosis may be detected only in nail beds or mucous membranes. Thus, although failure to see cyanosis does not rule out hypoxia, its presence is a strong positive sign of hypoxia.

Cyanosis is related to the degree of oxygen *unsaturation of capillary* blood perfusing body surfaces, and generally it requires the presence of about 5 g/dl of unsaturated hemoglobin to be detected. Obviously, the greater the concentration of unsaturated hemoglobin the deeper will be the cyanosis, since it is the reduced hemoglobin that gives to blood its bluish red "venous" appearance. Normally, capillary blood contains about 2.5 g *of reduced hemoglobin per deciliter of blood*, a value derived as follows: Since capillary blood represents blood continuously giving up oxygen as it passes from the arterial to the venous end of the capillary, its unsaturated Hb content may be considered the *average* of the unsaturation of the arterial blood entering the capillary and the venous blood leaving. At a normal $O_2$ saturation of 97%, 15 g/dl of arterial Hb has 3% unsaturated Hb, or 0.45 g/dl. Venous blood 70% saturated has 30% unsaturated Hb, or 4.5 g/dl. The average capillary unsaturation would thus equal:

$$\frac{0.45 + 4.5}{2} = 2.5\% \text{ of unsaturated hemoglobin}^{[74]}$$

Assuming a hemoglobin concentration of 15 g/dl and an a-v oxygen saturation difference of 24% (corresponding to an a-v oxygen content difference of 5 vol%, as described earlier), we can calculate that an arterial oxygen saturation of 79% will produce a mean capillary unsaturation of 5 g/dl (Appendix 11). Hypoxia below this level, which the oxygen dissociation curve shows to be the equivalent of about 45 mm Hg partial pressure of oxygen, will probably produce visible cyanosis. However, since cyanosis depends on a specific concentration of unsaturated capillary hemoglobin, in anemia, with its reduced quantity of available hemoglobin, there may not be enough unsaturated hemoglobin to produce cyanosis until the arterial saturation drops well below 80%. Conversely, polycythemia, with its increased supply of hemoglobin, may show cyanosis even though there is adequate circulating oxygen.

### Chronic hypoxia

If the onset of hypoxia is slowly progressive, the body may adjust to it without any acute reactions. Diseases most likely to cause chronic hypoxia include gradually destructive or fibrotic lung diseases, congenital or acquired heart diseases, and chronic blood loss. In general, a persistent state of chronic hypoxia simulates a condition of persistent mental and physical fatigue. Mental responses may become sluggish and acuity diminished, and patients frequently complain of inability to perform physical tasks with the same ease as formerly. As a rule, however, chronic hypoxia itself is not a common cause of disability; rather it is the underlying disease responsible for the hypoxia. Often, relief of the hypoxia only, with oxygen breathing, will have little effect on disability. In many patients with whom the respiratory therapist will have contact, it is the physical effort to maintain normal oxygen and carbon dioxide levels that is the real cause of disability. Just as in acute hypoxia, if the oxygen lack is severe enough chronically, cyanosis will be present.

People who are born at high altitudes and who continue to live for several years at those altitudes must physiologically adjust from the prenatal period to an environment with a lower oxygen tension than that which exists at sea level. Inhabitants of mountainous areas, especially those of the South American Andes and our own Rocky Mountains, have been extensively studied over many years, up to and including the present, to determine how the body adjusts to hypobaric conditions. Many people live normal and active lives at partial pressures of oxygen in the same range as that found in patients at atmosphere who are suffering from hypoxia due to disease. It is obvious that altitude residents must be endowed with some type of adaptation to their "hypoxic" environment; and although many of the details of their physiologic responses, cardiac as well as pulmonary, are still under investigation, a few pertinent facts have been established. These people have a larger "red cell mass" than do natives of lowlands. This means that the total mass (or volume) of all their circulating erythrocytes is greater than that of the average human population, generally accomplished by an increased number of such cells. In addition, altitude dwellers have significantly larger lung volumes. In a general way it may be safe to assume that mountain life has certain rigors not found at sea level, if for no other reason than the nature of the terrain itself and the fact that the economy of such areas has often been agrarian. The survival of generations in such an environment attests to the efficiency of natural adaptation. Indeed, extensive studies have failed to show any ill effects in the indigenous populations, as long as they remain at altitude. Apparently, however, if altitude dwellers leave their original environment for the lowlands for a certain period of time, they often lose their natural adaptation; and a return to low ambient oxygen tensions puts them at the same disadvantage as is experienced by any other transient from sea level. For the individual with a normal cardiorespiratory system, a period of several days may be required to acclimatize to the reduced oxygen partial pressure, during which time he may experience weakness and lassitude, headaches, and a marked impairment of his usual physical performance.

In a sense, the pulmonary hypoxic patient, with his low arterial oxygen tension, is in a situation much like that of the altitude dweller or visitor, with the important difference that he has a defective respiratory mechanism. Nevertheless, chronic hypoxia is accompanied by an attempt on the part of the body to accommodate to the limited amount of oxygen that is able to reach the arterial blood. Hypoxia stimulates the bone marrow to increase its production of erythrocytes (an action called *hematopoiesis*) so that, as in the altitude dweller, there is an increase in the number of circulating red cells or, more specifically, an increase in the red cell mass. This state is referred to as *secondary polycythemia*, meaning a more than normal number of red cells secondary to the underlying pulmonary disease. As may be expected, there is also a condition called primary polycythemia, or polycythemia vera, entirely unrelated to cardiopulmonary dysfunction. In secondary polycythemia there is no increase in the other cellular blood components. The presence of polycythemia is alway suspected in a chronically hypoxic patient, but its actual identification may not be apparent. In many patients it may be readily detected by examination of the blood and by noting an increase in the *hematocrit*, which is the ratio between the volume of cells (mostly red cells, of course) and plasma, in a centrifuged sample of blood that has been treated with an anticoagulant. Normally, this does not exceed about 45%, but in polycythemia it may be nearly double. The hemoglobin content is similarly elevated from its usual upper limit of 15 g/dl to perhaps 20 g/dl, and measurement of the circulating erythrocytes will often show an excess above the normal high of around 5 million per cubic millimeter of blood.

It has been demonstrated, however, that such simple measures do not always reflect the hypoxic hematopoiesis responsible for polycythemia.[75] There is usually an associated increase in plasma volume; and if this is of sufficient degree, those measurements that relate red cell numbers or hemoglobin content to blood volume may appear erroneously normal. The most definitive diagnostic technique is an actual measurement of circulating red cell mass, using procedures that employ the dilution of dye by the blood, or the "tagging" of red cells by radioactive substances, which permits evaluation of both the total circulating blood volume and the erythrocyte mass. It is felt that polycythemia is common in patients with chronic lung disease and, if such tests are performed, many who would not otherwise be detected will be revealed.

Enough patients show elevated hematocrits and hemoglobin contents to warrant a few remarks about the clinical significance of such findings. With a sufficient increase in the ratio of red cells to blood fluid, viscosity of the blood can be expected to rise, constituting a matter of concern in the management of this condition.[76] At least in principle, the retarding effect on blood velocity and ease of flow of increasing viscosity may outweigh the advantages of the additional oxygen-carrying capacity of the enlarged red cell mass, and cellular distribution of oxygen may be impaired by a slowing of or interference with perfusion of body cells. It has been suggested that viscosity is not physiologically significant until the hematocrit reaches 55% to 60%.[77] Still there is justified fear that the sluggish circulation of polycythemia may cause intravascular thromboses, especially in vessels that may already be damaged by sclerosis or narrowing from other causes, because slowly moving blood clots more readily than does swiftly moving blood.

The patient with overt polycythemia is usually cyanotic, despite an actual increase in the volume of oxygen carried by the blood. This is because the cyanosis depends upon the amount of circulating unsaturated hemoglobin, not saturated, and the patient with a greater than normal number of red cells can have a corresponding increase in the amount of hemoglobin that is unsaturated as well as saturated. There are often complaints of headache, fullness in the head, nasal stuffiness, lethargy, difficulty in taking a deep breath, and epistaxis (nosebleed). The small vessels of the sclera (the white of the eye) may be seen as grossly congested from an increased blood volume. Finally, the increased volume of circulating blood, especially if associated with significant viscosity, places an abnormal work load on the heart to overcome the resistance to flow. The less muscular right ventricle is especially affected; it becomes strained, enlarges in an attempt to sustain its increased load, and eventually fails. This produces the so-called *cor pulmonale*, "pulmonary heart," right-sided heart disease secondary to pulmonary disease.

The respiratory therapist will commonly encounter a physical sign in patients called *clubbing*. Although this condition is not exclusively associated with hypoxia, because of its frequency in this state, it is believed to be pertinent to the discussion here. Clubbing is one state of a more generalized process that affects bones and joints known as hypertrophic osteoarthropathy.[78, 79] The essential lesion of osteoarthropathy is a chronic inflammatory process with thickening of periosteum, especially of the long bones, accompanied by the deposition of new bone. By x-ray examination the bones are seen to be thickened, giving rise to the term *hypertrophic*.

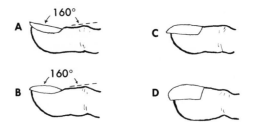

**Fig. 6-1.** Clubbing is characterized by marked curvature of the nail, a loss of the cuticular angle, an increase in the angle the surface of the nail makes with the terminal phalanx above the normal of 160 degrees, and a bulbous soft tissue swelling of the terminal phalanx. Sketches **A** and **B** show the contours of normal straight and curved nails; **C** and **D** represent increasing degrees of clubbing.

Joints may also be affected with swelling and inflammation. In a well-developed case many bones and joints may be affected with pain and disabling limitation of motion. Since the changes in the joints and long bones may frequently be detected by x-ray examination only and since lesser degrees are more frequently encountered in patients seen by the respiratory therapist, we will describe in greater detail that aspect of the process known as clubbing.

Clubbing may occur as an early stage of hypertrophic osteoarthropathy, or it may be found without subsequent long bone changes. It is manifested by a bulbous swelling of the terminal phalanges of the fingers and toes, which become enlarged and rounded, often but not always cyanotic. There is an increase in all diameters of the tips of the extremities, giving them a "drumstick" appearance. In contrast to the process found in long bones, pain is seldom a symptom of clubbing, although the soft tissue swelling at the ends of the digits may be considerable. A characteristic feature of clubbing is the contour of the nail, which becomes rounded both longitudinally and transversely. Curvature of the nail is not in itself necessarily a sign of disease and often is only a variation of the normal. In clubbing, however, the distortion of the nail is accompanied by a loss of the cuticular angle, the angle at the junction of the skin and nail as viewed from the side of the finger. This is shown in Fig. 6-1, illustrating a normal flat nail, a normal curved nail, and early and late clubbing. The marked cuticular angle in both normal nails is evident but is absent in clubbing. As the clubbing progresses from mild to severe, the degrees of curvature gradually increase. The first indication of imminent clubbing, before significant rounding is evident, is loss of the cuticular angle, associated with a "floating" nail base. This latter is characterized by a sponginess palpated under the base of the nail, which allows the nail to be moved up and down with compression.

Despite the frequency with which clubbing is seen, the specific etiology of clubbing, or the full osteoarthropathy, is unknown. It has been speculated that some or many of the following are responsible: chronic infection, unspecified toxins, capillary stasis from increased venous back pressure, arterial hypoxia, and local hypoxia. There is some disturbance in the circulation of the terminal portions of the digits, manifested by an increased blood flow. This has been demonstrated, through microphotography of a nail bed, as an increase in the width of the capillaries.[80] Nonetheless, this sign is an extremely important clinical one, even though it does not always indicate hypoxia, or even pulmonary disease. In adults approximately 75% to 85% of clubbing is due to pulmonary disease (lung tumors, bronchiectasis, fibrosis, empyema); 10% to 15% to cardiac disease (congenital right-to-left shunt, subacute bacterial endocarditis); 10% to liver or gastrointestinal disease (cirrhosis, chronic diarrhea conditions); 5% to miscellaneous causes (heredity, tumors of the thyroid or pharynx, aneurysms of large branches of the aorta). In children, clubbing is predominantly found with cystic fibrosis, bronchiectasis, empyema, and congenital heart disease.[81]

In summary, it can be said that clubbing suggests disease, first, of the respiratory tract, second, of the heart, and third, of the liver or gastrointestinal tract. It is of interest to note that the appearance of clubbing may antedate the x-ray signs of carcinoma of the lung by as many as 48 months. Finally, in many instances successful treatment of the underlying disease results in the resolution of the clubbing and a return of the digits to normal.

### Treatment of hypoxia

The obvious need in hypoxia is oxygen to preserve the life of body cells, but the details of its administration will be discussed elsewhere. It should be emphasized, however, that the objective of therapy is to restore arterial oxygen tension to normal, not to overload the blood with high pressures, except in very specific and limited circumstances. While hypoxia is being relieved, every effort must be made to correct the underlying pathology responsible for the hypoxia, for only when the latter is accomplished can we feel that the patient is improved. The therapist will see many patients in whom disease has left permanent lung damage of such a degree that sustained normal oxygenation is impossible to achieve, and the management of such patients will strain the ingenuity of physician and therapist alike. Again, to emphasize a point that cannot be overstressed, when hypoxia is associated with hypercapnia in the presence of an unresponsive respiratory center and the chemoreceptor hypoxic drive is active, ventilation must be supported mechanically during the administration of oxygen to prevent fatal apnea.

Where polycythemia is clinically significant, *phlebotomy* is often a useful procedure. Literally meaning "opening of a vein," phlebotomy entails the venous withdrawal of blood, in increments of about 300 ml, at intervals of 3 to 4 days. The objective of therapy is to lower the hematocrit to a maximum of about 50%, removing a segment of the red cell mass. Since blood water is restored by a shifting of the body fluids, the result is a reduction of blood viscosity. Some believe that the beneficial effects of phlebotomy are attributed to relief of the enlarged blood volume, not just to lowered viscosity. The clinical results are often very rewarding, as patients feel better both physically and mentally and the progress of cor pulmonale is retarded.[77] During an acute hospitalization, a patient may have several phlebotomies and then return as an outpatient for follow-up treatment as needed, usually with gradually decreasing frequency.

## AIRWAY OBSTRUCTION

Obstruction of the airways is one of the most common causes of cardiopulmonary disability and is almost always an important factor in the disease of patients treated by the respiratory therapist except for those with nonpulmonary ventilatory problems. Obstruction may be transient and reversible, or it may be permanent. We considered the effects of airway resistance on the mechanics of ventilation earlier and will now concern ourselves with a description of the physiologic and pathologic changes brought about by obstruction. For our purposes, we will not include gross obstruction, as from an inhaled foreign body or a large tumor, but rather will classify the causes of obstruction as *mucosal edema, bronchial spasm, increased secretions,* and *bronchiolar collapse.*

### Mucosal edema

Edema is an increase in the amount of interstitial fluid that bathes the body cells; pathologic changes cause a shift of body water from the plasma to the intercellular spaces, with resulting swelling of the affected area, which may be localized or extensive over larger areas of the body. The most common example of edema of the respiratory tract is the nasal swelling and inflammation (rhinitis) of the common cold, with the accompanying obstruction to breathing. This same reaction can be visualized in the lower portions of the respiratory passages. Severe edema of the larynx is well known as *croup,* and the same relative degree of airway narrowing can occur in the small bronchi and bronchioles.

Mucosal edema can be caused by:

1. Mechanical irritation or trauma to the respiratory mucosa, as from instrumentation, the presence of a foreign body, or the inhalation of caustic liquids or irritant fumes
2. Infection, bacterial or viral, in which the reaction represents a body defense against the invading organisms
3. Allergy to inhaled liquids or particulate matter, exemplified by the common allergic bronchial asthma

Respiratory mucosa becomes boggy in acute edema, soft, spongy, and waterlogged. There is usually an accompanying arteriolar and capillary congestion, which adds to the swelling. If of short duration, acute edema may be easily reversible following removal of its cause. However, if the edema is long lasting or frequently recurring, it may become *indurated,* giving to the tissue a permanent thickening and a firm, rather than soft, consistency. Such changes markedly interfere with mucosal function, especially through destruction of cilia, and the removal of the normal mucus blanket. Chronic respiratory infection aids in the perpetuation of such induration.

### Bronchial spasm

Spasm may be defined as an involuntary excessive contraction of a muscle. Common examples are found in extremity muscle cramps, spasm of neck muscles after injury, and intestinal cramps. Bronchial spasm is produced by excessive and prolonged contraction of the involuntary muscle fibers in the walls of the bronchi and bronchioles. Such contraction can seriously reduce airway lumens and may be localized or general. The causes of bronchial spasm are the same as those of edema listed above, but especially bronchial asthma, of which spasm is the major physiologic derangement.

## Increased secretions

By *increased bronchial secretions* we mean an actual increase in volume of secretions produced, an increase in their viscosity, or both. Although such reactions may follow exposure of the respiratory mucosa to many irritants, infection is the most frequent offender, and the common cold is again a familiar example with its abundance of sputum.

Bronchial secretions are composed of many ingredients[82]: *mucus*, secreted by the goblet cells and mucous glands of the bronchial mucosa; *DNA* (deoxyribonucleic acid, as a protein salt) and *RNA* (ribonucleic acid, as a protein salt), released from nuclei and cytoplasm of disintegrating cells; *plasma fluid* and *proteins*, including fibrinogen, escaping from pulmonary capillaries. The differentiation between normal and pathologic secretions depends on the relative concentrations of their components.

For purposes of discussion we can make a distinction between two broad types of sputum—mucoid and purulent. *Mucoid* secretions may be considered as a response by the airways to foreign matter invasion, infective or noninfective, in an attempt to remove the offending agent. One of the characteristics of a well-established chronic bronchitis is an actual increase in the number of mucous glands in the bronchial walls. The secretions so produced will consist of a high concentration of mucus, in respect to the other constituents. Mucus contains mucoproteins, a combination of any of several proteins with substances known as mucopolysaccharides, and long-chain carbohydrate-containing compounds, and it is these mucoproteins that are responsible for the viscosity of the secretions. Thus, when stimulated to overproduction of sputum by some irritative or pathologic process, the airways will contain larger amounts of fluid of a greater than normal viscosity. It should be added, because it is so important, that viscosity of normal secretions (normal relative concentrations of its components) can be raised to dangerous degrees simply by dehydration. This will be considered again later with the subject of humidification. *Purulent* secretions, on the other hand, are the result of invasion of the respiratory tract by pathogenic bacteria and the effect of such infection on the sputum. The natural inflammatory response to bacterial infection brings many leukocytes to the area, and they engage the organisms in destructive battle. The mucoid secretions, which are the first response, become grossly infiltrated with intact and fragmented bacteria, leukocytes, and tissue cells damaged by the process. Disruption of the cytoplasm and nuclei of the cells releases into the secretions a large amount of nucleoproteins, the DNA and RNA noted above. It is principally the deoxyribonucleic acid protein that gives to the secretions their purulent characteristics of viscosity to the point of tenacious stringiness and a yellow to green discoloration, in contrast to the colorless, clear or frothy, mucoid type. If the bronchial inflammation is acute, the sputum may have streaks of dark red or brown from extravasated blood. Finally, depending upon the offending bacteria or the presence of secondary or mixed infection, putrefactive organisms will often distinguish purulent sputum with a disagreeable odor.

The usually effective mucus blanket with its escalator cleansing action becomes less effective as its viscosity and volume increase, and these factors interfere with ciliary action. Often much of the cilia is destroyed, removing a valuable protective mechanism from the respiratory tract. As viscosity increases, the ordinary cough mechanism is less able to remove the secretions, and these plug airways, seriously interfering with ventilation. Parts of the lung may become airless, a condition referred to as *atelectasis*, with potentially grave consequences.

### Bronchiolar collapse

Usually associated with advanced bronchopulmonary disease, bronchiolar collapse is a clinically important form of small airway obstruction that, in many patients, becomes the most critical factor in ventilatory disability. The mechanism of its action is based on two components. First, there must be damage to the integrity of the bronchiolar walls so that they are unable to maintain patency in the face of the second factor, a pressure gradient across the bronchiolar walls. The conditions pre-

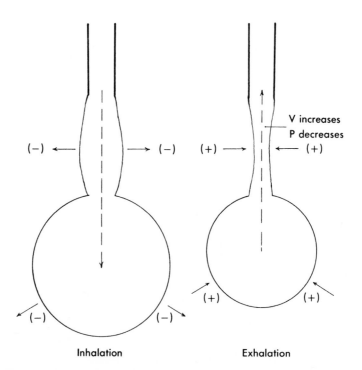

**Fig. 6-2.** A disease-weakened bronchiole is shown as thin walled and flaccid. Negative intrathoracic pressure inflates the alveolus with little difficulty. During exhalation, however, rising intrathoracic pressure compresses the diseased bronchiole as well as the alveolus, impeding airflow. In addition, the velocity of air through the bronchiolar restriction reduces intraluminal pressure, encouraging further collapse and worsening the obstruction.

disposing to bronchiolar collapse are most frequently found in the destructive lung diseases such as emphysema, bronchiectasis, and cystic disease; and, by far, emphysema is the predominant influence.

The bronchioles, devoid of cartilaginous support, are essentially highly pliable soft-walled tubes that depend for their patency on surrounding structures. Encompassed by masses of alveoli whose septa are arranged in a radial fashion apparently attached to their walls, the lumens of the bronchioles are kept from collapsing by the weblike support of these air sacs. During normal exhalation the rising intrathoracic pressure is exerted on the bronchiolar walls, as on all other thoracic structures, and does slightly narrow them; but the intact surrounding alveoli prevent further collapse. Fig. 6-2 illustrates diagrammatically what happens in the presence of bronchopulmonary disease. With destruction of alveoli and the loss of their supportive septa, the bronchiolar walls are responsive to pressure changes between the intrabronchiolar lumens and the pleural space. During inhalation the increasingly negative intrathoracic pressure and the inflow of air are sufficient to dilate the bronchioles to full patency. During exhalation, however, the rising thoracic pressure, unopposed by alveolar septal countertraction, compresses the resilient bronchioles and narrows them to the point of interference with airflow. At the same time, as the exhaled air is being forced through the narrowing bronchioles, its velocity progressively increases. In keeping with the Bernoulli principle, with the increase in intraluminal velocity, there is a drop in intraluminal pressure and the negative pressure gradient thus established across the bronchiole wall between the lumen and pleural space favors further narrowing. A vicious cycle is thereby set in motion that perpetuates the continuing airway collapse.[83]

The patients in whom this condition is clinically significant are usually those who already have expiratory difficulty from their underlying disease and must exert exceptionally great effort during exhalation. It is thus evident to what degree the element of bronchiolar collapse can contribute to a steadily worsening disability. In addition to its chronic influence on exhalation, bronchiolar collapse can produce an acute state referred to as *acute air trapping*. Frequently, without warning, a patient may suddenly find he is unable to complete a phase of exhalation he has already started. His chest is immobilized in a position of partial exhalation, and he is unable either to inhale or to empty his lungs further. He may struggle to move his chest and become severely cyanotic, especially in the face and neck. Such an episode may be triggered by an unnoticed early expiratory effort of greater force than usual; and as the sequence of events described above comes into play after the movement of part of his exhaled air, a number of his bronchioles completely collapse, trapping the remainder of his tidal volume. Although frightening to the point of panic to the patient and observers alike, these attacks are generally self-limiting. A series of sharp forceful lateral squeezes applied to both sides of the thorax will often supply spurts of air of sufficient pressure to overcome the collapse and empty the lungs. This is a technique learned by many patients and especially by members of their families. To prevent acute trapping and to accomplish the maximum exhalation with the minimum of effort, patients either learn spontaneously or are taught the technique of "pursed-lip breathing." In the maneuver the patient slightly purses his lips as he exhales, deliberately prolonging exhalation and trying to maintain an even flow of air. The moderate obstruction he effects at the mouth builds up a back pressure in his airways, not enough to make exhalation difficult but enough to retard air velocity and reduce the transbronchiolar pressure gradient to prevent collapse.

### Effect of obstruction on ventilation

Obstruction greatly increases the work of breathing because of the elevated resistance of smaller air passages and the retarding effect of air turbulence. Resistance to breathing may be more pronounced in one phase or the other of ventilation. For example, the laryngeal obstruction of childhood croup may necessitate such a strong inspiratory effort that there will be noticeable retraction of the sternum and epigastrium during inspiration, and the flow of air past the obstruction may produce a harsh sound known as a *stridor*. Most often, however, obstruction is a major problem in chronic bronchopulmonary diseases, and then exhalation is impeded. To a considerable degree the ventilatory muscles can overcome obstruction to inhalation, but the passive nature of normal exhalation is unable to deflate the lung to its resting position, and exhalation must employ muscular effort, at times very strenuous. The tremendous work involved in moving air against obstruction utilizes so much physical energy that it constitutes one of the major factors in the disability of chronic pulmonary diseases. Indeed, muscular fatigue may lead to ventilatory failure, hypercapnia, and respiratory acidosis.

Expiration time is usually prolonged beyond that of inhalation, and often contraction of the upper abdomen is evident during the latter part of exhalation. If bronchospasm is extensive or mobile secretions are present, characteristic breath sounds can be heard by the unaided ear or by the use of the stethoscope (auscultation) during exhalation. *Wheezes* are high-pitched squeaky noises produced by air passing with some velocity through passages narrowed by spasm or thick secretions. *Rhonchi* are coarser, lower pitched sounds caused by vibration of bronchial secretions in the airflow. *Rales* are fine bubbling or crackling sounds, usually noted during inhalation as air passes through fluid in the alveoli, and are not necessarily reflections of obstruction.

### Treatment of obstruction

Details of treatment will be considered elsewhere, but the general procedures will include the following.

*Aspiration.* Aspiration is the removal of secretions through the use of suctioning. It may be accomplished by means of *bronchoscopy*, the passage of a long, lighted tube, under direct vision, into the bronchi, allowing examination of these structures as well as extensive aspiration. Frequently employed is the insertion of a catheter into the main-stem bronchi in patients in whom a *tracheostomy* tube has been placed just below the larynx, or in whom an *endotracheal* tube has been passed through the mouth and larynx into the upper trachea. Small catheters, passed through needles inserted between the tracheal rings just below the larynx, are occasionally used for aspiration of thin secretions. These procedures will be described in more detail later.

*Aerosols.* The inhalation of very fine particles of liquids, in the form of a mist is extensively used and includes the following:

1. Water—to thin secretions by increasing their water content
2. Bronchodilators—agents that reduce bronchial spasm
3. Decongestants—agents that reduce vascular congestion
4. Liquefacients—agents that liquefy secretions by altering their physical or chemical characteristics

*Systemic liquefacients.* Some medications, taken by mouth or vein, make bronchial secretions more liquid and easier to raise.

*Postural drainage.* Physical therapeutic techniques that utilize gravity in mobilizing secretions, by positioning the patient, are an important part of both short-term and long-term therapy.

## PULMONARY DISTENTION

Pulmonary distention is a state of hyperinflation of the lung characterized by an increase in the functional residual capacity (FRC), and its two major causes are *airway obstruction* and *loss of lung elasticity.* As a rule, distention due to obstructed airways is generally of a temporary and reversible nature, exemplified by an attack of acute bronchial asthma. In this condition, diffuse bronchial spasm is the outstanding feature, and during such an episode the FRC may be markedly increased. On subsidence and in the absence of complications (especially bronchial infection), the resting thoracic level returns to normal and the FRC is reduced. It is also probable that some distention may accompany acute episodes of obstructive bronchitis, but this is apt to be variable and evanescent.

From a practical, respiratory therapy point of view, *pulmonary distention* usually refers to the hyperinflation of pulmonary emphysema. Although we have not considered the clinical and pathologic nature of this disease in a specific discussion, we have mentioned it so many times that the student may already be forming a mental picture of its characteristics. There are many excellent descriptions of emphysema (often called obstructive emphysema, bronchitis-emphysema, and chronic obstructive lung disease, among its many names) in any number of texts, and the student is encouraged to familiarize himself well with it, for it will probably be the most prevalent disease he will encounter. We will note only a few of its details here as they pertain to distention.

Basically, emphysema is a destructive disease characterized by disruption of variable numbers of alveolar walls; the more disruption, the more severe is the disease. This destructive process converts the lung from an organ with a large number of uniform-sized air spaces into one with a smaller number of variable-sized spaces and fewer gas diffusion surfaces. A consequence of the resulting architectural change in the lung is a marked unevenness of airflow and air distribution and, most serious, a great loss of elastic fibers.

Until fairly recently, it was generally believed that destructive distention was a sequela of progressive or persistent airway obstruction. It was postulated that because of any of the common causes of bronchial and bronchiolar obstruction, the resistance to expiratory airflow developed an intra-alveolar back pressure that eventually destroyed the alveolar walls. Somewhat oversimplified, it was like the rupture of a hyperinflated balloon. The continued expiratory resistance was then supposed to have trapped air in the enlarged air sacs. However, studies on normal individuals whose lungs are subjected to very high intrapulmonary pressures from back pressure for long periods of time (e.g., wind instrument musicians) have failed to show any adverse effects on lung function and no signs of distention.[84] Refined pathologic techniques that permit better correlation between pathology and function have demonstrated that in many if not most instances the distention precedes and causes the airway obstruction so frequently seen with it. It is speculated that some factors not yet clearly defined (sometimes infectious?) destroy the alveolar walls, with loss of diffusing surface and elasticity. Bronchiolar collapse, described above, causes obstruction, which is worsened by an ensuing chronic bronchitis subsequent to failure of cough-clearance of the airways.[83, 85] By this mechanism, following alveolar disruption the actual pulmonary distention is the result of loss of elasticity rather than of obstruction, since the thoracic expansile forces are now relatively unopposed.

Less well defined as a pathologic entity is the degenerative change that accompanies the aging process and that diminishes the tone of elastic tissue throughout the body. The loss of skin elasticity in the elderly is a common observation, and apparently a similar phenomenon takes place in the lung. The increase in FRC often seen with advancing age is sometimes unwisely referred to as *senile emphysema*, although there is no concrete evidence that this constitutes a true disease.

### Effect of distention on ventilation

The adverse effects of distention on ventilation can be described in the following three categories: reduced inspiratory capacity, low position of the diaphragm, and enlarged FRC.

*Reduced inspiratory capacity.* The elevated end-expiratory resting level of the thorax and the low, flat diaphragm (to be described next) produce the inspiratory position of the thorax. Thus at the resting level the lungs are already in a position of partial inspiration, since the lung-thorax relationship is unbalanced in the direction of the thoracic forces. The inspiratory capacity is encroached upon, and increase in tidal volume in response to exertional needs is limited. (See Fig. 3-22.)

*Low position of diaphragm.* Increase in the FRC forces the chest into the inspiratory position as the lung-thorax resting level rises, and the overdistention of the lung depresses and flattens the contour of the diaphragmatic domes. In a low position, contraction of the diaphragm, even though feeble, instead of lowering itself, pulls in the costal margin and reduces the volume of the thorax during inhalation, rather than enlarging it. With loss of effective use of the diaphragm, reduction in intrathoracic pressure is dependent upon contraction of the intercostals and the accessory ventilatory muscles. The pull of the accessory muscles causes an upward and outward displacement of the sternum, an increase in the sternal angle (the junction of the manubrium and body of the sternum, at the level of the second rib), and eventually an increase in the anteroposterior diameter of the chest. This produces the *barrel-chest* deformity common to long-standing distention. The thoracic negative pressure, generated at a tremendous energy cost to the patient, also acts upon the ineffective diaphragm, pulling it *upward* during inhalation, the so-called "paradoxical ventilation." Thus, while the intercostals and accessories are working hard to enlarge the thorax, the rising diaphragm, sucked upward by their action, partially negates their efforts, and the net gain in intrathoracic volume is small in proportion to the physical effort expended. When inspiratory efforts are strenuous enough, not only is the diaphragm elevated during inhalation but the abdominal wall is also retracted in a contrary manner. Exhalation, lacking the effective use of the abdominals, is a slow process, depending upon inadequate passive recoil and expiratory action of the intercostals; and during exhalation, rising intrathoracic pressure drives down the diaphragm as the abdominal wall balloons outward. The clinical picture is one of a short, gasping inhalation, with extensive use of accessory muscles of ventilation and epigastric retraction, followed by a prolonged exhalation accompanied by varying degrees of epigastric protrusion. The presence of a barrel-chest defect, with or without paradoxical ventilation, signifies serious disruption of the normal lung-thoracic architecture, and the attentive therapist should always be on the watch for it.

**Large functional residual capacity.** The physiologic significance of an enlarged FRC can be appreciated only if the part it plays in ventilation is visualized clearly. Since the FRC is a substantial volume of air remaining in the lung at the end of a quiet exhalation, the next tidal volume of inhaled air must mix with it to reach the alveoli. In other words, air that is ventilating the alveoli with each breath is a mixture of air already in the lung and new air entering. The larger the residual air volume the greater is the dilution of incoming tidal air. Since enlarged FRC is usually accompanied by airway obstruction, large and variable-sized air spaces, or both, an even distribution of tidal air to all alveoli is impossible. Thus *uneven distribution of inspired air* is a characteristic of severe pulmonary distention and results in nonuniform alveolar ventilation, a hazard to gas exchange, since it interferes with the normal ventilation-perfusion balance to be described below.

An estimate of the evenness with which inspired air is distributed among the alveoli can be made in the cardiopulmonary laboratory. One technique involves the breathing of pure oxygen for a number of minutes, gradually washing out nitrogen remaining in the lung from previous air breathing. The exhaled air is monitored by an analyzer that measures the gradually decreasing concentration of nitrogen removed, and the time-concentration relationship is noted. In a lung disrupted by severe obstruction or especially in which variable-sized air spaces empty in an irregular fashion, the relationship will be markedly abnormal. Another technique utilizes the inhalation of a known concentration of inert helium; by measurement of the time it takes for the lung air to reach equilibrium with the inhaled gas, the distribution characteristic of the lung can be determined.

**Treatment of distention**

The treatment of distention is nonspecific and is aimed to achieve the following.

*Reduce obstruction.* The methods employed to reduce obstruction are those described earlier, with emphasis on the use of aerosols and postural drainage.

*Improve pulmonary air distribution.* Closely related to the management of obstruction, treatment of distention employs the intermittent use of mechanical ventilators to assist air distribution by providing air under pressure. Aerosols to reduce obstruction, frequently delivered at the same time, help to maintain the integrity of the airways while ventilating alveoli that are otherwise poorly supplied with air.

*Improve mechanics of ventilation.* To help consolidate gains realized from the above two therapies, patients are retrained in the proper use of their ventilatory muscles through breathing exercises. Emphasis is placed upon restoration of effective use of the diaphragm and upon aiding the patient to limit his reliance on his accessory muscles. This approach is incorporated into the long-term management of the patient, and its techniques become part of his daily activities.

## PULMONARY RESTRICTION

Pulmonary restriction is defined as an interference with easy or adequate lung expansion and is often associated with a decrease in lung and/or thoracic compliance. There are many pathologic states that can restrict expansion of the lung, some of which will be briefly described in the following four groups: thoracic, intrathoracic (nonpulmonary), pulmonary, and abdominal.

*Thoracic causes.* Some of the thoracic causes of restriction are the result of structural changes in the chest, others of reduced flexibility:

1. Kyphoscoliosis is an abnormal curvature of the spine that, when it affects the dorsal segment, distorts the thoracic cage by compressing one side or the other. In general, it is produced by an imbalance between the bilateral skeletal muscle groups, weakness of one group allowing unopposed traction by the other, with eventual tilting and rotation of the spine and chest cage. Poliomyelitis is a frequent offender, as are developmental defects of childhood and adolescence from causes as yet unknown. The disfigured thorax may imprison portions of the lung, preventing normal expansion.

2. Destructive bone diseases of the spine and thorax, such as tuberculosis and osteoporosis, may produce restrictive distortion not classified as kyphoscoliosis.

3. Trauma, such as sternal and costal fractures, will cause severe although usually temporary restriction.

4. Reduced thoracic flexibility can result from such diseases as arthritis, scleroderma, and fibromyositis.

5. Paralysis of ventilatory muscles, as in poliomyelitis and myasthenia gravis, although not reflecting a decrease in compliance, markedly interferes with lung expansion.

*Intrathoracic (nonpulmonary) causes.* Diseases within the chest often impede lung expansion because of the following:

1. Pleurisy limits ventilation by restrictive pain or by subsequent restrictive pleural thickening.

2. Fluid in the pleural cavity restricts pulmonary expansion by direct compression of the lung. Such fluid may be *serous* in character, from pleural inflammation or heart failure; *purulent*, from pleural infection or extension of a lung infection into the pleural space or from infected chest trauma; or *hemorrhagic*, from trauma or destructive lung disease.

*Pulmonary causes.* Most of the pulmonary causes of lung restriction can be put into one of two categories:

1. Fibrosis or scarring of the lung accounts for most of the restrictive problems. It is a sequela of recurrent respiratory infections, often accompanying chronic bronchopulmonary disease such as emphysema, and follows such destructive diseases as tuberculosis, bronchiectasis, and many industrial or occupational diseases.

2. Intrapulmonary vascular congestion can significantly impair the compliance of the lung. Because of a failing heart, blood in the pulmonary circuit may back up, distending the vasculature of the lung with an increased blood volume. Since the total compliance of the lung depends on all structures in it, as the flexibility of the pulmonary vessels lessens with their congestion, the overall flexibility of the lung will be reduced. Mobility of the lung will be further impaired if the congestion is accompanied by pulmonary edema, with its increased fluid in the pulmonary intercellular spaces, and fluid in the alveoli.

*Abdominal causes.* Through immobilization of the diaphragm, abdominal pathology is a frequent cause of pulmonary restriction:

1. Abdominal splinting, a rigid contraction of the musculature of the abdominal wall, is usually an unconscious reaction to pain from intra-abdominal disease or postoperative discomfort. Ventilation can be seriously impeded, and the combination of restriction and hypoventilation comprises a common respiratory complication of abdominal disease.

2. Abdominal distention results from excessive accumulation of gas or air in the stomach or intestinal tract. This may be of such a degree that the abdominal wall is pushed outward into a rounded dome under great tension.

3. Abdominal fluid, referred to as *ascites*, usually the result of liver disease, heart failure, or some pathology causing widespread peritoneal irritation, increases intra-abdominal pressure to interfere with diaphragmatic descent.

## Effect of restriction on ventilation

Restriction reduces the vital capacity and in severe instances may limit it nearly to the resting tidal volume. In this case, as with distention, there may be little or no inspiratory reserve volume to accommodate the needs of exertion. The FRC may be normal in the absence of associated distention, but despite this, the measured residual volume is often enlarged, since the rigidity of the lung, or the lack of muscular effort, reduces the size of the forced expiratory reserve volume. More often than not, other ventilatory disturbances accompany restriction, especially in patients with chronic bronchopulmonary disease.

**Treatment of restriction**

Some specific objectives of treatment are obvious, such as the removal of pleural or abdominal fluid, the removal of pleural adhesions, the repair of structural defects of the thorax, and the improvement of circulation. In many patients, however, such corrective causes are absent, and relief of the restrictive agent is not possible. In general, the treatment is that outlined for pulmonary distention. The more specific techniques of maintaining controlled mechanical ventilation of the restricted patient in ventilatory failure will be discussed separately.

## VENTILATION-PERFUSION IMBALANCE

A disturbance in the ratio between ventilation and pulmonary perfusion is always secondary to some other disorder and is a condition that may be found with many types of diseases. In addition, this imbalance may also be the result of some of the disturbances already discussed in this chapter, but its clinical effects are so widespread and important that it deserves detailed consideration in any discussion of pathophysiology.

In terms of the body as a whole, with its myriad of individual cellular demands, the total exchange of oxygen for carbon dioxide is called the body *respiratory quotient (RQ)* and is expressed as the ratio of the quantity of carbon dioxide produced to oxygen consumed per unit of time, $\dot{V}_{CO_2}/\dot{V}_{O_2}$. Depending on the net metabolic needs of all parts of the body at a given moment, this ratio ranges from 0.7 to 1.0, with an average of 0.8. Because of biochemically limiting factors of metabolism, the RQ cannot exceed 1.0. Thus less carbon dioxide is produced by the body than oxygen is utilized, and to maintain necessary tissue gas exchange there must be a comparable exchange in the lung between alveoli and blood. For this the tidal flow of air into and out of the alveoli constitutes the pulmonary ventilation, and the pulmonary capillary blood flow, in direct contact with the alveolar walls, provides the perfusion of the lung. The relationship between the ventilation and perfusion is referred to as the *ventilation/perfusion ratio*, or the *respiratory/exchange ratio (R)*, symbolically designated as $\dot{V}_A/\dot{Q}_c$. It is the ratio between the minute flow of air into the alveoli and the minute flow of blood through the pulmonary capillaries. The respiratory exchange ratio of the whole lung is the same as the respiratory quotient, averaging 4:5, or 0.8[86] This means that for every 4 liters of alveolar ventilation, there are 5 liters of pulmonary capillary blood flow.

A normal R in itself, however, is not adequate assurance of effective gas exchange, since it does not tell us how the ventilation and perfusion are distributed throughout the lung. Consider the hypothetical example of all the ventilation going to one lung and all the perfusion to the other. In this situation, although the total amount of ventilation and perfusion may be normal, and R equal to 0.8, it is obvious that gas exchange will be absent and survival impossible. It is important to grasp the concept of a whole host of respiratory exchange ratios scattered throughout the lungs, the so-called "regional distribution of R's." Each lobule of the lung might well have its own ratio, depending on the local balance between ventilation and perfusion, but the overall lung R will be the same as the respiratory quotient. One can imagine generalized or localized disease or injury modifying both ventilation and perfusion so that the final functional effect on ventilation would depend on which was the more disturbed. Thus, when we attempt to classify the physiologic effects of disease as either ventilatory or circulatory imbalance of the ratio, we must recognize that either or both elements may be at fault.

Through the techniques of lung photo scanning it is possible to calculate ventilation/perfusion ratios and visually display regional distribution of ventilation and perfusion.[87-92] In principle, radioactive substances are injected intravenously to be carried to the pulmonary circulation or are introduced into the airway as gas or aerosol to penetrate the respiratory tract. A recording device, which may be a relatively simple rectilinear scanner or a highly sophisticated computer-assisted scintillation camera, by several techniques picks up the radiation emitted from the chest. The radiation "counts" are recorded on x-ray film or magnetic tape as up to 500,000 minute dots, in total producing a map of the lungs. In healthy lungs there is a normal distribution of density of the counts, indicating unimpaired pulmonary blood flow in perfusion scans and unobstructed airways in ventilation scans. Diseased lungs, in contrast, show areas of absent or low density radiation counts, so-called "cold spots," demonstrating lack of normal perfusion or ventilation. Interpretation of scans requires great skill and experience, but it should be apparent that these examinations are of tremendous value in detecting or evaluating pulmonary vessel blockage as from blood clots, cystic or emphysematous disease with loss of lung structure and vessels, through perfusion scanning, and airway obstruction with ventilation scanning.

**Perfusion scan.** The following inert radioactive substances may be used for perfusion scanning:

1. Microaggretated albumin (human) labeled with either radioactive iodine $^{133}$I, ($^{133}$I MAA), or technetium, $^{99m}$Tc ($^{99m}$Tc MAA)
2. Technetium–iron hydroxide aggregates ($^{99m}$Tc–iron hydroxide)
3. Indium particles ($^{113}$In)
4. Xenon gas dissolved in saline ($^{133}$Xe)

These are injected intravenously as boluses of less than 1 million particles with diameters between $25\mu$ and $50\mu$ (except the gas $^{133}$Xe). About one of each 250,000 precapillary pulmonary arterioles or pulmonary capillaries are temporarily blocked, allowing time for radiation counts to be recorded. Experimental evidence suggests that significant hemodynamic changes do not occur until 2000 times the usual image dose is used.

**Ventilation scan.** Ventilation scanning is generally performed shortly after perfusion studies if the patient is able to hold his breath at end-inspiration for at least 15 seconds. The two most currently popular techniques use the following materials:

1. *Technetium albuminate ($^{99m}$Tc MAA)*. Five microcuries (mc) in 5 to 10 ml saline are nebulized, and the aerosol is delivered by an inspiratory positive-pressure breathing (IPPB) machine until gone. Radiation counts are made at appropriate intervals.
2. *Xenon gas ($^{133}$Xe)*. Twenty-five microcuries of $^{133}$Xe gas are mixed with 5 liters of 100% oxygen in a closed spirometer system. End-inspiratory breath holding for at least 15 seconds is required for radiation counting. Easy breathing is

continued until equilibrium is reached between patient and reservoir; more counts are recorded; then the tracer gas is washed out with 100% oxygen.

Radioaerosol ventilation scans give accurate pictures in patients with normal airways and lung parenchyma, but they are apparently less dependable in patients with chronic obstructive airway disease. The general problems of aerosol penetration and retention, which is an important topic to be discussed later in this text, affect the efficiency of radioaerosol particles in evaluating ventilation. In contrast, inhalation of the gas $^{133}$Xe is more physiological than an artificial aerosol and gives good views of regional ventilation in both health and disease. It should be noted that obstruction of small airways, less than 2 mm in diameter, may not be evident in standard pulmonary function tests but may readily be detected by $^{133}$Xe ventilation scanning.

Let us now consider some of the implications of decreased and increased regional respiratory exchange ratios.

*Low $\dot{V}/\dot{Q}$.* A ratio less than the normal body respiratory quotient of 0.8 results from a decrease in regional alveolar ventilation, physiologically producing what is known as a *venous admixture.* Through some pathologic process, variable numbers of alveoli are subjected to differing degrees of underventilation. If they remain fully perfused, the blood leaving them will not be normally saturated with oxygen and will be at least partially venous in nature as it combines with the mixed arterial blood leaving areas of normal R. Fig. 6-3 schematically illustrates this mechanism with the complete obstruction of one alveolar unit.

The venous admixture is actually a *physiologic venous-arterial shunt,* although the term *admixture* is preferred in current terminology. It is a shunt because the effect, on mixed arterial oxygenation, of perfused blood denied its normal quota of oxygen is the same as that of blood bypassing the lung physically. It is termed *physiologic* because it is caused by a functional derangement of an organ that may have basically normal structure. We have already discussed how the natural human environment of ambient air at 1 atm pressure produces a small normal venous admixture because the distribution of ventilation throughout the lung is not even, and with any given breath some alveoli are incompletely ventilated. Thus the normal arterial oxygen saturation is about 97%. Fig. 6-4 diagrams the normal physiologic shunt, or venous admixture, showing the shunted blood as if it bypassed the lung.

We shall take some time to discuss the effect of a venous admixture on blood oxygenation. This will serve the double purpose of acquainting the student with a useful technique of evaluating cardiopulmonary function and at the same time enabling him to call upon some of the concepts of physiology that he has studied in an unavoidably isolated fashion so that he can put them to practical use. The important fact is not overlooked that our purpose is to educate the respiratory thrapist, not a professional postgraduate student, and although the detailed concepts of ventilation-perfusion relationships often tax the minds of the experienced physiologist, there is no reason why the therapist should not be stimulated to learn as much as he can about the patient he will be treating. We will use two hypothetical situations, with a graphic illustration of each, to show the clinical effect of a significant venous admixture. In the interest of simplicity, we will take some liberties with reality. First, the situations we will create will be exaggerated for emphasis, and as shown in Figs. 6-5 and 6-6, the lung in question will consist of only two alveoli, each with its own perfusing capillary. One alveolus will be completely nonventilated and will resemble a closed space; the other will ventilate under differing conditions. Second, in considering blood oxygen content, we will concern ourselves only with oxygen combined with hemoglobin, at 15 g/dl, ignoring the dissolved fraction. This facilitates calculation and, because of the minute

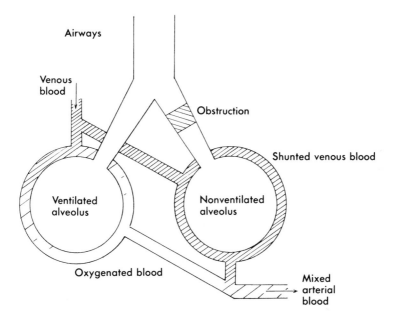

**Fig. 6-3.** *Venous admixture* is a term given to mixed arterial blood leaving the lung when it contains both fully oxygenated blood from normally ventilated alveoli and incompletely oxygenated "shunted venous blood" from poorly ventilated alveoli. In the sketch, ventilation to one alveolus is normal but is blocked to the other, and capillary shading represents a quantitative index of unsaturation. In the normal subject quietly breathing ambient air at 1 atm pressure, mixed arterial blood is approximately 97% saturated with oxygen.

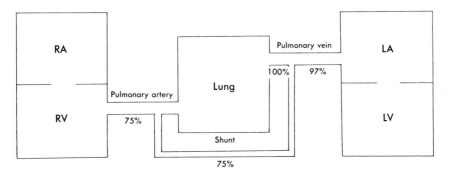

**Fig. 6-4.** This diagrams the normal physiologic shunt, or venous admixture, during tidal ventilation of air at 1 atm pressure. It shows some venous blood, with an $O_2$ saturation of 75%, as if it bypassed the lung as a result of perfusing scattered, nonventilated alveoli. The mixture of the shunted with the fully oxygenated blood gives arterial blood its usual saturation of about 97%.

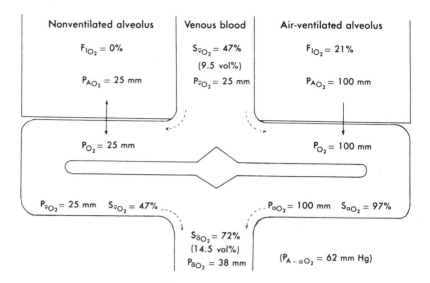

**Fig. 6-5.** The sketch represents an alveolus with no ventilation and one with normal air ventilation, each being perfused by one half the venous blood entering the system. The data are based on a hemoglobin content of 15 g/dl and an a-v oxygen difference of 5 vol%. Arterialized blood leaving the ventilated alveolus combines with shunted (venous) blood leaving the nonventilated alveolus, giving the mixed arterial blood a saturation of 72% and a $P_{O_2}$ of 38 mm Hg. There is thus an oxygen tension difference, or gradient, between the alveolar air and the mixed arterial blood of 62 mm Hg. This is called an A-$a_{O_2}$ gradient, symbolized as $P_{A-a_{O_2}}$.

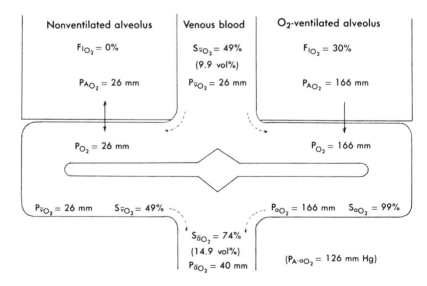

**Fig. 6-6.** This system is the same as that of Fig. 6-5, except that the functioning alveolus is ventilated with an inspired gas mixture containing 30% oxygen, resulting in a calculated $P_{A_{O_2}}$ of 166 mm Hg, and an A-$a_{O_2}$ gradient of 126 mm Hg. Thus, as long as blood is being shunted, an increase in $F_{I_{O_2}}$ will lead to a disproportionately smaller increase in $P_{a_{O_2}}$ and a widened A-$a_{O_2}$ gradient.

quantities of dissolved gas at atmosphere, introduces little error. We will further assume that, as the venous blood enters our simple systems, its flow divides so that equal volumes perfuse each alveolus and the arterial blood leaving is thus a mixture of equal parts from each alveolus. Finally, we will assume that in each instance the a-v oxygen difference (representing oxygen given up to body cells) will remain steady at 5 vol%. To accomplish this, we have calculated values that allow the fully arterialized blood from the ventilated alveolus, when diluted with the shunted blood of the nonventilated alveolus, to have an oxygen content 5 vol% greater than it has when it returns to the lung as venous blood after perfusing body cells. The student will notice that all values are exceedingly lower than the normals to which he has been exposed, but he must observe that these conditions represent what can be called a 50% shunt, in which half the circulating blood is denied oxygenation. Although they are grossly abnormal, there are clinical states that closely match them.

In Fig. 6-5, blood perfusing the air-ventilated alveolus, with its oxygen tension of 100 mm Hg, is fully oxygenated and approaches the outflow tract with a $P_{O_2}$ of 100 mm Hg and a saturation of 97%. On the other hand, blood perfusing the nonventilated alveolus picks up no oxygen. In fact, theoretically, there could be a diffusion of oxygen from the venous blood into the closed and oxygen-poor alveolus, maintaining a $P_{A_{O_2}}$ equal to the 25 mm Hg tension of the perfusing blood. This half of the blood volume thus reaches the outflow still as venous blood, with its $P_{O_2}$ of 25 mm Hg and a saturation of 47%. and here the two streams unite and thoroughly mix. The oxygen content of the *mixed* arterial blood depends on the degree of saturation of each of its two components, since saturation is volumetrically related to hemoglobin content. In this instance the final saturation is the average of the values of the two halves, or 72%, and by the normal oxygen dissociation curve this represents a partial pressure of 38 mm Hg. Note that a saturation of 72%, in this very hypoxic arterial blood, is the equivalent of a combined oxygen content of 14.5 vol% (72% of 20.1 = 14.5). On this basis the oxygen content of the venous blood was established as 9.5 vol%, at a partial pressure of 25 mm Hg.

If this were a subject under study and we were to get a sample of exhaled alveolar air to measure its oxygen content, or if we calculated it according to the alveolar air equation, we would find a $P_{A_{O_2}}$ of about 100 mm Hg.* The nonventilating alveolus, of course, contributes nothing to alveolar sampling. The difference between the oxygen tensions in the alveoli and in sampled arterial blood constitutes a gradient, called an *alveolar-arterial oxygen tension gradient*, or more simply an A-a$_{O_2}$ gradient, symbolized as $P_{A-a_{O_2}}$. Under normal conditions, with the small physiologic shunt usually present, the A-a gradient does not exceed 10 mm Hg. The gradient in our example is 62 mm Hg (100 − 38). A large gradient usually identifies a state of hypoxia as due to some cause other than an inadequate alveolar supply of oxygen and generally resolves the diagnosis to a differential between a venous admixture and a diffusion defect. Although we have illustrated the manner in which a gradient can be caused by shunting, a block to diffusion of oxygen across the A-C membrane theoretically

---

*See Appendix 12 for an explanation of the alveolar air equation.

could just as well have been responsible. Let us now describe a procedure that will help to differentiate between an $A-a_{O_2}$ gradient resulting from a shunt and one from a diffusion defect.

Fig. 6-6 represents the same general arrangement as described above, but now the ventilating alveolus carries a 30% oxygen mixture instead of the 21% of air. An a-v oxygen difference of 5 vol% is still assumed for uniformity. With this breathing mixture the alveolar oxygen tension is calculated to be approximately 166 mm Hg, and the perfusing blood leaving the ventilated alveolus equilibrates at this tension. The arterial oxygen saturation corresponding to a partial pressure of 166 mm Hg is difficult to read with accuracy from the flat upper portion of the dissociation curve, but according to a table designed to overcome this problem, it is approximately 99%.[93] Employing the same technique as before in determining the characteristics of the mixed arterial blood leaving the lung, we find a final arterial oxygen saturation of 74% and an oxygen tension of 40 mm Hg. If we now compare the alveolar and arterial oxygen partial pressures, we find an $A-a_{O_2}$ gradient of 126 mm Hg (166 − 40).

These two examples make it evident that, as we increase the oxygen concentration in the breathing mixture and as long as some of the blood is consistently bypassing ventilated alveoli, we will get a decreasing proportionate increase in the oxygen content of the mixed arterial blood. This should be expected, and if the student will examine the data carefully, he will see how the characteristics of the oxygen dissociation curve limit the value of increasing the oxygenation of the ventilated alveolus. We can thereby make the following generalization. If an alveolar-arterial oxygen tension gradient exists when room air is breathed and it is primarily due to a shunt, the gradient will widen with increasing concentrations of oxygen in the breathing mixture. It should be pointed out that this holds true for the normal subject since his negligible gradient will also increase as he breathes oxygen-enriched air. Finally, whereas an A-a oxygen gradient is characteristically present with a lowered $\dot{V}/\dot{Q}$, an arterial-alveolar $P_{CO_2}$ gradient or difference is not. The greater diffusibility of carbon dioxide permits its easy escape through ventilated alveoli, aided by the often present hyperventilation accompanying hypoxia.

In contrast to venous admixture, the hypoxia due to an impairment of oxygen diffusion is generally thought to be overcome by an elevation of the inspired oxygen concentration. With increasing alveolar oxygen partial pressure, enough additional oxygen molecules are diffused into the blood to bring the latter above the hypoxemic level, although at times breathing concentrations close to 100% may be necessary. Because of this, a subject with an A-a oxygen gradient from a diffusion defect will show a reduction in his gradient as he breathes an increased oxygen mixture, since the rise in his blood gas tension will be proportionately higher than that of his alveoli (although, of course, the former can never exceed the latter). It might be added that in both shunt and diffusion defect the hypoxia will worsen with exercise, and gradients will widen as the increased tissue use of oxygen lowers the venous gas content in the shunt and as the increased blood flow of exercise further reduces pulmonary gas exchange time of a diffusion defect.

The technique of subjecting a patient to two breathing mixtures with differing oxygen concentrations (often room air, and 30% to 40% oxygen) and calculating the two A-a gradients is termed a *double-gradient study*. It is a valuable diagnostic tool and, although by no means foolproof, gives a dynamic perspective to cardiopulmonary function hampered by hypoxia. Fig. 6-7 is a nonquantitative sketch showing the double oxygen–gradient characteristics of the normal state, shunt, and diffusion defect. The $P_{A-a_{O_2}}$, breathing air at 1 atm, in a given circumstance can be estimated by a simple equation.[94] With a normal mean $P_{A_{O_2}}$ of approximately 100 mm Hg and a mean $P_{A_{CO_2}}$ of 40 mm Hg, the sum of these two alveolar gases averages about 140 mm Hg. With such alveolar tensions it is felt that in the normal subject the sum of the arterial $PO_2$ and $P_{CO_2}$ should be at least 120 mm Hg. We can say, then, that the alveolar-arterial $P_{O_2}$ difference, if any, should be less than the difference between 140 mm Hg and the sum of the arterial gas tensions. This is expressed as

$$P_{A-a_{O_2}} = 140 - (P_{a_{O_2}} + P_{a_{CO_2}})$$

which tells us that the gradient should not exceed 20 mm Hg and that higher values are abnormal.

If desired, a practical working bedside estimate of the alveolar-arterial oxygen tension gradient can be calculated for any known combination of $F_{I_{O_2}}$, $P_{a_{O_2}}$, and $P_{a_{CO_2}}$. Sacrificing some accuracy in the interest of expediency, if we arbitrarily reduce the constant of 713 mm Hg in the alveolar air equation (which represents $P_B$ of 760 mm Hg minus saturated water vapor pressure of 47 mm Hg), to 700 mm Hg, and if the

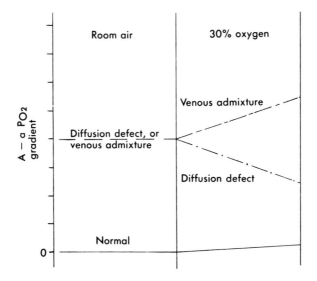

**Fig. 6-7.** Simplified schematic of differentiation between normal and abnormal A-a $P_{O_2}$ gradients, the latter shown in nonspecific arbitrary units, using the double gradient technique. Normal lungs show no significant gradient with air breathing but a slight one with 30% oxygen. Both diffusion defects and venous admixture produce gradients with air, but the gradient (*not* the absolute alveolar and arterial tensions) with 30% oxygen decreases with diffusion defects and worsens with shunting.

respiratory quotient R in the same equation is taken to be 1, then the difference between $P_{A_{O_2}}$ and $P_{a_{O_2}}$ will closely equal:

$$700(F_{I_{O_2}}) - (P_{a_{CO_2}} + P_{a_{O_2}})$$

We will look at a single-gradient procedure that permits the estimation of the degree of right-to-left shunt. The patient breathes *100% oxygen* for 15 to 20 minutes to assure equilibration between alveoli and capillaries and to allow maximum washout of alveolar nitrogen. At this point a normal lung will contain but three alveolar gases, $CO_2$, $H_2O$, and $O_2$. The easy equilibration of $CO_2$ lets us substitute its measured tension in arterial blood for alveolar, and water vapor pressure is a constant. Therefore, theoretically at least, under conditions of perfect alveolar-arterial equilibration, the $P_{a_{O_2}}$ should equal the difference between atmospheric pressure and the sum of 47 plus arterial $CO_2$ pressure. This can be expressed as:

$$P_{a_{O_2}} = P_B - (47 + P_{a_{CO_2}})$$

Using normal values, this translates to a $P_{a_{O_2}}$ of $760 - (47 + 40) = 673$ mm Hg. If measured arterial $P_{O_2}$ is less than 673 mm Hg, the inference is made that venous blood is mixing with arterial. For practical purposes it can be assumed that a *5% shunt* (5 parts venous blood to 95 parts arterial blood) is represented by every *100 mm Hg reduction in $P_{a_{O_2}}$* below that calculated in the above equation. Any difference between measured and calculated ideal $P_{a_{O_2}}$ is included in the rewritten equation

(1) Percent shunt (100% $O_2$) $= \dfrac{P_B - (47 + P_{a_{CO_2}} + P_{a_{O_2}})}{20}$

or, in its usual applied form,

(2) Percent shunt (100% $O_2$) $= \dfrac{673 - P_{a_{O_2}}}{20}$

***High V/Q.*** Regional elevations of the respiratory exchange ratio (R), which may reach 3.0 or more, result from the loss of adequate perfusion of ventilated alveoli; and when capillary flow to alveoli is reduced or absent, there is reduced or absent gas exchange even in the presence of normal or increased tidal alveolar airflow. As illustrated in Fig. 3-1, this constitutes *dead space ventilation.*

The basic effects of a highly localized elevated R are schematically illustrated in Fig. 6-8, which shows two normally ventilated alveoli, one *(A)* with normal perfusion and the other *(B)* unperfused because of a block in its perfusing capillary. Because alveolus *B* is not perfused, it receives no carbon dioxide and its $P_{CO_2}$ is zero. In the absence of carbon dioxide the gas of the alveolus consists of oxygen, nitrogen, and water vapor, and its oxygen partial pressure is approximately 150 mm Hg. With no component from the obstructed capillary, mixed arterial blood from the area has normal tensions of carbon dioxide and oxygen. The gas values of a mixed alveolar sample, however, are the averages of those of each alveolus, with a $P_{A_{CO_2}}$ of 20 mm Hg, and a $P_{A_{O_2}}$ of 125 mm Hg. Because of the perfusion defect, then, there are gas tension gradients present between the alveoli and arterial blood: an A-a oxygen gradient of 25 mm Hg and an a-A carbon dioxide gradient of 20 mm Hg. Again, this example is exag-

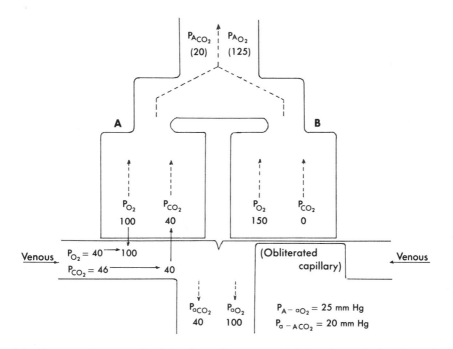

**Fig. 6-8.** Two normally air-ventilated alveoli are shown, one with full perfusion. **A**, the other without perfusion because of obstruction to (or destruction of) its capillary, **B**. Mixed arterial blood leaving the system has normal gas tensions, but sampled mixed alveolar air is high in $O_2$ and low in $CO_2$. This produces an $A$-$a_{O_2}$ gradient of 25 mm Hg and an $a$-$A_{CO_2}$ difference of 20 mm Hg. The latter normally does not exceed 5 mm Hg, and higher values indicate ventilation of nonperfused alveoli, or dead space breathing.

gerated, since one might expect to find a normal carbon dioxide gradient not in excess of 5 mm Hg, and a value of twice this would be considered highly significant. The only specific information that an elevated carbon dioxide gradient provides is to indicate that there is a general increase in pulmonary ventilation over pulmonary perfusion. This is dead space ventilation, but physiologically it means that there is a certain amount of work being invested in ventilation from which there is not a proportionate return in profitable blood gas exchange. The term *wasted ventilation* has been given to this uneconomical state.[95]

Clinically, this concept has a practical diagnostic application. Pulmonary embolism is a relatively common phenomenon and may express itself as a massive obstruction of a large branch of the pulmonary artery or as frequently recurring blockage of small arteries or arterioles. Within a few hours after the onset of such an episode, evidence of a high $\dot{V}/\dot{Q}$ may be noted. The terminal portion of the patient's tidal air, considered to be alveolar in quality, is analyzed for its carbon dioxide concentration and tension, while a sample of arterial blood is drawn for the same purpose. A significant difference between the carbon dioxide tensions of the two samples, indicating an elevated $\dot{V}/\dot{Q}$, is often helpful in complementing other data to support a diagnosis of embolism, although it obviously is not pathognomonic. The nature of the test has given it the familiar title of an *end-tidal $CO_2$ determination.*

In summary, two statements can be made:

1. A low $\dot{V}/\dot{Q}$ produces a venous admixture, with hypoxia and an A-a oxygen tension gradient resulting from a drop in arterial oxygen tension but with little effect on the carbon dioxide.

2. A high $\dot{V}/\dot{Q}$ produces alveolar dead space ventilation, with little hypoxia but with an A-a oxygen gradient due to an elevation of alveolar oxygen tension and an a-A carbon dioxide pressure difference.

It is important to remember that these concepts are to be used to explain *local* events in the lung, not necessarily the lung as a whole. Also, in disease all degrees of both ratio imbalances may be present, with the final state of lung function dependent on the net resulting mixed pathophysiology.

# Chapter 7

# AEROSOL AND HUMIDITY THERAPY

We will introduce the subject of clinical respiratory therapy with a discussion of aerosols and humidity. This deliberate pairing was chosen because the use of water in the treatment of bronchopulmonary disease requires an understanding of the principles of aerosols, and we will learn that of all the pharmacologically and physically active aerosols, water is the most important. From this point on, our attention will be directed primarily toward the patient—his needs and how we can best serve these needs. This does not mean that we will not frequently pause to consider some basic principle, but our thinking will be patient oriented, and we will lean heavily on the physical and chemical fundamentals covered in the preceding pages.

## PHYSICAL PROPERTIES OF AEROSOLS

The therapist will better understand the clinical use of medical aerosols, as well as the important health effects of atmospheric contaminants, if he has a background knowledge of the nature of aerosols in general. An aerosol is defined as a suspension of very fine particles (particulate matter) of liquid or solid in a gas. In general, aerosol particles are considered to fall within the size range of $0.005\mu$ to $50\mu$ in diameter, but from a practical point of view only those are important that are less than $3\mu$ in diameter, for it is at this mass size that gravity begins to lose its influence, a point of some importance, as we shall soon see.

Atmospheric aerosols can be considered to be either *natural* or *man made* and may consist of windblown dusts, bacteria, yeast, molds, water, dusts from explosions or earth-moving equipment, smoke, industrial wastes, and products of incomplete combustion of a large variety of commercial fuels, to list a few of the more prevalent. Another classification of atmospheric particulate matter, which is especially revealing in its relationship to disease production, is that which describes *neutral particles*, commonly referred to as dusts and "condensation nuclei." These are made up of hygroscopic substances (substances able to absorb water).[96] The neutral, dustlike particles range in size from $10^{-5}$ to $10^{-3}$ cm in diameter, have mostly a nuisance value, and are generally less harmful than the condensation nuclei. The latter are smaller, from $10^{-7}$ to $10^{-5}$ cm in diameter, and are composed mostly of chloride salts, sulfuric acid, phosphorus compounds, nitrogen oxides, and nitric acid. In the air such nuclei grow rapidly in size by the acquisition of water, as the relative humidity exceeds 70%, and easily produce haze and fog. It should be apparent also that any hygroscopic aerosol might undergo the same change during inhalation into the moist environment of the respiratory tract. Finally, although we are not studying the atmosphere as such, it is relevant to note that condensation nuclei, often consisting of toxic or irritant trace gases, tend to form on the most minute speck of matter, giving stability to these otherwise vaporous substances so that they are able to enter the respiratory tract, with harmful effects.[97] Their participation in the damaging action of contaminated urban air and smothering smogs is a matter of record.

To communicate clearly in a discussion of aerosol technology, we must learn some basic terms that are descriptive of the physical activity of particles. *Stability* of an aerosol refers to its ability to remain in suspension for significant periods of time or, in fact, to maintain its integrity as an aerosol. Such stability depends upon a number of characteristics, including size and nature of the particulate matter, concentration of particles, ambient humidity, and the degree of mobility of the carrier gas. *Instability* is the reverse of the above—the propensity of a suspended particle to remove itself, or be removed, from suspension. From a therapeutic point of view it is apparent that the stability or instability of a given aerosol will bear directly on the aerosol's effectiveness and be a matter of considerable concern to the manufacturer. It is not surprising that, among the many regulating mechanisms of nature and through a process almost like that of natural selection, a measure of stability is achieved among the atmospheric aerosols. Although the size range of particulate matter is great, as the myriad particles intermingle, some will condense on others, some will coalesce to form larger masses (agglomerate), and other will vanish through instability. A large population of aerosols thus undergoes a process of "aging," whereby there is a gradual increase in the number of particles of optimum size and concentration for maximum stability, with a reduction in the range of sizes. This *ideal* state consists of particles

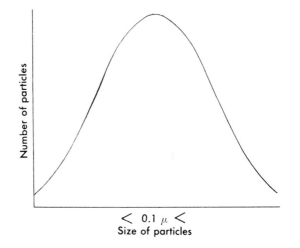

**Fig. 7-1.** This graph is a distribution curve of aerosol particle sizes. If a population of particles of many sizes is allowed to settle, the largest number will have diameters somewhere around $0.1\mu$, with decreasing frequency of sizes larger and smaller. (Modified from Lovejoy, F. W., and Morrow, P. E.: Anesthesiology **23:**460, 1962.)

from $0.2\mu$ to $0.7\mu$ in diameter, in concentrations of from 100 to 1000 particles per cubic centimeter of gas.[97] Fig. 7-1 is a graphic illustration of this phenomenon, showing the relationship among population, distribution of particulate diameters, and time.

Related to the characteristics of stability and instability, but especially pertinent to the therapeutic use of aerosols, are *penetration, deposition* or *retention*, and *clearance*, terms that are descriptive of the fate of particles once they have come into contact with the respiratory tract. *Penetration* refers to the maximum depth that suspended particles can be carried into the tract by the inhaled tidal air. *Deposition* is the result of an aerosol's eventual instability, permitting it to "fall out" on a nearby surface, whereas *retention* implies the deposition of a particle within the confines of a structure, such as the respiratory tract. Aerosol *clearance* is the opposite of retention and, depending upon its specific use, may have two meanings. Most authors refer to aerosol clearance as the process of removal of particles once deposited in the respiratory tissues by one of several biologic mechanisms that will be considered later. Occasionally the term implies the excretion of still-suspended particles in the exhaled air. Let us describe these activities in more detail.

### Penetration and deposition of aerosols

Because of their interrelation, penetration and deposition will be discussed together. Of significance is the location of the deposition of inhaled particles, for there is a considerable physiologic difference between particle contact with the relatively rugged and exposed nasal tissue and particle contact with the more secluded and reactive bronchial and alveolar cells. The latter areas are of more interest to us in the therapeutic use of aerosols. The depth of penetration of the respiratory tract increases as the particle size decreases. In fact, unless a particle is considerably less than $100\mu$ in diameter, it will not even gain entrance. The nasal filtering process (deposition in the nose) is so effective that it will remove completely particles down to $5\mu$ in diameter, whereas sizes below $1\mu$ can pass the upper tract and are retained in pulmonary tissue. We can make the generalization that the overall retention of particulate matter in the total respiratory tract is 100% for particles down to $5\mu$ in diameter, which are trapped in the nose, and about 25% for particles down to $0.25\mu$, which are deposited and retained along the rest of the tract. Deposition in the upper respiratory tract (conducting airways to the respiratory bronchioles) varies from 100% for large particles to 0% for particles of $1\mu$, whereas deposition in the alveoli is 90% to 100% for sizes down to $1\mu$.[98] There are five major factors that influence aerosol penetration and deposition—*gravity, kinetic activity of gas molecules, inertial impaction, physical nature of the particle*, and the *ventilatory pattern*.

**Gravity.** The speed with which a particle will "settle" is a measure of its ease of deposition. The settling rate is related to the force exerted by gravity on the particle mass or the combination of its density and size. The greater the mass of any body the greater will be the influence of gravity upon it. Suspended particles between $0.1\mu$ and $70\mu$ generally follow the prediction of Stoke's law of sedimentation.[99] In its entirety Stoke's law relates the velocity at which a small particle falls toward the

**Table 7-1.**  *Gravity deposition*

| Particle | Density | Diameter | Velocity |
|----------|---------|----------|----------|
| x | 1 | 2 | 4 |
| y | 1 | 4 | 16 |
| z | 2 | 2 | 8 |

earth with such physical factors as particle volume, density, acceleration of gravity, and viscous resistance of air. For our purposes, however, we can use it in a simplified proportionality and state that, within the above size range, the settling velocity of a particle is proportional to the product of its density and the square of its diameter. Thus:

$$\text{Settling rate} \cong \text{Density} \times \text{Diameter}^2$$

Table 7-1 compares the relative velocities with which the three hypothetical particles will deposit under the influence of gravity. Particle x, with a density of 1 unit and a diameter of 2 units, will settle with a velocity of 4 units. Particle y, of the same density but with twice the diameter, will settle four times as fast; whereas particle z, with the same diameter but twice the density, will settle twice as fast.

**Kinetic activity of gas molecules.** This interesting force of particle deposition is effective on sizes $0.1\mu$ or smaller. Because of their minute size, such aerosols are almost molecular in character and, as such, are subject to some of the physical activities attributed to molecules. They present the phenomenon of *Brownian movement* under the influence of the kinetic activity of the molecules of their carrier gas. The suspended particles are under constant bombardment from the gas molecules and are thus impelled into high-speed random movements for very short distances. The smaller the particles the greater will be their velocities. This transferred activity and mobility causes many of the particles to come into contact with nearby surfaces, and it is referred to as *diffusion* of the aerosol. The resulting surface impaction is called *diffusion deposition.* How much of the suspended material will deposit is a function of its *diffusion coefficient*, defined as the volume of particles that can diffuse a distance of $1\mu$ over an area of 1 cm$^2$ at a pressure of 1 atm and is inversely proportional to particle size. Whether a given particle will deposit or what fraction of a given volume of suspended particles will fall out is determined by the distance of the particles from the nearest suitable surface. The probability of deposition is related to time as well as to diffusibility and distance, and the average distance that the force of diffusion will move a minute particle is expressed by the following proportionality:

$$\text{Average distance traveled} \cong \sqrt{\text{Diffusion coefficient} \times \text{Time}}$$

We are not interested in quantitative values for such physical phenomena, but we should be aware that they play an important role in the efficiency of aerosol therapy, and we should recognize that consideration of these many factors in the design of aerosol generators can mean the difference between good and indifferent equipment. Fig. 7-2 illustrates gravity and diffusion deposition.

*Inertial impaction.* A particle being carried in an airstream tends to continue on a straight course when the stream undergoes a sudden change in direction[100], as shown by the large particles in Fig. 7-3. This divergence of the particle's path from that of the airstream is referred to as a "sideways slip." Because it occurs at angulations in the conducting channel, such a slip can precipitate a particle on a nearby surface. Whether a particle will deposit in such a manner depends partly on its loca-

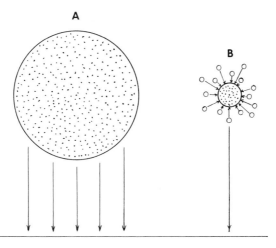

**Fig. 7-2.** The mass of the larger aerosol particle, **A,** makes it susceptible to the settling force of gravity. The smaller particle, **B,** is more affected by the bombardment of surrounding carrier gas molecules, eventually impinging on a nearby surface; this is called diffusion deposition.

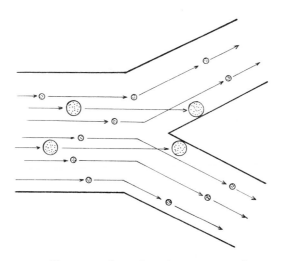

**Fig. 7-3.** Inertial impaction of large aerosol particles, whose masses tend to maintain their motion in straight lines. As airway direction changes, the particles deposit on nearby walls. Smaller particles are carried around corners by the airstream and fall out less readily.

tion within the airstream, the probability increasing with the particle's proximity to the periphery of the stream. Whether it will deposit also depends on the force of inertia, which opposes any change in direction of a moving particle, being great enough to free the particle from its fellows in the stream. To do this, inertia must overcome the resistance of air friction so that another probability of deposition depends upon the net effect of the two forces of inertia and friction. In summary, then, it can be said that inertial precipitation of aerosol particles of uniform density is related to particle velocity and size.

***Physical nature of particles.*** Of the many physical and chemical characteristics of minute matter, probably the most important in terms of deposition and retention is its hygroscopic nature, noted above. Initially small, a particle may absorb relatively large amounts of water from ambient air, especially in transit through the respiratory tract, and increase many times its diameter. This, of course, will alter its original probable point of impact. The solubility and chemical nature of particles, especially those in a heterogeneous atmospheric mixture, may play an important role. Very small particles may dissolve in or chemically react with aerosolized water or other solvents of a larger size and thus eventually deposit at levels different from those dictated by their original sizes. Finally, particle contour can influence deposition. Although we speak of aerosol particles as though they all had regular diameters like the spheroids of liquid particulates, some hard and brittle substances produce particles with many angulations and irregular plane surfaces. Such particles may follow transit and deposition paths considerably different from those predicted on the basis of physical laws we have been discussing. We might note here that our application of aerosol principles in the treatment of disease is somewhat simplified in that most therapeutic aerosols currently in use are liquids, and the aberrations that might be attributed to solid particles need not concern us.

***Ventilatory pattern.*** In general, deposition and retention of aerosol particles is directly related to inhaled volume and inversely related to respiratory rate. This generalization, however, is not applicable to sizes less than $1\mu$ in diameter. The character of air movement on particle behavior is significant down to the level of the terminal bronchiole, but air in the alveolar sacs is almost stagnant. Thus depth and frequency of ventilation have little influence on the deposition of particles once they have reached the alveolar level.[101, 102] The nature of ventilation higher in the tract does help to determine the volume of particles reaching alveoli and thus exerts an indirect influence. Deposition of particles is increased with both increasing tidal volume and decreasing frequency, and the effects of both are additive. Shallow breathing carries a reduced volume of aerosols per tidal volume, and a rapid breathing rate reduces the time available to the particles to settle.

If penetration and deposition are the objectives as in aerosol therapy, the ideal ventilatory pattern consists of slow, moderately deep breathing, with breath holding at end-inspiration. This facilitates the introduction into the respiratory tract of a significant volume of particles and allows adequate time for the smallest to enter the alveoli by diffusion and to settle by diffusion. This is a practical point that the therapist will have to keep in mind as he supervises and teaches patients the techniques of effective aerosol therapy.

## Clearance of aerosols

We will concern ourselves with the removal of particles from the respiratory tract by means other than the exhaled air and will discuss clearance of the upper and lower segments of the tract separately. The mechanism for cleansing the upper tract is referred to as the *ciliary mucus transport*, and there are several mechanisms to service the pulmonary areas.

*Ciliary mucus clearance.* It is assumed that the student already knows the anatomic structure of the airways and the pulmonary lobules. Of critical importance to the subject under discussion is the nature of the mucosal lining of the respiratory tract. We will recall that the mucosa is characterized by the presence of microscopic hairlike structures called cilia that extend from the beginning of the trachea through all the ramifications of the airways to the level of the terminal bronchioles. Approximately $3\mu$ to $4\mu$ long, the cilia are in constant wavelike motion called "beating," which goes on at a rate of some 1300 strokes per minute. The unique function of the cilia is made possible by more rapid upward strokes than downward recovery strokes. As the cilia wave cephalad (in the direction of the head), they propel an overlying thin layer of fluid called mucus. Respiratory mucus is a thin clear substance, produced by specialized cells *(goblet cells)* throughout the tract to the respiratory bronchioles, and is on the average $5\mu$ thick.[103, 104] Its function is to entrap foreign particles and, with the aid of the cilia, to remove them from the tract. Lying like a blanket over the cilia, the mucous layer is carried cephalad in an escalator fashion by the ciliary action at rates up to 13.5 mm/min. The mucus, with its captive particles, is brought into the trachea and then into the lower pharynx by a normal and almost imperceptible "throat clearing" action to be either expectorated or swallowed, depending on its volume. The system is extremely efficient as long as both cilia and mucus are in a healthy state. Should a pathologic process increase the depth of the mucous layer, its upward propulsion will gradually slow, becoming ineffective when the thickness of the fluid approaches four to five times the height of the cilia. Similarly, function will be impaired after damage to or destruction of the cilia. It is evident that airway obstruction from the prolific thick secretions accompanying bronchial irritation or infection can be self-perpetuating, as the increase in the secretory load retards its own removal.

*Pulmonary tissue clearance.* Particles in the lobular lung units can be removed by several routes. Some may be considered "functionally" removed in situ through encapsulation and immobilization by a deposit of fibrous tissue, remaining for the duration of the subject's life. It is not surprising that enough such reactions throughout wide areas of the lung might in themselves eventually present a problem. Other solid aerosols are picked up by wandering scavenger cells called *phagocytes*, whose mobility permits them to gather at sites of foreign matter deposition. After engulfing the particles within their own protoplasm, the phagocytes can transport them into the ciliary-mucous escalator for removal as described or into the interstitial lymphatics for incarceration in regional lymph nodes. Depending on solubility, some particles may dissolve in tissue fluid and diffuse into the general circulation to be disposed of by the body's metabolic processes.

Let us summarize the relation between particle size and deposition in the

**Table 7-2.**   *Particle size and site of deposition*

| Particle size ($\mu$) | Deposition in respiratory tract |
| :---: | :--- |
| 100 | Do not enter tract |
| 100-5 | Trapped in nose |
| 5-2 | Deposited somewhere proximal to alveoli |
| 2-1 | Can enter alveoli, with 95% to 100% retention of those down to $1\mu$ |
| 1-0.25 | Stable, with minimal settling |
| 0.25 | Increasing alveolar deposition |

respiratory tract and point out that although much of the research done on inhaled particulate matter has used nontherapeutic solid particles, the results give us a practical insight into the expected behavior of the liquid aerosols that we will have occasion to use. It is generally agreed that there is a particle size of *minimum* deposition, around $0.4\mu$ in diameter, and that above and below this size the incidence of deposition somewhere in the tract increases. The observed maximum particle diameter found in alveolar air never exceeds $1.2\mu$.[102] Thus the highest probability for pulmonary deposition is attributed to particles in the 1 to $2\mu$ range (gravity settling) and below $0.2\mu$ (diffusion precipitation); the lowest probability is found with particles 0.25 to $0.50\mu$, for which the effects of both gravity and diffusion are minimal.[105, 106] These data are summarized in Table 7-2.

As an aside from our specific topic of aerosol clearance, it should be emphasized to the student that these mechanisms are of great clinical importance in protecting the body from diseases caused by the inhalation of such pathogenic aerosols as bacteria and the toxic condensation nuclei described earlier. The ability of the respiratory tract to rid itself of foreign particles can be seriously hampered by such factors as smoke inhalation, exposure to cold air, ingestion of alcohol, and lack of adequate sleep.

The student should understand that in the above discussion of the properties of aerosols, many generalizations and assumptions are included that may or may not be valid. The current great interest in aerosols has produced many changes in investigative techniques, making it difficult to correlate data from one source to another. These differences in technique account for much of the variance found in the literature, especially pertaining to effective particle sizes[107] and to the degree of alveolar penetration by aerosols.[108] Nevertheless, we have reviewed the most widely accepted behavioral characteristics of aerosols as they apply to clinical medicine, and we can only be alert to new developments in this interesting field.

## CLINICAL USE OF AEROSOLS AND HUMIDITY

Aerosols and humidity are used to achieve the following four general objectives: *relief of bronchospasm and respiratory mucosal edema, mobilization of bronchial secretions for easier removal, administration of antibiotics,* and *humidification of the respiratory tract.* Without attempting to penetrate the field of pharmacology to any depth, we will describe some of the more commonly used medications, for although the respiratory therapist does not prescribe, he must be aware of the major effects of all therapy he administers. Only with such knowledge can he give safe and effective care to his patients, always on the alert for adverse reactions to treatment.

### Relief of bronchospasm and mucosal edema

Bronchospasm and mucosal edema are paired because not only are they frequently associated but many of the medications employed in therapy are effective against both. Those agents designed to reduce bronchospasm and edema are called, respectively, *bronchodilators* and *decongestants*. It should be emphasized that we are here referring only to those that are used as aerosols, for there are many bronchodilators and a few decongestants that can be administered parenterally (by injection) or orally.

Bronchodilators increase the lumen of the airways by relaxing the spasm of the bronchial muscle, which was triggered by disease or irritation. Decongestants (agents that relieve "congestion") function in one of two ways. Most cause a contraction of the muscle fibers of the arterioles and small arteries, thereby reducing blood flow to the affected area and lowering the hydrostatic pressure that permits fluid to move into the tissues. Others interfere with the natural defense mechanism that stimulates increased blood flow to an injured area and are called "anti-inflammatory" in action.

Recognizing that not all bronchodilators are also decongestants, in the interest of brevity we will confine our discussion to the more important of the two, the bronchodilators, and let the student acquaint himself with the characteristics of the individual drugs he uses. For purposes of discussion a bronchodilator can be classified as *autonomic-active, xanthine,* or *adrenocorticosteroid.* Awkward as they appear at first glance, these names have meanings that indicate either their origins or modes of action, features that are common to the terminology of many drugs with which the therapist will come into contact. The drugs in these categories are so important in the treatment of respiratory disorders that we are justified in taking time to review some of their pharmacologic backgrounds along with their clinical uses.

### Autonomic-active bronchodilators

The autonomic-active group of bronchodilators is clinically the most widely useful and contains the largest variety of drugs of the three categories. Bronchodilators whose actions either simulate or interfere with tissue stimulation by the autonomic nervous system have been effectively used for many years. Although our major interest in their physiologic actions is limited to the single function of bronchial dilatation, because of their extensive use and potency, it is essential that we understand their total effects. This necessitates a quick review of the autonomic division of the nervous system.

The nervous system is broadly separated into the *somatic* and *autonomic* divisions. The somatic division consists of those nerves that serve voluntary muscles and that transmit certain bodily sensations to the brain. The autonomic division, in contrast, functions beyond the level of our conscious control, does not respond to our voluntary demands, and is under the control of various centers of the brain. In short, the autonomic system performs its many duties, minute by minute, whether we are awake or asleep, according to impulses received by the higher centers that are transmitted to them automatically. The autonomic nerves, among other things, govern the activities of the cardiac muscle, the smooth or involuntary muscle of all bodily systems, the digestive and genitourinary systems, the sweat glands, and certain endocrine glands. In a general way it may be said that autonomic control maintains stability among the many interacting systems of the body, combatting any factor that would change the so-called "internal environment," much as our voluntary actions help us to adjust to the external environment. This internal balance is referred to as *homeostasis*.

The autonomic division is itself divided into two competitive subdivisions, *sympathetic* and *parasympathetic*, and most of the structures listed above are innervated (supplied with nerves) by both. Fig. 7-4 schematically shows the origin and distribution of each division. Sympathetic fibers arise in the thoracic and lumbar spinal cord segments and run to one of two types of ganglia, or relay points, where they can communicate with other fibers. One set of twenty-two ganglia, represented by (*1*) in Fig. 7-4, is close to the vertebral column, while another, (*2*), is made up of groups of ganglia throughout the abdomen. Parasympathetic fibers originate in the brain and sacral cord segment and differ from the sympathetic in that their ganglia, (*3*),

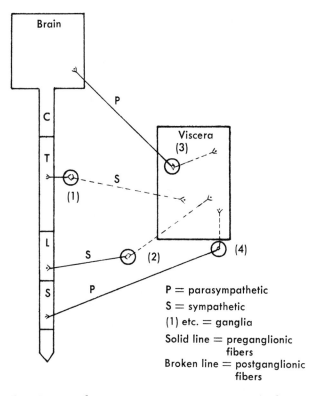

**Fig. 7-4.** Diagram of autonomic nervous system. (See text for description.)

and are located very near, on, or in the innervated viscera, *(4)*. Thus parasympathetic postganglionic fibers are much shorter than those of the sympathetic division.

The organ or cell receiving a nerve stimulus is called the *effector* or *receptor*, and the contact point between nerve and cell, the *neuroeffector junction*. Physiology of nerve conduction and stimulation is very complex, but for our purposes we can use the following simplified concept. An electrical process is responsible for the transmission of an impulse along a cablelike axon of a nerve, but response to stimulus at the neuroeffector junction is due to release by the nerve, at that point, of a chemical called a *mediator*. It is the nature of the mediator that identifies the type of nerve and its response. At the present it is believed that the mediator for transmission of sympathetic nerve stimulus to the cell is *norepinephrine* (levo-arterenol), possibly aided by small amounts of *epinephrine*, while the parasympathetic mediator is *acetylcholine*. Because the relationship between these mediators is so important, another digression in our discussion is pertinent, and we will comment briefly on them.

The medulla, or central portion, of the adrenal gland, synthesizes hormones known as *catecholamines*, two of the most important of which are the closely chemically related epinephrine and norepinephrine. They have many identical physiologic effects, but just as important, they have some significant differences, as listed in Table 7-3. When the effects of experimental stimulation of a sympathetic nerve are compared with the responses to injected norepinephrine and epinephrine, the former more closely simulates sympathetic nerve activity. It was thus inferred that norepinephrine, in addition to being produced in the adrenal medulla, is also released by sympathetic nerves as the neuroeffector sympathetic mediator. In contrast to the action of norepinephrine, which is limited to the neuroeffectors of postganglionic sympathetic nerves, the parasympathetic activator, acetylcholine, has a much wider influence. Without pursuing the subject in depth, we should note as a matter of interest that, in addition to its role as the parasympathetic mediator, acetylcholine is also responsible for nerve impulse transmission at many other receptor sites, including all the autonomic ganglia (sympathetic and parasympathetic), the adrenal medulla itself (for production of epinephrine and norepinephrine), and somatic nerve junctions with skeletal muscle. As a final point, the quantity of mediators available at any given time is the net result of production by their respective autonomic nerves and destruction by appropriate metabolic agents. Acetylcholine

**Table 7-3.** *Different responses of epinephrine and norepinephrine*

|  | Epinephrine | Norepinephrine |
| --- | --- | --- |
| Blood pressure | + | +++ |
| Cardiac output | + | 0 |
| Central nervous system stimulation | + | 0 |
| Pulse rate | + | ± |
| Renal blood flow | − | 0 |
| Skeletal and cardiac vessels | Dilate | 0 |
| Splanchnic vessels | Constrict | Dilate |

is destroyed by the enzyme *acetylcholinesterase*, while norepinephrine and epinephrine are inactivated in the liver and bowel and by the enzyme *amine oxidase*.

Broadly speaking, we say the effects of each subdivision on a given receptor organ are antagonistic to the other; inactivity of one allows the action of the other to dominate the organ response. Each thus exerts a constant action against the other, like two forces maintaining a steady pull on each end of a rope. This action is called *tone*, and it establishes a balance of influence on receptor function, assuring fine control over function and rapid response. Generally, the sympathetic division is designed to protect the integrity and maintain the safety of the organism, which involves the expenditure of energy. The parasympathetic division, on the other hand, is less kinetic in its objectives and is more concerned with conservation and restoration of function.

We can begin to compact this information for practical use in our special area of interest by introducing two new terms that describe these opposing autonomic divisions. *Adrenergic* nerves act through the release of norepinephrine (or epinephrine), and *cholinergic* nerves release acetylcholine at their receptor terminals. Table 7-4 lists a few selected functions that differentiate adrenergic from cholinergic stimulation. Opposing responses of some blood vessels to adrenergic stimulation are due to variations that will be described shortly. Using this nomenclature, drugs can be designated as adrenergics or cholinergics, depending upon which neuroeffector responses they simulate. Also, drugs interfering with these responses can be referred to as blocking or anti-agents. We will consider two types of bronchodilators based on this classification.

**Adrenergic bronchodilators.** On the basis of antagonistic responses within the group, two primary types of adrenergic receptors have been identified, designated as *alpha* and *beta*, and their characteristic effects are shown in Table 7-5. It can be seen that beta receptor stimulators combine bronchodilatation with undesirable

**Table 7-4.**   *Comparison of adrenergic and cholinergic innervation*

| Receptor | Target | Adrenergic | Cholinergic |
|----------|--------|------------|-------------|
| Bronchi | Glands | – – – – – – – – | Stimulation |
| | Muscle | Relaxation | Contraction |
| Eye | Ciliary muscle | Relaxation | Contraction |
| | Iris | Contraction | – – – – – |
| Heart | Contraction | Increase | Decrease |
| | Rate | Increase | Decrease |
| Intestine | Motility | Decrease | Increase |
| | Sphincters | Contraction | Relaxation |
| Salivary glands | Secretion | Viscid | Profuse, watery |
| Vessels | Abdominal | Constriction/dilatation | – – – – – |
| | Cerebral | Constriction | Dilatation |
| | Coronary | Constriction/dilatation | Dilatation |
| | Pulmonary | Constriction/dilatation | Dilatation |
| | Skeletal muscle | Constriction/dilatation | Dilatation |
| | Skin/mucosa | Constriction | Dilatation |

elevation of blood pressure and cardiac rate. As the search continued for agents with effective bronchial relaxation, but with minimal cardiac stimulation, it was discovered that some beta stimulators could be differentiated into two distinct groups according to their abilities to (1) hydrolyze fatty acids; (2) stimulate the heart; (3) dilate bronchi; and (4) relax arterioles.[109, 110] The major effects of the agents included one of two pairs of these four parameters. Thus some beta stimulators were strong in fatty acid lysis and cardiac stimulation and less effective in dilating bronchi and arterioles. Others responded conversely. It was deduced that there are two subtypes of beta receptors, one found in the heart and digestive tract, the other in the bronchi and vascular bed, and they were designated *beta₁* and *beta₂*, respectively. Substances that elevate blood pressure and increase cardiac rate more than they dilate bronchi are called *beta₁ stimulators*, and those that dilate bronchi more than they raise blood pressure or heart rate are *beta₂ stimulators*. Other agents elicit both types of responses. Obviously, the ideal bronchodilator should be a beta₂ stimulator.

It is worth noting here for completeness that at least some of the adrenergic bronchodilators perform the additional valuable role of increasing the transport of airway mucus. Studies following the parenteral use of the beta stimulant, terbutaline, showed up to 110% of average tracheal mucus velocity in patients with chronic obstructive airway disease.[111] There was no apparent increase in flow in normal subjects. It is thus possible that the effectiveness of catecholamines in the treatment of obstruc-

**Table 7-5.**  *Adrenergic receptor effects*

| Alpha | Beta |
|---|---|
| Vasoconstriction (skin, mucosa, skeletal muscle, brain, bronchi, abdominal viscera) | Vasodilatation (coronary, skeletal muscle, abdominal viscera) |
| Uterine contraction | Uterine relaxation |
| Intestinal relaxation* | Intestinal relaxation |
| Gastrointestinal sphincter contraction | Bronchodilatation |
| Pupillary dilatation | Increased cardiac contraction* |
| Ureteral contraction | Increased cardiac rate* |

*Generally, alpha stimulation produces excitation and beta produces relaxation, except as noted. Intestinal smooth muscle responds in the same way to both.

**Table 7-6.**  *Receptor site stimulation of some adrenergic drugs*

| | Alpha | Beta₁ | Beta₂ |
|---|---|---|---|
| Epinephrine (Adrenaline, Suprarenin) | × | × | × |
| Ephedrine | × | × | × |
| Isoproterenol (Isuprel, Norisodrine, Aludrine) | | × | × |
| *l*-Norepinephrine; levarterenol (Levophed) | × | | |
| Isoetharine (Dilabron) | | | × |
| Metaproterenol sulfate (Alupent, Metaprel) | | | × |
| Solbutamol | | | × |

tive disease is due to the dual action of bronchodilatation and increased mucus transport. Although the mechanism for the latter is not apparent, it may account for instances of subjective evidence of increased mucus removal even though tests of airway patency show no improvement.

There is a large number of commercially available sympathetic-like drugs (sympathomimetics), and the properties of most of them are amply described in pharmacology texts and promotional literature. We will comment on only a few that are more or less representative of the major characteristics of the group. Table 7-6 lists six adrenergics according to their principal neuroeffector actions.

*Epinephrine.* Epinephrine is the standard against which most sympathomimetics are judged. Epinephrine is a potent drug, and since it stimulates all three adrenergic receptors, its use carries with it the risk of serious unwanted side effects. It performs important functions in regulating the body's metabolism and maintaining a state of alertness to cope with the environment. The therapist will see this drug used frequently in the hospital for its effect on the circulation and to combat allergic reactions, for which purposes it will be administered by injection under the skin, into muscle, or into superficial veins. It is almost completely inactivated in the stomach; thus oral use is not feasible, but it has been used parenterally for many years for the relief of acute bronchial asthma.

Epinephrine is one of the most powerful bronchodilators and decongestants, whether given by injection or by aerosol. Indeed, its action by aerosol is both *topical* (local, by application to a surface) and *systemic* (distributed to many parts of the body), since the small particles act by direct contact with the bronchial mucosa and are also absorbed into the circulation by way of the pulmonary flow. Thus inhalation generally affords quicker response than does subcutaneous or intramuscular injection, although not exceeding the intravenous route. There are two major hazards to aerosolized epinephrine. First, the unwanted side effects may be a danger as well as a nuisance, and the effect on the cardiovascular system may outweigh its benefits. This is especially true in elderly patients or those with known heart or vascular disease. Second, repeated use of epinephrine often leads to a condition of "fastness," in which there is a progressive decreasing response to the drug and dangerously larger doses are required for therapeutic effect. A patient exhibiting this phenomenon is considered to be epinephrine-fast. Less commonly seen but worthy of note is a third complication apparently attributable to any of the sympathomimetic compounds by which the symptoms of acute bronchial asthma are made worse by these aerosols. It is felt that this adverse effect is due to the development of an allergy to some of the metabolic end products of the drugs.[112]

If epinephrine is to be used as a bronchodilator-decongestant aerosol, nothing stronger than a 1% aqueous solution (1:100) should be considered safe. Two effective inhalations from 30 to 60 seconds apart are sufficient, and treatments should be spaced at least 4 hours apart. Because of the development of safer preparations, some of which are described below, the use of epinephrine aerosol has rapidly declined in recent years.

*Ephedrine.* Although ephedrine is not used as an aerosol, its close similarity to the action of epinephrine and its frequency of use warrants its mention at this time. Ephedrine is an alkaloid (nitrogen-containing organic compound with physiologic action) derived from a plant, with a less intense but longer lasting bronchodilating effect than epinephrine, and unlike epinephrine, it is a strong cerebral stimulant. A major advantage of ephedrine is its oral effectiveness, and most commonly it is used in conjunction with other bronchodilators, expectorants, or sedatives. Excessive use, as by patient self-administration, can cause serious mental excitation.

*Isoproterenol.* A powerful beta stimulator with negligible alpha effects, isoproterenol has enjoyed wide use as an aerosol bronchodilator. Although much more selective in its effects than are epinephrine and ephedrine, its role as a bronchodilator is somewhat limited by its stimulation of beta$_1$ receptors. Cardiac output increase may reduce the ventilation/perfusion ratio by raising pulmonary perfusion more than bronchodilatation improves ventilation, and thus worsen hypoxia. Further, the risk of cardiac arrhythmias is increased by beta$_1$ stimulation in the presence of hypoxia.[113] However, clinical experience with it is extensive enough that it can still be used effectively as an inhalant, with a wide range of safety. A major advantage of this aerosol is its somewhat better bronchodilating effect than that of epinephrine, with nearly complete absence of vasopressor action. In contrast to epinephrine, isoproterenol produces vasodilatation and thus has negligible decongestant value. It tends to lower diastolic and not systolic blood pressure but may encourage a sinus tachycardia. Its symptomatic side effects are infrequent, tend to be mild, and include nausea, excitement, tremors, and rapid heart action.[114]

Although available in aqueous concentrations of 1:100 and 1:200, for routine aerosol use the *1:200 strength is recommended.* For intermittent short-term therapy, as in self-administration, two to four well-spaced inhalations at 4-hour intervals is a conservative program, although the general safety of the drug allows for considerable flexibility according to clinical need. It can be noted here that, since all aerosols are, in a sense, foreign bodies, overuse of them often causes severe pharyngeal and laryngeal irritation, further aggravating the very condition being treated. Warning of this possibility should be included in instructions given to all patients who are to treat themselves. For prolonged bronchodilatation, especially as administered with mechanical ventilators, the isoproterenol should be further diluted to concentrations of 1:400 or 1:600.

*l-Norepinephrine; levarterenol.* The major sympathetic nerve stimulus mediator, when administered therapeutically, is very limited in its action and, although not a bronchodilator, is included here for completeness. Levarterenol is exclusively an alpha receptor stimulant, with its primary effector the cardiovascular system. Given intravenously, its only clinical use is the support of blood pressure in certain types of shock.

*Isoetharine.* Although its bronchodilating effect is somewhat less than that of isoproterenol, cardiovascular side effects of isoetharine have also been noted to be less intense.[115] It is claimed to be mostly a beta$_2$ stimulator, with clinically insignificant beta$_1$ activity. In one test of cardiovascular responses to a strong exposure to the drug, intravenous administration of isoetharine to anesthetized patients caused a decrease in systolic and diastolic blood pressures (beta$_2$ effect) and an increase in heart rate (beta$_1$ effect) but no arrhythmias.[116] Isoetharine can be administered orally as well as by aerosol, and is reportedly more effective in conditions characterized by diffuse bronchospasm, as in bronchial asthma, than in those with obstructing secretions, as chronic bronchitis.[117]

*Solbutamol.* Not yet available for general clinical use, solbutamol is reported to have even less beta$_1$ activity than isoetharine and beta$_2$ bronchodilatation comparable to isoproterenol.[117a] In clinical doses it apparently has little effect on heart rate or circulation time. Metabolism of solbutamol is slower than that of the other adrenergics, giving it prolonged action. A major asset is its effectiveness by mouth as well as by aerosol.

*Metaproterenol.* One of the more recently available bronchodilators, metaproterenol is inhaled as an aerosolized powder or taken orally. It is primarily a beta$_2$ stimulator, although tachycardia and blood pressure elevation may occasionally occur.

It should be emphasized that adverse effects, or at least failure to achieve or sustain benefit, are commonly seen with most of the adrenergics now in use. Such results may not always be due to stimulation of unwanted effector sites but are often the result of local airway mucosal irritation or the blockade of beta receptors by accumulated adrenergic metabolites.[118] Isoproterenol is especially susceptible to the latter reaction, particularly if used too frequently or over too long a period of time. Metabolic products of the breakdown of isoproterenol can accumulate faster than enzymatic degradation can destroy them. Some of the metabolites block the beta receptor from bronchodilator action, and further administration of isoproterenol increases bronchospasm. Also, the student will find that there is a wide variety of adrenergic bronchodilators commercially available that differ chemically from one another, and many are combined with other agents for supposed multiple effect.[119]

It is not our purpose to comment on the relative virtues of these varied compounds, but the respiratory therapist may have occasion to note the presence of *propylene glycol* in many preparations, and its function might just as well be explained at this time. Propylene glycol is a fairly simple organic compound, related to glycerin but less irritating, that is frequently used as a vehicle or solvent for active substances to be administered by intramuscular injection and is itself completely inert physiologically. In liquids designed for aerosol use, advantage is taken of another characteristic of propylene glycol: It is hygroscopic, and through its ability to absorb water, it supposedly will minimize shrinkage of aerosol particles by evaporation as the particles enter the warmth of the respiratory tract. However, the probability is just as great that aerosol size may so increase through hygroscopic growth that penetration will be hampered; and it is sometimes suspected that aerosol particles may become so stable that they exert no therapeutic effect in the respiratory tract and are exhaled intact.

**Anticholinergic bronchodilators.** Reference to plural agents in this category is actually unwarranted at the present, since there is only one that justifies consideration as a clinical bronchodilator. *Atropine* is an alkaloid found in the plants *Atropa belladonna* and *Datura stramonium*, and it has been used for many years in the treatment of airway disease. Inhalation of the smoke of stramonium leaves was a favorite remedy for asthma, but the increased use of adrenergic drugs gradually displaced atropine therapy until, at present, little reference to it can be found in modern treatment regimens. Yet, because we frequently encounter patients who are resistant to the common drugs, we should at least keep it in mind as a potential agent.

Related to other drugs such as scopolamine and hyoscyamine, atropine blocks the effect of parasympathetic stimuli by increasing the threshold of response of effector cells to acetylcholine. It thereby depresses the reactions of structures supplied by the parasympathetic division, and its action generally resembles stimulation of adrenergic receptors, since these are freed of competing and counteracting cholinergic stimulus. The most extensive of the cranial nerves are the paired vagus nerves, large conveyors of parasympathetic fibers. Coursing from the brain, the vagi pass through the neck, supplying all the organs in the thorax, and continue into the abdomen, where they innervate the digestive system and other abdominal viscera. Thus in our area of interest, the action of atropine inhibits vagal stimulation of the heart and respiratory tract, elevating blood pressure and cardiac rate and dilating bronchi by paralyzing the terminals of the vagal parasympathetic nerve endings. In addition, atropine is believed to have action in the central nervous system, stimulating the cerebral respiratory center to generate rapid, deep breathing.[120]

Relative to the patient with airway obstruction, the two most important actions of atropine can be summarized as follows.

1. *Reduction of secretions.* Atropine inhibits secretions of nose, mouth, pharynx, and bronchi, and by reducing their fluid volumes, increases their viscosities. This property made atropine and related derivatives popular in compounds prescribed to relieve symptoms of the common cold and in preoperative medication to reduce the mucus-producing stimulus of anesthetics and airway instrumentation. However, this effect of atropine poses a potential threat to the patient already handicapped by thick bronchial exudates and subjects him to the risk of serious aggravation of his obstruction. This hazard has probably been the major impediment to the continued use of atropine in respiratory problems.

2. *Bronchodilatation.* By blocking cholinergic constricting influences on bronchial muscle, atropine potentiates beta adrenergic dilatation, and widens the airways. Because there is no evidence that acetylcholine plays an active role in generating bronchospasms, atropine is a less effective dilator than either epinephrine or isoproterenol in therapeutic doses, yet the beneficial effect of atropine on bronchoconstriction has been well demonstrated in airways that were subjected to dust inhalation and protected by the drug parenterally administered.[121] Aerosol studies have employed 1.0% and 0.2% concentrations of atropine in equal parts of propylene glycol and water.[122] It has been emphasized that the medication must be microaerosolized, with mean particle diameters from $0.03\mu$ to $0.05\mu$. This avoids potential toxic effects from the powerful drug by assuring maximal deposition in the alveoli and minimizing absorption from the upper tract. Through the use of very small particle size, total dosage of the alkaloid is kept within safe limits, but microaerosolization to such a controlled degree can be achieved only with specialized equipment, to be described later. With the

proper administration of atropine aerosol, airway resistance can be significantly reduced in normal subjects as well as in obstructed patients. Bronchi are also protected against the induced bronchospasm of inhaled irritants such as carbachol and aluminum dust. It was also found that results were equally satisfactory with the 0.2% as with the 1.0% solution. It has been suggested that atropine in small amounts be added to sympathomimetic mixtures, and one study demonstrated that an aerosol of isoproterenol and atropine methonitrate gave better bronchodilatation than either alone, combining the rapid onset and short duration of isoproterenol with the slower but more prolonged effect of atropine.[123]

Currently undergoing study in Europe and the United States, and not yet available for clinical use, is a derivative of atropine, *N*-isopropyl nortropine, for experimental use designated as Sch 1000.[124, 125] Administered as an aerosol in doses of 10 to 20 $\mu$g, it produces bronchodilatation about as effectively as does isoproterenol. Onset of its action is three to six times as long as isoproterenol's, but its duration is four times greater. The major effect of Sch 1000 seems to be in large rather than peripheral airways, and apparently no subjective drying of oral or ocular secretions has been noted. Finally, bronchodilatation is better in patients with chronic bronchitis than with asthma, an observation consistent with the theory that bronchitics are more sensitive to vagal activity than are asthmatics. It is to be hoped that Sch 1000 soon becomes clinically available, giving us an effective alternative bronchodilator to the many adrenergics that now dominate the market.

### Xanthine

There is a group of vegetable organic compounds called the xanthines, of which the three most important are *caffeine, theophylline,* and *theobromine.* We are all familiar with caffeine as the important ingredient of coffee, tea, and cocoa, but the xanthine group as a whole has some specific physiologic actions that make them valuable as pharmacologics. Although the degree to which these three react varies, in general their activities include the following: central nervous system stimulation, respiratory stimulation, smooth muscle relaxation, diuresis (increased production of urine), coronary artery dilatation, cardiac stimulation, and skeletal muscle stimulation. It is evident that there is a great potential for the medical use of these substances. Frequently used in the past for cardiac stimulation (caffeine) and diuresis (theobromine), for the most part they have been replaced by more effective agents, with the exception of theophylline. This agent, used plain or compounded as theophylline ethylenediamine (aminophylline), still plays an important role in therapeutics. It is useful in certain types and stages of congestive heart failure and is especially valuable in correcting Cheyne-Stokes ventilation, but we will confine our discussion to its use as a bronchodilator.

The therapist will see aminophylline frequently used for patients with diffuse bronchospasm, and in cases of intractable bronchial asthma, especially when there is refractoriness to the sympathomimetics. The usual mode of administration is intravenous, adding to a saline infusion the contents of a 20 ml ampule of the drug, containing 0.5 g. Intramuscular and rectal routes are sometimes used, but these are less effective, and theophylline can be irritating to the gastric mucosa unless given as a specially coated tablet. Rapid administration may produce such side effects as headache, rapid heart action, dizziness, hyperventilation, nausea, and hypotension; but with care, these are usually not a significant problem.[126]

As an aerosol, aminophylline has not enjoyed as widespread usage as the sympathomimetic agents, although the effectiveness of this technique has been recognized for many years.[127] The intravenous preparation is used for aerosolization, by any convenient method available. Continuous nebulization has been used until relief is obtained, often requiring as much as 0.5 to 0.7 g of aminophylline. Intermittent therapy, with positive pressure or an aerosol mask, alone or in conjunction with sympathomimetics, is also effective in bronchial asthma. Because of the relatively small amounts of the drug absorbed, side effects of aerosol administration are very rare.[128, 129] It seems practical to consider aerosolized aminophylline in those patients with diffuse bronchospasm who no longer respond to safe doses of sympathomimetics, for the speed of action and economy of the latter still justify their consideration as first-line drugs.

## Adrenocorticosteroid

Adrenocorticosteroids have assumed a position of great importance in the therapy of almost all branches of medicine. Again, although we are interested in a relatively limited aspect of their use at present, some general background knowledge of them is essential because the therapist will encounter them throughout his patient care experience. For the sake of convenience, we will use the commonly employed abbreviated expression "steroid," with the understanding that we mean adrenocorticosteroid. We must understand also that, like many familiar terms, it is not really correct, for steroids comprise a large group of organic compounds, many of which have other physiologic properties than those in which we are interested. The steroids that concern us are potent hormones secreted by the *cortex* (outer layer) of the adrenal glands, as opposed to the sympathomimetic products of the adrenal medulla, already described. There are some five general groups of complex organic compounds produced in the adrenal cortex, of which the only one of importance to our present needs is the *glucocorticoids*. The name of this group derives from its involvement in carbohydrate metabolism, and its two most clinically useful members are *cortisol* and *cortisone*. There are available many commercial preparations and modifications of these two, with variable potencies and supposed specific responses.

The adrenal steroids exert a tremendous influence on the body physiology, touching all organ systems. They have been referred to as "stress hormones" because they are secreted in excessive amounts when the body is put under stress, and severe trauma or prolonged grave illness may cause a depletion of their supply. In a complex way the steroids give support to the body to aid it through a crisis, and if they are acutely depleted or if their production is interrupted by abrupt destruction of the adrenals, the body functions deteriorate rapidly. On the other hand, a slow, chronic increase of cortical function does not produce a catastrophic picture but rather a multiplicity of signs and symptoms described as *Cushing's syndrome*. A patient beginning to show evidence of excessive steroid action is often referred to as "Cushinoid." We will describe some of the more common and important effects of hyperadrenalism to illustrate the wide range of steroid action. The glucocorticoids have the following effects.[130-132]

*Formation of glucose from body protein.* When excessive, the formation of glucose from body protein can raise the blood sugar level high enough to produce "steroid diabetes" or to activate a latent, subclinical true diabetes. There can be associated protein loss with muscle wasting and weakness.

*Depletion of bone calcium.* Through a process of resorption, calcium is removed from bone, so thinning its consistency that fractures are frequent. This state of the bone is called *osteoporosis.*

*Increase in fat production.* Excessive amounts of fat are produced, also from body protein, and are characteristically deposited in the subcutaneous tissues of the head and trunk. This results in a rounding of the facial contour, referred to as *moon face,* and an accumulation of fat at the base of the neck and upper back, called *buffalo hump* These are two of the most prominent visible signs of a Cushinoid state.

*Impairment of immunologic response.* Steroids inactivate circulating antibodies and thus can protect the body against the harmful effects of severe allergies. By the same token, however, this function lowers the body's resistance to infection, a point of significance in the therapeutic use of steroids.

*Reduction of inflammatory response.* Steroids decrease the local vascular congestion and cellular infiltration that is the natural response to injury or infection. In addition, the deposition of fibrous tissue as part of the reparative process is inhibited. Of use in controlling the adverse effects of inflammation, this function also facilitates the spread of infection, since it interferes with the usual process of localization. This is a serious threat to the patient with quiescent tuberculosis.

*Increase of gastric acidity.* An increase in gastric acidity predisposes to the development of stomach ulcer, or the worsening of one already present. Bleeding and rupture are ever-present risks.

*Elevation of blood pressure.* Steroids, through the mediation of certain electrolytes and other hormones, elevate the blood pressure. Of therapeutic significance, in state of shock, when the cardiovascular system no longer responds to sympathomimetics, steroids often aid the vasoconstrictors to regain their pressor effects on the arterioles.

To complete the review of steroid action, mention should be made of the pituitary gland. The adrenal cortex is directly controlled by the anterior division of the pituitary gland, through a pituitary hormone called *adrenocorticotropic hormone.* The name itself describes a substance that stimulates *(-tropic)* the adrenal cortex and, not surprisingly, is almost always referred to as ACTH. Administration of ACTH can be expected to elicit the same response as cortisol and cortisone, by stimulating the adrenal production of these substances. This presupposes that the adrenal cortex is in a functioning state, able to respond. Because the adrenals are likely to slacken in their activity during the therapeutic administration of steroids (the body is receiving adequate hormone from its outside source), there is risk of adrenal atrophy with prolonged loss of function. Under such circumstances, ACTH may be given for periods of time to stimulate the adrenals to function and to prevent their atrophy.

For the most part, in the treatment of respiratory diseases, steroids are administered orally and parenterally. They are used for their potent anti-inflammatory and antifibrogenic effects in acute and chronic obstructive diseases and in resistant allergies of the respiratory tract. The therapist will witness dramatic responses to steroid therapy, especially in the patient acutely obstructed by intractable bronchospasm and mucosal edema. However, because of the almost inevitable development of some side effects or because so many patients have conditions that contraindicate the use of these drugs, it has been hoped that aerosol administration might offer a safer route for prolonged therapy. It was thought that such a topical application directly to the target organ might give enhanced action with a smaller total dose. So far, no unanimity of opinion has brought this hope to reality, and although steroid aerosol enjoys moderate acceptance, it has not yet become a major agent. Among the many steroids that have been aerosolized, the following deserve special mention.

*Dexamethasone sodium phosphate* is available in a gas-propelled pressurized capsule and can be used alone or mixed with isoproterenol. It is the consensus of its users that this steroid is therapeutically active and effective throughout the entire respiratory tract from the nose to the bronchioles in the treatment of nasal allergies, allergic asthma, and some chronic obstructive states.[133,134] However, with no doubt concerning its local effects, dexamethasone has been found to have definite systemic effects, readily detected by special urinary excretion tests. Some investigators believe that the local responses in the respiratory tract are significantly greater than the systemic responses and thus justify its use.[135] Others have found a safe dosage difficult to control by aerosol administration, with Cushinoid symptoms of prior oral administration unrelieved by the change to aerosol, and believe that it has no place in therapy at this time.[136] Still other users have found therapeutic results with aerosol application as effective as the oral route, but they warn of the risk of complications of self-administered medication.[137] This is always a hazard inherent in any procedure when the patient is responsible for his own therapy on a home-treatment program. The risk is increased with use of a drug whose unfavorable side effects may develop insidiously rather than acutely.

Other steroids have been investigated for their therapeutic potential as aerosols. *Prednisone* (as the acetate), a popular oral form of this group, has been found to have satisfactory physiologic effects, but it apparently tends to produce bronchospasm.[138] Although the addition of bronchodilators to the program alleviates the spasm, the irritant effects of the steroid are not completely eliminated. *Triamcinolone acetonide* is a poorly soluble compound with good local and negligible systemic effects, which can be aerosolized for respiratory tract action. It is packaged as a suspension for intramuscular, intra-articular, or intrabursal injection but not intravenous. One dilution that is especially useful for our purposes contains 40 mg/ml of steroid in 1, 5, and 10 ml vials. Starting aerosolization with 10 mg, dosage can be titrated for each patient by clinical response and serum cortisol levels. After several years of use in Europe, the inhalant steroid, *beclamethasone dipropionate* became available in the United States in mid-

1976. At this writing it can only be purchased in a Freon-propelled dispenser for self-administration. It is purported to invoke negligible adverse steroid side effects within recommended dose ranges. Beclamethasone dipropionate aerosol is indicated in patients over 6 years of age with intrinsic, extrinsic, or mixed asthma who need chronic steroid therapy. We will know if it lives up to its highly heralded reputation in Europe only after further experience with it in this country.

Determination of the actual dose of steroid aerosol to be administered is a matter of professional judgment and is the responsibility of the attending physician. By and large, since steroid aerosols are usually packaged in self-administered gas-propelled units, the physician gives directions for the use directly to his patient. However, should the therapist be assigned to oversee the patient's treatment program, he should make certain that the physician is specific in his orders. Whereas this should be the practice for any treatment, there are many instances in which established routines can be used, allowing the therapist some flexibility to adjust techniques to individual needs. The great potency of the steroids and the possibility of adverse reactions mitigate against their administration by anything less than specific instructions for each patient. The many variables that influence the efficiency of aerosol treatment, such as function of the nebulizer, depth of ventilation, and ventilatory rate, make it impossible to predict the systemic absorption of the drug. The physician must "play it by ear," judging total dosage necessary by clinical response.

Although it is not a bronchodilator, *cromolyn sodium* is described here because it is often part of a treatment program for asthma, used cooperatively with bronchodilators. It is a powder packaged in 20 mg doses in capsules, administered only as an aerosol with a special inhaling device that punctures the capsule, releasing the powdered drug for transport to the lung during inhalation.

Cromolyn apparently interferes with the release of mediators that result from contact, in allergic persons, between allergen (substance to which an individual is allergic) and antibody (a protein mobilized by the body to inactivate allergen). Such mediators as histamine and SRS-A (slow-reacting substance of anaphylaxis) can cause severe bronchospasm, and although their exact roles are not known, they are felt to participate in initiating or propagating asthmatic attacks. It must be emphasized very strongly that cromolyn is only of value in *preventing* or *moderating* asthmatic attacks and is completely ineffective once bronchospasm is established. It has made two important contributions to asthma management. The regular use of cromolyn inhalations during remission of symptoms may reduce the frequency and severity of attacks and lessen the amount of adrenocorticosteroids previously needed to control symptoms.[139]

*Summary.* We have considered those bronchodilators that are now standard in the treatment of spastic and edematous airway obstruction, and the sequence in which they were discussed generally parallels the priority given to their use. All of the agents noted are effective, but with variation among patients, and in the same patient at different times.

New products are constantly being evaluated for safe and effective treatment of obstruction. Currently of interest, although yet in the investigative stage, is a bronchodilator of an entirely different type. A group of biologics called *prostaglandins* is found chiefly in seminal plasma but also in other organs. There are six primary prostaglandins, designated $PGE_1$, $PGE_2$, $PGE_3$, $PGF_{1a}$, $PGF_{2a}$, and $PGF_{3a}$, and they elicit many and varied responses from several organ systems. Because of the experimental nature of prostaglandins, a detailed description of their actions is unjustified in this text, and the interested student can find many good references in the literature.[140-143] Both $PGE_1$ and $PGE_2$ produce bronchodilatation, while $PGF_{2a}$ constricts bronchial smooth muscle. Aerosolized $PGE_1$ has been shown to decrease airway resistance in asthmatic patients to a greater degree than isoproterenol, and $PGE_2$ has an additive effect to beta-adrenergic stimulation. Approaching the problem from a different direction, bronchodilatation can also be achieved experimentally by the action of a substance known as polyphloretin phosphate, which inhibits the constrictor effect of $PGF_{2a}$. It is expected that the future will see the prostaglandins revealing previously unknown mechanisms in the production of bronchospasm and at the same time increasing our arsenal against airway obstruction.

### Mobilization of bronchial secretions

Of all the agents used to modify the character of respiratory tract secretions, rendering them more fluid for easier removal, none is more important than water; but the very importance of water justifies a separate discussion, which will be undertaken below. Our concern here will be with those physical and chemical substances that are used with water for sputum mobilization. We are already well aware of the great hazard to health and life from airway obstruction, and the relief of bronchospasm and mucosal edema corrects only a part of this serious defect. In a large percentage of patients suffering from chronic bronchopulmonary disease, the presence of increased amounts of sputum, or increased viscosity of the sputum, is a major cause of ventilatory disability. We will describe the aerosols most frequently used for removal of bronchial secretions, arbitrarily dividing them into the two groups of *mucolytics* and *proteolytics*. The former are most effective against sputum that is predominantly mucoid, and the latter, against purulent sputum with its high protein content. Some products are claimed to be of equal value against both.

**Mucolytics.** Although *mucolysis* means the disruption of the long chains of organic compounds that constitute mucoid sputum, fragmenting them into smaller more mobile molecules, we will include here, for convenience, *wetting agents*. These substances do not break molecular bonds and thus are better referred to as *mucoevacuants* than mucolytics, but through their surface-active effects they lessen the integrity of secretions and aid in their separation from airway walls.

*Wetting agents (detergents).* The commercially trademarked product Alevaire contains 0.125% aqueous solution of the wetting agent tyloxapol (also known as Superinone), 2% sodium bicarbonate, and 5% glycerine for stability. Sodium bicarbonate in this concentration has itself mucolytic properties, since some of the polysaccharides will separate in a sufficiently alkaline medium. In vitro studies of the action of tyloxapol on homogenized specimens of sputum demonstrated its surfactant action. The sputum, with a measured surface tension of 52 dynes/cm, was not altered in the addition of water, but when subjected to the action of tyloxapol, the surface tension dropped

20%.[144] It was concluded that a second major function of the wetting agent took place at the wet surface interface between the respiratory mucosa and the mucoid layer, breaking the adherence of the mucus to the bronchial wall. This allowed the mucoid layer to be separated and then removed by cough.

Tyloxapol has been used for several years, and although the mechanical effect of its detergent on mucoid specimens in the laboratory is unquestioned, there is still not a uniform opinion as to its value in clinical application. Many believe that it is effective in removing secretions from both sinuses and bronchi and can be used continuously for long periods of time for its humidifying effects as well as its mucoevacuation.[145, 146] In the treatment of acute infections of the respiratory tract, tyloxapol has been found to increase the effectiveness of simultaneously administered antibiotics.[147] Other users feel strongly that the value of tyloxapol lies in the humidifying effects of its water-glycerin solvent and that the wetting agent does not influence viscosity or amount of sputum or clinical improvement.[148] It has been suggested that subjecting the bronchioles and alveoli to detergent action may produce such histologic changes in the lung as membrane damage and interstitial infiltration, sometimes seen in postmortem examination of patients succumbing to ventilatory failure. Such diverse opinions are usual concerning any type of treatment. When a new therapy is proposed, there is typically great enthusiasm for its hoped-for success, much of which is generated by its promoter, and it is only after considerable practical experience that exaggerated claims are disproved, more specific indications for its use are recognized, and effective techniques for its application are developed. Then its proper role in clinical medicine can be evaluated. It might be opportune to note here that the anticipated results of any treatment are usually in direct proportion to the skill with which the treatment is administered. This is especially pertinent to respiratory therapy, in which, because of its rapid growth and extensive use, we can never be certain that uniformly efficient techniques are employed in a given circumstance. This point must be kept in mind when we try to reconcile conflicting clinical data.

The therapeutic use of wetting agents might be summarized by saying that they do have a limited effect on bronchial secretions and, by rendering these secretions less viscid, will supplement the efforts of an existing effective cough mechanism. They are physiologically nontoxic and, when employed as a vehicle for other active substances, enhance the latter's probability of contact with respiratory tissue. It should be emphasized, however, that detergents have little value against frankly purulent sputum.

*Acetylcysteine (N-acetyl-L-cysteine, Mucomyst).* In the search for agents other than detergents effective in breaking the mucoproteins responsible for the viscosity of sputum in chronic respiratory diseases, the action of the naturally occurring amino acid, L-cysteine, was studied. Although it was found to be a potent mucolytic, it had irritating properties that could be eliminated by modifying the acid into an acetyl form, as it is now employed. The chemical reaction between acetylcysteine and bronchial mucus has been extensively studied,[149] and basically it consists of a disruption of chemical bonds holding together segments of the long-chain mucoproteins by the direct action of specific groups of the amino acid. It is thus a true mucolytic and reduces the viscosity of mucoid sputum in direct proportion to its concentration. Some claim is made for a liquefying action on purulent sputum, but since acetylcysteine has no specificity for the ribonucleic acids characteristic of purulency, such action is probably indirect and mediated through associated mucoid components.

Some studies have indicated that mucolysis is as effective with a 10% as with a 20% concentration and, whereas the stronger preparation tends to induce bronchospasm in some patients, the lesser strength is a negligible hazard.[150] Other studies have found both 10% and 20% to be harmless, neither producing significant bronchospasm.[151] The possibility of damage to alveolar surfactant has been of concern with the inhalation of microaerosols of any kind, and especially with one of potent lytic qualities. Examination of both human and animal lung tissue after use of 10% acetylcysteine aerosol showed no change in surface activity.[152] Serious complications are rare. A burning sensation in the upper passages is occasionally reported, and nausea may be experienced. Some patients complain of the rotten-egg odor, but most become adjusted to it quickly and appear to ignore it.

In general, the clinical response to this aerosol for the removal of mucoid secretions has been favorable, with indications for its use covering a wide range, from the cystic fibrosis of childhood (in which it seems to have scored considerable success), through the suppurative lung diseases, to the chronic bronchitis-emphysema of late adulthood.[153, 154] Nevertheless, a small minority have felt that acetylcysteine, though effective in vitro, has not shown any benefit in patients and is of no clinical value.[155] Of interest, in reference to comments made above, one source felt that the aerosol was effective in cleansing the upper airways but did not aid the lower regions and expressed the opinion that this is probably the fault of inadequate equipment or techniques currently available.[156] We shall see shortly that there are aerosol generators able to supply particles of a tremendous size range for the deposition of medication to any level of the respiratory tract. Failure of particles to reach the target area should not be a reason for lack of anticipated response.

A practical point to note is the chemical reactivity between acetylcysteine and certain component parts of nebulization equipment, especially iron, copper, and rubber. To avoid the loss of potency of such reactions, parts coming in contact with the amino acid (liquid or aerosol) should be made of glass, plastic, aluminum, chromed metal, silver, or stainless steel.

There is no critical dosage schedule for administering acetylcysteine aerosol; it is used according to individual needs. It can be administered by hand nebulizer, pump, or aerosol mask, and in positive-pressure breathing devices, but the drug itself should not be put in a heated nebulizer. In addition to the aerosol route, acetylcysteine is often effectively used by direct instillation, especially to facilitate bronchial aspiration through tracheostomy or endotracheal tubes.

*Ethyl alcohol (ethanol).* With an indication, real or optional, in almost all aspects of man's activities, we should not be surprised to find alcohol included among the therapeutic aerosols. In contrast to most of its uses, however, its virtue as an aerosol depends upon its local action in the respiratory tract. As a matter of convenience, alcohol is included with the mucolytics, although not without some justification, for it is used to modify surface tension of pulmonary fluids. More often, however, it is referred to as an antifoaming agent. Its action is not directed primarily to abnormal mucoid substances but rather to the thinner but equally hazardous edema fluid that frequently obstructs bronchioles and alveoli. Aerosolized alcohol performs a valuable service in the treatment of acute pulmonary edema and can often be helpful in cases of low-grade edema.

From whatever cause, acute pulmonary edema is characterized by the accumulation in the alveoli and bronchioles of a thin watery fluid, often containing some blood. There is enough protein in edema fluid to produce froth as air passes through it with tidal ventilation. A relatively small volume of fluid can thus be increased to a much larger volume of massed bubbles that severely obstruct the small airways and alveoli. It is this foamy edema fluid that so seriously compromises the alveolar ventilation/perfusion ratio and in a sense drowns the patient in his own water.

The function of aerosolized alcohol is to mix with the edema fluid, where its ability to reduce the mass of suffocating, frothy foam had been observed long before the advent of current respiratory therapy techniques.[157] Delivered by the force of inspiratory positive-pressure breathing instruments, alcohol aerosolized by oxygen has become part of the standard treatment of acute pulmonary edema. Frothy fluid is converted to a liquid state that not only occupies less bronchiolar and alveolar space, with relief of obstruction, but is more readily removed by the cough mechanism and the perfusing pulmonary circulation. Despite the observed benefit of this therapy, there is no uniform agreement on, or clear-cut explanation of, the exact mechanism by which alcohol disperses pulmonary foam. Most authorities attribute the action to a modification of edema fluid surface tension but differ as to what direction this change takes.

The surface tension, in dynes per centimeter, of four alcohol concentrations are: 100% = 22; 50% = 28; 30% = 32; 25% = 34. If, for the sake of discussion, we could assume edema fluid to be composed of approximately equal parts of tissue fluid and blood plasma, we might give to the froth a surface tension of about 60 dynes/cm. It would then be convenient to consider ethanol mist, with a relatively low surface tension, as exerting a simple dilutional effect on the froth, lowering its surface tension so that gas trapped in its bubbles expand, rupturing the bubbles. However, should edema surface tension exceed that of alcohol aerosol, then obviously bubble tension would increase.[158] Even here, the result might be the same, since trapped gas could well diffuse out of the contracting bubbles, under an increasing pressure gradient. It would seem that too little is known of the degree of uniformity of the surface-active properties characterizing edema fluid.

Perhaps either of these mechanism is effective in disrupting pulmonary edema froth, but an explanation involving two possible actions in exact opposition is difficult to accept without supporting experimental data. A more reasonable theory takes a different point of view.[159, 160] The stability of edema bubbles, like that of alveoli, is due to the action of normal surfactant, which increases or decreases surface tension with bubble size. Ethanol, in contrast, maintains a uniform surface tension regardless of the area over which it is distributed (i.e., the size of the bubble). When aerosolized, ethanol is thought to replace normal surfactant and thus deny edema fluid the special surface-active forces necessary for the formation of stable froth. Only those substances that do not show variation in their surface tensions with change in surface area are classified as antifoaming agents.

Concentrations between 25% and 50% are suitable for therapeutic effect, without undue risk of local airway irritation. Although absorption does occur in the alveoli, the actual amounts of alcohol in the bloodstream at any one time are well within the limits of sobriety. Alcohol can be given by any standard aerosol generator by way of oropharyngeal catheter, mask, or positive pressure. The latter two applications are preferred for the treatment of acute episodes. More will be said of therapy in the discussion of mechanical ventilation, for a respiratory therapist on night duty in an active general hospital will have many opportunities to treat acute pulmonary edema in his emergency room.

*Sodium bicarbonate (baking soda).* Reference was made to the mucolytic effect of this common household commodity in the above discussion of the action of tyloxapol. Large mucoid molecular chains tend to break as the pH of their environment rises, and local bronchial alkalinity can reach a pH of 8.3 without untoward irritation or damage.[144] Indeed, the treatment of acutely obstructive episodes of cystic fibrosis often includes, along with other modalities, the deliberate production of systemic alkalosis by the intravenous and oral administration of bicarbonate to make full use of its mucolytic properties. Although this regimen is less necessary with the availability of more potent mucolytics, such as acetylcysteine and proteolytics (to be discussed next), sodium bicarbonate aerosol still has a place not only in this disease but also in chronic states of the adult. It is not uncommon to encounter patients in whom mucolysis from the usually effective agents lessens, and for such patients it is occasionally beneficial to switch to aerosolized 2% sodium bicarbonate to see whether mucus flow can be stimulated. For home use a teaspoonful of the soda in a cup of water makes a readily available solution.

*Proteolytics.* As the name indicates, members of this group lyse the protein material found in purulent sputum, and although there is only one commercial preparation, for all practical purposes, enjoying widespread use, a brief description of the development of this therapy is felt to be pertinent here. Because the effectiveness of mucolytics decreases with increasing purulency of bronchial secretions, the early efforts to find an adjuvant agent centered on *trypsin*, a proteinase (enzyme active against protein) of the pancreas. Trypsin plays an important role in the natural digestion of ingested protein, but it is most effective on protein that is already partially digested. It also acts on respiratory and intestinal mucin and on fibrin. The use of trypsin as an aerosol demonstrated its effectiveness in cleansing the upper airways of proteinaceous accumulations, apparently without damage to living cells or impairment of ciliary function. Some early investigators were disappointed with its results, feeling that it sometimes worsened the obstruction. Hoarseness was a frequent and troublesome complication, attributed to too high concentrations of the drug or too rapid administration.[161-163] Aerosolized trypsin was used for several years, and in my opinion produced fairly satisfactory results, superior to other products then available. There were a few febrile reactions noted, and because of the real or imagined risk of an allergic reaction, it was common to include an antihistamine in the treatment program. The effectiveness of a proteolytic aerosol was enough to prompt further search for better products, and trypsin has now been replaced by dornase.

*Dornase (pancreatic dornase, pancreatic deoxyribonuclease, Dornavac).* Dornase is not a digestant in the same manner as trypsin, although it, too, is an important natural proteolytic. It is more specific in its action than is trypsin, since it depolymerizes (breaks long chains into smaller ones) deoxyribonucleic acid (DNA).[164] Therapeutically, this is most important, since it has been determined that from 30% to 70% of the solid matter of purulent secretions is composed of DNA.[165] The principle source of dornase is beef pancreas, but dornase is also produced by the pathogenic bacterium hemolytic streptococcus. Indeed, the filtrate of a culture of hemolytic streptococcus contains two active enzymes, streptococcal fibrinolysin (streptokinase) and streptococcal deoxyribonuclease (streptodornase). We might infer from its name that streptokinase acts mostly on fibrous tissue and as such is not particularly relevant to our present needs. A combination of these two enzymes is commercially prepared as Varidase, and although it is rather widely used for local application and intracavitary instillation, it has had limited use as an aerosol.[166, 167]

Clinically, dornase is indicated in any bronchopulmonary condition in which the accumulation of purulent sputum interferes with ventilation or with the resolution of an infection. It is thus of use in pneumonia, pulmonary abscess, bronchiectasis, cystic fibrosis, and especially in an acute respiratory infection superimposed on chronic lung disease.[168] As might be expected, there are some who believe that enzyme aerosols have no useful role in clinical medicine.[169] However, after using pancreatic dornase for many years, I believe it to be one of the most valuable of available aerosols for *specific* use. It is effective only against infected sputum, and indications for its use can be determined by visual examination of the sputum for color and consistency. For predominantly mucoid secretions it is of little value. No significant side reactions have been noted, and the only common patient complaint is posttreatment burning of the mouth, easily prevented by a vigorous mouthwash immediately following therapy. Inhalation of 100,000 units two to three times daily for no more than 4 consecutive days is generally sufficient. More prolonged use in one sequence is inadvisable because of the possible appearance of an inhibiting antideoxyribonuclease, which inactivates proteolytic action.[170] A course of therapy may be repeated after an interval of a week or more. Dornase is also useful for intraluminal instillation, as an adjunct to aerosol therapy, when gross airway obstruction is present. During dornase therapy, the attending therapist must always be ready to aspirate the liquefied secretions if the patient's cough is inadequate, a precaution of great importance in the unresponsive patient being supported by mechanical ventilation.

### Administration of antibiotics

When it became apparent that a new effective route was available for the administration of drugs, interest soon developed in the use of this new route in treating respiratory tract infections, especially such localized bronchopulmonary diseases as lung abscess, necrotizing pneumonia, and bronchiectasis, which were especially resistant to conventional therapy. In the mid-1940s sulfonamides were aerosolized, but the advent of penicillin and subsequent antibiotics stimulated extensive use of aerosols and the accumulation of a significant background of experience.[171-176]

The rationale for aerosol therapy was based on the speculation that, even with adequate blood levels of systemically administered antibiotics, the diffusion of the drug from blood into infected tissue for its direct antibacterial action was blocked by tissue reaction to the infection. In localized lesions, especially, it was believed that the presence of thick bronchial and alveolar exudates comprised a formidable diffusion barrier. Also, it was thought probable that interstitial edema and fibrosis of the diseased area were additional factors in preventing therapeutic antibiotic tissue levels. These observations were borne out by the frequent observation of active microbial growth in sputum while intensive systemic therapy was being administered.

The ideal antibiotic for aerosol use is one with effective topical action and which is poorly absorbed. Further, it is necessary that the infection being treated is accessible from the respiratory tract surface. From a practical point of view it can be generalized that aerosolized antibotics play their greatest role in the treatment of stubborn gram-negative respiratory tract infections, where the nature of the infection and the frequently accompanying airway obstruction require long-term therapy. Large doses of effective antibiotics can be used, self-administered at home if desired, with minimal hazard of untoward reactions. In the interest of economy, antibiotics should be aerosolized during inhalation only, using either a simple pump or gas-powered hand nebulizer or an ultrasonic nebulizer.

Table 7-7 lists those antibiotics that have been found suitable for aerosolization, with suggested doses for their use.

The reported results make it apparent that there is no magic cure in the technique of aerosolization and that although some patients respond dramatically, others show little or no benefit.[177, 178] In view of the modifying factors listed above and with the variability of bacterial susceptibility encountered in systemic therapy, this is not

**Table 7-7.** *Antibiotics for aerosol use\**

| Antibiotic | Aerosol dose |
|---|---|
| Carbenicillin | 1-3 g |
| Neomycin† | 50-400 mg |
| Bacitracin† | 5000-200,000 units |
| Streptomycin | 750-1000 mg |
| Chloramphenicol | 200-400 mg |
| Kanamycin† | 100-400 mg |
| Colymycin-M | 25-150 mg |
| Polymyxin† | 10-50 mg |
| Gentamicin† | 40-120 mg |
| Amphotericin† | 5-20 mg |
| Mycostatin† | 100,000-400,000 units |

\*From Miller, W. F.: Fundamental principles of aerosol therapy, Respir. Care **17**:295, 1972.
†Poorly or nonabsorbed in aerosol state.

surprising. However, the efficacy of aerosolized antibiotics can be significantly increased by using a technique that deserves special mention.[179] The same exudates and secretions that impair drug diffusion from blood to tissue are able to interfere with the action of aerosolized particles, and they are probably responsible for many instances of therapeutic failure. The prior or concomitant use of bronchodilators will aid penetration of antibiotic particles but will not bring them into bacterial contact in the presence of thick secretions. Often, extensive therapy with heated water aerosol, to be described next, and chest physical therapy, to be explained later, are essential to clear the airways for penetration and deposition of antibiotic aerosols. If a secretion's barrier still blocks contact of antibiotic with the infected area, the antibiotic may be combined with pancreatic dornase. The latter reduces viscosity of purulent sputum and, while so doing, exposes the infecting organism to the action of the inhaled antibiotic. Assuming that the antibiotic has significant potency against the organism, therapeutic bactericidal levels of the drug can be delivered directly to the diseased tissue. The choice of antibiotic is a matter of professional medical judgment, not in the province of the respiratory therapist, and is based on clinical experience, identification of the offending bacteria, and sensitivity tests of several antibiotics against bacterial cultures. Since most patients with these resistant infections are seriously ill, they are usually treated with a combination of systemic and aerosol antibiotics of the same or different type. In all probability, the effectiveness of the systemically administered drug is enhanced by liquefaction of the intrapulmonary diffusion barrier through the action of the proteolytic alone, but in several reported instances clinical and bacteriologic improvement was delayed until aerosol antibiotic was added. Soluble or intravenous preparations of the drugs are used, and their dose-calibrated solutions can be conveniently mixed with the dissolved dornase for joint administration, or, if desired, the two may be used sequentially.

In summary, we can say that, for the most part, aerosolized antibiotics are not intended to supplant the systemic but rather to supplement them in treating diseases characterized by copious purulent sputum. The respiratory therapy reduces the amount of secretions and clears it of bacterial growth, but we must remember that the risk of distant spread of infection to other parts of the body can best be controlled by maintaining therapeutic blood levels by systemic antibiotics. Of special interest to the therapist is the frequent appearance of *Pseudomonas aeruginosa (Bacillus pyocyaneus)* in the respiratory tract of patients suffering from chronic respiratory disease or who have been receiving treatment from poorly maintained respiratory therapy equipment, especially patients who have been tracheotomized and require frequent tracheobronchial suctioning. A potentially serious infection, it is notoriously resistant to systemic therapy, even by those drugs which sensitivity tests would indicate to be effective. The most encouraging results appear to follow the combined therapy of pancreatic dornase and gentamicin, which, because systemic absorption from the aerosol is so slight, can be used safely.

### Humidification of the respiratory tract

Water is a major therapeutic agent in the treatment of bronchopulmonary disease and the most important of all the aerosols. In an earlier chapter we considered some of the physical properties of water in the atmosphere, but we will now discuss water and its relation to respiratory hygiene, defining some terms and general principles with which the respiratory therapist should be familiar.[180] Unfortunately, the inhalational use of water is associated with a variety of terms and expressions, and it is helpful to have an understanding of some precise definitions to avoid confusion of meaning. Inhaled water fits into two categories, and we must differentiate between humidity and vapor, on the one hand, and mist, aerosol, "cold steam," and fog, on the other. We will use *vapor* to refer to the first classification and *aerosol* to the second. Recall that water vapor is water in a gaseous form, sometimes referred to as "molecular water," and as such is invisible. By definition, on the other hand, aerosolized water is water in a very fine particulate form, suspended in the air. Thus water aerosol is "liquid water" and exerts no partial pressure as does the vapor. Depending on the size of its particles, water aerosol is visible or reveals its presence by light diffraction, giving rise to the terms *mist*, *fog*, and the descriptive but inaccurate *cold steam* used in water aerosol therapy. The following defines in simple expressions some of the common terms used in respiratory water therapy. (See Chapter 1 also.)

**aerosol**   Particles of liquid or solid suspended in a carrier gas.
**atomization**   Production of an aerosol with a wide range of particle diameters.
**fog**   Water condensed into fine, visible particles, suspended in air; an aerosol of water.
**humidity, absolute**   Amount of water in gas, or weight per volume.
**humidity, relative**   Ratio of actual content of water vapor in gas to the capacity of the gas for vapor at a given temperature.
**mist**   Similar to fog but less dense and with a greater tendency to precipitate.
**nebulization**   Atomization, with baffling to remove particles above and below specified diameters.
**water vapor**   Invisible, gaseous state of water, exerting temperature-dependent pressure.

The amount of water vapor in a given volume of gas is measured according to the principles of absolute and relative humidity, with which we are acquainted. For evaluation of respiratory humidity the convenient term *percent body humidity* is sometimes used.[181] It refers to the amount of water vapor in a volume of gas as the percent of the water in gas saturated at body temperature. For example, air at 20° C, saturated with vapor, contains 18.5 mg of water per liter, whereas saturated air at body temperature contains 43.8 mg/$\ell$. The room air could be said to have 42% body humidity.

Liquid water particles can be measured, as any aerosol, by particle size. Less frequently they are measured as the number of particles per cubic millimeter of gas. Finally, aerosolized water production is calibrated in the number of milliliters of water aerosolized per minute, especially useful in comparing the performances of large-volume aerosol generators.

The therapist will recognize that there is considerable overlapping in the therapeutic use of water vapor and water aerosol, but it is still convenient to describe their indications separately for clarity and to emphasize their basic differences.

**Water vapor.** Water vapor is used specifically to prevent or correct a "humidity deficit" in the respiratory tract (Table 7-8). Normally, the tracheobronchial tree can maintain saturation of inspired gas at body temperature by evaporation from the respiratory mucosa, most of which probably occurs proximal to the carina. Gas thus reaching the pulmonary tissue contains 44 mg of water vapor per liter of gas. If the

**Table 7-8.** *Humidity deficit*

| | |
|---|---|
| Air 37° C, saturated | 44 mg $H_2O/\ell$ |
| 21° C, saturated | 18 mg $H_2O/\ell$ |
| | (deficit = 26 mg/$\ell$) |
| 21° C, 50% relative humidity | 9 mg $H_2O/\ell$ |
| | (deficit = 35 mg/$\ell$) |

inspired gas contains less than this amount of water, its vapor pressure will be less than the 47 mm Hg of body humidity, and a vapor pressure gradient will be established between the inspired gas and the respiratory mucosa. Evaporation of body water from the mucosa into the gas brings the latter to full humidification. When the respiratory tract and the general body hydration are in good health, this humidifying mechanism works efficiently, but a humidity deficit of pathologic degree, which the body may have difficulty in compensating, can be produced under two circumstances.

*Breathing dry gas.* The administration of therapeutic gases from a tank or central supply subjects the respiratory tract to large volumes of vapor-free gas. The normal humidification process may be inadequate to cope with this load and may have to draw on the water content of the entire mucosal surface. Such failure will be hastened or aggravated by an associated dehydration incident to systemic disease. Depletion of mucosal moisture increases the viscosity of the mucus blanket of the tract and slows its escalator movement. At the same time ciliary action is adversely affected. The increased or abnormal secretions, so often present in patients requiring gas therapy, become dehydrated and less mobile, contributing significantly to airway resistance.

*Mucosal crusting.* The same secretions noted above, resulting from bronchopulmonary infection and irritation or systemic disease, can cover the mucosal surface with a dry and crusted coat. Impervious to the diffusion of moisture, it blocks the normal humidification process from the underlying mucosa, and its own desiccation may be perpetrated by the inhalation of therapeutic gases that are inadequately humidified.

**Water aerosol.** Water aerosol serves a double function. Its principle duty is to deliver liquid water, in minute particle form, to the mucosal surface. The site of its maximum deposition is determined by factors that we already know, particle size and ventilatory pattern. The water that "rains out" in the airways is intended to dilute thick secretions or moisten dry crusts for easier removal by cough or aspiration. In addition to this local effect of physical water particles contacting the airway surfaces, aerosols provide an important source of moisture for humidifying the inspired carrier gas. As the gas enters the warmth of the body and its vapor *capacity* increases, suspended water particles evaporate into the gas, raising its vapor tension to that of body humidity. Humidification can be increased by heating the water to be aerosolized so that it reaches the respiratory tract with no humidity deficit, not only increasing the inhaled water content but also sparing the respiratory tract its duty of humidifying the air. Reference will be made again to this maneuver when equipment is discussed.

The use of bland aerosol is extremely valuable in patients with mucosal crusting, thick secretions, or plugging of small airways with inspissated mucus. Bland means soothing or nonirritating and, in reference to therapeutic aerosols, means a solution lacking strong chemically or physically active ingredients. A useful bland solution is one that contains 3% propylene glycol in normal saline, although normal saline alone can be used. For patients with respiratory tract soreness, as from frequent unproductive coughing, delivering the aerosol warmed by an immersion heater aerosol generator adds a welcome factor of comfort. Also, humidification of the airways by evaporation is enhanced by the increased water vapor carried in heated inspired air. Unless poorly tolerated, bland mist generally should be used heated. An alternative is delivery by an ultrasonic nebulizer, the output of which is at or slightly above room temperature. Details of aerosol generators will be discussed a few pages on. Propylene glycol gives stability to water particles so that fewer evaporate, leaving more to deposit and dilute viscid mucus. It also enhances particle density of the aerosol mass.

Administration of bland aerosol should be preceded by a bronchodilator aerosol to assure maximal penetration of the heated particles. The mist should be inhaled through the mouth, not the nose, using a mouthpiece or mask with careful instructions in mouth breathing. To avoid tiring the patient treatments are best limited to a maximum of 30 minutes at intervals of 2 to 4 hours, or as tolerated. During dense mist therapy, patients should frequently be asked if they are comfortable because some will experience feelings of suffocation as well as fatigue. Soon both patient and therapist will learn the patient's threshold of comfort, making treatment schedules progressively easier.

The clinical indications for water therapy are many, and the therapist is responsible for seeing that it is properly administered. It is an old therapy, going back through many generations, as man has often used inhaled steam to relieve his respiratory distress. Our current techniques are more efficient, but the objectives are the same. The therapist will use aerosolized water to treat laryngeal croup of childhood, the thick secretions of cystic fibrosis, and chronic bronchial infections, and he will routinely include it with the administration of all therapeutic gases. Unless otherwise specified, distilled water is preferred to tap water because its cleanliness and freedom from solutes are a protection for both the patient and the equipment.

There is one special use of water aerosol therapy that deserves individual attention because of its widespread use and importance—the induction of sputum specimens for laboratory examinations. Such examinations are done for two general reasons. First, specimens are prepared by skilled technicians called cytotechnologists and are carefully examined under the microscope for the presence of malignant cells in suspected cases of cancer of the respiratory tract. Often, if such disease is in communication with the airway, cells from the surface of the tumor will desquamate, mix with bronchial secretions, and be expectorated. Although the absence of malignant cells in this test, called a *cytologic* sputum examination, does not eliminate the possibility of cancer, their presence is strong evidence of the existence of cancer somewhere in the bronchi or lungs and necessitates a careful search for its location or for some other explanation for the abnormal cells. Second, a *bacteriologic* sputum examination attempts to determine the presence or absence of bacteria in the secretions and to identify those present. Initially the specimen is smeared on a glass slide, stained with a dye, and microscopically examined for organisms. This often gives a good idea of the general type of microbe present and permits the start of therapy. The rest of the specimen is mixed with several kinds of culture media (nutrients that promote bacterial growth) and incubated from a few hours to several days or weeks to allow maximum growth. Examination of the culture allows specific identification of the bacteria.

Most of the patients treated by the respiratory therapist will have little trouble providing sputum specimens for analysis, and no special procedures will be required. On the other hand, patients with suspected malignancy or nonacute tuberculosis may have very scanty sputum or none at all, and to obtain specimens from them may be critical. For these patients techniques are available to procure an *induced sputum* specimen, so called because agents are used by inhalation to promote an increased flow of bronchial secretion and to stimulate a cough. It has been indicated earlier that bronchial secretions will respond to almost any inhaled irritant, and for induction many have been tried, including 10% sodium chloride, dornase, acetylcysteine, sterile distilled water aerosols, and sulfur dioxide gas.[182] The last, although effective, has been found too irritating and is not generally recommended, and the mucolytics and proteolytics have little value in the absence of secretions. The salt-and-water aerosols, when delivered by standard aerosolization, are preheated to 140° to 185° F by any suitable means, but usually by an immersion heating unit in the aerosol generator.[183] This "superheated" aerosol is well saturated with humidity as the patient inhales it, and it also contains large numbers of particles for deposition throughout the bronchial tree.

The distilled water particles condense on the bronchial mucosa and mix with and increase the volume of the normal thin layer of mucus present. The abundance of fine particles also has an irritant effect, stimulating a cough that expectorates the diluted secretions. Sodium chloride aerosols have the same effect, and one additional: because a 10% concentration is more saline than the average body fluids (approximately 0.9%), this aerosol is hypertonic, and as it contacts the bronchial wall, its osmolarity draws fluid from the mucosal layer into the bronchial lumen, increasing the volume of secretions available for expectoration. With both fluid aerosols the stimulated cough causes the secretions thus moved to carry with them loose or superficial cells from the mucosal surface as well as any available bacteria close to the bronchial lumen. Cells and bacteria, which the subject would be unable to produce by voluntary cough, can thereby be examined.

When the technique of sputum induction became accepted, it was customary to use a 20% solution of propylene glycol as the saline solvent because of the stabilizing properties attributed to this agent. It was believed that the inclusion of propylene in the mixture assured the penetration and deposition of a maximum number of particles in the respiratory tract. However, further experience demonstrated that propylene glycol itself had an inhibiting effect on the causative organism of tuberculosis (*Mycobacterium tuberculosis*), destroying it or preventing its growth in culture.[182] This was a serious handicap, since the recovery of tubercle bacilli is an important function of sputum induction. From a practical point of view of the overall use of this technique, since it is diagnostic and the condition of the subject to be examined is therefore not known, it is advisable to omit propylene glycol from induced sputum mixtures and to use simply 10% sodium chloride in water. The units especially available for administration of heated aerosol are compact and easily portable, lending themselves well to private office and outpatient use and to general hospital use. However, some hospitals have found ultrasonic aerosol generators, which will be described later, to be most effective in inducing cough. Using distilled water at room temperature, these generators produce finely uniform particles that stimulate a heavy cough, usually after only a few breaths. As yet there are no available data comparing the relative amounts of secretions produced by ultrasonic aerosols as against the standard heated hypertonic saline aerosols. Precautions should be taken to protect medical personnel from possible contamination, especially when they are obtaining specimens suspected of containing tubercle bacilli. The use of a specially ventilated hooded table has been suggested and appears to be as practical a method as any.[184]

The usefulness of this procedure is widely recognized. For many years it was a common practice to aspirate the stomach through a long tube swallowed by the patient and to examine the gastric secretions for tubercle bacilli that the patient had inadvertently swallowed after unnoticed small coughs. Although not a difficult procedure, it was a nuisance that has been replaced by the much more convenient induced cough, which most investigators find to have a far greater bacterial yield.[185, 186] It has proved to be a great boon to cancer detection, at times eliminating diagnostic procedures that are much more hazardous.[187, 188] In addition to its diagnostic value, sputum induction often affords excellent symptomatic relief of airway obstruction by removing inspissated mucus, and not infrequently this technique of heated supersaturated aerosolization is used for its therapeutic benefit. The duration of exposure to the aerosol, for diagnosis or therapy, can be varied to suit each individual. The patient is instructed to inhale the aerosol through his mouth in an easy and comfortable manner, resting as often as necessary, and at most the session should not exceed 15 minutes. Samples of sputum should be collected over the ensuing 30 minutes, and care should be taken not to collect saliva but only secretions that obviously arise from the depths of the airways. Sterile containers should be available for all specimens. If sputum is to be examined for malignant cells, it *must* be free of foreign particles. This is best accomplished by having hospitalized patients wash their teeth and thoroughly rinse their mouths prior to collection, and outpatients at least to rinse. As a maximum precaution against contamination, it is helpful to collect as many cytology specimens as possible before breakfast; sputum yields are usually most abundant at that time.

The pharmaceutical and physical agents described in this section are by no means an all-inclusive list of potential aerosols, and it is probable that other substances will be found suitable for this dosage form. Some work was done to determine the usefulness of aerosolized dipalmitoyl-lecithin, a synthetic form of one of the active ingredients of pulmonary surfactant. It was hoped that its administration would help negate the often disastrous effects of surfactant deficiency, but so far the results are scarcely more than slightly promising.[189] Some felt that aerosolization might lend itself well to nonpulmonary medication, and heparin was given a trial. An anticoagulant, widely used to prevent and treat vascular thromboses and emboli, heparin is given by an inconvenient parenteral schedule. However, its administration by aerosol does not yet appear to have won acceptance.[190] Such apparently unlikely substances as dyes have a limited aerosol use. The respiratory therapist will have occasion to note the concern caused by finding heavy sputum cultures of a yeastlike fungus called *Candida albicans*, and he will learn of the dispute centered about the question of whether or not this organism is a true pathogen. A frequent normal inhabitant of the mouth, throat, and upper respiratory tract, *C. albicans* is usually considered to be pathogenic in its own right if it is accompanied by a sufficient overgrowth. A clinical infection with it is often called *moniliasis*. Moniliasis frequently accompanies chronic or debilitating diseases and can be very resistant to treatment. Some of the coal-tar dyes, especially *brilliant green* and *methylene blue*, have been found to be effective by aerosol. Treatment is carried out for several weeks, with either a 0.2% solution of brilliant green or a 0.1% solution of methylene blue, in 50% propylene glycol, aerosolizing 2 ml five times daily. Repeated courses of 10 days each until clinical improvement is evident have proved satisfactory.[191, 192] Staining of skin and linens poses nonmedical complications, but the effectiveness and freedom from toxicity of these drugs justifies their consideration whenever clinical moniliasis is a threat.

With the improved aerosol equipment and techniques of the past few years and especially with the development of skilled technical personnel to administer them, it is hoped that increasing advantage will be taken of this relatively easy and painless method of treating disease.

## AEROSOL AND HUMIDITY GENERATORS

This section is not intended to be a technical manual, describing the details of specific equipment or comparing the characteristics of competitive products, for such information is available through the commercial brochures and specification tables provided by all manufacturers. We will discuss principles involved in the design and operation of aerosol and humidity generators so that the therapist will recognize and understand the features of any piece of equipment with which he will have to work. He will develop his own criteria for judging equipment, based on his experience, and will soon learn that he must thoroughly read all descriptive literature provided with each item before he attempts to put that item to clinical use. He will make it a point to disassemble the parts, familiarizing himself with the location and function of each component, with an eye to the ever-present problems of maintenance and repair. Although most ethical manufacturers of quality medical equipment are straightforward in their advertising, their objective is to sell, whereas the main interest of the therapist is the welfare of patients under his care. Thus the therapist will try to determine for himself such features of his equipment as safety, probable patient acceptance, quality of performance, ease of cleaning, durability, and economy. This type of critical appraisal is the mark of a safe and effective therapist.

Instruments used to generate aerosols are called *nebulizers* (from "nebula," meaning a cloud or mist), and those that increase water vapor content, *humidifiers*, although there is a considerable overlap between them both in function and in application and they sometimes differ only in degree or in the use to which they are put. It may be generalized, however, that nebulizers are designed to deliver a maximum number of particles of desired size, of pharmaceutics or water, for penetration and deposition in the respiratory tract, and that humidifiers are designed to deliver a maximum amount of water vapor with a minimum of particulate water. Some humidifiers produce varying amounts of aerosolized water, but the prime difference between them and nebulizers is the tremendous volume of particles of the latter. This difference may be a consideration when possible spread of infection is of concern. Bacteria, in general, are of the same magnitude of size as aerosol particles and can thus attach themselves to the particles for transport directly into the lungs. In contrast, the absence of water mass of humidity provides bacteria with no mobile nuclei to carry them. Humidifiers therefore pose less of a threat of bacterial contamination to the patient than do nebulizers. From a practical point of view this difference is probably only significant, if at all, when the patient is breathing for a long time through a piece of equipment that may be difficult to maintain hygienically clean, such as a ventilator. Moistening the inspired gas with a humidifier rather than a nebulizer will at least deny bacteria easy access to the respiratory tract.

Nebulizers and humidifiers are both available for use with water at room temperature or, by the inclusion of heating devices, with water at elevated temperatures. By raising the water temperature far above that of the body (up to 60° C), some humidifiers can add enough vapor to the inspired gas so that, despite the drop in temperature in transit from instrument to patient, when gas enters the body it will be at or near body humidity. Some nebulizers, when used to deliver liquid water to the respiratory tract, employ the same principle so the carrier gas will have its quota of vapor and will not "steal" it from the suspended particles intended for deposition.[193] To help us keep in mind that there is a basic therapeutic difference between humidification and nebulization, let us employ the following rough classification of the types of equipment used for each: *humidifiers*—jet (aerosol), Hydro-Sphere, pass-over, and bubble-diffusion; *nebulizers*—jet, impeller, and ultrasonic. We will describe some of the characteristics of each of the five different types.

## Jet aerosol-humidifier

Although the jet instruments can be used for both aerosol generation and humidification, for the sake of simplicity we will refer to them as nebulizers and differentiate between their specific uses when indicated. The jet nebulizer is the most versatile of all this group of instruments and enjoys the most widespread usage. It is simple, can function without moving parts, and is based on the Bernoulli effect as illustrated in the simplified sketch of Fig. 7-5. Although jet nebulizers assume many shapes and sizes, they all have the fundamental features shown in the illustration. A source of gas pressure must be provided that may be a simple hand-operated rubber bulb, a motorized compressor, or tanked gas. The gas enters the nebulizer chamber through a restricted orifice, providing a jet stream of high velocity (*A*). The jet is directed across

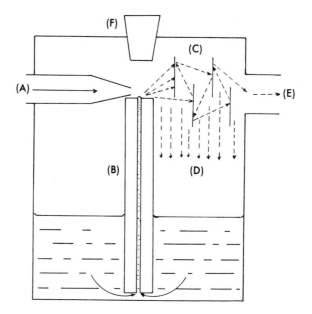

**Fig. 7-5.**   Principle of jet nebulization. (See text for explanation.) (Modified from Egan, D. F.: Conn. Med. **31:**353, 1967.)

the end of a fine capillary tube *(B)*, the other end of which is immersed in the solution to be nebulized. The high velocity of the gas produces a local drop in pressure immediately adjacent to the capillary ostium (Bernoulli effect), and because the reservoir surface is subjected to atmospheric pressure, liquid is forced up the capillary (solid arrows). As it reaches the top of the tube, the liquid is continuously blown off by the gas jets as small particles and thrown against one or more barriers called baffles *(C)*. Again, these baffles can be of many shapes such as small spheres, rods, or plates, or the configuration of the nebulizer chamber may function as a baffle. Here the particles are further fragmented, and many coalesce into masses too large to transport; these return to the reservoir as a condensate *(D)*. The outflow gas to the patient *(E)* contains aerosol particles of the desired therapeutic size. Many chambers provide an optional opening for the introduction of air into the gas-particle mixture *(F)*. When opened, a venturi is created as the jet gas draws room air into the chamber (termed *air entrainment*), providing an increased flow through the nebulizer to the patient, increasing the rate of nebulization of the reservoir, and thus administering more liquid per unit of time. The need for such an additional source of gas varies with the instrument and its specific use, a matter to which we will have occasion to refer later. However, it must be remembered that changing the physical environment of a nebulization chamber may alter the character of the aerosol output, especially in terms of the effect of the turbulence of higher flows on particle stability. These are influences that the interested therapist can determine for himself by carefully controlled measurements of equipment performance under various conditions.

Essentially, the structure of the baffle system of a jet instrument determines

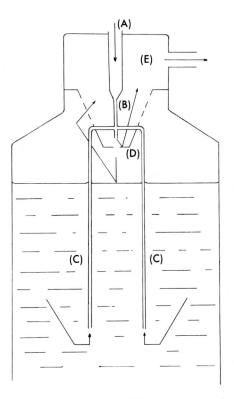

**Fig. 7-6.** Components of a jet humidifier. (See text for description.)

whether it is to function as a nebulizer or as a jet humidifier. Fig. 7-6 depicts the jet principle employed in humidification. The power gas enters at *A*, passing through a restriction *(B)* into which twin capillary tubes *(C)* open. The venturi at *B* produces a foaming mixture of liquid and gas that meets a baffle *(D)* as it emerges from the jet orifice. The baffle may be a perforated plate against which some liquid particles impinge, fracture, and are reflected into the vapor chamber *(E)*. Other particles penetrate the plate and are further baffled by the reservoir surface, which retains the larger ones; the remainder are screened once more as they enter the vapor chamber through the plate baffle. Baffled particles condense and return to the reservoir. The minute water particles that continue into the chamber evaporate into the gas to raise its vapor content, supplemented by water of evaporation from the reservoir surface. Gas issuing from the unit will thus have a maximum amount of water vapor and a minimum of liquid water particles, and it is with this type of humidifier that electric immersion heaters are most frequently used. The amount of humidity can be easily increased, but the output temperature must be monitored to avoid overheating in case of malfunction of the thermostatic control of the unit, and special attention must be paid to prevent the reservoir of water from being depleted.

There are two interesting variations of the jet nebulization principle that deserve comment—liquid filtration and self-propulsion.

*Liquid filtration nebulizers.* [194] Nebulizers of this type are reportedly able to produce aerosol particles consistently less than $0.5\mu$ in diameter, the so-called "microaerosols," or submicronic particles. Technically, they are classified according to a "D" series, such as D.10, etc., up to D.37, depending on size, particular structure, and other specifications. The basic feature of these nebulizers is the use of the nebulized solution as the baffling system of the units. The principle depends on the observation that if a mass of aerosolized liquid particles of heterogeneous sizes is brought into contact with successive volumes of the liquid, particles of increasingly smaller size will be removed from the aerosol until only completely stable particles of a very small size remain in suspension. Fig. 7-7 demonstrates this in the simplest fashion. Container $A$ represents a typical air jet, nebulizing a dye-colored solution, whereas containers $B$ to $E$ are a variable number of glass flasks containing, initially, volumes of the uncolored solvent used to prepare the nebulizing solution. The flasks are connected in series so that the total output of the nebulizer will pass through each one in succession. In operation it will be noted that the solvent in each flask becomes decreasingly colored, until one flask will show none. Thus relatively large numbers of large particles are trapped by the solvent in flask $A$, deeply staining the fluid, but by the time the aerosol issues from the last flask (at $F$), the particles are of such a uniformly small and stable size that none are baffled.

The use of this "scrubbing" process for the removal of unwanted large liquid particles in commercial nebulizers is modified according to the need of space economy and is illustrated in Fig. 7-8. A heterogeneous aerosol is generated by an air jet immersed in solution at $A$ and passes upward through a series of constrictions $(B)$. Turbulent flow removes from the stream all but the smallest and most stable particles, condensing them so that they return to the reservoir. Those particles leaving the ports $(C)$, in order to have escaped the scrubbing turbulence, are submicronic in size.

*Inert gas-powered nebulizers.* Popular because of their compactness and ease of operation, nebulizers with a self-contained power supply are in widespread use. They are made of a small vial containing the solution (or powder) to be nebulized and a physiologically inert gas under pressure as a propellant. With the supplied mouthpiece in place, a slight squeeze releases a small valve allowing the gas to nebulize the medication and deliver it in self-limited premeasured doses.

There is an unresolved controversy as to just how inert are the propellant gases of these units (and household commercial aerosols, as well). [195-199] The gases are of a chemical group known as fluorocarbons, with many members, but of which Freon 11 is one of the most widely used. Animal experiments suggest that fluorocarbons may cause cardiac arrhythmias and death if inhaled in the presence of hypoxemia, and there have been reports of rhythm disturbances in humans. It is speculated that instances of sudden or unexpected deaths in asthmatic patients may be due to fluorocarbon-induced cardiac arrest. This view is by no means unanimous, and some investigators question the evidence on which the claims of propellant hazards are based. Much of the dispute centers on the validity of projecting experimental animal data to humans and on the duration of fluorocarbon blood and tissue levels following

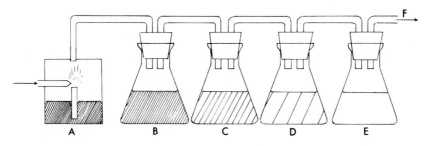

**Fig. 7-7.** Demonstration of the principle of liquid filtration in the production of microaerosols. Shading of the liquid represents the concentration of dye. (See text for further explanation.)

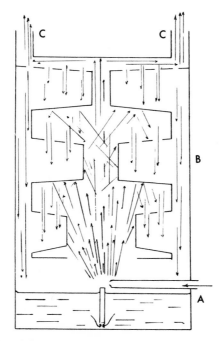

**Fig. 7-8.** Utilization of liquid filtration in an aerosol generator. Turbulent flow through the constrictions removes all but the smallest particles. (See text for description.)

inhalation. Despite the unsettled question of safety, gas-powered aerosol units are very popular, and as long as they will be used, patients should be instructed in their proper use and advised strongly to keep exposure to a minimum.

For the purpose of discussing the clinical use of jet nebulizers, we can arbitrarily divide them into two classes—intermittent nebulizers and reservoir nebulizers—although it will be obvious that there is no clear-cut line of demarcation between the two.

*Intermittent nebulizers.* This group comprises the relatively small instruments with a capacity of about 5 ml used for limited periods of time on an intermittent basis, mostly for the administration of pharmaceutical aerosols rather than water or humidity. The prototype is the so-called "hand nebulizer," which combines a simple glass or plastic air jet powered by a hand-operated rubber squeeze bulb and is especially suited to the short-term administration of sympathomimetic bronchodilators, for which it was originally designed. The therapist should acquaint himself with the energy required to operate a hand bulb so that he will appreciate the difficulty experienced by a patient attempting to use such a nebulizer for a long period of time. Most units of this type have air ports that permit two velocities of airflow and nebulization. In general, the slower rate without air entrainment is satisfactory, but the option permits adjusting therapy to individual needs. Simple though the instrument is, proper technique in its usage is essential for good results. All patients should be instructed in the nebulizer's use, with a demonstration by the therapist, and should not be permitted to rely only on the manufacturer's directions. Two major points should be emphasized. First, the patient should be instructed to open his mouth widely so that the lips and teeth will not obstruct the aerosol flow, then hold the nebulizer so that its delivery port is directed toward the mouth but is about 1 inch away from the lips. This allows the aerosol to be entrained in the inspiratory airflow, but if the nebulizer tube is inserted into the mouth and the lips tightly pursed about it, much of the aerosol will be deposited in the mouth. Second, the patient should be taught to inhale as slowly and deeply as possible and to deliver the first charge of aerosol just after he starts his inhalation. The therapist will observe that many patients release the aerosol at, or even before, the start of inhalation, depositing much of it outside the respiratory tract. Depending on the length of inhalation, two or three aerosol doses may be delivered in one breath. At end-inspiration the breath should be held for 2 or 3 seconds to allow maximum aerosol distribution and deposition.

Usually two to four good inhalations of a sympathomimetic at one time, repeated in 2 to 4 hours, are adequate. The therapist will see many patients for whom this schedule is not completely satisfactory, and he will be asked how often the patient can use the nebulizer. In cases of severe bronchospasm it may be necessary to allow more frequent treatments, but it must always be kept in mind that bronchodilator drugs are potent, with possible serious side effects. Sympathomimetics are locally irritating to the respiratory tract, and too frequent use can actually aggravate the very condition for which they are being used. If relief cannot be obtained with a safe conservative schedule, some other or additional therapy may be indicated, but unrestrained use of the bronchodilator is not. In this regard, the very convenience of the gas-powered nebulizer, described above, is a hazard. In principle, such units are both effective and safe as they deliver measured doses well within limits of tolerance. However, their ready availability and the ease with which they can be used leads to frequent patient abuse and disregard for advised schedules. It is not unusual to see patients using these nebulizers every 5 or 10 minutes. One can imagine the chemical irritation of the respiratory mucosa added to the disability of the underlying disease, and appreciate the possible harm from excessive exposure to fluorocarbon propellants, as noted earlier. Overuse of the hand bulb nebulizer is apt to be less harmful because of the work involved in its operation, which may be considerable for the patient with respiratory distress. It is often prudent to prescribe this type of instrument for the patient suspected of a tendency to self-medication.

For the administration of mucolytic, proteolytic, or antibiotic aerosols, or for longer therapy with dilute bronchodilators, the small-volume nebulizers can be adapted to a power source. A small compressor is most practical, since it does not need the pressure regulator or flowmeter of tanked gas and is safe for home use. For treatments that may last up to 30 or 60 minutes, the use of an aerosol mask is advisable. Not only is the patient spared the nuisance and fatigue of holding a nebulizer to his face, but the design of such a mask holds a mass of aerosol particles about the mouth as a reservoir from which the patient can inhale. Since nebulization during the exhalation is wasteful of medication, a simple Y-connector can be inserted in the tubing from the pump to the nebulizer, with the stem of the Y connected to the pump and one of the arms to the nebulizer. The other arm, left free, can be obstructed by the finger during inhalation to permit nebulization and can be released during exhalation to shunt the airflow away from the nebulizer. Although the same general pattern of slow deep breathing is advised for prolonged therapy, as was described earlier, the patient should be warned about overbreathing to the point of discomfort from either the effort involved or possible hypocapnia. In addition to directions included in the original medication prescription, specific dose measurements should be given to the patient, in drops or milliliters, depending on the technique used in filling the nebulizer, and he should be taught not to flood the capillary tube by overfilling. Finally, the patient should be instructed to rinse his nebulizer after use by nebulizing a small amount of water to prevent clogging of the capillary or jet with dried medication.

*Reservoir nebulizers.* As the name implies, these nebulizers have a large capacity for the solution to be nebulized and are intended for prolonged intermittent or continuous use. Thus they are predominantly used for aerosolized water or humidity therapy, although occasionally for more active agents such as mucolytic detergents. For purposes of discussion we can consider the use of reservoir jet nebulizers in the two categories of prolonged intermittent and continuous.

PROLONGED INTERMITTENT USE. Prolonged intermittent use refers to the administration of water (usually) aerosol for periods longer than would be practical with a small-volume nebulizer to avoid the inconvenience of repeated replenishment of the latter. The use of heated aerosol of hypertonic saline, with or without propylene glycol, for sputum induction or for the removal of thick bronchial plugs is a common example. This technique was discussed in the previous section of this chapter and needs no further amplification except to stress its therapeutic as well as its diagnostic value. Intermittent water aerosol is not new in the treatment of acute laryngitis, since several generations have taken advantage of the relief afforded by the inhalation of steam. Aerosol generators, however, are more efficient than the heated tea kettle, providing a steady volume of particles of more uniform size than can be found in steam. Water aerosol can be generated for prolonged periods of time at room temperature ("cold steam") or warmed by an immersion heater or by setting the reservoir in a container of water on a hot plate. Jet humidifiers (or aerosol generators) are effective in the daily management of patients with permanent tracheostomies, for whom high humidity should be added to the inspired air at regular intervals to maintain the integrity of the respiratory tract mucosa. This procedure can easily be carried out at home with a tracheostomy mask to direct the maximum amount of humid air directly into the trachea.

CONTINUOUS USE. Continuous use implies an uninterrupted administration of humidity or water particles for long periods of time. Probably the most common and important example is the humidification of therapeutic oxygen, since, except during short-term emergency use, oxygen (or any other compressed gas) should never be given without adequate humidification. Inhalation of the bone-dry gas not only is uncomfortable to the patient after a few minutes, but its desiccating effect on the respiratory mucosa can be critically harmful. For most patients receiving oxygen, unless bronchial secretions are a major problem, a simple jet humidifier is effective and easy to set up. The patient with an "acute trach" must have continuous humidification until his underlying disease has become stabilized. This is the patient whose acute respiratory problem required a tracheotomy operation and whose resultant tracheostomy is used either to ease his spontaneous breathing or to assist him with mechanical ventilation. Details of the management of the tracheotomized patient will be discussed later, and at this point we will only emphasize that the life of the patient may be in jeopardy if adequate water is not provided for his respiratory tract. Aerosolized water is a standard part of therapy for childhood croup, or acute laryngotracheobronchitis. The laryngeal edema, characteristic of this condition, can rapidly and fatally obstruct the airways of small children but often is dramatically relieved by water-saturated inspired air or oxygen. As noted above in reference to the treatment of laryngitis, steam has long been used for croup, but because the benefit of mist therapy is directly proportional to the concentration of water particles and the length of patient exposure, boiling water as a source of aerosol has limitations. Many hospitals have special "croup rooms" equipped with jets that fill the temperature-controlled room with a dense fog or use a more elaborate combination of air and live steam to create "natural fog."[200] Although effective, these units waste valuable hospital space when not in use. Large-volume jet nebulizers have had extensive use in the past few years, since when combined with a bed or crib canopy, they constitute a personal croup room about the individual patient. They are most effective when used with a temperature-controlled oxygen tent, which we will describe in another section; such a unit is then called a mist tent. Instruments designed for just this type of therapy are available, the most recent innovation being the ultrasonic nebulizer, which will also be described later in this chapter. The ultrasonic nebulizer produces a large volume of water aerosol and has thus gained great popularity over the jet nebulizer for prolonged high-humidity therapy. However, some of the most recent jet models have nearly the same mist production as the ultrasonic, and the simplicity, lower initial cost, and minimal maintenance of the jet nebulizers make them still the front-line instruments for humidity and mist. Finally, patients hospitalized with chronic bronchopulmonary disease frequently have serious problems with obstructive secretions, and the aerosol deposition of water in the respiratory tract is an important part of their therapy. It should be repeated here for emphasis that, for this type of patient, the most important of all the aerosol medications is water, a point we will have occasion to note more than once when we consider other therapeutic techniques.

One of the virtues of a skilled respiratory therapist is his versatility. With his knowledge of equipment and the objectives of therapy, he is able to choose the right instrument, or combination of instruments, to accomplish these objectives. He will frequently be called upon to use imagination and ingenuity in setting up equipment to suit the needs of patients with special problems. Because of the great variety and numbers of jet aerosol-humidifiers, it would be impractical as well as needless to attempt to describe the idiosyncrasies of each, but we will mention a few operational principles common to all which the therapist should bear in mind. To begin with, the relationship between the output of the jet nebulizer and the main flow of gas being humidified is important, and it may be described in one of two ways, *sidestream* nebulization and *mainstream* nebulization.[201] In sidestream nebulization the aerosol is discharged into the therapeutic gas flow between the delivery instrument and the patient, as shown in Fig. 7-9. The nebulizer has its own separate gas power supply, which is smaller than the therapeutic gas flow, and when the aerosol mixes with the greater volume of dry gas in the patient delivery tube, it is too diluted to raise the humidity of the gas to maximum. The sidestream method is mostly used with mechani-

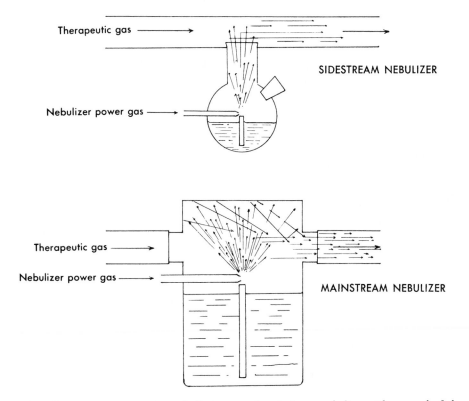

**Fig. 7-9.** Diagrammatic comparison of sidestream and mainstream nebulizers. The aerosol of the sidestream unit is considerably diluted by the large volume of dry therapeutic gas and provides limited humidity. It is used primarily to administer medication. The entire therapeutic gas flow passes through the mainstream nebulizer chamber and is able to pick up significant moisture. The effectiveness of this nebulizer can be increased by heating the fluid reservoir.

cal ventilators of the inspiratory positive-pressure type, and although it is limited in the humidity it contributes, the moisture is usually sufficient for short-term therapy; but for prolonged ventilator therapy the humidity is not adequate, and frequent refilling is necessary. Primarily, it is an effective way of administering medication during a treatment, and all the pharmaceutical agents described in the last section of this chapter can be given by this route. In mainstream nebulization the entire gas flow to the patient passes through the chamber of the nebulizer. These units are reservoir nebulizers, and with the high aerosol production the outflow gas to the patient can be supplied with a therapeutic level of humidity, up to 100% if a heating element is included. The importance of a heated water reservoir cannot be overstated if the goal is 100% humidification. It has been demonstrated that, in unheated nebulizers, either jet or bubble (to be described shortly), as oxygen flows through the unit the water temperature drops significantly.[202] At flows up to 12 liters per minute, the temperature of the reservoir water may drop as much as 13° C below its starting ambient temperature within 1 hour. Even the small-volume sidestream nebulizer will show a temperature drop of up to 5° C in 10 minutes. The temperature of the water thus becomes the limiting factor in the final humidity of the delivered gas. Even if the gas in the nebulizer chamber is saturated at its temperature, at the end of the gas delivery tube the humidity may fall to 50%, at the temperature of that point. The use of a heating device in the nebulizer to raise the water temperature to 53° C (125° F), in conjunction with a delivery tube of 1.9 cm internal diameter to prevent water clogging, will permit vapor saturation at body temperature. The jet oxygen humidifiers, as illustrated in Fig. 7-6, are theoretically mainstream units when the oxygen supply powers the jet; but oxygen concentrations can be varied by diluting the oxygen with air either in the nebulizing unit or at the patient end of the delivery tube, and the added volume of inspired gas at room temperature and humidity can lower the net humidity of the total inhaled gas. Combinations of sidestream and mainstream nebulization are often used together, especially during mechanical ventilation. The ventilator output is directed through the large reservoir nebulizer, and a small sidestream nebulizer is added to the flow just before it reaches the patient. Such a combination

**Table 7-9.**  *Influence of tubing on vapor temperature*\*†

| Distance from reservoir | | Temperature in tube (°C) |
|---|---|---|
| *(cm)* | *(ft)* | |
| 30.5 | 1 | 48.5 |
| 60.9 | 2 | 40.5 |
| 91.4 | 3 | 37.0 |
| 121.9 | 4 | 35.0 |
| 152.4 | 5 | 34.5 |

*From Wells, R. E., Jr., et al.: Humidification of oxygen during inhalational therapy, N. Engl. J. Med. **268:**644, 1963.
†Reservoir temperature = 53° C; tube length = 153 cm; internal diameter = 1.9 cm.

allows a continuous humidification of the main gas flow and the continuous or intermittent addition of medication. However, the therapist should remember to shut off
the mainstream nebulizer while administering medication through the sidestream unit
to avoid diluting the medication in the latter and perhaps negating its effect. If the
reservoir nebulizer is heated for maximum humidity, there will be a drop in temperature as the gas traverses the delivery tube, with precipitation of excess water in the
tube. Table 7-9 shows the magnitude of temperature drop in an aerosol tube at varying distances from its origin. In addition, the considerable volume of gas powering
the sidestream nebulizer, which is not heated, will further lower the final delivery
temperature, and although theoretically the inhaled gas might be saturated at its given
temperature, the volume of vapor it contains may be lower than 100% body humidity.
If the therapist thoroughly understands his equipment, he may be able to modify
it to deliver heated gas to the medication nebulizer and increase the delivered
humidity.

Attention should be given to the effect of the air jet on flow in the reservoir nebulizers, especially when they are used as mainstream humidifiers. Most units are designed to operate at power gas pressures of 50 pounds per square inch (50 psi) delivered
through a flowmeter that regulates the number of liters per minute available to the
nebulizer. Because the jet through which the gas must pass is a restricted orifice, a
considerable back pressure develops at the jet, according to the principles of pressure,
resistance, and flow discussed in earlier chapters. There will thus be a limit to the
amount of gas per unit of time that can go through a given nebulizer under operating
conditions. This is information that every therapist should know about his equipment,
either through information supplied by the manufacturer or by the process of testing
the equipment himself, measuring and recording the data.

Jet nebulizers are frequently used with canopy tents or other enclosures for high-
humidity or mist therapy, and care must be taken to see that there is adequate airflow
for the patient's needs. Some jet nebulizers may not be able to exceed an output of
more than 8 lpm and if used with tent oxygen therapy requiring a minute turnover
of 12 liters, will be inadequate. Separate oxygen supply lines will be needed for nebulization and ventilation. If an air compressor is used to power a nebulizer, the flow output of the pump must be known, not when functioning unrestricted but when attached
to the nebulizer. Thus a pump may be rated 20 lpm but when attached to an instrument may deliver only 10 lpm, and if this is the sole ventilatory supply to a mist tent,
additional sources of air must be made available either through air-entrainment ports
in the nebulizer or through the canopy itself.

Many of the large nebulizers have provisions for diluting the oxygen they deliver.
These consist of a port with variable openings to draw in room air, calibrated for concentrations of oxygen at various settings. This added air increases the total flow output
from the nebulizer. The lower the concentration of oxygen in the delivered mixture the
greater will be the volume of ambient air added, and the greater the total flow. Some
manufacturers provide data that relate the flowmeter reading with the oxygen concentration and the total output, but if these are not available, the therapist must determine them himself. The air-dilution ports are closed when heated nebulization is

used because the inflow of diluting air cools the air-mist mixture and negates the purpose of the instrument. With the output of the nebulizer functioning at its lowest level, there are many times when the flow will not be adequate for the patient's need, and full advantage cannot be taken of the 100% humidity potential of the nebulizer.

Safety pressure release valves are necessary in the large jet nebulizers, and they should be periodically checked. There is always the risk of compression or kinking of the output line, and the buildup of pressure in the unit is potentially dangerous. Also, because such an event would stop the therapy, relief valves usually have audible signals to warn of the shutoff of gas supply to the patient.

### Hydro-Sphere nebulizer-humidifier

To some degree the Hydro-Sphere is a modification of the jet nebulizer with same indications for its use. The basic difference between the two is the mechanism by which pressured gas is brought into contact with the liquid to be aerosolized. Instead of a capillary tube-jet complex, the Hydro-Sphere uses gravity flow over a glass sphere, as demonstrated in Fig. 7-10. A pumping mechanism (not shown) carries solution from the reservoir (*A*) through tube (*B*) to the top of a hollow glass sphere (*C*). The solution is continuously and gently poured onto the upper pole of the sphere at (*D*), where it distributes itself by gravity as a very thin film (*E*) over the spherical surface. The film is greatly exaggerated in the sketch for illustration purposes. A gas source, at pressures

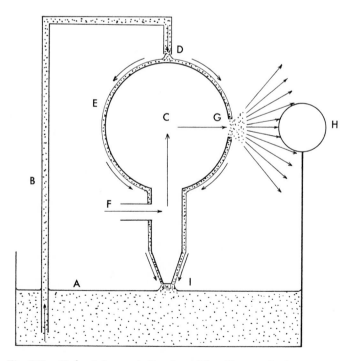

**Fig. 7-10.** Hydro-Sphere nebulizer-humidifier. (See text for description.)

between 10 and 50 psi, enters the hollow sphere at $(F)$, pressurizing the interior of the sphere $(G)$, rupturing the overlying liquid film and dispersing it as small particles. An impactor baffle $(H)$ removes the large droplets, permitting the outflow only of those within the therapeutic range. Excess, unnebulized fluid flows down the sphere and is directed by the sphere's tapered base back into the reservoir for recirculation $(I)$.

Among the virtues claimed for this aerosol generator are (1) the absence of moving parts minimizes maintenance; (2) 97% of its aerosol output is said to be within the $1\mu$ to $10\mu$ diameter range, and 50% below $5\mu$; (3) aerosol is delivered at a temperature of $6°$ to $10°$ F below ambient; and (4) there is an apparent consistent aerosol density over a wide range of airflows. Several published reports support the efficacy of the Hydro-Sphere's performance, and only the test of time is needed for final confirmation.[203, 204]

### Pass-over humidifier

The pass-over humidifier is the simplest of all and depends on evaporation to supply humidity to air directed across its surface. Although its efficiency can be increased by heating either the water or the air, this type of humidifier has been replaced, for the most part, by the other humidifiers and nebulizers under discussion.

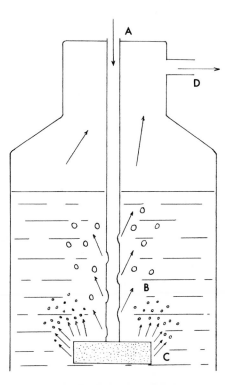

**Fig. 7-11.** The bubble-diffusion humidifier bubbles therapeutic gas, A, through a perforated tube, B, or a porous diffusion head, C. The larger the number of small bubbles the greater will be the evaporation area to humidify the gas leaving outflow port, D.

### Bubble-diffusion humidifier

One of the oldest methods of humidifying oxygen consists of bubbling it through a reservoir of water, thus providing a large number of gas-liquid surfaces to enhance evaporation. Fig. 7-11 illustrates two commonly employed techniques. Gas enters the unit at *A* and passes through a tube immersed nearly to the bottom of a jar containing water. Sometimes the tube contains multiple perforations *(B)* through which the gas escapes as bubbles of a size determined by the size of the openings. The relatively small amount of gas in each bubble, surrounded by a large amount of water, picks up water of evaporation to varying degrees of humidity and leaves the outflow port *(D)*. Instead of the holes, the immersed oxygen tube may be fitted with a porous stonelike *diffusion head (C)* at its lower tip. This breaks the gas into much smaller bubbles than the perforated tube, thus increasing the total gas surface for evaporation of water among the much larger number of small bubbles. At best, humidity of between 40% and 50% is all that can be expected at the outflow, and this probably drops to less than 20% in the warm respiratory tract. Although the old "bubble bottles" have been replaced by more effective humidifiers, the bubble-diffusion principle has not been altogether discarded, and there are some new designs of this instrument that have proved to be effective. Made especially for adaptation to mechanical ventilators, one such unit, known as a "cascade" humidifier, effectively breaks the inspired gas into minute bubbles and passes them through water heated by an adjustable immersion heater. The temperature of the humidifier can be raised to such a level that the moist gas will still be humid when it reaches the patient, and 100% saturation can be achieved.

### Impeller nebulizer

Physical force of a rapidly rotating disc is used to break up water into fine particles and to emit it as a heavy mist. The disc, driven by an electric motor, sucks water from a reservoir and literally throws it through a meshed or slotted baffle. Of less uniform size than the particles from a well-constructed jet nebulizer, the aerosol does produce a grossly visible fog and affords the inspired air a good supply of water particles for evaporation, although, with the heterogeneous particle sizes, there tends to be more "rain out" about a patient enclosed in a tent. Because there is no need for a compressed gas source and the units are compact and easy to operate, the impeller nebulizer is popular for home use. It is available in a number of sizes and output capacities, some decorator styled for room size humidification.

### Ultrasonic nebulizer

The ultrasonic nebulizer is a complex electronic instrument that has been adequately described elsewhere, and we will only briefly review its major features and applications.[205, 206] An ultrasonic nebulizer consists of two compartments—a power chamber and a nebulizing chamber. The heart of the unit is a transducer, a device that is activated by one form of energy and relays it in another form. The transducer is ceramic and is classified as *piezoelectric* because it is able to change pressure *(piezo-)* energy into electric, and vice versa. Thus, when electrical energy is applied to a piezoelectric transducer, the latter responds by a rapidly oscillating change in shape, manifested by physical vibration, a form of pressure energy. Conversely, if the transducer is subjected to pressure, it will convert such energy to electrical.

In the ultrasonic nebulizer, alternating current is applied to the transducer and electrical energy is transformed into vibrational energy at frequencies beyond the range of human hearing. Commercial units operate at frequencies of from 1.3 to 1.4 megacycles/sec, truly remarkable rates. The rapid vibrations are carried through water (called a couplant), and are focused on a flexible diaphragm supporting the liquid to be nebulized, in the aerosol chamber. The diaphragm vibrates in sympathy and literally shakes the liquid into a mass of small particles. The transfer of energy is accompanied by the production of a small amount of heat, varying from 3° to 10° C above ambient. The aerosol particles can be carried to the patient by a small blower provided with the instrument, by oxygen as a carrier gas, or by the patient's own ventilation. Depending upon the make and model of nebulizer, there are adjustments for variable aerosol concentrations, and up to 6 ml of water can be nebulized per minute. Because of the high aerosol output, heating is not necessary and the therapy can be given at room temperature.

Fig. 7-12 demonstrates some of the important characteristics of ultrasonic nebulization. Each model is a rough representation of a nebulizer, showing the electrical input to the piezoelectric transducer at the bottom, the resulting vibrational wave transmission through a couplant liquid to a responsive diaphragm in the center, and the effect of diaphragm vibrations on the aerosol chamber target liquid.[207] Vibrational frequency determines the response of the liquid surface to vertical oscillations. Fig.

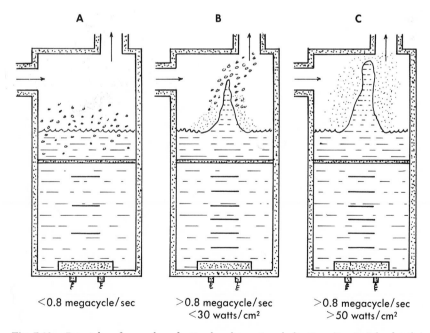

|  A | B | C |
|---|---|---|
| <0.8 megacycle/sec | >0.8 megacycle/sec <br> <30 watts/cm² | >0.8 megacycle/sec <br> >50 watts/cm² |

**Fig. 7-12.** Principles of aerosol production by ultrasonic nebulization. (See text for details.)

7-12, *A*, shows that low-frequency energy, less than 0.8 megacycle/sec, produces surface waves, the crests of which break into droplets greater than 25$\mu$ in diameter, but no fine mist. As the frequency increases above 0.8 megacycle/sec, we see from Fig. 7-12, *B*, that the liquid surface is pushed up into a column, like a fountain, emitting fine particles from its base and coarser droplets from its top. Let us now consider the influence of electrical power on aerosol production. At low power levels, such as 30 watts applied per square centimeter of liquid surface, the effect is pulsatile, and the high-frequency–generated column breaks discontinuously into a wide range of particle sizes. As power increases to about 50 watts/cm$^2$, with continued high frequency, pulsed fog emission becomes continuous, and as demonstrated in Fig. 7-12, *C*, there is a steady production of high-density mist of fine particles, ideal for water aerosol therapy. The final control over particle size of aerosol delivered to the patient is a function of baffling, often by a flow of air directed at the fountain. The higher the velocity of the impinging air stream, the smaller the emergent aerosol particles.

Clinical response testifies to the efficacy of ultrasonic nebulization and its ability to deposit water in the respiratory tract, but there is little specific information regarding mean particle size produced. On the one hand, it is asserted that measured mean values varied from 1$\mu$ to 10$\mu$ in diameter but with a narrow distribution range,[208] and on the other, it is claimed that the mass of particles falls within the 0.8$\mu$ to 1.0$\mu$ range with probable 80% deposition within the lung.[209] The lack of condensation of moisture on a piece of glass held in the aerosol steam indicates an effective stability of particle size. In the process of determining the degree of humidity actually delivered to the respiratory tract, a revealing experiment was conducted on dogs.[209] Very small humidity transducers were introduced into the primary division of the bronchi and were attached to recorders responsive to the amount of water vapor with which the transducers were in contact. Calibrations were in arbitrary "humidity units," depending upon the deflection of the recorder with known humidity. This permitted the comparison of the amount of moisture delivered to the airway with air-activated and ultrasonic nebulizers. Standard nebulizers increased bronchial vapor content an average of 0.18 units, whereas the ultrasonic achieved 0.71 and 4.03 units, on two volume settings. In addition, the duration of maintained humidity was longer with the ultrasonic than with the air-generated instruments.

With the large aerosol production of which the ultrasonic nebulizer is capable and the obvious penetration of water into the respiratory tract, the question of possible harm to the lung arose. Washing the lung with water or saline is known to disrupt its surface tension stability, presumably by the removal of pulmonary surfactant, and because it was important to know whether ultrasonic aerosolization posed the same risk, animal experimentations were carried out.[210, 211] The lungs of dogs subjected to nebulization of isotonic saline and distilled water were examined, and no evidence of interference with surface tension stability was detected, even after 72 hours of aerosols. It was speculated that the small particle size and the total low fluid volume were not harmful, in this respect. On the other hand, it was noted that after prolonged aerosol exposure all animals receiving saline mist, and a few of those on distilled water, showed microscopic pulmonary changes consistent with bronchopneumonia. The deposition of hypertonic saline, the result of water evaporating from normal saline, was felt to be responsible. It was concluded that continuous wetting of the lung with ultrasonic mist for long periods of time might be deleterious, although no time-limit safety guides were suggested.

In addition to its large aerosol volume, the ultrasonic nebulizer has other physical virtues. Of importance is the independence of the aerosol production from the flow of the breathing gas. Whereas the output of the jet nebulizer depends on the flow of its power gas, the ultrasonic nebulizer can dispense a steady particle volume regardless of the flow. This is an advantage when the nebulizer is incorporated into an oxygen therapy or mechanical ventilation procedure, since it will not materially disturb the therapeutic gas flow pattern. Because the only grossly moving part of the instrument is the small blower, operation is quiet and inoffensive. Parts are easily cleaned and sterilized, and the inflow can be filtered.

The clinical use of the ultrasonic nebulizer is extensive, but it is of prime value when the actual deposition of water in the respiratory tract is desired. The basic indication therefore is the liquefaction by dilution of bronchial secretions, and a secondary use is the maximum humidification of inhaled air. It is effective in stimulating cough for both therapeutic and diagnostic purposes, when its full output volume is held close to the mouth and slowly inhaled. Water aerosol is usually more irritating than saline for this purpose and is valuable in inducing a sputum specimen for laboratory examination, but it is equally useful in wetting thick bronchial secretions and stimulating expectoration. In general, the ability of the adult patient to cooperate with the techniques employing simpler and less expensive, heated or unheated, aerosol generators and humidifiers obviates the need for the ultrasonic instrument except for unusual circumstances. However, if mobilization of secretions by other methods is unsatisfactory, and it is thought that the problem can be corrected by an increase in the density of inhaled water particles, then an ultrasonic unit should be used. Unfortunately, there are no good data based on sound scientific principles that let us set up objective criteria for using aerosol therapy. Techniques employed in a specific instance generally depend on the personal experience and bias of the responsible attending physician. This is a branch of therapeutics desperately in need of practical basic and clinical research.

Ultrasonic nebulization has been used in all the usual pediatric diseases characterized by obstructive secretions, but its most outstanding success has been in the treatment of cystic fibrosis (cystic fibrosis of the pancreas, mucoviscidosis). Of unknown etiology, cystic fibrosis is a complex hereditary disease involving several organ systems, characterized by a malfunction of mucus-secreting glands with the production of markedly viscid mucus. Early descriptions of the disease emphasized cystic destruction of the pancreas secondary to plugging of its excretory ducts by thick secretions and gave the disease its not quite accurate name. Because this disease is not uncommon, the student is encouraged to familiarize himself with its many clinical features, but we will concern ourselves here with its pulmonary complications. Fatalities are usually due to respiratory failure from pulmonary mucoviscidosis. Along with secretions elsewhere in the body, bronchial mucus is remarkably thick and tenacious, severely obstructing airways and leading to secondary bronchitis, bronchiectasis, emphysema, and repeated pulmonary infections. Although the total treatment program involves many aspects, none is more important than the constant effort to maintain airway patency. To this end the prolonged inhalation of aerosolized water has long been standard therapy, either on an intermittent basis when secretions develop acutely or on a regular regimen of a prescribed number of daily hours in a mist tent. In these situations ultrasonic nebulization has become a valuable tool.

The deposition of water in the respiratory tract is able to thin secretions by dilution and to facilitate their removal by the natural cough mechanism, by vigorous postural drainage, and occasionally by aspiration. This requires subjecting the small patient to an atmosphere filled to as near capacity as possible with water particles able to penetrate the depths of the respiratory tract, assuring not only 100% humidity but also a significant excess of particulate water for intrabronchial deposition. Such a "supersaturated" state of therapeutic effectiveness is difficult to attain with jet or impeller nebulizers, without using two or three at a time, but it is possible with the high aerosol output of the ultrasonic nebulizer. With a minimum of appliances and noise, the smallest child can rest undisturbed in a mist tent served by this unit, and the particle stability prevents any significant external wetting from fallout. The small infant in a dense water aerosol atmosphere must be watched carefully for overhydration, since relatively large amounts of water can be absorbed from the lung into the circulation. Infants are weighed frequently to assess water uptake, and the amount supplied by nebulization is deducted from the daily total dietary source. For prolonged nebulization there is no universal agreement as to the relative values of water (preferably sterile) or isotonic saline. Some believe that water is safer because the immature kidney of infants and small children has difficulty in excreting the added sodium load of saline, retention of which might seriously disturb water and electrolyte balance.[212] Others prefer normal saline because of the irritating effects of such a large volume of water particles.[213] For safety's sake, even during an acute obstructive exacerbation, patients are removed from the mist tent at intervals. During "normal" or nonacute phases of cystic fibrosis, as a prophylactic measure many patients are placed in a mist tent during the sleeping hours, a technique employed as part of home care that often reduces the number of hospitalizations for acute obstruction.

It should be evident that, in addition to cystic fibrosis, ultrasonic nebulization is valuable in the treatment of the acute obstruction of croup, as described earlier. Although water and saline are the two most frequently used media in the ultrasonic nebulizer, there is increasing interest in the use of other substances, with pharmacologic action. There has been concern about using substances with pharmacologic action because of the fear that the vibrational energy of ultrasonic nebulization might degrade or disrupt the structure of chemical substances and either destroy their specific action or produce harmful by-products.[212] However, studies of the complex relationships between high-frequency vibrations and mist production have resolved this apprehension. The power, or energy, applied to the target surface of an ultrasonic aerosol generator, and measured in watts per square centimeter rather than the sonic frequency, determines both fog output and the degree of particle damage. It has been shown that instruments with an acoustic power output of less than 20 watts/cm$^2$ and an aerosol production less than 2.0 ml/min will not degrade substances aerosolized. These are known as *drug nebulizers* and can safely dispense pharmaceuticals. Power outputs greater than 50 watts/cm$^2$ required to generate flows exceeding 2.0 ml/min are apt to disrupt the chemical structure of aerosolized particles. Such instruments produce large volumes of particles and are used as *fog nebulizers*.[214] Another major limitation to drug nebulization is viscosity, and in general, liquids with viscosities greater than 10 centipoises are difficult to aerosolize. There still are no dependable guidelines for ultrasonic nebulization, but to date at least water, normal saline, saline propylene glycol, acetylcysteine, and some antibiotics have been so aerosolized. We have no way of knowing, however, whether or not the use of jet nebulization might have been just as effective.

Let us summarize ultrasonic nebulization with the following statements: (1) it is effective in producing a large volume of high density mist; (2) sonic frequencies above 0.8 megacycle/sec prepare the necessary column or fountain of the liquid to be nebulized, while 20 to 50 watts/cm$^2$ power input to the transducer determines the volume of fog output; (3) delivered aerosol particle size is controlled by baffling; (4) solutes may be degraded by power levels of 50 watts/cm$^2$ needed for high-volume fog production but not by power at or below 20 watts/cm$^2$; (5) solutions with viscosities above 10 centipoises are difficult to nebulize with ultrasound.

Before closing the subject of aerosol therapy, note should be made of a hazard of potential clinical importance. During the baffling and recycling of solutions undergoing nebulization, as droplets are continuously returned to the fluid reservoir, there has been observed a gradual increase in the concentration of the solution yet to be nebulized. The risk of drug toxicity is evident, as the patient is subjected to increasingly higher concentrations during the course of therapy. It was at first believed that this phenomenon was primarily a characteristic of jet nebulizers, but an excellent study has demonstrated that *drug reconcentration* is a function of both jet and ultrasonic nebulizers.[215]

One of the drugs used was acetylcysteine, and when subjected to 30 minutes of ultrasonic nebulization using ambient air as the carrier gas, concentrations of the drug

**Table 7-10.**  *Drug reconcentration during ultrasonic nebulization**

| Aerosolization time | Percent acetylcysteine | |
| --- | --- | --- |
| Minutes | Ambient air | Humidified air |
| 0 | 20.5 | 20.5 |
| 5 | 21.7 | 20.4 |
| 10 | 23.0 | 20.2 |
| 15 | 26.4 | 20.1 |
| 20 | 29.0 | 20.2 |
| 25 | 32.8 | 20.6 |
| 30 | 40.1 | 20.5 |

*Modified from Glick, R. V.: Drug reconcentration in aerosol generators, Inhal. Ther. **15**:179, 1970.

rose from 20.5% to 40.1%. The experiment then demonstrated that when control of temperature and humidity assured full water vapor saturation of the carrier gas, reconcentration did not occur. Table 7-10 vividly illustrates the effect of this humidification. The conclusion drawn was that, in the presence of a humidity deficit of the carrier gas, the greater ease of evaporation of water solvent molecules than of the heavier drug solute progressively raised the concentration of the shrinking residual solution.

In summary, with the widespread indications for aerosol therapy and the increasing variety of equipment appearing on the market, the respiratory therapist who has supervisory responsibility is faced with a difficult test of judgment. The medical director of a department of respiratory therapy and the hospital administrator will often rely on his recommendations as to type and quality of equipment to be purchased and he must weigh the therapeutic value of each proposed addition to his inventory against its expected use and cost. His objective will be to provide the maximum service to a heterogeneous hospital patient population, within the limits of his budget, and he will have to consider the initial cost of new equipment, the service required to maintain it in workable condition, and the probability that all members of his department will not use it with the same degree of efficiency and uniformity. The decision may be a compromise between what the therapist would like to have and what is practical. He will find from experience that it is generally unwise to disburse a large fraction of his budget for the purchase of a few expensive items which, although desirable, may be essential for only a few patients when the same expenditure could provide more less sophisticated items that would be satisfactory for many. Again, this underscores the need for a competent therapist to understand fully the merits of his equipment and the general therapeutic needs of his hospital's patients.

Chapter 8

# GAS THERAPY

## MEDICAL GASES

The administration of therapeutic gases is the most important function of the respiratory therapist. Indeed, it is from the humble beginning of the so-called "oxygen service" of the average general hospital that the present skilled technology of respiratory therapy evolved, and even though the therapist has now assumed a host of duties and responsibilities, gas therapy is the foundation of his work. We have covered many aspects of gases—something of their behavior and characteristics, the mechanics of introducing them into the body through ventilation, and the activities of some of them as they participate in bodily functions. In this chapter we will consider the packaging and distribution of compressed therapy gases and the clinical equipment and techniques for using them to treat patients. We will call upon some previously discussed principles as we describe both the gaseous and liquid forms of gases. Much of the data in this section of the chapter are drawn from two sources with which all respiratory therapists should be familiar, the codes of the National Fire Protection Association[216] and pamphlets of the Compressed Gas Association, Inc., especially those that describe the common medical gases and the many important safety measures for which the therapist must be held responsible.[217] In addition, the student will find useful information in the many good brochures and other publications of the manufacturers of gases and gas equipment.

As noted in Chapter 1, the commercial gas industry and the various fields of related engineering use the English system of measurement almost exclusively, and the student must familiarize himself with the necessary units when considering the packaging of gases; but he will find himself back in the metric system when discussing their application to the patient. Before we attempt to discuss the matter at hand, there is one variation of measurement we have not had occasion to use in the past but which is essential in considering gas therapy. Pressure in the English system is expressed as pounds per square inch and, in the parlance of commercial gases, is abbreviated *psi*. However, it is often necessary to be more specific and to denote whether a given pressure includes that of the atmosphere or is in excess of atmospheric. This need arises because of the use of calibrated gauges to measure and record pressures. A pressure gauge, which usually consists of a numbered circular dial with a centrally pivoted needle indicator, registers zero pressure under atmospheric conditions. In other words, at zero gauge pressure there is already 1 atm of pressure (14.7 psi) active, and any deviation above zero by the gauge indicates pressure above atmospheric. Therefore the recorded pressure is referred to as *pounds per square inch, gauge* (psig). Less commonly used in ordinary gas therapy, but widely used in hyperbaric medicine, is the concept of absolute pressure. This means the actual total pressure of a gas, including that exerted by the atmosphere, and is called *pounds per square inch, absolute* (psia). To orient his thinking, the student can remember that psia is always 1 atm, or 14.7 $lb/in^2$, greater than psig. Thus 14.7 psig = 29.4 psia; 371.2 psig = 385.9 psia. For completeness it should be noted that hyperbaric terminology frequently employs units of atmospheres and refers to so many atmospheres, gauge (atg), or atmospheres, absolute (ata), with the same relationship described for pounds per square inch. By common usage, in compressed gas data, gauge pressure is implied unless otherwise specified, and psi and psig are used interchangeably, although the latter is more correct.

### Cylinder gases

Of all the many gases that are compressed into cylinders for distribution, we will be interested in the few that are called medical gases. Even of these, we will discuss in detail only some because a few are used mainly in the laboratory and others are anesthetics, which are not in the province of the respiratory therapist. Initially, we will include in our discussion the groups of gases listed in Table 8-1. These, prepared and packaged for medical use, will give us a wide scope to discuss techniques involved and characteristics of compressed gases; then our clinical discussions will be limited to the therapy gases.

From a safety point of view, compressed gases are classified as nonflammable (will not burn), nonflammable but will support combustion, and flammable (will burn readily). The above gases can be grouped according to their flammability as follows:

*Nonflammable:* $N_2$, $CO_2$, He
*Support combustion:* $O_2$, $N_2O$, air, $O_2/N_2$, $O_2/CO_2$, $He/O_2$
*Flammable:* $(CH_2)_3$, $C_2H_4$

***Gas cylinders.*** The containers used to hold and ship compressed or liquid medical gases are high-pressure units, carefully controlled in their specifications by regulations, both federal and industrial. They are made of seamless steel, finely tempered and nonreactive with their gaseous or liquid contents, and are classified as type 3A or

**Table 8-1.**  *Therapy and anesthetic gases*

| Limited therapy, laboratory gases | Therapy gases | Anesthetics |
|---|---|---|
| Nitrogen ($N_2$) | Air | Cyclopropane ($(CH_2)_3$) |
| Carbon dioxide ($CO_2$) | Oxygen ($O_2$) | Nitrous oxide ($N_2O$) |
| Helium (He) | Oxygen-nitrogen ($O_2/N_2$) | Ethylene ($C_2H_4$) |
| | Oxygen-carbon dioxide ($O_2/CO_2$) | |
| | Helium-oxygen ($He/O_2$) | |

3AA cylinders. We will compare various pressures used in medical gas cylinders; but regardless of the cylinder pressure, all tanks used for therapy have valves that in clinical use are fitted with devices to reduce the pressure going to the patient to a "working pressure" of 50 psig. The valves also have safety releases that will give way before the cylinders burst should exposure to sudden heat dangerously elevate the gas pressure.

Cylinders are given a letter designation according to size. Following is a list of most of the common sizes, in inches of diameter and height including valve, with an asterisk indicating the relatively few with which the respiratory therapist can expect to have frequent contact:

| A | B | D* | E* | F | M | G* | H&K* |
|---|---|----|----|---|---|----|------|
| 3·× 10 | 3½ × 16 | 4¼ × 20 | 4¼ × 30 | 5½ × 55 | 7⅛ × 46 | 8½ × 55 | 9 × 55 |

Sizes A through E are referred to as small cylinders and are used most often for anesthetic gases and portable emergency oxygen supply. These small tanks differ from the larger ones in the mechanism by which they attach to the appliances they serve. They employ a connector called a *yoke*, whereas the large cylinders (F to H&K) have a threaded outlet from their valves to which a nut attaches a pressure reducer. Fig. 8-1 illustrates the general structure of the cylinder valves and the yoke used with small cylinders. A represents a small cylinder valve, but the principle of the large valves is similar. *1* is the stem on which a handgrip is placed when in use; *2* is the valve plunger with its threaded lower end; *3* is the outlet of the valve, a recess in the small valves but a projecting threaded nipple in the large ones; *4* is the valve seat; *5* is an emergency

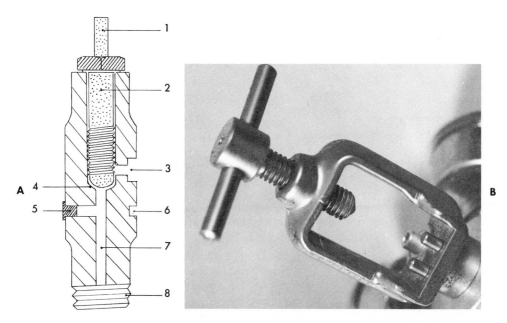

**Fig. 8-1.** **A,** Diagrammatic sectional sketch of a small cylinder valve. **B,** Photograph of the yoke connector used with small cylinders. (See text for description.)

pressure release; *6* is one of a pair of borings in the valve body of the small cylinders only, part of the Pin-Index Safety System, to be described later; *7* is the gas channel into the valve; *8* is the threaded connection between the valve and the cylinder. *B* is an illustration of a yoke connector for the A to E cylinders that fits about the cylinder valve, showing the aperture that is slipped about the valve; a screw that holds the yoke firmly onto the valve; the small receiving nipple that fits snugly into the gas outlet (*3*, in *A*); and the pins of the Index System noted above.

Medical gas cylinders are marked by metal stampings on their shoulders that are supposed to supply specific information. The letters ICC (Interstate Commerce Commission) on cylinders manufactured before 1967 or DOT (Department of Transportation) on cylinders new since then, are followed by the designation of the cylinder as a 3A or 3AA type and then by the maximum working pressure of the cylinder in psi. This is the filling pressure of the tank, which can generally be exceeded by 10%. For example, a frequently encountered cylinder has a marked pressure of 2015 psi but is usually filled to about 2200 psi. Below these data the letter size of the cylinder is marked (E, G, etc.) followed by the serial number of the cylinder. A third line of stampings includes the initials of the company that owns the cylinder, and as a fourth line there is a mark identifying the inspecting authority. On the opposite surface of the tank there is another set of stampings the first line of which indicates the method by which the cylinder was manufactured, often noted as "Spun Cr-Mo," indicating the use of chrome-molybdenum. Below are a series of symbols that include the identification of the manufacturer of the cylinder, the data of its original safety test, dates of all subsequent tests as prescribed by regulation, and frequently the notation "E.E.," followed by a number that indicates the cubic centimeter elastic expansion of the cylinder under test conditions. In addition to these permanent marks, all tanks should have securely attached to them labels clearly identifying the contents and their concentrations, and some will tell the cubic feet or gallon measurement of the gas.

As an aid to the easy identification of medical gases, Table 8-2 lists the color code for the size E cylinders, specifically those intended for use on anesthesia machines, that has been adopted by the Bureau of Standards of the United States Department of Commerce.

It is strongly emphasized that the color of a cylinder is to be used only as a rough guide, and the therapist *must always check* the cylinder contents by *carefully reading its label.* Many of the larger cylinders employ essentially the same color scale, but there is enough variation among the many tanks the therapist may have occasion to handle to make the color identification unreliable. It is hoped that soon there will be a fully uniform international color marking system.

Every 5 to 10 years compressed gas cylinders must be subjected to a safety inspection and testing as specified in DOT regulations. Under compression such factors as leaks, cylinder expansion, and wall stress are determined, and the cylinders are inspected internally and cleaned. The date of each such testing is stamped on the cylinder shoulder.

Because of the many ways of expressing gas volume measurements, it is helpful to be able to convert from one to the other by the use of the factors in Table 8-3.

**Table 8-2.** *Color code for size E gas cylinders*

| Gas | Color |
|---|---|
| Oxygen | Green |
| Carbon dioxide | Gray |
| Nitrous oxide | Light blue |
| Cyclopropane | Orange |
| Helium | Brown |
| Ethylene | Red |
| Carbon dioxide and oxygen | Gray and green |
| Helium and oxygen | Brown and green |

**Table 8-3.** *Gas volumes conversion factors*

| Cubic feet | Liters | Gallons |
|---|---|---|
| 1.0 | 28.316 | 7.481 |
| 0.03531 | 1.0 | 0.2642 |
| 0.1337 | 3.785 | 1.0 |

**Table 8-4.** *Pressure ranges of medical gases*

| Gas | Physical state | psig | Gas | Physical state | psig |
|---|---|---|---|---|---|
| Air | G | 1800 | $CO_2$ | L | 825 |
| $O_2$ | G | 1800-2400 | He | G | 1650-2000 |
| $O_2/N_2$ | G | 1800-2200 | $(CH_2)_3$ | L | 75 |
| $O_2/CO_2$ | G | 1500-2200 | $N_2O$ | L | 745 |
| $He/O_2$ | G | 1650-2000 | $C_2H_4$ | G | 1250 |
| $N_2$ | G | 1800-2200 | | | |

It should be kept in mind that, because of the different filling pressures of gases, volumes of different gases in the same size cylinder will vary. For example, a G cylinder contains about 187 cubic feet of oxygen but only about 147 cubic feet of helium. Table 8-4 gives an idea of the approximate filling pressure ranges of medical gases, depending on the types of cylinders used, calibrated at 70° F.

*Filling (charging) cylinders.* We will differentiate between gases and liquid gases.

*Gases.* The general rule is that gas cylinders will be filled at a temperature of 70° F to the pressure specified for a given cylinder, as stamped on its shoulder. However, certain gases, including oxygen, helium, helium-oxygen, and oxygen–carbon dioxide, may be filled to 10% in excess of the stated pressure. Thus a cylinder certified for 2015 psi may be filled to a pressure of 2217 psi and is generally referred to as a 2200 lb tank.

*Liquid gases.* For those gases that are packaged in liquid form, there is a limiting "filling density" that determines how much may be put in each cylinder. The filling density is the ratio between the weight of liquid gas put in a cylinder and the weight of water that the cylinder can contain. Thus the carbon dioxide filling density of 68%

means that the weight of the liquid gas allowable to charge a cylinder is equal to 68% of the weight of water that the cylinder has the capacity to hold. The filling densities of cyclopropane and nitrous oxide are 55% and 68%, respectively.

It should be noted that cylinder pressures for liquid gases are considerably lower than those for vaporous gases, and the critical temperatures of the three liquid gases under consideration are all above average room temperature ($CO_2 = 88°$ F; $[CH_2]_3 = 256°$ F; $N_2O = 98°$ F). Because liquid gas does not fill the entire volume of a given cylinder, the space above the liquid surface contains vapor of the gas in equilibrium with the liquid, and the measured pressure in the cylinder is the pressure of the *vapor* at any given temperature. Thus, although the pressure of a tank of carbon dioxide at its critical temperature of 88° F would be 1071 psig (critical pressure) and would rise with continued elevation of temperature, at room temperature of 70° F it is only about 825 psig. Similarly, the pressure of cyclopropane at its critical temperature of 256° F is 797 psig but is only 75 psig at room temperature. To compare vapor gas cylinders with liquid gas, we can say that the pressure in the former represents the force required to squeeze into a cylinder a given volume of gas; whereas in the latter it is the vapor pressure of the gas over the surface of a given weight of liquid poured into the closed container. The liquid gas pressure is dependent upon the temperature and is the result of the filling of the cylinder, not the cause.

### Measuring cylinder contents

*Gas cylinders.* The volume of gas in a cylinder is directly related to the cylinder pressure at a constant temperature. If a tank is full at 2200 psig, it will be but half full as usage drops the pressure to 1100 psig. The usual method of monitoring the depletion of cylinder contents is by the use of gauges. If greater accuracy is needed, weighing the cylinder when the weight of the empty cylinder and the density of the gas are known is more precise.

*Liquid gas cylinders.* Since the pressure in a liquid gas cylinder is that of the gas vapor in balance with the liquid at a given temperature, it gives no indication of how much liquid remains in the cylinder at any one time. As long as there is liquid in the cylinder, the vapor pressure and thus the recorded gauge pressure will remain unchanged even though gas is being drawn off. When the liquid is finally gone and the cylinder contains only vapor, then the pressure will fall in proportion to the reduction in the remaining gas volume until the tank is empty. Thus gauge pressure is of use in monitoring cylinder contents only terminally; if contents must be determined, the cylinder must be weighed. Fig. 8-2 compares the pressure behavior of gas and liquid gas cylinders. Of course, the vapor pressure of liquid gas cylinders will vary with the temperature of their contents. Whereas carbon dioxide has a cylinder pressure of 838 psig at 70° F, at 60° F it has a cylinder pressure of only 733 psig. Then, as the temperature rises and approaches the critical point, more liquid will vaporize in the cylinder with an accompanying rise in pressure. Should a tank of carbon dioxide warm up to 88° F, the entire liquid contents will convert to gas; and if the temperature does not drop, as the gas is withdrawn, the cylinder gauge pressure will fall proportionately. Ethylene, on the other hand, is a gas at room temperature but with a relatively high critical temperature of 49° F; should it cool below this value, it will liquefy and its gauge pressure will stabilize as long as liquid remains in the cylinder.

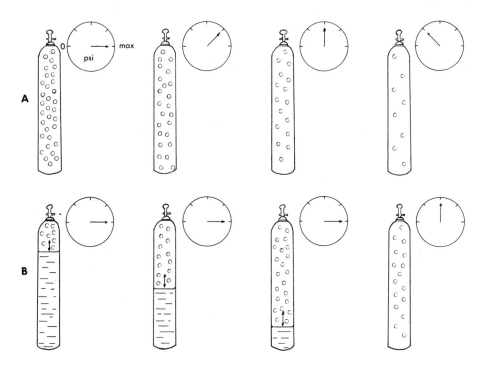

**Fig. 8-2.** The content of a gas-filled cylinder, **A,** is directly proportional to the gas pressure. As gas is withdrawn, for example, a pressure drop of 50% indicates a loss of 50% of the contained gas. In a liquid-gas cylinder, **B,** gauge pressure measures only the vapor pressure of gas in equilibrium with the liquid phase, and this remains constant at a given temperature as long as liquid is present. Only when all the liquid phase has vaporized, as the cylinder nears depletion, does the gauge pressure drop proportionately to the terminal volume of remaining gas.

***Estimating duration of cylinder flow.*** When we set up a therapeutic procedure that utilizes cylinder vapor gas and that is expected to cover an extended period of time, it is a matter of both safety and convenience to be able to predict the approximate time to prepare for the replacement of the cylinder. Although this cannot be done with unerring accuracy because of the possibility of irregular flow, a practical rough estimate can be made on the basis of the average anticipated gas flows, the cylinder size, and the cylinder pressure at the start of therapy. Factors that can be used to convert these data into a time estimate can be calculated from the information on commonly used gases and cylinder sizes in Table 8-5.

Here is an example of the cumbersome combination of both the English and metric systems of measurement. Commercial gas cylinder calibrations and values are usually recorded in the English system; but once a therapeutic gas leaves the cylinder pressure reducing gauge, it is subject to the medical custom of using metric measurements. In essence, we wish to determine the length of time a given number of liters of gas per minute (lpm) will flow from a source of a given cubic footage of gas under a measurable pressure in psig. We now know that at a given temperature the cylinder gas volume will decrease in proportion to the drop in gauge pressure; therefore each reduction in pounds per square inch or pressure represents a specific volume of gas loss

**Table 8-5.** *Pressures and volumes of commonly used cylinders*

| Gas | Full cylinder pressure | Cubic feet of gas | | | |
|-----|------------------------|-------|-------|-------|--------|
| | | D | E | G | H&K |
| $O_2$ | 2200 | 12.7 | 22 | 187 | 244 |
| $O_2/CO_2$ | 1800 | 12.7 | 22 | 187 | 244 |
| $He/O_2$ | 2200 | 10.8 | 17.7 | 150 | 194 |
| $O_2/N_2$ | 2200 | | | 187 | 244 |
| Air | 2200 | | | 187 | 244 |

**Table 8-6.** *Factors to calculate duration of cylinder flow in minutes*

| Gas | Cylinder size | | | |
|-----|------|------|------|--------|
| | D | E | G | H&K |
| $O_2$, $O_2/N_2$, air | 0.16 | 0.28 | 2.41 | 3.14 |
| $O_2/CO_2$ | 0.20 | 0.35 | 2.94 | 3.84 |
| $He/O_2$ | 0.14 | 0.23 | 1.93 | 2.50 |

from the cylinder. This factor, relating pressure drop to gas volume, is calculated as follows:

$$\frac{\text{Cubic feet of gas in full cylinder} \times \text{Factor to convert from cubic feet to liters}}{\text{Pressure of full cylinder in psig}}$$

For example, an oxygen G cylinder contains about 187 cubic feet of gas under a filling pressure of 2200 psig. Therefore the volume of gas leaving the cylinder for every psig drop in pressure would be $(187 \times 28.3) \div 2200 = 2.41$ liters per psig ($\ell$/psig).

Factors, so calculated for the gases and cylinders listed above, are shown in Table 8-6.

The principle employing the use of these factors is based on the relationship that tells us: liter loss in cylinder volume per drop in each pound per square inch of cylinder pressure, multiplied by the observed cylinder gauge pressure and divided by the liter per minute gas flow delivered to the patient, equals the number of minutes the gas will flow until the cylinder is empty. Thus:

$$\frac{\text{Duration of flow}}{\text{in minutes}} = \frac{\text{Gauge pressure in psi} \times \text{Factor}}{\text{Liter flow}}$$

As an example, let us estimate the duration of a G cylinder of oxygen with a gauge pressure of 800 psi if we use a flow of 8 lpm. Referring to Table 8-6, we find the oxygen G cylinder factor of 2.41 and set up the simple fraction:

$$\frac{800 \times 2.41}{8} = 241 \text{ minutes, or approximately 4 hours}$$

## Bulk oxygen

Because of the tremendous volume of oxygen used in the average general hospital, a separate discussion of special large bulk storage systems is warranted. Bulk oxygen storage consists of any system capable of accommodating more than 12,000 cubic feet of the gas ready for use or more than 25,000 cubic feet including unconnected reserves. Such systems may be located out of doors or in a special building set aside for the purpose. Strict regulations for locating and maintaining bulk oxygen systems have been established by the National Fire Protection Association, subject to further control by local community fire and building codes. The supervision and maintenance of bulk oxygen units are not always functions of the respiratory therapist but often are responsibilities of oxygen service companies and hospital departments of engineering and maintenance. Nevertheless, the therapist should be acquainted with the systems, since they concern his most important therapeutic tool and because he should be knowledgeable enough to be able to participate in dealing with emergency interruption of gas supply.

Bulk oxygen systems may provide either gaseous or liquid oxygen, and these will be discussed separately below. Bulk oxygen is used as a "central supply," or "piped-in system," in which the gas is carried from its station to the hospital divisions by a system of pipes built into the walls of new construction or often added to the wall surfaces of older buildings. It is thus possible to have an oxygen outlet conveniently located by each patient's bed and any other area desired. The great values of such a centrally located oxygen supply should be obvious. There is almost no risk of a depletion of oxygen during therapy, and the inconvenience and hazard of transporting and storing individual tanks are obviated. Finally, pressure reduction of oxygen is accomplished at the central station, and the gas is piped to the clinical areas already reduced to the standard working pressure of 50 psig. This eliminates the need for pressure-reducing valves at the patient outlets and requires the use of only flowmeters. As opposed to cylinder gas supply, a central system is referred to as a low-pressure system.

***Gaseous bulk oxygen.*** There are three general systems that employ large central supplies of the gas form of oxygen.

*Standard cylinders.* Large-sized standard cylinders can be banked together, usually pressurized at 2400 psig. Numbers of them can be tied together by a *manifold*, which, essentially, converts the individual units into one continuous supply. The manifold mechanism contains pressure-reduction valving and flow-control and alarm systems that warn of impending depletion or malfunction. As tanks empty, they are replaced by others. Sometimes packages of six or more tanks are manifolded together, each package replaced as needed.

*Fixed cylinders.* In contrast to the cylinders just described, fixed cylinders consist of large banks of up to seventy-five cylinders permanently fixed at a stationary site. When empty, they are refilled on location from a truck that contains liquid oxygen and converts the liquid to gas for pumping into the cylinders.

*Trailer units.* Mounted on trailers, tanks of a variety of sizes can be towed to the central area and connected to the distribution circuit. For heavy oxygen consumption there are available large trailers with up to thirty permanently attached long horizontal tubes. Replacement is a simple matter of switching trailers. Like the other tank systems, trailer gas is also at 2400 psig pressure.

***Liquid bulk oxygen.*** An extremely economical method of transporting and storing oxygen, liquid gas systems are widely used where the demand justifies their installation. Although we have already discussed the liquid form of some medical gases packaged in standard cylinders, because of its physical characteristics, liquid oxygen deserves special consideration. The major physical difference between oxygen and those liquid gases noted above is its very low critical temperature $(-181.1°$ F) and boiling point $(-297.3°$ F). The mechanisms for producing and maintaining the liquid state of oxygen are much more complex than are those for other medical liquid gases, but the practical returns justify the effort. Of prime importance is the fact that, at its boiling point, 1 cubic foot of liquid oxygen is the equivalent of 860.6 cubic feet of gaseous oxygen at ambient temperature and pressure.

Brief reference has been made earlier to the method of producing liquid oxygen from the compression and cooling of air. To prevent the liquid from reverting to gas, the liquid must be kept below $-297°$ F, both in transportation and storage. This is accomplished by keeping it in special containers, under a pressure not to exceed 250 psig. All such containers for liquid oxygen, whether trucks for transporting the substance or hospital supply stations, are constructed on the principle of a large thermos bottle with which we are all acquainted. They consist of inner and outer steel shells, separated by a vacuum, which effectively blocks the transfer of heat into the liquid. This evacuated space is filled with a noncombustible insulation, and the inner shell is silvered to aid in repelling heat. The containers are vented so that vaporized liquid oxygen can escape if warming occurs. It should be apparent that when liquid oxygen is kept below its boiling point, it can be exposed to atmospheric pressure, at least for short periods of time, without immediately vaporizing. Otherwise, transferring the material from supply truck to bulk container, for example, would be difficult. There are two types of containers for hospital use of liquid oxygen—the liquid oxygen cylinder and the permanent station.

*Liquid oxygen cylinder.* This unit is not necessarily classified as part of a bulk system because individual tanks of liquid gas can be used. These cylinders measure 58 inches high and 20 inches in diameter and hold the equivalent of 3000 cubic feet of gas at ambient temperature and pressure, matching the contents of more than twelve

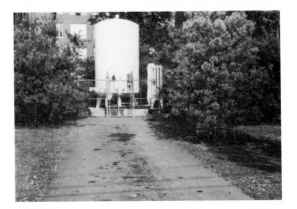

**Fig. 8-3.** Typical liquid oxygen storage facility in a hospital setting.

large gas cylinders. As with the gas tanks, the liquid cylinders can be banked by manifold to provide a space-saving supply of oxygen.

*Fixed station.* These units are cylindrical or spherical containers with capacities up to a gaseous equivalent of 130,000 cubic feet. The liquid is converted to usable gas by a heating unit called a *vaporizer*, which may be heated by steam, hot air, electricity, or hot water. Elaborately controlled to assure a steady, even conversion of liquid to gas according to need, these systems assure an unlimited gas supply no matter what the peak demand load may be. They are refilled from service tank trucks according to schedules suited to each hospital. All liquid gas sources reduce their already low pressure to the 50 psig hospital line pressure. Fig. 8-3 illustrates a typical unit.

## Regulation of gas flow

Whatever the source of medical gas, a device is needed to regulate its flow as it is administered to a patient. This ensures that the gas will be given at a safe pressure and allows adjustment of the volume of gas to suit the patient's needs. Such a device is called a *regulator,* and it performs two functions: it reduces the high pressure of the gas in the cylinder to a safe working pressure, about 50 psig, and it allows the controlled release of gas over a narrow range of flows, usually from 1 to 15 $\ell$/min. The student may wonder why this would be necessary for central oxygen supply, when the outlet pressure already has been reduced to 50 psig. In such instances the entire regulator mechanism is not needed, and only the flow control is used. We will discuss separately the following four topics: regulation of high-pressure cylinder gas, regulation of low-pressure centrally supplied systems, pressure compensation, and safety indexed connector systems.

*High-pressure cylinder gas regulators.* There are three types of cylinder regulators, and though they function on the same basic principle, they deserve individual description. They may be designated as preset, adjustable, and multiple-stage regulators.

*Preset regulator.* Fig. 8-4 shows a schematic illustration of the preset regulator. Attached to the cylinder outlet, high-pressure gas enters the regulators through *A*, with cylinder pressure (and thus contents) recorded on the presure gauge *(B)*. The body of the regulator is divided into a pressure chamber *(C)* and an ambient pressure chamber *(D)* by a flexible diaphragm *(E)*. Attached to the diaphragm, in the atmospheric chamber, is a spring *(F)* fixed to the other side of the chamber. Also attached to the diaphragm, but in the pressure chamber, is a valve stem *(G)*, the other end of which controls the flow of gas through a valve *(H)*. Gas goes to the patient through the outflow *(I)*, passing through a Thorpe-tube flowmeter *(J)*. The amount of gas released to the patient is regulated by the needle valve *(K)* and is read on a calibrated scale as liters per minute according to the height at which the ball is elevated in the Thorpe-tube flowmeter. The pressure chamber is supplied with a safety vent *(L)* that prevents an accidental buildup of pressure beyond 200 psig in the event of malfunction. This regulator is called *preset* because it is so constructed that the spring *F* will give if pressure on the diaphragm *E* exceeds 50 psig. When this happens, the valve stem *G* will be pulled back and the valve *H* will close, preventing further entry of gas into the

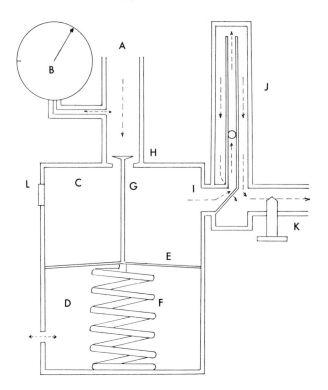

**Fig. 8-4.** Diagram of preset, high-pressure gas regulator. (See text for details.)

regulator. As long as the needle valve *K* is open, allowing the escape of gas from the pressure chamber, the valve at *H* will remain open and permit gas flow. Thus a balance will be established so that the valve at *H* is open just enough to meet the demand of valve *K* and the automatic adjustment of the diaphragm-spring combination will prevent excessive pressures from building up in chamber *C*.

*Adjustable regulator.* The adjustable regulator is one of the most commonly encountered regulators, differing from the preset type in two aspects, as shown in Fig. 8-5. The identifying feature of this regulator is the threaded hand control on its face *(K)*. This is attached to the end of the spring and allows displacement of the diaphragm. Whereas the valve *(H)* in the preset regulator is open until gas enters the pressure chamber and closes it by pressure against the diaphragm, in the adjustable regulator the valve *(H)* is closed until the hand screw advances the whole mechanism and opens it to allow gas flow. The valve can thus be opened to permit a wide range of flows, and the pressures in chamber *C* will vary according to the relation between the amount of high-pressure gas entering and the amount leaving the regulator, but the spring will prevent the pressure from exceeding 50 psig. In the preset one, pressure in the chamber is always 50 psig, but in the adjustable regulator it can be anything up to 50 psig. A second characteristic of the adjustable regulator is the use of a Bourdon flow gauge *(J)* instead of a Thorpe. In reality, the Bourdon meter is a pressure gauge, like that at the regulator inflow *(B)*, and functions on the principle crudely schematicized

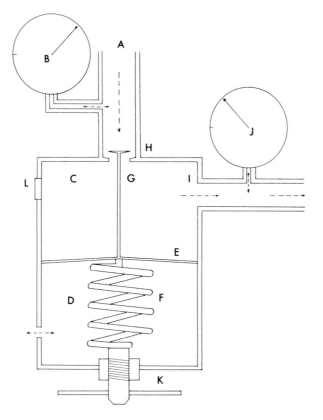

**Fig. 8-5.**   Diagram of an adjustable, high-pressure gas regulator. (See text for details.)

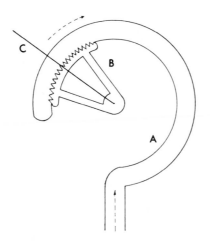

**Fig. 8-6.**   Crude diagram of the principle of a gas-pressure gauge. (See text for description.)

in Fig. 8-6. The heart of the gauge is a curved flexible closed tube *(A)* that responds to the pressure of gas entering it by changing shape. The force of the gas tends to straighten the tube, causing its distal end to move as indicated by the arrow; and through a gear mechanism *(B)* this motion is transmitted to an indicating needle *(C)*. A numbered scale is calibrated by its manufacturer to read the needle movement either as pressure or liter flow, and gauges are constructed to varying degrees of sensitivity according to the ranges of pressure to which they are to be subjected. The Bourdon gauge is a low-pressure device (less than 50 psig) that meters the gas leaving the regulator, with a scale that converts pressure to flow in liters per minute (see below).

*Multiple-stage regulator.* As the name implies, this instrument accomplishes pressure reduction in two or three steps instead of one and is essentially one or two valves in one. Therapists may have occasion to use two-stage reducing valves, but rarely three. The first stage of high-pressure reduction is preset at the factory and lowers cylinder pressure to an intermediate level, somewhere around 700 psig; in three-stage units the second stage lowers it to about half the first. The final stages, second or third as the case may be, therefore work off a lower pressure than does a single stage valve and presumably are able to effect somewhat more precision and smoothness in flow control. A multiple-stage reducing valve may be provided with either a Bourdon or a Thorpe-tube metering device. It is larger and more costly than a single stage and is indicated where minimal fluctuations in pressure and flow are critical factors. For routine hospital work the simpler single-stage regulators are satisfactory. The number of stages in a reducing valve can be easily determined by noting the number of safety vents present; there will be one for each pressure chamber.

*Low-pressure gas regulators.* It was emphasized earlier that one of the assets of a central gas supply system is the reduction of pressure at the central location so that the gas is at its working pressure when it reaches the outlets. This eliminates the need for pressure-reducing devices for patient administration and requires only a simple flowmeter. The Thorpe-tube flowmeter is used for this purpose, since it is calibrated to work off a pressure of 50 psig, as shown in Fig. 8-4. With outlets of a low pressure–oxygen or compressed-air system located by the patient's bed, therapy can be instituted in moments merely by plugging in a flowmeter and adjusting its flow as desired.

*Pressure compensation.* The term *pressure compensation* refers to a design in the Thorpe-tube flowmeter to prevent changes in gas pressure flowing through it from affecting its liter flow calibration. Although all standard manufacturers of these devices now supply them pressure compensated, the therapist should understand the importance of this and be on the alert for old equipment still in use that might not conform to present standards.

The problem of pressure compensation is the result of the effect of back pressure on a flowmeter, when the gas outlet of the meter is connected with a therapeutic instrument. Practically all gas-administering equipment contains some restrictions in its circuits, and in some, such as jet aerosol generators, these restrictions are acute. When gas flow encounters a restriction, a back pressure is generated. At this point we might define back pressure as a pressure drop across a restriction, according to concepts considered in some detail earlier, when we learned of Bernoulli's principle and the relations among pressure, flow, and resistance. Therapeutically, we are interested in the delivered pressure distal to an obstruction, and if this is lower than the line pressure entering the restriction, we have a back pressure proximal to the restriction. Let us now compare three flow-measuring devices, a Bourdon flow (pressure) gauge, an uncompensated flowmeter (Thorpe-tube), and a compensated flowmeter.

*Bourdon gauge.* As just described and illustrated in Figs. 8-5 and 8-6, the Bourdon gauge measures pressure and is thus not a flowmeter. It measures the pressure of gas flowing from the pressure chamber of an adjustable reducing valve, and at the factory it is calibrated to indicate given flow volumes of gas at different pressures with its outflow *open to the atmosphere.* Thus the face of the valve shows supposed flows. In clinical use, however, the gauge output is faced with the back pressure resistance of therapeutic appliances, and it responds to this pressure, indicating a flow higher than the patient actually receives. At low flows the pressure drop across an obstruction may be slight, but if the patient needs higher flows, the reducing valve must be opened further to supply gas at a higher pressure. At these increased rates there will be more of a pressure drop across the obstruction, and the gauge-indicated flow may be considerably greater than that which actually reaches the patient. Indeed, because the gauge records reducing valve chamber pressure, it will register (flow on its printed face) with the valve open and *the output completely blocked.* Remember, the Bourdon gauge is in direct communication with a pressurized chamber, which may be either part of a reducing valve or the cavity of a gas cylinder. If outflow is blocked and the valve opened, the gauge and chamber will immediately equilibrate, and pressure will be recorded by the gauge. If the gauge face is calibrated in units of flow, then flow will be indicated although no gas is moving.

*Uncompensated flowmeter.* The uncompensated flowmeter is also calibrated in liters per minute against the atmosphere, without restriction. Gas flow at 50 psig into the meter is controlled by a needle valve *proximal* to the meter, as shown in Fig. 8-7, A. The heart of the meter consists of a tapered transparent tube with a float, as shown much exaggerated in Fig. 8-8, with its diameter increasing from below upward. The float is suspended in the tube by the flow of gas past it, and its position is noted against an adjacent scale, which indicates the flow. Because the tube is part of the gas conduction system, the float cannot occlude it and must depend for its support on the Bernoulli effect. The space between the float and the inner surface of the tube constitutes a restriction, and the increased velocity of gas through this restriction produces a pressure drop immediately above the float. In Fig. 8-8, pressure above the float $(P_2)$ is less than that below it $(P_1)$, and the float rises in the tube until its own weight equals the lifting force. When therapy equipment is attached distal to the meter, back pressure is generated in the atmosphere-equilibrated circuit, from the point of restriction in the equipment back through the flow tube to the needle valve, Fig. 8-7, A. As long as the back pressure does not exceed the source pressure of 50 psig, gas will continue to flow into the tube, but the back pressure does increase the pressure distal to the float ($P_2$ in Fig. 8-8). This reduces the pressure differential from $P_1$ to $P_2$, lessens the lift effect, and lets the float drop to a lower position. Therefore a flowmeter that does not compen-

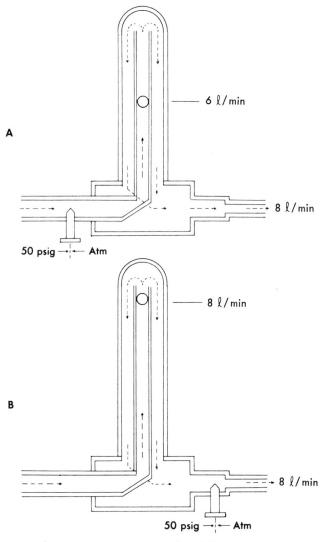

**Fig. 8-7.** Comparison of, **A**, pressure-uncompensated, and **B**, pressure-compensated flowmeters. In the former, the flow-control valve is proximal to the meter, and the gauge records less than the actual output. In the latter, location of the valve distal to the meter correlates the gauge reading with the output. (See text for detailed explanation.)

sate for back pressure, when faced with a restriction, records less gas flow than the patient actually receives.

*Compensated flowmeter.* In contrast to the preceding two instruments, the scale of the compensated flowmeter is calibrated against a constant pressure of 50 psig instead of the atmosphere, and its major structural feature, shown in Fig. 8-7, *B*, is a flow control needle valve *distal* to the flow tube. Thus the entire meter, including the tube, to the needle valve is at a constant pressure of 50 psig, whereas in an uncompensated meter the 50 psig inlet pressure stops at the needle valve proximal to the

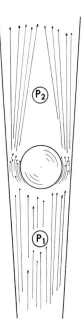

**Fig. 8-8.**   The position of a flowmeter float depends upon a Bernoulli-generated pressure differential across it so that $P_1 > P_2$. Back pressure on the float increases $P_2$, reducing the differential and permitting the float to drop even though actual flow may be maintained.

tube. With a restriction distal to the meter, back pressure will develop in the atmosphere-equilibrated portion of the circuit, from the restriction back to the needle valve. However, as long as the back pressure does not exceed 50 psig, it can have no effect in the tube and will not alter the flow kinetics, which are responsible for the lifting force on the float. Such a pressure-compensated flowmeter, regardless of restrictions, will accurately record the flow to the patient and is the preferred instrument for clinical use.

*Safety indexed connector systems.*  With the tremendous number of compressed gases in current commercial, medical, and scientific use, one of the greatest risks in medical gas therapy is the inadvertent administration of a wrong gas to a patient. Certainly, care on the part of the medical attendant in reading labels or other identifying marks is the most important deterrent to such an accident. The human error, however, must always be considered a potential risk, and to compensate for this there have been developed specially designed connectors for compressed gas tanks and their accessories. The purpose of an indexed connector system is to make impossible certain connections between cylinders and delivery systems. When properly used, for example, a cylinder of any gas other than oxygen could not be functionally attached to any system for which only oxygen is specified. The importance of such a precaution for anesthetic gases is obvious. The systems commonly in use will be briefly described, but the therapist is encouraged to familiarize himself with their details as set forth in publications of the Compressed Gas Association. There are three basic indexed connector systems:

the American Standard Compressed Gas Cylinder Outlet and Inlet Connections, the Diameter-Index Safety System (DISS), and the Pin-Index Safety System.

*American standard compressed gas cylinder valve outlet and inlet connections.* In the United States and Canada the specifications for threaded connections between compressed gas cylinders and their attached tubing have been standardized according to the type of gas concerned and are explained in detail in one of the publications of the Compressed Gas Association, Inc.[218] This system is confined to cylinders with threaded outlets from their valves and includes specifications for the mating nipples and hexagonal nuts by which an appliance (usually a pressure regulator) is attached to the valve. Fig. 8-9 illustrates a cutaway of a joined threaded outlet and nipple. The gas channel through the nipple of the regulator is aligned with the channel through the threaded outlet, and the two parts are secured by a wrench-tightened hexagonal nut that is held loosely on the nipple by a shoulder and flange mechanism.

The Standard system is based on varying dimensions of the cylinder outlet and nipple to limit the introduction of cylinders into a gas circuit specific to certain groups of gases. There are four fundamental divisions of the calibrated system—internal and external threads and right-handed and left-handed threads. Each division is further segmented by varying the number, pitch, and diameter of the threads. In general, left-handed threads are used for fuel gases, and right-handed threads are used for non-fuel. Most of the valve outlets have external threads, and their corresponding nipples internal threads. The threads of the Standard system are usually classified as NGO (National Gas Outlet), but a few are NGT (National Gas Taper). Each gas does not have its own specific connection, but one to thirteen gases may share the same one since there are some twenty-six different connections for about sixty-two listed gases. The Standard system of classification is not binding on manufacturers, and the respiratory therapist must certainly read the specifications of cylinders supplied to his hospital so that he will be completely familiar with any deviations from standard design.

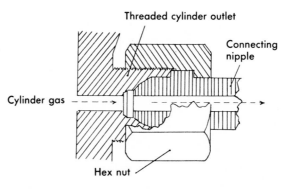

**Fig. 8-9.**   This sketch illustrates the structure of a typical American Standard connection, such as might be used to attach a reducing valve to a large high-pressure cylinder. The hexagonal nut is held onto the nipple of the reducing valve by a circular collar, seen as a cross-sectional projection on the nipple. As the hex nut is tightened on the threaded cylinder outlet, the end of the nipple is snugly seated into the conical outlet. (Modified from CGA Pamphlet V-1, connection no. 540, Compressed Gas Association, Inc., New York.)

In catalogues of cylinder gas dealers, the therapist will see the connection specifications listed for each type of cylinder and gas. A typical description is as follows for a large cylinder of oxygen:

CGA-540  0.903-14NGO-RH-Ext

This tells us that the connection for the threaded outlet of this cylinder is listed by the Compressed Gas Association as connection no. 540, that the outlet has a thread diameter of 0.903 inch, that there are fourteen threads per inch of the National Gas Outlet type, and that the threads are right handed and external.

Generally, the respiratory therapist will use but one or two outlet connections, since most of the relatively small number of different gases he employs are grouped within a few connector sizes. He should be familiar with the classifications, however, since expanding instrumentation and scope of services may bring him into increasing contact with gases and tubing systems in the future.

*Diameter-Index Safety System (DISS).* As a sequential companion to the American Standard system described above, the DISS was established to prevent accidental interchanging among the removable threaded connectors used for medical gas–administering equipment at pressures of *200 psig or less.* Specifically, DISS in respiratory therapy is utilized in effecting safe union between pressure regulators or flowmeters and any threaded connectors that are frequently engaged or disengaged in routine use. Such connections will also be used with therapy equipment and anesthesia apparatus. It should be noted that the standard removable threaded oxygen connector that has been in long use, 0.5625 inch in diameter, eighteen threads per inch, has been given a DISS number (1240) and included in the system.

The system is designed as follows: Each connection consists of an externally threaded body (like the threaded outlet of a cylinder but smaller) and a mated nipple with hex nut, illustrated in Fig. 8-10. The body of the connector has two concentric borings, a primary bore, noted as *Bore 1,* and a counterbore, *Bore 2.* The accompanying nipple has two shoulders, identified as *1* and *2,* and a loose hex nut secured by a

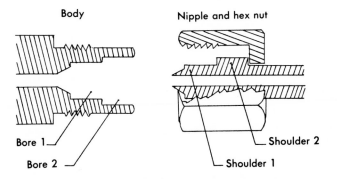

**Fig. 8-10.** Schematic illustration of components of a representative DISS connection. The two shoulders of the nipple allow the nipple to unite only with a body having corresponding borings. If the match is incorrect, the hex nut will not engage the body threads. (Modified from CGA Pamphlet V-5, DISS connection no. 1100, Compressed Gas Association, Inc., New York.)

**Table 8-7.** *DISS connection numbers and assigned gases*

| Connection number | Gas | Connection number | Gas |
|---|---|---|---|
| 1020 | Unassigned | 1140 | $C_2H_4$ |
| 1040 | $N_2O$ | 1160 | Air |
| 1060 | He | 1180 | He/$O_2$ (He 80% or less) |
| | He/$O_2$ ($O_2 < 20\%$) | 1200 | $O_2$/$CO_2$ ($CO_2$ 7% or less) |
| 1080 | $CO_2$ | 1220 | Suction |
| | $O_2$/$CO_2$ ($CO_2 > 7\%$) | 1240 | $O_2$ (standard) |
| 1100 | $(CH_2)_3$ | | |
| 1120 | Unassigned | | |

flange behind *Shoulder 2.* It can be seen that, as the two parts are joined, the corresponding shoulders and bores mate and the union is held by the tightened hex nut. Indexing is achieved by varying the dimensions of the borings and shoulders; starting with a basic set of dimensions, bore 1 is increased and bore 2 decreased in increments of 0.012 inch. The nipple shoulders are changed accordingly. The final connection is a smooth-bored body and a nipple of regular diameter. There are eleven indexed connections, which accommodate eleven gases or gas mixtures, and Table 8-7 lists the DISS connection numbers with the gases assigned to each from data of the Compressed Gas Association, Inc.[219]

To illustrate the use of the DISS, let us imagine an equipment catalogue listing the specifications of a pressure regulator to be used on a cylinder of 100% carbon dioxide. The *inlet* (inlet of regulator, which mates with the threaded outlet of the cylinder) will require an American Standard connection designated as CGA-320. According to CGA data this will be a 0.825-inch 14NGO-RH-Ext cylinder outlet for which there is a specific regulator nipple.[218] The *outlet* (of the regulator, to which a low-pressure line is attached to supply an appliance) will require a DISS connection CGA-1080.

Most of the time the therapist will use oxygen from a regulator, utilizing the standard removable connection designated as CGA-1240, which is not a DISS unit; but he will frequently have occasion to administer helium-oxygen mixtures and oxygen–carbon dioxide mixtures, both of which have DISS connections. To avoid the cumbersome stocking of a large variety of pressure regulators and to make economical use of those on hand, he can use adapters to convert the outlets of the common oxygen regulators to suitable DISS dimensions for special gas use.

*Pin-Index Safety System (PISS).* Pin-Indexing is incorporated in the specifications of the American Standard listing just described but as a special section applicable only to the flush valve outlets of the small cylinders, up to and including size E, which use a yoke connection. These valves do not have a threaded outlet but, rather, a recess in a flat face of the valve into which fits a nipple on the yoke to receive the gas (Fig. 8-1). The Pin-Index is intended for use on anesthesia machines or similar equipment, where fixed yokes are attached to internal gas circuitry, and is designed to prevent the wrong cylinder from being attached to a given yoke.

Two holes are drilled in the face of the valve, their exact position varying with the gas in the cylinder. There are two pins in corresponding positions on the yoke, and

**Table 8-8.** *Pin-Indexed gases*

| Gas | Index hole position |
|---|---|
| $O_2$ | 2-5 |
| $O_2/CO_2$ ($CO_2$ not over 7%) | 2-6 |
| $He/O_2$ (He not over 80%) | 2-4 |
| $C_2H_4$ | 1-3 |
| $N_2O$ | 3-5 |
| $(CH_2)_3$ | 3-6 |
| $He/O_2$ (He over 80%) | 4-6 |
| $O_2/CO_2$ ($CO_2$ over 7%) | 1-6 |
| Air | 1-5 |

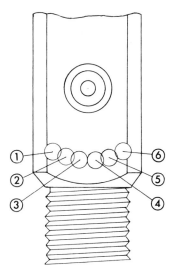

**Fig. 8-11.** Location of the Pin-Index Safety System holes in the cylinder valve face, various pairs of which constitute indices for different gases. (See text for the complete pairings.) (Modified from CGA Pamphlet V-1, Pin-Index Safety System, Compressed Gas Association, Inc., New York.)

unless the pins and holes align perfectly, the yoke nipple will not seat in the recess of the valve. Six hole-pin combinations comprise the total system, but because of overlapping, adjacent holes cannot be used, and there are thus ten possible combinations, of which nine are now in use. Fig. 8-11 is a composite illustration of the location of all six possible holes and the numbers by which they are indexed. Table 8-8 is based on Compressed Gas Association information and lists the gases now in Pin-Indexed cylinders, with their index positions.

## OXYGEN THERAPY

The single most important need of the human organism, as an earth surface dweller, is oxygen; and the therapist, now well versed in the hazards of hypoxia, can understand that the effective administration of oxygen is his most vital function.

Indeed, most of the techniques he employs in patient care are designed to facilitate the adequate distribution of oxygen to pulmonary capillary blood. As a technical expert in the clinical use of this essential gas, the therapist should learn as much about it as he can through independent study, and to give him a start, we will consider some of the basic characteristics of oxygen that specifically relate to its medical use.

In the cosmos as a whole, the three most abundant elements in order are hydrogen, helium, and oxygen; in and about the earth oxygen is the most prevalent and widely distributed. In view of our great dependence upon oxygen, the presence of which we take so for granted, it is interesting to note that countless millions of years ago oxygen was completely missing from the atmosphere of earth. In those first hours of time, earth's atmosphere probably consisted entirely of hydrogen.[220] The evolution of our common air was a complex sequence of physical-chemical reactions spanning eons of time and involving the production and consumption of energy, the magnitude of which defies the imagination. It is theorized that the great energy of the stars was produced by the burning of hydrogen, with its eventual conversion to helium and other elements heavier than itself. Under conditions of extraordinary temperature, helium can transform to carbon and can even react with some of this carbon to produce the element oxygen along with gamma radiation. Such reactions, slowly progressing over millions of years, gradually shifted the composition of the earth's atmosphere, increasing the concentrations of oxygen. Other contributing phenomena included the ultraviolet energy of the sun, which dissociated water into hydrogen and hydroxyl radicals, further breaking the latter into hydrogen and oxygen, and finally, when life on earth was represented by algae in the sea, the significant chemical reactions of photosynthesis. It has been estimated that there was a great increase in the amount of oxygen in the atmosphere about $5.5 \times 10^8$ years ago, coincidental with a surge in evolution of life forms. As oxygen established itself among the earth's elements, the lighter hydrogen gradually diffused outward into space. Thus, since its origin, earth's atmosphere has been in a process of continuous change, and it is interesting to ask ourselves whether we should consider our present atmosphere any more permanent than the atmosphere of 10 million or 100 million years ago and to speculate that the familiar composition of our air may be but a momentary step in the evolution of nature, gradually to give way to other as yet unguessed-at gases. However, faced with survival in a breathing mixture, of which oxygen comprises some 21%, let us examine some of the features of this element and then discuss the therapeutic uses of the "number one medicine."

## Characteristics of oxygen

Oxygen is a colorless, transparent, tasteless, and odorless gas occurring in nature as free molecular $O_2$ and as a component of a host of chemical compounds, both organic and inorganic. It comprises almost 50% of the weight of the earth's crust and occurs in all living matter as water and in combination with elements other than hydrogen. At 0° C and 1 atm pressure, oxygen has a density of 1.429 g/$\ell$, compared with the density of air, 1.30 g/$\ell$. It is only slightly soluble in water; at room temperature and 1 atm pressure 3.3 volumes of oxygen dissolve in 100 volumes of water. Nonetheless, this small amount is essential to aquatic life, both plant and animal.

Oxygen does not burn. However, it does support combustion, a matter of considerable importance to its widespread use in hospitals. A minute spark can become a large hot flame in an enriched oxygen environment, or a glowing ember can burst into open flame. The relationship between the burning intensity of a combustible substance and the amount of ambient oxygen is direct but not simple. Burning speed increases with an increase in the partial pressure of oxygen in the environment. Thus either an increase in concentration of oxygen at a fixed total pressure or an increase in total pressure of a constant gas concentration will augment the kinetics of combustion. However, burning speed will also increase if only oxygen concentrations are raised, and the partial pressure of the various oxygen percentages is kept constant by suitably lowering the total pressure.[221] These data demonstrate that both oxygen concentration and partial pressure influence rate of burning. Another factor to consider in the relation between burning and the amount of oxygen is the self-perpetuating effect of combustion in oxygen. The reaction of oxygen with other elements is markedly enhanced at elevated temperatures, and once combustion starts in a high-oxygen atmosphere, the heat produced potentiates further combustion and is not wasted on the relatively inert nitrogen content of ordinary air.

Although oxygen can be produced by many chemical reactions and the electrolysis of water, as noted in Chapter 1, its main source is compressed air. Under the influence of tremendous pressure followed by the cooling effect of sudden expansion combined with heat exchangers, the components of air are converted to liquid. Through the process of fractional distillation, as the liquefied air is allowed to heat slowly, nitrogen, with its boiling point of $-195.8°$ C ($-320.5°$ F), escapes first; then the trace gases of argon, krypton, and xenon are removed. Standards require that the final remaining oxygen have a purity of at least 99%, a value that is usually exceeded. The liquid oxygen is stored in special containers or converted to gas under high pressure in tanks.

## Hazards in the use of oxygen

We have emphasized the importance of oxygen in the treatment of disease and have considered in some detail the seriousness of oxygen deprivation, but it must not be thought to be a completely innocuous agent. The respiratory therapist must familiarize himself with all aspects of the physiologic action of oxygen, the harmful as well as the beneficial. He must be aware of those conditions in which oxygen is not indicated, when it may even be a threat to life, for such caution will make him a safe as well as effective therapist. Before discussing the equipment and techniques for administering oxygen, we will consider some of the risks of its use and explore a bit its pathologic potential. First we will discuss the effects of oxygen on ventilation, then oxygen toxicity, both at 1 atm pressure.

### Ventilatory effects of oxygen

*Oxygen-induced hypoventilation.* This is not a new topic, for in the study of cardiopulmonary physiology earlier, we covered oxygen-induced hypoventilation superficially in discussions of ventilatory control and the role of the peripheral chemoreceptors. Here, we will be interested not only in the specific academic relationship between oxygen and the ventilatory control mechanisms but also in the practical clinical use of oxygen in patients suffering from failure of these mechanisms. For example, for the patient who is in ventilatory failure with its accompanying hypercapnia, we may usually assume that oxygen can be safely administered at concentrations slightly above ambient, at 1 atm pressure. Flows of 1 to 2 $\ell$/min carry little risk and can be achieved by techniques to be discussed subsequently. Even so, the arterial carbon dioxide level may rise slightly but, after a period of perhaps 1 hour, will usually plateau at a level still within the bounds of safety. It has often been noted that if the oxygen administration is stopped, oxygen tension in arterial blood may fall below pretreatment levels.[222] In such a situation it is evident that intermittent use of the gas may be dangerous to the patient's respiratory equilibrium, and to assure adequate oxygenation, oxygen should be given constantly with mechanical suport of ventilation if necessary. This latter aspect will be dealt with in detail in another chapter.[223] As a guide for the use of oxygen in patients with ventilatory failure, it has been suggested that an arterial oxygen tension of about 50 mm Hg will prevent immediate death from hypoxia while keeping the adverse effects of oxygen to a minimum. This does not imply that such a level is therapeutically desirable as definitive therapy but that this tension will prevent rapid deterioration of the patient's state while other measures are being prepared.[224]

The effect of oxygen administration on ventilation is well documented in a study of several patients with chronic respiratory disease who were tested for their response to concentrations of oxygen in the 90% to 100% range.[225] When a normal subject breathes 100% oxygen, his chemoreceptors remain inactive, and because of the increased oxygen in the blood, there is less reduced hemoglobin available for carbon dioxide transportation and arterial $P_{CO_2}$ tends to rise. To maintain a normal acid-base balance, the increased $P_{aCO_2}$ acting on the chemoreceptors, plus the irritating effect of the high concentration of oxygen on the respiratory mucosa, can produce a 5% to 20% increase in ventilation and correct the hypercapnia. In the presence of hypoxia, the arterial unsaturation stimulates the chemoreceptors, and if there is no airway obstruction to carbon dioxide excretion, the augmented ventilation may produce hypocapnia. This reaction is not uncommon in patients at high altitude, with venous-arterial shunts, and with alveolar-capillary block. Of course, this sensitive response implies a normally functioning respiratory center. In contrast, when hypoxia exists with the hypercapnia of ventilatory failure, because the latter denotes an unresponsive respiratory center, oxygen administration suppresses the chemoreceptors and produces a hypoventilation that is not compensated.

It was observed that, on the average, when the arterial carbon dioxide tension was greater than 50 mm Hg, the risk of oxygen-induced hypoventilation increased, and this value seemed more significant than the pH level. This substantiates the observation, which the respiratory therapist will have frequent occasion to make, that the obstructed patient with hypoxia presents the greatest hypoventilation risk and that not far behind is the patient whose respiratory center is obtunded by sedation or narcosis.

This hazard of oxygen therapy does not militate against its use when indicated, for the relief of hypoxia is the most critical therapeutic need, and even for the most unresponsive patient there are methods of giving oxygen. It does mean, however, that the therapist assigned to administer oxygen must never assume such administration to be a "routine" procedure. He should take the time to acquaint himself with the basic disease problem under treatment so that he will be alert to potential danger. This point is important enough that we will return to it again when we specifically discuss the management of ventilatory failure.

*Atelectasis.* The collapse of alveoli as the result of high concentrations of oxygen in the inhaled air is due to the elimination of nitrogen from the lung and the effect of oxygen on pulmonary surfactant. We will consider the first here and the second below. Normally, the most prevalent gas in the alveoli is nitrogen, the bulk of which comes from the inspired air, with a much smaller amount coming from the general body metabolism. Breathing pure oxygen depletes the circulating nitrogen within several minutes as each tidal air excursion washes it out of the alveoli, into which the gas has diffused from the blood. The patient who is excessively relaxed and ventilating at a minimal tidal level, especially if he has some degree of airway obstruction as from retained secretions, is liable to suffer ill consequences of 100% oxygen breathing. As the patient breathes the oxygen, should the easy tidal flow be impeded to and from a partially blocked alveolus or one somewhat hampered by a dependent location, the oxygen that gains access to the alveolus may diffuse into the pulmonary circulation faster than it can be replaced by ventilation. This results in a gradual shrinking of the alveolus and, when aided by other factors, may lead to complete collapse. In the alert patient this is not as great a risk, since the natural "sigh" mechanism periodically hyperinflates the lung, ventilating those alveoli that may be considered sluggish in their tidal exchange.

It is of historical interest only that, in the past, the nitrogen-washout effect of 100% oxygen was used to relieve intestinal distention.[226] Nitrogen is one of the major intestinal gases causing distention, especially postoperatively. Because of its diffusibility into the lungs, 100% oxygen was used to remove it from the blood, thereby creating a gradient that allowed the nitrogen to move from the bowel into the circulation, thence to the lung, and out. It was shown that a given amount of nitrogen could be reduced 62% in 24 hours by this method, as against 10% by breathing room air. It is interesting to note that breathing 95% oxygen for no longer than 10 hours was one recommended technique; and we can only wonder how often recovery may have been retarded by pulmonary complications, even though bowel distress may have been relieved.

**Oxygen toxicity.** The adverse effects of oxygen described above can be considered local in nature and, although serious, do not cause the widespread destruction that is classified as toxicity. The scope of injury to the organism varies from the mild and transient to the overwhelmingly fatal, and we will describe the more important clinical and pathologic changes characterizing oxygen toxicity. Before we get into the subject matter, it may stimulate the student's interest to consider oxygen toxicity as one of nature's most remarkable phenomena.

The emergence of oxygen, as described a few pages back, in a universe consisting mostly of hydrogen was an event of great magnitude. However, its initial production had little direct influence on earth's biologic activity, since concentrations of the new gas close to earth's surface were very limited. The great impact of oxygen was delayed until the appearance of the blue-green algae as a significant segment of the biological population. Using solar energy in the process of photosynthesis, these primitive living cells were able to split water molecules and release oxygen directly into the atmosphere. Life on earth, such as it was at the time, probably consisted of primordial amino acids that could not have survived in an oxygen environment. Thus, as atmospheric oxygen concentrations grew, organisms that had existed since their inception in an anaerobic world were faced with two major challenges. First was the need to survive the destructive combustion engendered by an oxygen environment, and second, to learn how to use oxygen as a fuel for high energy-yielding reactions that could accelerate evolution and development of these same organisms. A critical milestone was reached when oxygen comprised a significant concentration of earth's atmosphere, and from then on the evolutionary process of selective adaptability depended on mechanisms of survival and profitable use of oxygen.

The human, as an example of all aerobes, finds himself fully dependent for existence upon a gas basically lethal to him, a fascinating biological paradox. No substitute energy source for metabolic machinery has yet been found, and the poisonous gas remains man's most indispensable need. The fact of aerobic survival is testimony that somewhere along the evolutionary course man developed effective defenses against the toxic actions of oxygen.[227] We will review the important manifestations of oxygen toxicity as outlined:

*Somatic*
1. Substernal distress
2. Cough
3. Nausea and vomiting
4. Paresthesias

*Metabolic*
1. Inhibition of tissue cultures
2. Inactivation of enzymes
3. Damage to capillary endothelium
4. Destruction of Type I pneumocytes

*Morphologic*
1. Reduced mucociliary mobility
2. Interference with pulmonary surfactant
3. Oxygen pneumonia
4. Bronchopulmonary dysplasia
5. Alveolar membrane formation
6. Retrolental fibroplasia

*Somatic effects.* Early signs and symptoms of oxygen toxicity such as substernal distress, cough, nausea and vomiting, and paresthesias of the extremities may go unrecognized because of their nonspecific nature, but under hyperbaric conditions serious reactions such as convulsions may occur. The onset of discomfort beneath the sternum has been suggested as a significant indication of actual or impending toxicity.[228] The time necessary to produce toxic symptoms in human volunteers breathing 100% oxygen is reported to range from 6 to 30 hours, in one study, with the maximum limit of tolerance at 110 hours.[228] However, the voluntary limit of tolerance to 100% oxygen has been estimated to be between 53 and 75 hours.[229] As a rough guide, it has been suggested in the past that the risk of toxicity was minimized if the partial pressure of the inspired oxygen did not exceed 425 mm Hg, which is the equivalent of an oxygen concentration of 56% at 1 atm pressure. It is now believed that, given enough of a time exposure, toxic symptoms can appear at partial pressures much lower but that, because it is not known at what tension level man has unlimited tolerance, there are no sure rules to follow in the administration of oxygen. These so-called early signs and symptoms may progress to severe structural lung damage and to injury to other systems.

*Metabolic effects.* This aspect of oxygen toxicity is complex and in some details very speculative, for it includes biological responses to oxygen that may be apparent only to molecular scientists or theoretical biochemists. Much of the information comes from laboratory animal experiments, and one can question how much animal data can justifiably be projected to the human. Nevertheless, some of the reported work is convincing, and the implications that oxygen can adversely affect our basic life processes are so awesome that we cannot ignore them. As has been our custom with so many other topics, we will simplify this discussion to highlight the few most important relationships between oxygen and cellular integrity.

It is felt that oxygen toxicity is mediated through the actions of chemical units known as *free radicals*. These are extremely reactive atoms or groups of atoms, which have half-lives in aqueous solution of $10^{-5}$ seconds or less and which carry at least one unpaired electron. They can exist "free" for only the merest moment and then must stabilize themselves by chemically combining with other atoms. Detailed consideration of the chemistry of free radicals is much too involved for us here, but we should be aware that three of them are believed to be involved in oxygen toxicity—the hydroxyl, perhydroxyl, and superoxide free radicals, of which the last is of the greatest interest to us.

We know that plus and minus superscripts denote ions. In contrast, a free radical is identified by a small dot representing the unpaired electron. Two of the radicals noted above are written with the dot, thus: hydroxyl radical $= OH^{\cdot}$, and perhydroxyl radical $= HO_2^{\cdot}$. The unpaired electron gives to superoxide an extra negative charge so that it is both an anion and a free radical. Theoretically, therefore, superoxide could be written $O_2^{\overline{\cdot}}$ showing its dual designation, but by custom it is symbolized as an ion, $O_2^{-}$, implying the presence of an unpaired electron and its free radical role.

As oxygen participates in cellular biochemical actions, it takes on electrons and is reduced, while its electron donors are oxidized. It is this intracellular reduction of oxygen that is responsible for producing the superoxide radical. In its electron structure, oxygen has two single, or unpaired, electrons in its outer orbit, and during reduction tends to accept electrons one at a time. This is called *univalent reduction,* and as a result there is a brief moment when one of the electrons is unpaired and the oxygen is a superoxide radical. Superoxide thus is referred to as an intermediate product of oxygen reduction. As metabolic reactions continue, superoxide is converted to another free radical, perhydroxyl, and this in turn reacts with additional superoxide to produce the powerful hydroxyl radical. We are not interested in the details of such reactions, and this sequence is noted only to emphasize the metabolic interactions that generate a continuous supply of these potent substances.

INHIBITION OF TISSUE CULTURES. It has been known that 100% oxygen at atmosphere is able to inhibit growth of living tissue cultures, apparently by interfering with the synthesis of DNA and RNA. It is now believed that free radicals are responsible for this action, possibly by blocking the metaphase stage of cellular mitotic reproduction or through mechanisms still undefined. If any substance can be considered the basic matter of life, in our present state of knowledge it is certainly the DNA-RNA complex. We can scarcely help but wonder at the circumstance of chemical reactants manufactured in the body from the gas on which we are so dependent that can imperil our own cellular survival. As yet there are no direct clinical implications of this action of free radicals.

INACTIVATION OF ENZYMES. Free radicals are also able to inactivate some enzyme systems that regulate the efficiency of our metabolism. Especially vulnerable are those enzymes whose functions are dependent upon sulfhydryl groups. These are highly reactive paired SH atoms present in many biologically active compounds, such as proteins, enzymes, and co-enzymes. In addition, the sulfhydryl group is needed to help maintain the exact state of cytoplasmic fluidity, referred to as the gel/sol relationship. Again, interference in these areas by free radicals puts at great risk some very critical and delicate metabolic mechanisms.

DAMAGE TO CAPILLARIES AND PNEUMOCYTES. Specifically related to our sphere of interest are two targets of free radical activity in the lung—the pulmonary capillary endothelium and the Type I alveolar cell. Integrity of the capillary wall is damaged by toxic action of oxygen, allowing the escape of fluid from capillary into lung interstitium and parenchyma. We will see that this can present an acute and difficult clinical problem to manage. The alveoli are composed of two kinds of cells, called pneumocytes, and designated Types I and II. Type I pneumocytes are flat, elongated, membranous cells that cover most of the alveolar surface, while Type II cells are more cuboidal, contain many inclusion bodies (implying diverse cellular functions), and produce the important lipoprotein surfactant. The free radicals, and apparently especially superoxide, destroy Type I pneumocytes and threaten disruption of alveolar walls.

*Morphologic effects.* Our primary interest in oxygen toxicity is its varied clinical manifestations, and these are related to the pathology of the toxic reactions, the abnormal structural changes that occur in tissues and organs. We will review a half dozen examples of tissue responses to high tensions of oxygen.

REDUCED MUCOCILIARY ACTION. Feline experiments have shown that the rate of cephalad movement of minute particles deposited on the distal tracheal mucosa is markedly slowed in the presence of 100% oxygen.[230] If this unwelcome action of oxygen can be extrapolated to the human airway, serious clinical implications are obvious. It is of considerable interest, however, that administration of low concentrations of oxygen also slow mucus transport time. Apparently the system will not work if it is not fueled with sufficient oxygen and can be inactivated by too much.

Perhaps it is clinically important to note that the retarding action of high-tension oxygen can be prevented or reversed by parenteral or aerosol administration of epinephrine, isoproterenol, and adenosine triphosphate.

INTERFERENCE WITH PULMONARY SURFACTANT. Further animal experiments have established that prolonged exposure to high oxygen concentrations can interfere with the function of pulmonary surfactant.[231] It has been postulated that the surfactant probably is not destroyed because it can still be demonstrated in extractions of affected lungs. More than likely the oxygen causes a redistribution of the surfactant, removing it from close contact with alveolar walls. The potential for this toxic reaction of oxygen to produce atelectasis is very evident, and when coupled with the risk of oxygen absorption from poorly communicating alveoli, subjects the patient to a double hazard.

OXYGEN PNEUMONIA. Prolonged exposure to inspired oxygen concentrations in excess of 50% can give the lung an x-ray picture identical to that of a diffuse broncho-pneumonia.[232] Patchy infiltrates tend to be most prominent in the lower lung fields, but all areas may be involved. Pulmonary pathology includes alveolar wall edema and an intra-alveolar exudate of large cells. Polymorphonuclear leukocytes, white blood cells that protect us against infection by destroying bacteria, are not prominent, and bacteria are few in number. As with any pneumonia, because of alveolar exudate, patients with oxygen toxicity pneumonia suffer increasing hypoxemia. If patient survival can be maintained while inspired oxygen concentrations are lowered, the pulmonary lesion may resolve.

BRONCHOPULMONARY DYSPLASIA. To some extent this pathological state carries lung damage beyond the stage of the oxygen pneumonia just described and depicts the destructive healing that accompanies chronicity.[233] Two microscopic pathological stages have been identified, defined by one study as exudative and proliferative.[234]

The following excellent description needs no amplification:

> The lungs in the *exudative phase* showed capillary congestion, an alveolar proteinaceous exudate, intra-alveolar hemorrhage, and a fibrinous exudate. Prominent "hyaline" membranes lined the alveolar walls, alveolar ducts, and respiratory bronchioles. Only a sparse chronic inflammatory component was present. The striking features of the lungs in the *proliferative phase* were marked alveolar and inter-lobular septal edema, fibroblastic proliferation with early fibrosis, prominent hyperplasia of the alveolar lining cells, and a variable component of the alterations characteristic of the exudative phase. It is our impression that these 2 categories are stages of a progressive deterioration, with the exudative phase representing an earlier change that progresses, if survival is sufficiently prolonged, to the proliferative or fibrotic phase.[234]

An additional tissue response sometimes accompanying the proliferative phase is referred to as *capillary tufting*.[235] From the thickened alveolar septa, proliferated (overgrown) pulmonary capillaries project as tufts or small masses into alveolar spaces. These capillary tufts probably resolve and disappear in surviving patients, but while present they are intra-alveolar, space-occupying lesions that add to existing problems of ventilation and gas exchange.

Finally, it has been noted that the damaging effect of oxygen on the lungs tends to be less in patients with well-established lung disease than in those without intrinsic disease. The implication is that preexisting exudate, fibrosis, edema, and the like from chronic disease protects the pulmonary tissue from a direct assault by oxygen. The validity of this conclusion may need additional support.

ALVEOLAR MEMBRANE FORMATION. Alveolar membrane was referred to above, but its clinical importance as one of the major manifestations of oxygen toxicity justifies a detailed description. To introduce the topic, we will digress just a bit and describe a relevant pediatric disease.[236, 237]

Many infants born prematurely suffer from a condition called *hyaline membrane disease*, or respiratory distress syndrome of the newborn (RDS). The major defect in this disease is a severely noncompliant lung, placing a tremendous physical strain on the ventilatory mechanics of the underdeveloped child. Many of these patients succumb in their early postnatal life, and others may survive only after intensive mechanical ventilatory support. The alveoli of the victims are lined with a thin but definite membrane, which because of its clear, transparent homogeneity is referred to as a "hyaline membrane." Such a structure is a normal prenatal component of the lung, but one that disappears prior to birth, and premature birth often does not allow time for its natural disappearance. One of the more serious complications of high concentration–oxygen therapy is the appearance of a hyaline membrane, in adults as well as children. As a demonstration of the ease with which a membrane can be formed, 75% of a group of guinea pigs exposed to 98% oxygen at atmosphere from 40 to 100 hours developed such a defect. Interestingly, if a subject survives despite this injury, there is apparently no residual damage. The hyaline membrane produced experimentally with high oxygen concentrations appears to be structurally identical with that which occurs in RDS and seems to be the result of injury to the alveolar duct and terminal bronchiole. If the experimental animal is given high doses of adrenocorticosteroids with the elevated oxygen concentration, it deteriorates rapidly and dies from fulminating pulmonary vascular damage. Human postmortem lung specimens demonstrated reactions similar to the experimental response if the patients had been treated with high oxygen concentrations. The membranes noted consisted of layers of fibrin on the alveolar walls, extending into the alveolar ducts and respiratory bronchioles. Many patients succumbing to oxygen toxicity not only had received oxygen concentrations in the 90% to 100% range but had also had this delivered by mechanical ventilators. However, there is little correlation between the pulmonary pathologic changes and the mechanical ventilation, per se, but there is close correlation with the oxygen therapy. As yet, no dependable safety limits have been determined for oxygen administration, but it is evident that both factors of gas concentration and duration of treatment are critical. There is some evidence that prolonged administration of oxygen concentrations above 70% will increase the risk of membranous toxicity and that levels above 90% are dangerous.

**RETROLENTAL FIBROPLASIA.** The term *retrolental* means "behind the lens" and refers to an ocular condition of premature infants associated with oxygen administration. The disease was established as a specific entity in the 1950s, when it was observed that some premature infants given oxygen therapy developed damage to the eyes that was severe enough to produce permanent blindness. The pathology is basically a fibrotic process behind the ocular lenses, which impairs light penetration to the retina. Apparently excessive blood oxygen levels produce retinal vasoconstriction, and if this is severe enough to persist after the cessation of oxygen therapy, permanent damage is likely.[238] This risk poses a serious management problem, for the premature infant is often in great need of supplementary oxygen, and as in the infant with a lung expansion defect, sometimes large amounts of oxygen are necessary for survival. Experience has demonstrated that if the concentration of inspired oxygen delivered to the small patient does not exceed 40%, the risk of retrolental fibroplasia is significantly reduced. Using the alveolar air equation (Appendix 12), and assuming a $P_{a_{CO_2}}$ of 40 mm Hg and a respiratory quotient (R) of 0.8, it can be calculated that inhalation of 40% oxygen will produce an alveolar oxygen tension of about 237 mm Hg.

Since $P_{a_{O_2}}$ cannot exceed $P_{A_{O_2}}$, this value may be considered to represent the blood oxygen level above which ocular integrity is at risk. In infants with lung disease, it is difficult to raise $P_{a_{O_2}}$ much above 200 mm Hg, and thus the risk of eye damage is slight in hypoxic infants. Most incubators, which provide the proper environment for premature infants, have devices that limit the oxygen concentration to 40%. However, more experience will be needed to determine more precisely the critical arterial oxygen tension level that is associated with oxygen damage to the eyes. As a final note, it should be mentioned that oxygen-induced eye damage has not been considered an adult hazard, but in what might be the first such recorded incident, near total blindness was reported in a 32-year-old man. The apparent cause of visual loss was retinal arterial constriction following prolonged arterial oxygen tensions of 250 to 300 mm Hg.[239]

*Defense against oxygen toxicity.* It was pointed out earlier that evolution of the human being had to include built-in protection against the harmful effects of oxygen, or survival would have been short indeed. Research in this field is relatively new, and as yet only the surface has been scratched. An organism as complex as the human body doubtless has many mechanisms that prevent oxygen damage, but at the present the one attracting the most interest is the enzyme *superoxide dismutase (SOD)*.[239a-239c] By definition, a dismutase is an enzyme able to effect simultaneous oxidation-reduction. SOD specifically catalyzes the following reaction

$$O_2^- + O_2^- + 2H^+ \longrightarrow H_2O_2 + O_2$$

whereby dangerous superoxide is transformed into hydrogen peroxide and molecular oxygen. Hydrogen peroxide, in turn, is metabolized into water and more oxygen by enzymes, peroxidases and catalases. There are four kinds of SOD, differing in their sources and the metals contained in their formulas. We are not concerned with their chemical structure, but we are interested in what they do.

Most experimental rats exposed to 100% oxygen die within 72 hours. However, if they are first exposed to 85% oxygen for a week, they can then survive 100% oxygen for a long time. This phenomenon is called *tolerance* to 100% oxygen, and while it is developing, lung content of SOD increases by about 50%. Apparently SOD production is stimulated by inhalation of moderately elevated oxygen concentrations, and the body subsequently can tolerate 100% oxygen, since SOD controls the levels of superoxide.

It has been established that while experimental oxygen tolerance is being generated and pulmonary SOD levels are rising, alveolar Type II pneumocytes increase in number up to 300%. This tremendous proliferation of alveolar cells is obviously related to the increasing SOD. It probably represents a high initial dismutase cell content, allowing cell survival in the face of high oxygen tension, or stimulation of

sed SOD production by the pneumocytes. It thus seems that Type II alveolar
e an important source of superoxide dismutase and the primary defense against
..monary oxygen toxicity.

Before leaving this section, it is only just to point out that the villain is not all bad. Scavenging granulocytes, comprising a major body defense against infection, manufacture and release superoxide and the other free radicals to kill invading bacteria.[240, 241] The lethal potential of these substances are thus directed in chemical warfare against other threats to our survival.

*Summary.* There are important clinical implications in the available data concerning the scope and mechanisms of oxygen toxicity. We frequently encounter patients whose hypoxia demands oxygen therapy, often with mechanically assisted ventilation, but who show a progressive downhill course while increasing concentrations of oxygen are administered in a vain attempt to maintain adequate blood levels. Not only is alveolar-capillary diffusion impaired but obstruction of small airways and alveoli by edema, hemorrhage, and capillary proliferation produces an increasing venous admixture, demonstrated in the laboratory by a widening alveolar-arterial oxygen tension gradient.[242] We appreciate that this can be the direct result of the topical action of high-concentration oxygen on the pulmonary tissue, with the creation of a chaotic disturbance of physiology as the lung is beset, simultaneously, with shunting and atelectasis. Because the relation between pure oxygen breathing and absorption atelectasis was recognized before the more deep-seated oxygen damage to the lung was known, it was frequently assumed that the morbidity and mortality of oxygen-breathing was associated with atelectasis. On this basis, it has been suggested that prevention of lung injury might be accomplished by alternating periods of oxygen breathing with the breathing of air, permitting expansion of alveoli by the nitrogen content of the latter. Studies of this maneuver, however, have failed to substantiate its predicted virtue.[243]

We can summarize the topic of the dangers of oxygen by emphasizing again, strongly, that when oxygen is needed, it must be given, even though we recognize its potential risk. After all, the patient might not suffer toxic reactions, since these are not predictable with any precision, but failure to supply oxygen may well cause irreversible tissue damage. Nevertheless, oxygen, like any potent medicine, should be used with reason and according to indications. If high concentrations of oxygen are necessary, the duration of administration should be kept to a minimum and reduced as soon as possible. In general, the objective of therapy is to administer oxygen sufficient to maintain arterial oxygen tension between 80 and 100 mm Hg, not 150 or 200 mm Hg. The exceptions are those circumstances in which delivery to the pulmonary blood is normal but the oxygen-carrying capacity of the hemoglobin is impaired. Anemia and carbon monoxide inhalation are two common clinical conditions needing high blood gas tensions to increase dissolved plasma oxygen, compensating for the deficient hemoglobin transport. Frequent arterial blood monitoring is a mandatory safety measure when concentrations above 50% are used. Also, the exact concentration of inspired oxygen should be measured, especially when the gas is used in mechanical ventilators, and if air-diluting mechanisms cannot be depended upon to deliver desired concentrations, then premixed gases should be used. The safe and effective administration of oxygen to suit any individual need is one of the most important services that a knowledgeable and skilled respiratory therapist can offer, a service matched by few other technical members of the hospital health team.

### Oxygen equipment and techniques

*Masks.* Oxygen masks are of many different types, varying in style of construction, materials, and specific purpose. Not too long ago most masks were of rubber, but now many are made of plastic and can be discarded after use, minimizing the risk of cross contamination, work of sterilizing, and storage space. Although we will discuss some critical differences among them, oxygen masks have some important common characteristics. The therapist will note variation in the use of masks, as with other pieces of equipment, among the hospitals with which he may have contact; but in general, we can say that the oxygen mask is used where oxygen is needed quickly and for relatively short periods of time. It is the emergency equipment of choice, and some type of a mask should be available wherever patients are being treated. A mask may be used for up to several hours, but other techniques are more appropriate for prolonged constant therapy.

Masks can be uncomfortable as a result of the frequent need for a tight seal between the unit and the patient's face, and the head strap or harness necessary to hold it in place adds to the discomfort. They are often quite hot, as they confine heat radiating from the face about the nose and mouth. The therapist must ever be aware of the risk of producing pressure necrosis of the skin when he attempts a tight fit of the mask to the face. Constant pressure of the edge of the mask over areas where little subcutaneous tissue separates skin from underlying bone, such as the bridge of the nose and the malar eminences of the cheeks, can readily interrupt cutaneous blood flow. Within a short time the skin may become devitalized, with the risk of permanent scarring. A snugly fitted mask should be removed frequently and dried, and the face should be dried and gently massaged over the pressure areas to stimulate circulation, then powdered to minimize the accumulation of moisture, which tends to soften the skin and to augment danger of pressure damage. An oxygen mask can be hazardous on a patient who is prone to vomit, for it can block the flow of vomitus and subject the patient to dangerous aspiration. Because of this risk of aspiration, and the possibility of airway obstruction by a flaccid tongue, a mask should never be strapped onto an unconscious patient. If mask therapy is indicated in such a patient, an oral airway should be inserted to prevent the tongue from retracting into the pharynx, and the oxygen mask should either be held in place by an attendant or loosely set on the face.

Finally, the therapist must recognize that by the nature of their construction face masks add dead space to the patient's airway, which may be considerable with some appliances. The space under the mask, about the nose and mouth, is functionally an extension of anatomic dead space and, depending on the location of the exhalation ports, may cause a significant accumulation of carbon dioxide. Assuming a normally responsive respiratory center, the dead space of many masks produces a hyperventilation that may add to the patient's work of breathing, and in the patient with an obtunded center and hypercapnia, such dead space can be an added hazard.

Despite these shortcomings, however, oxygen masks have a wide use in therapy and are often lifesaving. We will describe some of the characteristics of the following five general types of masks: simple, rebreathing, partial rebreathing, nonrebreathing, and venturi.

*Simple mask.* The usual simple mask, shown in Fig. 8-12, is a disposable plastic unit with neither valves nor reservoir bag, exhaled air being vented through holes in its body. Generally, it is relatively loosely fitted without the capability of close molding to facial contours possible with more elaborate types. In the event of an interrupted oxygen supply, air is drawn in through the exhalation ports as well as around the edge of the mask. The mask dead space and its "reservoir effect" influence the relationship between oxygen flow and the resulting alveolar oxygen concentration.[244] A minimal flow is necessary to flush the dead space for removal of carbon dioxide, but beyond a given flow, since the oxygen supply is continuous throughout the ventilatory cycle, the reservoir or dead space is filled with oxygen at the end of exhalation. The oxygen enrichment of inhaled air depends on the balance between the patient's ventilatory need and the oxygen supply during inhalation. The deeper the tidal volume or the greater the inspiratory flow of the patient the more will the oxy-

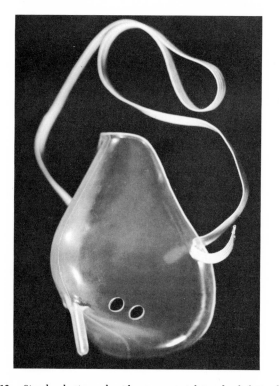

**Fig. 8-12.**   Simple plastic mask with an oxygen inlet and exhalation holes.

gen be diluted by supplementary air drawn in through the ports or around the mask, since at any given instant the inspiratory flow may exceed many times the delivered oxygen flow. The more oxygen supplied during inhalation the greater will be its alveolar concentration.

Because of its convenience and relative comfort, the simple mask is widely used whenever moderate oxygen concentrations are desired for short periods of time. This includes the postoperative recovery state, temporary therapy while awaiting definitive plans, and interim therapy while weaning a patient from continuous oxygen administration. The crudeness of a simple mask makes it impossible to predict exact amounts of oxygen going to the patient, but in general the delivered concentrations vary from 35% to 55% at gas flows of 6 to 10 $\ell$/min.[245] It must be kept in mind that such values give no indication of the alveolar or arterial oxygen levels.

A special problem is presented by the very small infant, for whom the standard masks are often ineffective. There is available a custom-made and fitted mask that is molded from a very malleable plastic compound inside a shell, contoured like an infant's nose.[246] When partially set, the mask is molded about the patient's nose for a perfect fit, allowed to harden, and then cemented to the face. The dead space of such an appliance ranges from 0.3 to 0.5 ml, as compared to the tidal volume of newborn infants, which measures from 7 to 15 ml. This mask can withstand delivered gas pressures over 40 cm of water and can be used with mechanical ventilators. The infant's skin is reported to be undamaged after the continuous use of the mask for as long as 4 days.

*Rebreathing mask.* The rebreathing mask is not used for clinical respiratory therapy and will be only briefly described. It consists of a mask tightly covering the mouth and nose, with an attached reservoir bag into which the breathing mixture flows and from which the patient inhales. The bag and mask are used in a closed system whereby the exhaled gas is circulated through a carbon dioxide absorber and additional breathing gas is added to replace that metabolized by the patient. The chief use for a rebreathing circuit is the administration of anesthesia, since it prevents waste of anesthetic agents and permits the addition of desired amounts of oxygen to the breathing mixture.

*Partial rebreathing mask.* Like the rebreathing mask, the partial mask is a combined face mask and reservoir bag, but unlike the rebreathing mask, it is an open circuit without a carbon dioxide absorber. The purpose of the partial rebreathing mask is to conserve oxygen by a technique that, as the name implies, permits the patient to rebreathe some of his exhaled air. Fig. 8-13, A, schematically illustrates the basic parts and function of such an appliance. Source oxygen flows into the neck of the mask and during the inhalation phase passes directly into the mask proper, but during exhalation it enters the reservoir bag. As the patient exhales, approximately the first third of his exhaled air is returned to the reservoir bag to mix with source oxygen. This fraction of the exhaled volume essentially represents the pulmonary dead space, which contains mostly oxygen, and it is flushed into the bag to be reinhaled. As the bag distends with both source oxygen and exhaled air, pressure in the system then directs the terminal two thirds of exhaled air, with its carbon dioxide load,

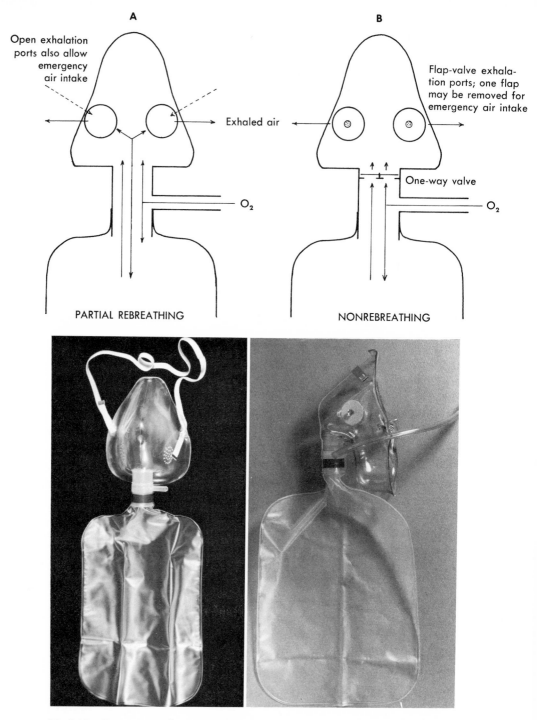

**Fig. 8-13.** Diagrammatic illustrations of the difference between, **A,** partial rebreathing oxygen mask and, **B,** nonrebreathing mask. In both, oxygen flows directly into the mask during inspiration and into the reservoir bag during exhalation. However, the early portion of exhaled air in **A** returns to the bag to be rebreathed with incoming oxygen in the next breath. Terminal air escapes through exhalation ports. In **B** all exhaled air is vented through a port in the mask, and a one-way valve between the bag and mask prevents rebreathing.

out the exhalation ports. If the oxygen inflow is adjusted so that the bag does not collapse during inhalation and the rate is over 4 $\ell$/min, the amount of carbon dioxide contaminating the reservoir is negligible.[247] The exhalation ports of many masks are only vents in the facepiece, and they also serve as emergency inlets for room air in the event of a failure of source oxygen. With a well-fitted partial rebreathing mask, adjusted so that the patient's inhalation does not deflate the bag, inspired oxygen concentrations of from 35% to 60% can usually be achieved at delivered flows between 6 and 10 $\ell$/min.[248]

*Nonrebreathing mask.* Also a mask and reservoir bag device, the name of the nonrebreathing mask indicates that there is no exhaled gas rebreathing. Fig. 8-13, *B*, depicts the essential differences between the partial and nonrebreathing masks. The one major characteristic of the nonrebreathing mask is a one-way valve placed between the bag and the mask. As in the partial rebreather, source oxygen flows either into the bag only (during exhalation) or into the mask and bag (during inhalation). However, the valve between bag and mask prevents exhaled air from returning to the bag and diverts it into the atmosphere through a flap valve in the facepiece. Somewhere, either in the neck as illustrated or in the mask itself, flap- or spring-loaded valves permit the intake of room air should source oxygen fail or the patient's needs suddenly exceed the available oxygen flow.

Because the patient inhales only the gas present in the bag, the nonrebreathing technique is the most precise method of administering a specific gas concentration, but to be effective there must be no significant leakage about the face or elsewhere in the system. This is the type of apparatus used to deliver 100% oxygen or tanked gases of precise composition such as oxygen-nitrogen, helium-oxygen, and carbon dioxide–oxygen mixtures. Care must be taken to provide suitable humidification, and some reservoir bags have drain plugs for removal of accumulated moisture. By and large, the nonrebreathing mask and bag is one of the most useful and practical tools for short-term precision administration of respiratory gases.

*Venturi, or dilution, mask.* This mask, strictly speaking, should be called a dilution mask rather than venturi, since it is not provided with a true venturi but operates on the principle of Bernoulli. As shown in Fig. 8-14, oxygen is delivered through a jet orifice and is diluted by the entrainment of ambient air through ports in the surrounding housing. Depending on the design of the jet-entrainment complex, oxygen concentrations of 24%, 28%, 35%, 40%, and 50% are available. A theoretically predictable oxygen concentration can be delivered, which is especially advantageous in the management of patients experiencing ventilatory failure.

Dilution masks are in widespread use, but concern is frequently expressed about their accuracy. Manufacturers usually recommend operating oxygen flows, since each unit is designed to maintain a given oxygen/air entrainment ratio to deliver its specified oxygen concentration. Apparently many users are hesitant to deviate from the advised oxygen flows, fearing unpredictable delivered oxygen levels. A short but excellent report of a study of this problem should be reassuring.[249] The oxygen concentration output of several masks of various dilutions was tested at oxygen flows of 1 to 15 $\ell$/min. When operating against no resistance, the predicted oxygen levels were

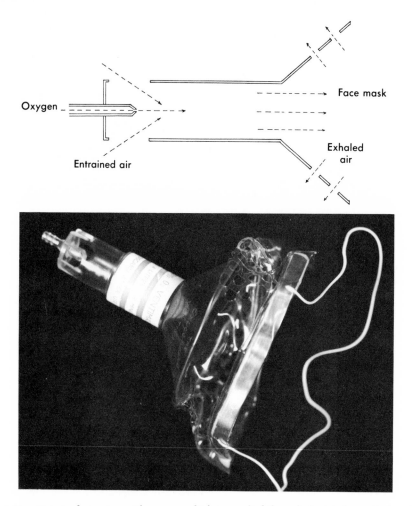

**Fig. 8-14.** Entrained air mixes with oxygen, which is supplied through the jet of a venturi mask. Construction design maintains a constant air/oxygen ratio, ensuring a fixed concentration of inhaled oxygen over a wide range of oxygen flows.

delivered for all masks above a flow of 2 $\ell$/min. Downstream resistance, on the other hand, through its back pressure, impeded air entrainment more than oxygen flow so that increasing flows resulted in the delivery of higher than predicted oxygen concentrations.

The report pointed out an important clinical consideration. It is not enough for us to be concerned only about delivered oxygen concentrations, for we must also be sure that the total airflow, oxygen plus air, is adequate for the patient's ventilatory needs. If total flow is too low, carbon dioxide may build up in the mask of an obtunded patient. If the patient is alert and aware of his total air needs, he will draw in supplementary air through exhalation ports and around the perimeter of the mask, diluting the oxygen he is getting. The important conclusion of the study is that we can give oxygen at flows exceeding those recommended by the manufacturer and not affect the

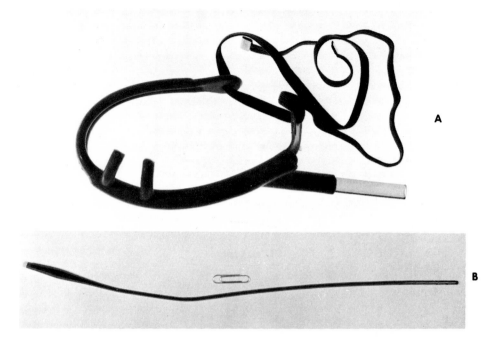

**Fig. 8-15.** **A,** Nasal oxygen cannula. **B,** Oropharyngeal catheter.

delivered oxygen concentration if there is relatively little obstructive back pressure. In the presence of significant obstruction, we should be aware of the risk of increased delivered oxygen concentration, use different masks, if needed, and observe the patient's oxygenation state with exceptional care.

*Cannulas and catheters.* We will discuss these two similar items together, for their general principles of function are the same. Their proper designations are *nasal cannula* and *oropharyngeal catheter*.

The *nasal cannula* (Fig. 8-15, *A*) is a plastic appliance (formerly made of metal) consisting of two tips about ½ inch long arising from an oxygen supply tube and inserting into the nostrils. It is held in place by looping over the ears and snugging under the chin like a lariat. The cannula has the advantages of ease of application, lightness of weight, economy, and disposability. It has the disadvantage of instability, being easily dislodged from a restless or unobservant patient. It is a common experience, while making medical rounds, to note open oxygen flowmeters with cannulas so twisted out of place that the patients could not possibly get any significant therapy. It is also necessary to pay attention to the patient's comfort when instituting treatment, since excessive flows (variable among patients) can produce considerable pain in the frontal sinuses. Finally, such nasal pathology as a deviated septum, mucosal edema, mucus drainage, and polyps may interfere with adequate oxygen intake.

The *oropharyngeal catheter* (most commonly called *nasal catheter*) is so named because it is placed with its tip in the oropharynx (Fig. 8-15, *B*). Made of soft flexible rubber or plastic, the catheter has several holes in its terminal 1 inch. Success in catheter therapy depends on its proper insertion and maintenance, techniques with which every respiratory therapist should be familiar.

Prior to introduction, the distal one third to one half of the catheter is lubricated with either a water-soluble lubricant or a thin layer of petrolatum. The latter is a better and longer lasting lubricant and, if used sparingly, poses little risk of oil aspiration. A low flow of oxygen is started to ensure patency of the tube and its apertures and continued during the insertion. The catheter is gently slid along the floor of either naris into the oropharynx until, in the cooperative patient, direct viewing into the mouth while the tongue is depressed shows the tip of the catheter just below the uvula. It is then retracted out of sight and fastened to the bridge of the nose with adhesive tape. If direct vision is not possible, there are two "blind" procedures that can be used. The catheter can be placed on the side of the patient's face and the distance from the nose to the ear measured off; this length of the catheter is then inserted through the nose into the pharynx. Alternatively, with a moderate oxygen flow, the catheter can be introduced into the pharynx until the patient starts to gulp air and can then be retracted approximately 1 inch and fastened. Under no circumstances must force be used to advance the catheter through the nose, and if significant resistance is encountered, the opposite naris should be used. Nasal disorders as enumerated above may block passage of the tube, and attempts to ram it through will only produce mucosal edema and worsen the condition. There are patients in whom this therapy cannot be used. Catheters should be removed and fresh ones inserted in the opposite nostril at least every 8 hours, since because they are foreign bodies in the nose, nasal secretions will cause them to adhere to the nasal mucosa if they are not changed periodically and their removal is a painful event. Generally, a well-placed catheter is not uncomfortable and allows at least a bit of bed mobility for the patient.

This therapy should be used with some caution in a deeply comatose patient with completely obtunded reflexes and in a patient who is elderly and debilitated, such as in a post-stroke state. With ineffective epiglottal reflexes or epiglottal paralysis, the administered oxygen stream may be directed down the esophagus and seriously distend the stomach. The risk of gastric rupture is real, and distention will further handicap ventilation that is already impaired. After inserting a catheter in such a patient, the therapist should observe and palpate the epigastrium for several minutes to see whether distention develops and, if present, he should remove the catheter and employ some other technique. Finally, because oxygen is delivered as a blast in the pharynx, its desiccating effect on the respiratory tract must be prevented by adequate humidification. For this a good humidifier is safe and effective because it provides good water vaporization with a minimal amount of particulate water to deposit in and obstruct the oxygen tubing.

There has been considerable controversy over the relative merits and efficiency of the nasal cannula versus the oropharyngeal catheter. The issue has been clouded by failure of partisan advocates to apply uniform criteria in evaluating these appliances. Some have studied their performance in healthy subjects, others in patients; some have used the delivered oxygen concentration as a gauge, others have used arterial oxygen tension. Nevertheless, there seems to be enough available data to make at least some valid generalizations. With oxygen flows up to 6 $\ell$/min, concentrations of 40% can probably be achieved with a well-placed nasal cannula; with flows to 8 $\ell$/min, concentrations up to 50% can be delivered by an oropharyngeal catheter. It has been suggested that for the mouth-breathing patient a catheter is preferable to a cannula on the grounds that mouth breathing would dilute the nasal flow of oxygen below a therapeutic level. Studies have shown, however, that the eventual delivery of oxygen to the blood is not significantly different when either a cannula or catheter is used and whether the mouth is open or closed.[248,250] We may conclude therefore that the choice between a cannula and a catheter will rest more on convenience than on significant differences in performance. Both techniques are useful in those instances when low oxygen concentrations are desirable and are thus interchangeable with the venturi mask, described above. There is little doubt that the cannula is more comfortable or less of a nuisance than the catheter, but patient acceptance as a determinant must be weighed against the reliability of each technique. It might be practical to suggest that a cannula be considered for the cooperative and alert patient who can be depended on to keep the appliance in its proper position, and the catheter for the restless or less dependable patient.

*Tents.* In hospitals with modern respiratory care services, the use of oxygen tents has diminished nearly to the vanishing point, with the possible exception of special needs they sometimes meet in pediatric therapy. Nevertheless, because there are significant numbers of them still in operation throughout the United States, it was decided to retain this section and postpone its reduction or deletion to a later edition. The trained therapist should still understand their functions and operations.

There are many styles of tents commercially available, of which two are shown in Fig. 8-16, but we will describe what might be termed a typical unit and emphasize some of the features with which both physicians and therapists should be familiar. The term *oxygen tent* implies an electrically operated, recirculating, canopied appliance

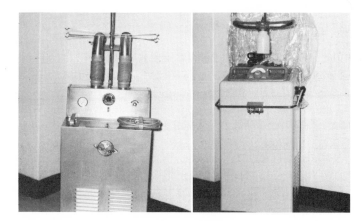

**Fig. 8-16.** Two typical oxygen tents.

designed to provide a patient with an oxygen-enriched, temperature-controlled, humid environment. The mechanism and controls are housed in a console placed by the bedside, attached to which is a plastic canopy enclosing the upper half of the patient's body. A well-maintained and well-operated unit may be expected to provide a canopy atmosphere of no more than 50% oxygen. Because there are far more economical ways of supplying oxygen, the tent is usually employed where oxygen and humidity, or humidity alone, are the therapeutic needs at a comfortable and constant temperature.

With these general indications for tent therapy as a start and before we consider the more technical aspects of treatment, three precautions should be emphasized. First, along with mechanical efficiency of the tent, success of treatment depends on the proper application of the tent to the patient. The key is a tightly fitted canopy. The therapist will learn by experience the best methods of attaching a canopy to the patient's bed so that leaks are kept to a minimum. Unless a maximum seal can be attained between canopy and bed, leaks will negate any therapeutic effect. Maintaining a canopy in its proper operational state can be a problem with a restless or uncooperative patient. Second, and related to the first, is the need to leave the patient and his tent as undisturbed as possible. Every time the canopy is opened for any reason, the enclosed atmosphere is disrupted. An informal rule-of-thumb guide is to reserve the use of a canopy tent for those patients who can be left alone for periods of 3 to 4 hours at a time. If a patient is so ill that medical and nursing attention must be given every 10 or 15 minutes, he will not enjoy the benefits of the tent and will do much better with some other technique of oxygen or humidity administration. Third, if it is ever necessary to operate a canopy tent from cylinder oxygen, the therapist must be sure to have at least two cylinders in manifold and to replace tanks as soon as they are emptied. Should the oxygen supply be depleted, the patient may suffocate in his plastic enclosure.

The canopy atmosphere is recirculated through the console, where excess moisture is removed, and heat exchange keeps it at the desired, thermostatically controlled temperature. The cooling unit is often of the compressor-Freon-12 type, which allows circulation of the canopy air about cooling coils or which itself cools water to circulate through coils in the tent. Removal of carbon dioxide is no problem as long as there is an adequate inflow of oxygen into the tent, since carbon dioxide readily diffuses through the plastic canopy into the atmosphere. All therapists should read the excellent description of gas exchange in oxygen tents by Jahn.[251] Despite the airtightness of a well-placed canopy, there is tremendous escape of gas from the tent. This explains why high-liter flows are required to maintain a steady concentration although no patient ever consumes more than 0.5 $\ell$/min of oxygen. Tent oxygen is lost by displacement of incoming gas at the junction of canopy and bed and around the console and by diffusion of gas molecules through minute leaks. Formulas are available to allow calculation of oxygen flow into canopies of various sizes that will provide specific oxygen concentrations and prevent the accumulation of carbon dioxide above specific limits. For practical purposes this is unnecessary, and with the popular size tents, liter flows of source oxygen of 12 to 15 $\ell$/min will keep oxygen concentration to a maximum and carbon dioxide to a minimum. The initial filling of a canopy requires flushing for several minutes with very high flows until the desired concentration is reached. For safe operation the atmosphere of all tents should be measured with an oximeter every 4 hours. This not only monitors the oxygen concentration but also allows the therapist to check the level in the water overflow pan, to look for signs of mechanical overheating, and in general to assure himself of the operating efficiency.

As noted above, an oxygen tent may often be used primarily for the administration of high humidity, and most units have very effective aerosol generators for this purpose. If oxygen is used to power the aerosol generator, the therapist must remember that back pressure of the nebulizer jet may reduce the liter flow into the tent below the safe value to wash out carbon dioxide. A second oxygen line must be attached to the gas inlet to provide the necessary ventilation. If oxygen therapy is not indicated and the tent's aerosol generator is powered by a compressor, canopy ventilation will also be inadequate unless the compressor is able to deliver 15 $\ell$/min from the nebulizer. With some equipment this may not be possible, and another source of ventilation must be provided. Many tents have an air intake venturi as part of the aerosol generator, and with this open, entrained room air will make up the needed liter flow.

There are many variations of the canopy tent designed for pediatric use. The incubator (Fig. 8-17) is a controlled-environment unit with special provisions for steady elevated temperature and humidity. A special feature of the incubator is an oxygen-limiter, which unless specifically adjusted otherwise, limits the concentration of the oxygen in the unit to a maximum of 40%, as a precaution against the dangers of elevated

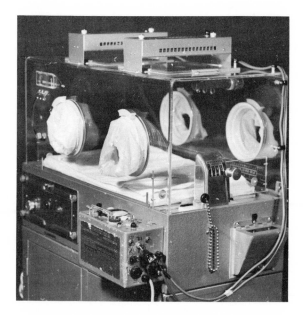

**Fig. 8-17.** Incubator to provide the premature or newborn infant with an environment of controlled oxygen concentration, temperature, and humidity.

oxygen in the newborn or premature infant. Accessories are available to monitor the infant's skin temperature and regulate the incubator accordingly. For the older child the "croup tent" is frequently used (Fig. 8-18). Designed to be used in a crib or small bed, it provides high humidity through a nebulizer powered either by oxygen or by a compressor. Cooling of the unit is by ice, which lowers the temperature not more than 8° F below ambient. A venturi in the aerosol generator circulates the canopy atmosphere through the ice and mixes it with freshly generated aerosol.

Reference was made above to the necessity of frequent measurement of the oxygen concentration of all tents, and it should be obvious that the need is even greater with incubators. The therapist can acquaint himself with the details of testing equipment through information supplied by manufacturers, but a brief résumé of the principles upon which the three most commonly used types depend will be noted at this time. The older chemical analyzers have given way to those that operate on either "thermal conductivity" (commonly called electric analyzers), "paramagnetic susceptibility" (also called physical analyzers), or "galvanic electrochemical sensing" (fuel cell analyzers).

The *electric analyzer* consists of a battery-powered Wheatstone bridge of platinum wires, two arms of which are subjected to the test gas, the other two exposed to air, functioning as references. The instrument is designed only to measure differences in concentrations in a mixture of oxygen and nitrogen and is *not* to be used with any other gas or gas mixture. A physical property of oxygen is its ability to remove heat from a warmed object faster than can nitrogen; so the higher the concentration of oxygen, the cooler will be the object (the platinum wires in this instance). Since the electrical

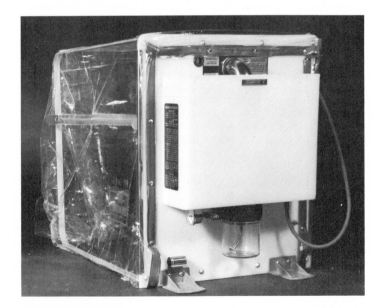

**Fig. 8-18.**  Croup tent, an ice-cooled unit that provides high humidity and aerosolized water, powered either by compressed air or oxygen.

resistance of a wire varies directly with the temperature, the resistance will reflect the oxygen concentration. The instrument is calibrated before use by the drawing of room air into it and balancing the Wheatstone bridge by adjusting the scale to read 21%. The test gas is then entered, and variations in oxygen concentration will upset the balance of the Wheatstone bridge through the effect on electrical conductivity, an event noted by an ammeter whose indicating needle reads out on a scale calibrated in oxygen percent.

The *physical analyzer* uses a small glass dumbbell suspended on a taut quartz fiber in the field of a permanent magnet. In the absence of oxygen, the forces of the torque of the quartz fiber and the magnetic field are equal and in balance. If oxygen is introduced into the system, because of its unique capability among all the gases, of being magnetized, it is drawn into and augments the magnetic field. This upsets the balance, as the torque of the quartz fiber is overcome,and the glass dumbbell rotates in response to the new magnetic force. A small mirror attached to the fiber reflects a beam of battery-powered light onto a translucent scale calibrated to translate motion into oxygen percent. A major advantage of this oximeter is its ability to detect and measure concentrations of oxygen in any mixture of gases, and the instrument can safely be used with flammable and explosive gases.

The *fuel cell analyzer* is an electric cell activated by oxygen, which like a fuel is consumed in the ensuing chemical reaction. The sensor consists of a gold cathode, a lead anode surrounded by an electrolyte bath of potassium hydroxide, a Teflon membrane, and an electrical load resistor. Oxygen diffuses through the Teflon membrane, and its molecules are reduced into hydroxyl ions. The hydroxyl ions react with the lead anode to form lead oxide and release electrons. The electrons flow between anode and cathode, through the resistor, and generate a voltage that varies directly with the number of oxygen molecules undergoing reduction, and thus with the amount of oxygen in the ambient atmosphere. The cell output is calibrated in percentage of oxygen and portrayed as such on a needle gauge or by digital readout. It uses no batteries or electrical power and is safe in an inflammable environment.

A few comments must be made concerning the fire hazard of oxygen tents, a question that the therapist may expect to encounter occasionally. A frequent source of worry is the presence of static electrical sparks often generated by the friction of movements of the patient in bed or by uniforms of personnel rubbing against bed clothing. This subject has been studied in some detail, and the respiratory therapist should be aware of the following data. To start any fire three conditions must be met: flammable material must be present; oxygen must be present; the flammable material must be heated above its flash or igniting temperature and kept there by some external heat or the heat of its own combustion. Thus for any spark to ignite flammable material, the spark must be able to generate enough heat energy to start the process. In relation to the patient in bed, it was determined that the maximum energy capacity was to be found in the ungrounded bed itself (estimated to be less than 100 micromicrofarads); and it was further estimated that the electrical potential of a hospital bed is about 20,000 volts. Theoretically, such a combination could produce a spark some $7/10$ inch long with a maximum energy of 0.02 joule. The likelihood of a casual, random static spark of this magnitude was thought to be very remote. Under conditions of oxygen concentrations varying from 21% to 100%, sparks exceeding this potential were applied to such fabrics as vinyl plastic canopy material, tissue paper, nylon, wool, cotton, muslin, and dacron-cotton. With a barrage of sparks at a frequency of 60 per minute, ignition was achieved with elevated oxygen concentrations, but under no circumstances was a single spark able to produce fire.[252] Further experiments were conducted with fabrics impregnated with petroleum jelly or lanolin, simulating conditions that might be expected in the presence of surgical dressings. Again, even with high concentrations and frequent sparking, few ignitions occurred. The conservative conclusions were drawn that the overall hazard from static sparks with the fabrics in common use, even in high oxygen concentrations, is very low but not nonexistent.[253] The static sparks just do not have sufficient heat energy to raise the material to their flash points. The minimal risk that may be present can be further reduced by maintaining a relative humidity in the tent of 60% or greater.

It should be strongly emphasized that the above refers only to static sparking *not* sparks from electrical equipment such as meters or exposed switches, which are very dangerous. All appliances that transmit house current should be kept out of oxygen tents. The energy of battery-operated current, such as might be found in the many applicances being developed for cardiac support, probably is of too small a magnitude to constitute a risk, especially if well grounded, but the specifications of these appliances should include this information. Recording equipment, such as cardiac monitors, are not hazards, since they pick up only minute physiologic currents and amplify them for inspection outside the high oxygen environment. It is expected that the therapist is fully aware of the precautions to take against the presence of open flames about a tent and the prohibition of smoking in the room with an operating tent. One last note of caution should be made, more for completeness than for anything else. With an attached appliance an oxygen cylinder should be opened slowly to avoid a rush of gas downstream into the appliance. The heat of compression of rapidly flowing oxygen carries the potential risk of elevating to their ignition points such materials as valve seat packing and contaminants in the system. Gradual dissipation of this heat by slow opening of the valve will avoid this hazard.[254]

***Miscellaneous oxygen equipment.*** Although most therapeutic oxygen is administered by the mask, cannula, catheter, and tent techniques described above, there are a few others that deserve mention. The *face tent* is a popular item for short-term use because it is economical and easy to apply. With a plastic enclosure open at the top, the face tent is held by head straps in such a manner that encompasses a space about the chin, mouth, and nose. By means of a simple attachment at the bottom, oxygen flows into the enclosure supplying a reservoir from which the patient can inhale. Exhalation simply diffuses out the open top. At oxygen flows of 6 to 10 $\ell$/min, delivered concentrations up to 45% may be realized. The chief disadvantages of the face tent are, first, the nuisance of the appliance attached to the face and, second, the heat retained about the face by the plastic. The *head tent* is no longer frequently used because of its inherant clumsiness. It consists of a transparent, hard, plastic box without a bottom and with a cutout in one end to fit over the neck. With the patient supine the appliance covers the entire head. An adjustable vent in the top allows the escape of exhaled air, and an inner receptacle is provided for ice. A modification of this principle is available, utilizing a container completely open at the top for the removal of both carbon dioxide and heat, with provisions for adequate continual flushing of the unit by oxygen. Finally, oxygen is frequently given by inspiratory positive-pressure devices, but these will be dealt with later.

## SUMMARY

Because of the wide variety of techniques of administering oxygen, it is obvious that there is no one best method, and although the decision to give oxygen to a patient is a medical one, determined by the physician, it is not always easy for him to know which procedure will be the most effective in a given instance. Clinical observation of the patient, coupled with experience, will often suffice for the physician to initiate treatment, and in the not too distant past these were his only guides. More recently, however, improved technology in both instrumentation and diagnosis have made the therapeutic use of oxygen much more rational and precise.

In our discussion of oxygen equipment, it will be noted that values of oxygen concentration were suggested for each type. Such data certainly have merit, but only in a very general way, for the delivered concentration of gas from any appliance is subjected to many modifying influences such as condition of the equipment, technique of application, cooperation of the patient, and the ventilatory pattern of the patient. It is probably necessary to know only, for example, that the delivery of high oxygen concentrations can best be accomplished by a nonrebreathing mask; intermediate concentrations by a simple mask, tent, or high flows with a cannula or catheter; and low concentrations with cannula, catheter, and venturi mask. It is much more important to recognize that complete relief of hypoxia may be easily achieved by low-flow cannula oxygen in one patient and be impossible by mask therapy in another. Indeed, there may be instances in which, at least for a period of time, full correction of hypoxia may not even be desirable. The point to be grasped here is that the pathology of the disease under treatment is the major determinant of the effectiveness of oxygen administration. Except for short-term therapy such as prophylaxis or for conditions felt to be very transient, safe and rational treatment must depend on the actual measurement of blood oxygenation. At the present time, in view of current techniques, this means the determination of oxygen tension of arterial blood. We have considered the major pathologic and physiologic changes that disease can effect in ventilatory and gas exchange functions of the lung, and it is easy to visualize that there may be little correlation between the fractional concentration of inhaled oxygen and the realization of a normal arterial oxygen content. Unless the initial degree of hypoxia is quantitated by direct measurement and such measurements continued through therapy until stability is reached, treatment can be based on little more than guesswork.

The correction of hypoxia as part of the management of patients with acute or chronic ventilatory failure requires special care because of the disturbance in the acid-base balance. Because of the risk of untoward reactions to oxygen in acute failure, many techniques of oxygen administration have been suggested that are based on the use of low concentrations of oxygen or oxygen with supporting mechanical ventilation. Although the latter is usually required in severe circumstances and will be discussed in detail later, oxygen alone may be indicated. We know the great hazard of hypercapnia if therapeutic oxygen obliterates the hypoxic drive mechanism, and to minimize this risk, the use of cannulas or the venturi mask on continuous or intermittent schedules has had various advocates.[249, 255-257] Similarly, continuous low-flow oxygen in the treatment of chronic hypoxia has received much attention. However, the criteria for the choice of patients for such therapy, as well as an evaluation of its success, are always dependent upon the effective arterial oxygen tensions achieved and the response of the acid-base balance. Thus, after the degree of hypoxia has been determined, the choice of technique may require some trials and errors, guided by blood oxygen levels, with thought given to patient comfort as well as the avoidance of over-oxygenation.

## HELIUM THERAPY

In an earlier chapter, reference was made to the use of helium in the treatment of obstructive disease, and we will now discuss this technique in more detail. Helium is second only to the highly inflammable hydrogen as the lightest of all gases, with an atomic weight of 4.003 and a density of only $0.1785$ g/$\ell$. Limited in supply, the source of most commercial helium is deep mines in the Southwest, produced under control of the federal government. Chemically, it is an inert element, and thus physiologically it neither participates in nor interferes with any biochemical process in the body. It is odorless, tasteless, noncombustible, nonexplosive, poorly soluble, and a good conductor of heat, sound, and electricity.

It is the low-density property of helium that makes the gas a valuable therapeutic tool, and its only medical indication is the management of airway obstruction. We know from previous discussions that turbulence characterizes the gas flow pattern through an obstruction and that in such a circumstance the most influential property of a moving gas is its density. With no technical background, we should be able to perceive that the less dense a gas is the easier it can negotiate an obstruction, but for clarity let us look at the process from two slightly different viewpoints. First, it should be noted that as a flow of gas passes from a relatively wide passage into one that is relatively narrow, if the driving force is constant, the gas velocity must increase to maintain the same volume leaving as entering the restriction. As Bernoulli's principle demonstrates a decrease in pressure with an increase in gas velocity, there is thus a pressure drop across an obstruction. However, since less driving pressure is required to move a light (low-density) gas than a heavy one, at the same velocity there would be less of a pressure drop. In ventilation this would mean greater efficiency and less work expended in breathing. Second, the movement of a gas through the narrow aperture of an obstruction subjects it to some of the principles of diffusion, or the passage of a gas across an obstruction in response to a pressure gradient. In Chapter 4 we learned that the rate of diffusion of a gas follows Graham's law and is inversely proportional to the square root of the density of the gas. Obviously, the speed (or ease) of such movement is greater for low- than for high-density gases.

Currently, helium is the only low-density gas acceptable for medical use, and since it is inert and unable to support life, it cannot be used alone but must always be mixed with oxygen. The therapist should keep in mind that helium has no curative properties of its own, in a pharmacologic sense, and that its sole purpose is to lower the total density of any mixture of which it is a part so that such a mixture can ventilate the lungs with minimal effort. All helium-oxygen mixtures must have at least 20% oxygen to supply basic metabolic needs, and a popular combination is the so-called 80-20 mixture, with 80% helium and 20% oxygen. For practical purposes such a mixture is comparable to air, with helium substituted for nitrogen. A patient breathing 80-20 helium is not being provided with any more oxygen than would be provided by air, but because of the low density of the helium mixture, he is effectively getting more; the helium more readily reaches the alveoli through obstructed passages and thus more oxygen actually is available for diffusion into the blood. For a more specific comparison it should be noted that the density of air is 1.293 g/$\ell$, whereas that of 80-20 helium is 0.429 g/$\ell$. It may be said that with the same effort three times as much of the helium mixture as of air will ventilate the lungs or that the same volume of helium-oxygen ventilation as of air can be moved with one third the effort. In either case the tremendous advantage of a helium mixture is evident to a patient struggling, often to the point of physical exhaustion, to breathe against severely obstructed air-ways. It should be noted that the viscosities of oxygen and helium are almost identical, although both are slightly greater than that of air. The mixing of the two gases therefore does not alter the laminar flow patterns of pure oxygen breathing, and only insignificantly those of air-oxygen mixtures. Table 8-9 lists the densities and relative diffusibilities of air, helium, oxygen, and certain combinations of these and nitrogen, frequently used in therapy.

It is possible to mix pure helium and oxygen at the bedside, but the hazards of error and mechanical failure are so great that it is much safer, as well as more convenient, to use commercially prepared cylinders of premixed gases. In addition to the 80-20 combination, discussed above, another commonly used mixture is a 70-30. This gives an additional quantity of oxygen, often helpful in correcting severe hypoxia associated with obstruction, and although it does so at a slight cost of low density, as noted in Table 8-9, it is probably the most generally useful mixture.

Completely safe to use, helium-oxygen is one of the most valuable therapeutic tools in the treatment of respiratory disorders and should be available in all hospitals caring for pulmonary patients, even though it may be put to only occasional use. For reasons that are not clear, the use of helium-oxygen has not been popular in the past 20 years. I have used it frequently, sometimes with dramatic results, yet I have never encountered a colleague who uses it. In several years I have seen only one report in the literature supporting its use.[259] Helium-oxygen is specifically indicated for the patient with diffuse airway obstruction, especially when due to bronchospasm, as in status asthmaticus, or following instrumentation or other traumatic bronchial irritation. It is also useful in obstruction from extensive secretions, although in this case the

**Table 8-9.** *Densities and relative diffusion rates of selected gases (rate of diffusion varies inversely with square root of density)* [258]

| Gas | Percentage | Density | $\sqrt{Density}$ | Relative diffusibility |
|---|---|---|---|---|
| Helium | 100 | 0.179 | 0.423 | |
| Air | 100 | 1.293 | 1.135 | |
| Oxygen | 100 | 1.429 | 1.182 | |
| Oxygen-nitrogen | 40/60 | 1.321 | 1.105 | |
| Helium-oxygen | 80/20 | 0.429 | 0.655 | |
| Helium-oxygen | 70/30 | 0.554 | 0.745 | |
| $\dfrac{Oxygen}{Air}$ | $\dfrac{100}{100}$ | | $\dfrac{1.135}{1.182}$ | 0.960 |
| $\dfrac{Oxygen\text{-}nitrogen}{Air}$ | $\dfrac{40\text{-}60}{100}$ | | $\dfrac{1.135}{1.105}$ | 1.027 |
| $\dfrac{Helium\text{-}oxygen}{Air}$ | $\dfrac{80\text{-}20}{100}$ | | $\dfrac{1.135}{0.655}$ | 1.743 |
| $\dfrac{Helium\text{-}oxygen}{Oxygen}$ | $\dfrac{80\text{-}20}{100}$ | | $\dfrac{1.182}{0.655}$ | 1.805 |
| $\dfrac{Helium\text{-}oxygen}{Oxygen}$ | $\dfrac{70\text{-}30}{100}$ | | $\dfrac{1.182}{0.745}$ | 1.586 |

major effort should be directed toward airway cleansing. More ordinary therapy is usually employed first, to achieve bronchial patency, and then oxygen administration by conventional techniques next, to combat hypoxia. However, if the obstructive process is unresponsive or the patient is in risk of weakening from fatigue, helium-oxygen should be promptly started before the patient deteriorates to a critical state. There are four points of practical importance to consider in giving helium-oxygen:

1. Helium mixtures must always be given in a tightly closed system because their high diffusibilities will allow them to escape from even small leaks. Tents, catheters, and cannulas are not satisfactory and the gases should be given by a tightly fitted nonrebreathing mask and bag or through cuffed endotracheal or tracheostomy tubes. They are frequently administered to great advantage by inspiratory positive-pressure ventilators.

2. The average hospital gas flowmeter is calibrated for oxygen, and since it depends on the kinetic support of a float by the metered gas, gauge readings will not be accurate for the lighter helium-oxygen mixtures. Special meters, calibrated for the helium mixtures, can be used, but they are not necessary because correction can be made for the scales of the oxygen meters. Table 8-9 shows that an 80-20 helium-oxygen mixture is 1.8 times as diffusible as 100% oxygen, and a 70-30 mixture 1.6 times. This means that for every 10 lmp gas flow recorded on the meter, 18 lmp and 16 lmp, respectively, of the above helium gases would flow. To deliver a desired flow, the flowmeter is adjusted to a reading equal to the desired rate divided by either 1.8 or 1.6, depending

with variable success is their one common factor: they all withhold carbon dioxide and produce some degree of hypercapnia. This is what stops the hiccups. Subjecting the respiratory center to excessive stimulation of hypercapnia supposedly initiates a rhythmic discharge of impulses to the diaphragm so strong that they override the interposed spasmodic contractions and restore a normal cycle. The administration of low concentrations of carbon dioxide usually accomplishes this more quickly and smoothly and in most instances is effective in stopping the hiccups. Sometimes simple mechanical stimulation of the pharynx, with a catheter, will stop the attack through a reflex mediated by way of the vagus nerve. This technique has been used with success by anesthesiologists on patients suffering from postanesthesia hiccups. For some patients combined therapy, including tranquilization, is necessary to bring relief.

Because carbon dioxide, like helium, does not support life, it must be used in combination with oxygen. In addition to its action as an asphyxiant, carbon dioxide produces toxic effects in excess dosage, and it *must be given with great care.* During its administration the therapist must remain in constant attendance and watch the patient closely because there is variation among individuals in their responses to the gas. It is suggested that each department of respiratory care establish its own rules governing the use of carbon dioxide and that these include such items as the following: (1) unless otherwise specified, all treatments will use a mixture no stronger than 5% carbon dioxide and 95% oxygen; (2) no treatment will exceed a period of 10 minutes in duration; (3) if higher concentrations or longer periods of treatment are ordered, a physician must be present. The carbon dioxide mixture should be given with a well-fitted nonrebreathing mask and bag, and the mask should be held to the patient's face by an attendant rather than strapped on so that it can be removed in an instant if necessary.

The potential side effects are many and include headache, dizziness shortly after start of treatment as diastolic blood pressure makes an initial drop, dyspnea, nasal irritation, palpitation, dimming of vision, muscle tremors, paresthesias, sensation of cold, and mental depression. The toxic symptoms indicate serious physiologic injury and should be watched for because they can appear any time after 15 minutes of treatment. Toxicity is manifested by severe dyspnea, nausea and vomiting, disorientation, and a dangerous elevation of blood pressure. When the pressure reaches 200 mm Hg, systolic convulsions and cardiac collapse are apt to occur. It is recommended that carbon dioxide be contraindicated in patients with significant airway obstruction for two reasons. First, it is this type of patient who is most likely to have a less than normally responsive respiratory center and run the risk of hypercapnia. Second, with an active respiratory center the increased work of breathing under carbon dioxide stimulation against obstruction may more than negate any positive value of therapy.

# Chapter 9

# MECHANICAL VENTILATION

It should be emphasized at the start that this chapter is not a technical manual of ventilators, nor is it intended to supplement commercial material supplied by manufacturers of equipment. There is an unquestioned need for a well-composed, comprehensive technical textbook, describing structural and operational details of all commonly used ventilators, with emphasis on preventative maintenance and repair. Our objective is to discuss the basic principles of mechanical ventilation, relating them to patient care; and we will note the characteristics of specific instruments, as needed, to illustrate topics under discussion.

Before discussing the principles and function of mechanical ventilators, we should understand the nature of the conditions for which they are used. Unfortunately, there are several terms used to describe these clinical states, such as pulmonary or respiratory failure, pulmonary or respiratory insufficiency, and ventilatory insufficiency or failure. Lack of clear-cut definitions of and differentiation between these terms has seriously hampered both communication and education in this critical segment of respiratory care. Observation continues to show us that both physicians and therapists often do not grasp the fundamental principles of ventilatory therapy and the limited but specific indications for its use.

To help the student fit mechanical ventilation into the total picture of respiratory care, let us take advantage of our increasing experience and look at this subject from the following viewpoint. Reducing the indications for mechanical ventilation to the simplest terms, we can say that it can be used in those conditions that directly cause either or both of the following.

1. *Alveolar hypoventilation*, through interference with neural control of breathing, neuromusculoskeletal ventilatory performance, or expiratory airway conductance. The characteristics defining this category are *ineffective minute alveolar rinsing, hypercapnia, acidemia*, and *hypoxemia*. The last is often a product of the hypoventilation rather than the primary disease, since an air exchange inadequate for carbon dioxide removal will not satisfy oxygen demands. It might broaden the student's thinking to note, although somewhat irrelevantly at this point, that we are discussing indications, and an indication is not a mandate for therapy, since the decision to treat or not is a matter of professional clinical judgment. There is a wide variety of diseases that can cause hypoventilation, and they may roughly be grouped as follows[261]: (1) alveolar hypoventilation associated with normal lungs—respiratory

centers damaged by disease, trauma, drugs; paralysis of ventilatory muscles from neurologic diseases; thoracic skeletal deformities as from kyphoscoliosis, trauma, and mutilating surgery; (2) diffuse fibrosis or pulmonary granulomatosis—asbestosis, scleroderma, beryllosis, sarcoidosis, recurrent or chronic infections, and healed destructive turberculosis; (3) chronic bronchitis-emphysema—combinations of distention, destruction, expiratory obstruction with air-trapping, and fibrosis.

2. *Shunt hypoxia*, through decreased ventilation/perfusion ratios (physiologic shunting) not corrected by the unassisted breathing of high concentrations of ambient oxygen. In contrast to the hypoxia secondary to hypoventilation, which reflects a reduced oxygen delivery into the respiratory tract, shunt hypoxia implies a normal, or even an above-normal, air supply and adequate ventilatory mechanics, but with some pathologic process preventing an even intrapulmonary distribution of the inspired air. Consequently, the ventilation/perfusion ratios are reduced in some pulmonary units, producing local areas of physiologic veno-arterial shunting. The resulting hypoxia stimulates increased ventilation of unaffected areas, increasing their ventilation/perfusion ratios. However, the additional oxygen uptake of perfusing pulmonary capillary blood is limited more by the oxygen tension in the ventilated alveoli, which is a function of inspired oxygen tension, than it is by the amount of alveolar hyperventilation. In other words, overventilating one alveolus to make up for another that is underventilated does not necessarily compensate for the oxygen deficiency of the latter, but the increased ventilation will remove from the blood large amounts of easily diffusible carbon dioxide. The characteristics of shunt hypoxia, then, are *hyperventilation, hypoxemia, hypocapnia,* and *alkalemia.* It may be found with small airway obstruction (i.e., bronchiolitis), pneumonia, pulmonary edema or congestion, the so-called shock lung syndrome, and loss of surfactant, or any other condition that causes increase in alveolar opening pressures in scattered lung areas.

Two points should be emphasized. First, many patients will have both of the above, and it is thus essential that we watch for elements of each so that we can better judge the need for mechanical ventilation, the time to initiate it, and once started, understand the varying clinical picture that so many of these patients show. Second, although alveolar hypoventilation and shunt hypoxia may present markedly different manifestations, both etiologic and clinical, they have one important common denominator. In both, the basic functional defect is an impaired ventilation, an inadequate or unbalanced movement of air into and out of the pulmonary lobules. In alveolar hypoventilation this deficit is absolute, with low alveolar minute volumes; in shunt hypoxia it is relative because, while the total alveolar airflow may be normal or above, it still fails to satisfy respiratory needs. Thus, in relation to gas exchange needs, there is ventilatory failure in both conditions. In summary, we can simplify terminology by stating that mechanical ventilation is used to support patients suffering from *ventilatory failure,* manifested by *alveolar hypoventilation,* or *shunt hypoxia,* or a combination of the two. These terms will be used in the remainder of the text.

The severity of failure runs the gamut from questionable to rapidly fatal, and the decision to designate such a condition as significant is a responsibility of the attending physician, a task that is not always easy. With the techniques now available to treat this condition, the diagnosis of acute ventilatory failure implies a course of therapy that may be drastic as well as intensive, and yet it is a state that cannot long go un-attended without subjecting the patient to increasing risk. Although, as in most aspects of medicine, there are no hard and fast criteria for judging a patient to be in or approaching a critical level of ventilatory failure, there are guidelines available to the physician, with some of which the respiratory therapist treating this type of patient should be familiar. The fundamental evaluation of the patient is a clinical one, involving the physician's knowledge of the patient's past history, physical findings, and careful observation of the disease progress for signs of a compromised ventilatory system. It is important that the physician determine whether his patient's condition can be reasonably explained on a purely respiratory basis or whether it is also influenced by some metabolic disorder. With this background the physiologic measurements of arterial blood pH and carbon dioxide and oxygen tensions will be meaningful and in most instances decisive in the evaluation. However, even though these laboratory data are objective and accurate in themselves, each physician must interpret them according to his own standards, and although there will be little disagreement with values that are grossly abnormal, those that vary but slightly from normal are often difficult to judge. It has been suggested that acute ventilatory failure is present, and deserving of intensive therapy, if there is clinical evidence for it supported by findings of an *arterial blood pH less than 7.25, arterial blood carbon dioxide tension greater than 55 mm Hg, and/or arterial blood oxygen tension of less than 60 mm Hg.* [262] Such data are more significant if they represent acute changes, and there could be no criticism of using less severe values than these. This matter is being emphasized to underscore the importance of employing both clinical and physiologic evaluation, for treatment, after all, is directed toward a patient and not a laboratory report.

Objectives of the respiratory care of ventilatory failure are thus twofold: (1) the correction of hypoxia and (2) the improvement of alveolar ventilation, with stabilization of acid-base balance. We have discussed the latter in the last chapter and will refer again to oxygen therapy in relation to its role in management of the patient in failure, but our prime attention now will be directed to the correction or compensation of *alveolar hypoventilation,* using mechanical devices to accomplish that which the patient is unable to do for himself. Mechanical support of ventilation ranges from the relatively simple use of a breathing gas driven by positive pressure, on an intermittent basis, to the full maintenance of a helpless apneic patient, and such support is divided into the two descriptive categories of *assisted* and *controlled* ventilation. For our purposes we will define assisted ventilation as mechanically generated airflow that augments the patient's spontaneous, but inadequate, breathing and that is initiated by his own inspiratory effort. Controlled ventilation is mechanically generated airflow delivered according to a predetermined cycling pattern, completely without patient influence. It must be used to support an apneic patient, but the choice of either mode is available to the patient with spontaneous breathing, according to clinical need and circumstance. Assisted ventilation may be administered on a continuous or intermittent basis, but controlled ventilation is usually continuous. Therapeutic details will be discussed below, but it should take little imagination for the therapist to appreciate that controlled ventilation imposes an awesome responsibility upon all members of the managing medical team. Whenever he is given such an assignment, the therapist must always be aware that the patient is completely dependent upon the skill and integrity of the medical attendants and the effective function of the equipment used. It is the responsibility of the patient's physician to judge the clinical status and prescribe therapy, but it is the respiratory therapist's responsibility to see that the therapy is properly and safely instituted, maintained, and monitored. Only those therapists with a sound physiologic background and mature dedicated interest are qualified to participate in this dramatic and rewarding aspect of medical care. Finally, it should be recognized by all members of the medical team that *the performance of a ventilator is no better than the skill of its operator*. The simplest apparatus is safer and more effective in the hands of an expert therapist than the most sophisticated in the hands of an amateur.

## VENTILATORS: CLASSIFICATION AND PRINCIPLES
### Classification

There are many available references describing the origin and development of mechanical ventilators, classifying them according to different criteria, structural and functional.[263-265] Such classifications tend to be based on technical characteristics that are not necessarily clinically oriented, and the continued development of ventilators of increasing complexity, with overlapping principles and features, makes classification difficult. Actually, a rigid classification of equipment is not essential, but some type of grouping according to similar characteristics allows an orderly approach to the study of ventilators and helps to keep in mind the physical features by which they function. We will classify ventilators according to characteristics that are easy to differentiate and that lend themselves to description and illustration using the outline below. Fig. 9-1 pictures several commonly used instruments.

    I. Negative-pressure, time-cycled ventilators
        a. Controller
            (1) Body tank (iron lung) (Drinker)
            (2) Cuirass (Monaghan)
        b. Assistor-controller: cuirass, modified (Emerson)
    II. Positive-pressure ventilators
      A. Volume-cycled (pressure-limited)
        1. Electric
        a. Controller
            (1) Piston, rotary drive, single-circuit (Emerson)
            (2) Piston, rotary drive, double-circuit (Engström)
        b. Assistor-controller
            (1) Piston, linear drive, single-circuit (Bourns)
            (2) Compressor-bellows, double-circuit (Bennett)
        2. Pneumatic, assistor-controller
            (1) Fluidic, double-circuit (Monaghan)
      B. Pressure-cycled, pneumatic, assistor-controller
            (1) Flow-adjustable (Bird)
            (2) Flow-sensitive, time-cycled control (Bennett)

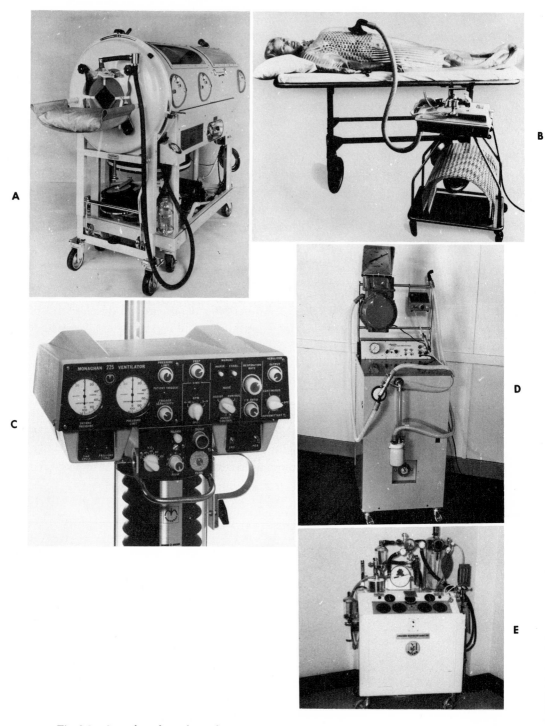

**Fig. 9-1.**　Several mechanical ventilators representing a variety of operating and functional principles, details of which will be discussed in the text. **A,** Drinker. **B,** Emerson cuirass. **C,** Monaghan 225. **D,** Emerson Post-Operative. **E,** Engström. **F,** Bourns. **G,** Bird. **H,** Bennett. **I,** Ohio Critical Care.

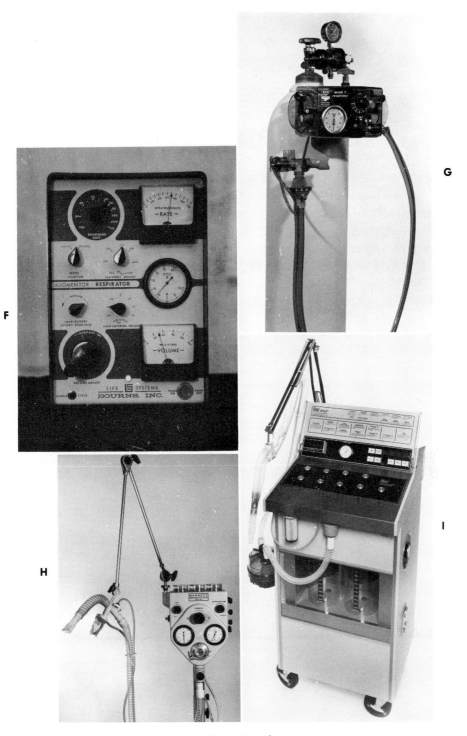

**Fig. 9-1, cont'd.** For legend see opposite page.

It should be noted that some of the ventilators are designated as controllers and others as assistor-controllers. The former are limited only to complete control of the patient's ventilation; if spontaneous respiration is present, it must adjust to the operation of the machine, the machine must be adjusted to it, or the machine may override the patient's voluntary efforts. Assistor-controllers can either assist spontaneous ventilation or control breathing completely, depending on how they are operated. There are appliances that can be classified as only assistors, but in a practical clinical sense they are not considered as true mechanical ventilators, since they are not suited for maintaining the patient in severe failure, and reference will be made to them later in a discussion of inspiratory positive-pressure breathing treatments. The student should also note that the ventilators are divided into two major groups—those classified as negative-pressure ventilators and those as positive-pressure ventilators.

Fig. 9-2 schematically illustrates the basic difference in function of these two types of machines during the inspiratory phase of airflow. The negative-pressure ventilator generates a negative pressure (more precisely, a subatmospheric or gauge-negative pressure), or suction, on the external surface of the thorax, as shown by the arrows in Fig. 9-2, *A*. This negative pressure is transmitted to the interior of the thorax, creating a pressure gradient with the atmosphere, and air flows into the lung. In contrast, the positive-pressure ventilator, using a power source, forces air into the lungs, developing an intrathoracic positive pressure that expands lungs and chest, as depicted in Fig. 9-2, *B*. Perhaps the student will observe that the negative-pressure ventilator is more physiologic in its function than is the positive-pressure, since normal ventilation is the product of negative pressure generated in the thorax by the action of the ventilatory muscles. Reference will be made to this important point later.

Let us make two observations here that may help the student avoid later confusion in terminology. First, by custom, unless otherwise specified, the expression *mechanical ventilator* or *mechanical ventilation*, refers to the use of positive-pressure

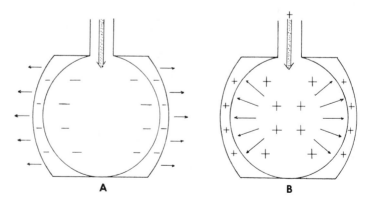

**Fig. 9-2.**   Diagrammatic illustration of the difference between inspiratory forces of, **A,** negative-pressure and, **B,** positive-pressure ventilators.

ventilators. Reasons for this will become apparent in the following description of equipment and techniques of their use. Second, regardless of the differences in their operating principles or machine design, positive-pressure ventilators all deliver breathing gas to the patient with positive pressure during inspiration. They thus provide the patient with *inspiratory positive-pressure breathing* (IPPB). For several years IPPB has been the abbreviation of *intermittent* positive-pressure breathing, but many users believe that the adjective "intermittent" is inadequate, since it does not describe the phase of ventilation during which positive pressure is applied, only that it is not continuous. Use of "inspiratory" has recently been recommended as being more realistic, since it specifically separates inspiratory positive pressure from expiratory, a discrimination of considerable importance.[32] Although the new terminology has no official acceptance yet, in this text inspiratory will replace intermittent in the interpretation of IPPB.

Two additional observations are appropriate regarding IPPB. First, and again by custom and habit, IPPB has a definite connotation, referring in respiratory therapy to a short-term treatment procedure by which a patient is subjected to inspiratory positive pressure, usually for the purpose of aerosol administration. Also, the instrument by which IPPB is given is always a type classified as a pneumatic pressure-cycled assistor, frequently a greatly simplified version. In other words, IPPB therapy is not given by any of the time-cycled or volume-cycled machines listed in the classification above. The topic of IPPB will be discussed in detail separately later in the text. Second, to differentiate between the uses of the ventilation equipment to be described next, the term *IPPB* will be understood to relate to the treatment defined above using the equipment noted. *IPPV* (ventilation or ventilator) will refer to the mechanical support of a patient and/or the equipment used, regardless of type, as long as it delivers an inspiratory positive pressure. While IPPV admittedly is not an official designation and was not included in the terminology recommendations referred to, it enjoys wide general use and is a helpful term.

Attention of the student should be drawn to the three different control modes of ventilators—time cycling, volume cycling, and pressure cycling. It might occur to him that volume cycling, whereby the functioning of an instrument depends upon the delivery of a volume of air to the patient, is the most reasonable, since after all, the act of breathing is designed to bring into the lungs a volume of air adequate to satisfy physiologic needs. In other words, we breathe a volume of air rather than a pressure or time. Perhaps the student can see, however, that whether we talk about pressure, volume, flow (volume per time), or time, we are talking about the same thing. It is somewhat like using any one of several doors to enter a house. Spontaneous ventilation is a summation of the effect of muscular activity (pressure), delivering air at a rapid enough rate, to bring into the lungs the correct volume of air within the time limit set by metabolic demand. A healthy, normally controlled respiratory system is able to integrate all these factors on an instant-to-instant basis to achieve effortless resting gas exchange and to expand this function to accommodate the needs of severe exertion. An appliance that attempts to substitute for the damaged normal mechanism, on the other hand, is limited in its ability to coordinate as efficiently and must confine its operation to one major function. The more sophisticated the apparatus, the better able it is to influence the remaining elements of ventilation. The plain fact of the matter is that there is no "best" mechanical ventilator or else there would not be the large variety now available on the market. Each type or style of machine is an attempt to exploit some facet of physiology that seems to lend itself well to manipulation by a mechanical principle or, conversely, to exploit some mechanical principle that holds promise of better regulating ventilatory physiology. None of them are particularly good, in the sense that they can safely and predictably replace normal breathing; but to the patient in ventilatory failure for whom death is soon inevitable without assistance, they are infinitely better than nothing.

Let us now consider some of the structural and functional features of representative ventilators listed earlier. It is strongly emphasized that the choice of instruments used as a basis for our discussion in no way implies a rejection of competitive models by omission. Those chosen are believed to be such familiar examples of their respective classes that they lend themselves well to description.

**Negative-pressure, time-cycled ventilator.** The exponent of this type of ventilator is the time-honored body tank respirator, known for so long as the "iron lung."* First described in 1929, the tank respirator saw widespread, lifesaving use through many poliomyelitis epidemics.[266] The body respirator is an airtight cylinder that accommodates the patient up to his neck, leaving his head exposed to atmosphere. At the opposite end, or underneath the tank, is a large bellows powered by an electric motor, with a handle for manual operation in the event of electrical failure. Expansion of the bellows creates an intracylinder negative pressure, the magnitude of which is indicated by a pressure gauge calibrated in centimeters of water. Under the influence of the pressure gradient between the interior of the respirator and the atmosphere, air flows into the patient's lungs, and subatmospheric pressures of up to 15 cm $H_2O$ are frequently employed.

This respirator has the advantages of ruggedness and durability and relative ease of operation. However, it has many disadvantages and in most institutions has been replaced by equipment of more recent design. The unit is large and cumbersome, requiring considerable space to compensate not only for its physical size but also for its operational noise. From both nursing and medical viewpoints it makes patient care difficult and awkward. A patient ill enough to require respirator care generally needs much personal attention, and yet he is isolated from his surroundings, accessible only through arm ports in the wall of the tank or by being removed from the machine for hurried care. Monitoring of physiologic functions and the administration of intravenous infusions are done under handicaps. Even more important than these inconveniences is the inflexibility of the tank respirator's function. It is a controller with an adjustable negative pressure that moves the thorax at set, predetermined intervals, with no provisions for the patient to use whatever spontaneous ventilation he may possess. There is no way of controlling or regulating

---

*Drinker-Collins respirator, Warren E. Collins Co., Boston, Mass.

flows—a feature that is less important in ventilating patients with normal lungs, such as those with poliomyelitis (with whom the tank had its initial experience), than it is in ventilating the larger number of patients who are disabled with obstructive pulmonary disease. In the latter, flow control may be critical to successful ventilation. A generalization may be inserted at this point by stating that a patient in ventilatory failure, but with normal airways and lungs (neuromuscular or central nervous system disease), can usually be ventilated adequately with any of the standard ventilators now available. It is the patient with obstructive or restrictive pulmonary disease who presents the greatest maintenance problems. Finally, the negative pressure by which the tank respirator functions can, itself, be a hazard to the patient. The negative pressure is applied not only to the semirigid thorax but also to the much more pliant abdomen and is, accordingly, transmitted to the abdominal cavity. Here it tends to cause the venous blood on its return to the right atrium to pool in the large vascular abdominal reservoirs, with a resulting decrease in venous return and cardiac output. The so-called "tank shock" was not an uncommon complication, as peripheral vascular collapse followed the interference with cardiovascular dynamics. This effect will be dealt with in a little more detail, later in this section, in relation to the physiology of positive-pressure breathing.

In an attempt to retain the benefits of negative-pressure ventilation while minimizing the disadvantages of the large tank respirator, the *cuirass*, a shieldlike appliance, was developed.* Basically, this consists of a rigid shell (available in a number of sizes) with its edges designed to conform to the lateral surfaces of the thorax, base of the neck, and hip-pubic area. From the top of the shell a flexible hose leads to an electric pump. In operation the cuirass functions as does the full body respirator, but the negative pressure is confined only to the thorax, avoiding the undesirable effect upon the abdomen as described above. At the same time, however, it is less efficient than the tank; and with its own inherent deficiencies, it cannot be relied upon to give the support to an apneic patient that is possible with the larger unit. It is frequently difficult to effect the necessary close fit of the shell to the great variety of body contours, and unless it is applied properly, it is undependable. A loose contact between patient and shell not only reduces the available ventilating pressure but can also produce serious chafing of the skin. Like the tank respirator the cuirass is a controller, and it can "assist" only if its cycling pattern can be adjusted exactly to the patient's spontaneous breathing, although this is not true assisted ventilation by our definition. The main use of the chest respirator, as it is commonly called, is to wean a patient from the body tank. This was especially helpful in the treatment of poliomyelitis, since it allowed access to the patient's extremities for the much needed physical therapy of that disease. Many patients with residual, permanent, partial paralysis of the respiratory muscles who could function adequately during their waking hours have used the chest respirator regularly upon retiring to prevent the occurrence of hypoventilation during sleep.

Although use of the cuirass, along with that of the body respirator, has declined

---

*Portable respirator (chest), J. J. Monaghan Co., Denver, Colo.

in recent years, an improvement in design has made available a chest respirator that is an assistor as well as a controller.* Instead of the heavy and rigid chest piece of the original style, the new model uses a lightweight fenestrated plastic shell that sits loosely over the patient's trunk, with no close skin contact. An airtight seal is achieved by a plastic wrapping that encloses the shell and the patient's back and is snugly applied around the legs. A vacuum cleaner–type power unit supplies the negative pressure and can be adjusted for various settings of the control mode. The major feature, however, is a triggering device that permits the patient to initiate the powered inspiratory phase of ventilation at his own rate and to support his own voluntary breathing. An electronic sensor, attached in front of the patient's nostril, responds with high sensitivity to the slight airflow of the start of his spontaneous inspiration and activates the respirator to assist the rest of inspiration.

We can summarize the status of the negative-pressure ventilators by making a few final comments about the group as a whole. Shortly, we will discuss details of the use of *intubation* of the airway in mechanical ventilation, which entails passing a tube through the mouth and larynx into the trachea or through a surgical opening beneath the larynx directly into the trachea. This is a procedure usually necessary for the application of positive-pressure ventilators but is not ordinarily required for negative-pressure ventilators. The ability to ventilate a patient without the need for intubation is certainly an advantage in favor of the negative-pressure machines, but it is an advantage that must be viewed with some reservation. First, patients with chronic bronchopulmonary disease in ventilatory failure need frequent aspiration of secretions, done most effectively through an airway. Second, many patients in failure without pulmonary disease, in whom pathologic secretions are not a problem, may have paralyzed or obtunded epiglottal reflexes, and normal oral secretions may pool in the mouth or hypopharynx. In such instances the strong inspiratory suction of a negative-pressure ventilator may draw these fluids into the bronchial tree, with resulting atelectasis or pulmonary infection. Intubation is usually necessary to prevent such complications.

In addition to the problems of size and patient isolation posed by the negative-pressure machines, the much greater versatility of the positive-pressure generators, which have developed in recent years, has placed these machines in the foreground of the therapy of ventilatory failure. The original indication for the big tanks was the large number of patients with bulbar, or respiratory paralytic, poliomyelitis, but effective prophylactic medicine has reduced the incidence of this disease to a negligible quantity. At the same time there has been a steady increase in the number of patients with failure due to airway obstructive disease, and in this group the negative-pressure ventilators are generally less effective than the positive. Nonetheless, because there are some patients who can benefit from the use of negative-pressure support of their ventilation, and especially if the avoidance of intubation is felt to be advisable for some valid reason, ventilators of this group should be available in hospitals with a heavy load of respiratory care patients.

---

*U-Cyclit chest respirator, J. H. Emerson Co., Cambridge, Mass.

***Positive-pressure, volume-cycled, electric controller ventilator.*** Ventilators in the positive-pressure, volume-cycled class that are electrically operated depend on a motor-driven piston to deliver a predetermined volume of air from a cylinder. Volume, rather than time, is the cycling monitor, with pressure, as in the time-cycled machines, exerting a limiting effect beyond an established safety level. Adjustable gearing allows changing the travel distance of the piston to vary the volume of air displaced from the cylinder, and this constitutes the tidal volume delivered to the patient.

This type of ventilator is powered by a wheel-and-piston mechanism that might be called a rotary drive. The electric motor turns a wheel to which is attached a connecting rod, which in turn is attached to the shaft of the piston. Such an arrangement produces forward movement of the piston that can be plotted graphically as a so-called *sine curve*. The student, in reading the literature and advertising media, will frequently encounter reference to a sine curve pattern and certain benefits attributed to it. Although the importance of this phenomenon in the daily practical application of mechanical ventilation is probably overemphasized, the sine curve pattern is at least of academic interest as a characteristic of one type of ventilator; thus the student should understand its meaning and the influence it may have in therapy. Without straying too far afield, we can describe a sine curve, which is a trigonometric term,

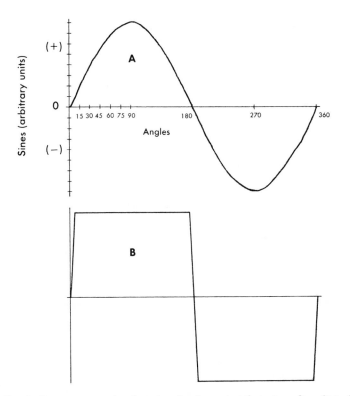

**Fig. 9-3.** **A,** Sketch of a *sine wave*, a plot of a series of angles against their sine values. Note that for angles greater than 180 and less than 360 degrees the curve is negative. **B,** Contrasts a "square wave" with the sine. (See text for significance of these graphs.)

as a graph obtained when one plots the sine values of a series of angles against the angles. A complete sine curve results from recording the values of a full circle of angles, and it has the configuration shown in Fig. 9-3, *A*, an undulating, reciprocal curve with equal positive and negative components above and below a base line. The sine curve is a natural function in that it occurs in many natural phenomena, where it is given the name of periodic or harmonic motion, and it is characteristic of the behavior of alternating electrical current, the vibration of a stretched string, and the movements of electrons within atoms.

The relevance of the sine wave to ventilation may come into focus if we recognize that, as a given point travels around a circle, at any instant its position represents an angle to the center of the circle, for which there is a corresponding sine value. Thus its circular route can be plotted as the sine wave of an infinite number of angles. Let us now consider Fig. 9-6, which schematically represents a wheel driving a piston (not shown), ignoring the legend, which pertains to a later topic. Half the circumference of the wheel is marked off in eighteen equal arbitrary units of time ($t_0$, $t_1$, $t_2$, etc.), indicating uniform velocity of the wheel; the time markers are projected by dashed lines onto the horizontal diameter of the wheel. A connecting rod, from wheel to piston shaft, is attached to the wheel at point $A$, which corresponds to a time marker, and the diameter of the wheel is divided into ten equal arbitrary units of horizontal travel of point $A$, also the travel of the piston. With the wheel turning at a fixed rate, the forward velocity (distance per time) of point $A$, and the piston gradually increases from its starting position at distance *0*, and time point $t_0$, to a maximum at distance *5*, and time $t_9$, one quarter of a turn, or 90 degrees of travel. Beyond this the velocities of point $A$ and the piston decrease to zero again at distance *10*. This increase and decrease of velocity is shown by the relative numbers of distance intervals per time markers on the horizontal scale. At both ends there is only a fraction of a distance unit per time, whereas in the center there is almost a one-to-one ratio. In the piston ventilator the forward motion, delivering a tidal volume, represents the inspiratory phase. Obviously, the distance-time relationships will be the same during the exhalation phase return of the piston to its starting point, but since this half of the cycle does not involve airflow to the patient, we need not consider it at this time.

It is evident that the forward travel of the piston, represented in Fig. 9-6 by point $A$, conforms to the first or upright half of the full sine curve shown in Fig. 9-3, *A*. This is what is meant by the sine wave characteristics of this type of volume-cycled piston ventilator. The significance of the sine wave is related to its effects on the kinetics of inspiratory airflow. Because the piston gradually picks up speed in its forward motion during the first half of inspiration (90 degrees of travel) then progressively slows down, the gas it delivers into the patient's airways must follow the same pattern. Therefore, from a point of no airflow prior to inhalation, the velocity of the breathing gas increases to midinspiration, then decreases to zero at end-inspiration. The slowly increasing airflow, with its minimal turbulent effect, theoretically is better able to overcome the initial inertia of the lung-thorax system and the resistance of decompressed bronchi than if the flow were of sudden high velocity, following a pattern like that of Fig. 9-3, *B*. The sine wave pattern facilitates maximum flow at midinspiration, when the bronchial tree is best able to accommodate it, and finally, toward the end of inspiration, the slowing flow supposedly enhances an even distribution of gas among the alveoli.

Two ventilators of this category will be described—one employing a single gas circuit and the other a double circuit.

*Single-circuit (Emerson\*).* This ventilator is relatively simple in its construction, durable, and easy to use. The essentials of its circuitry are diagrammed in Fig. 9-4. The electric motor acts through a belt to turn a large wheel, shown as dashed lines, but the basic parts directly concerned with air delivery are solidly sketched. The piston drive wheel *(1)* is eccentrically contoured and attached to the hub of the large wheel. It moves the piston *(2)* through the action of a connecting rod *(3)* that is fixed to a pivoting arm *(4)*. The piston rod *(5)* attaches to the pivoting arm by a screw-

---

\*Post-Operative ventilator, J. H. Emerson Co., Cambridge, Mass.

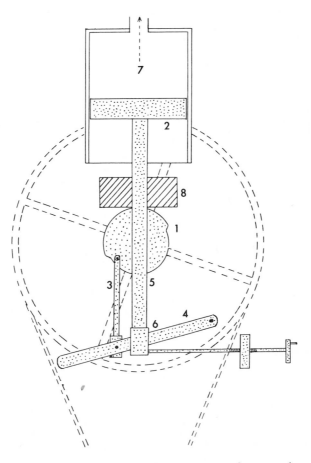

**Fig. 9-4.** Positive-pressure, volume-cycled, single-circuit, rotary-drive ventilator. (See text for description.)

adjusted slide block *(6)*. It can be seen that the position of the slide block in relation to the pivot point of the arm will determine the extent of the vertical travel of the piston and thus the amount of air delivered from the cylinder *(7)* per stroke. Air intake into the cylinder is not shown, but because the power of the machine is exerted directly on the breathing gas going to the patient, this apparatus is designated as a single-circuit unit.

Phasing of the ventilatory cycle is possible through independent controls of inspiratory and expiratory times, activated by a special switching mechanism *(8)* and the eccentric drive wheel. Through a mechanical sensor the wide arc of the wheel triggers the inspiratory cycle, and the narrow arc the expiratory cycle, the timing of both of which can be adjusted by the operator. Humidification, automatic deep sighing, excessive pressure release, and the addition of oxygen are all provided for. Although the screw mechanism that sets the piston to deliver a desired tidal volume has a calibrated scale, the volume must be measured by one of several meters available for this purpose. The measurement of exhaled air is usually accurate enough for clinical purposes and eliminates the need to account for the effect of gas compression in the system. As the student considers the function of this ventilator, he may begin to understand why it is difficult to formulate a hard-and-fast classification of ventilators. Although it is designated as a volume-cycled machine, timing through phasing control, certainly plays a role in its function.

*Double-circuit (Engström\*).* Much more complex than the Emerson ventilator just described, the double-circuit, time-cycled piston machine embodies the same principles but utilizes them in a more elaborate manner. By its designation, the Engström has separate pneumatic circuits for power and ventilation. A motor-driven piston moves back and forth in a cylinder, alternately creating positive and negative pressure. The cylinder is connected to a large transparent pressure chamber in which is suspended a breathing bag. When negative pressure is generated in the power cylinder, it is transmitted to the chamber and air flows into the suspended bag, which is valved to the atmosphere. During the positive-pressure cycle, pressure transmitted to the chamber empties the breathing bag into the patient circuit. Fig. 9-5 illustrates the general relationships and function of the two circuits and needs little further explanation. Not indicated in the sketch is the safety water lock and the rest of the valve control system, including the manner in which oxygen or anesthetic gases can be added to the breathing mixture. A feature of this instrument not found in its single-circuit counterpart is a mechanism for creating a negative pressure in the patient's airways if desired, the physiologic and clinical indications for which will be discussed in detail later. Suffice to point out here that the intake-output port of the power cylinder can be used to activate a venturi in the patient's exhalation line and drop the pressure in the respiratory tract to subatmospheric.

One of the major characteristics of the Engström ventilator is the pattern by which its flow is delivered to the patient, and to describe it, we will refer to Fig. 9-6. The ventilator has a fixed inspiratory/expiratory ratio of 1:2, which means that one third

---

\*Engström respirator, LKB Instruments, Inc., Rockville, Md.

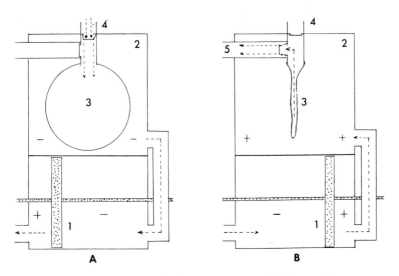

**Fig. 9-5.** Positive-pressure, volume-cycled, double-circuit, rotary-drive ventilator. **A,** During expiration, travel of the piston, *1,* to the left creates subatmospheric pressure in the chamber, *2,* filling the breathing bag, *3,* with air through the intake valve, *4,* in preparation for the next inhalation. **B,** During inspiration, travel of the piston to the right pressurizes the chamber, driving air from the breathing bag into the patient circuit, *5.*

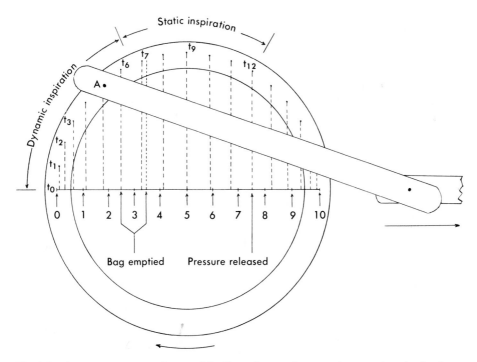

**Fig. 9-6.** Some inspiratory mechanics of the Engström ventilator are shown in this wheel and piston–drive shaft sketch. Half the circumference of the wheel is marked off in equal *time units,* and the diameter of the wheel is divided into 10 *distant units* of forward travel of point A. With a fixed I/E ratio of 1:2, inspiration must be complete when point A reaches time marker $t_{12}$. (See text for detailed description.)

the total ventilatory cycle is used for inspiration and two thirds for exhalation, regardless of the minute breathing rate. A range of frequencies is available from 10 to 30 per minute, and once a given rate is chosen, the predetermined tidal volume is delivered according to the machine's specifications. To maintain its inspiratory/expiratory ratio of 1:2, the ventilator must complete its inspiratory function by the time point $A$ reaches time marker $t_{12}$, for this represents one third the full cycle. Inspiration is thus completed by the time the piston has reached three fourths its forward stroke distance, for time $t_{12}$ corresponds to 7.5 distance units of a total of 10. Under conditions of normal lung-thorax compliance and minimal airway resistance, the tidal volume in the breathing bag will empty into the patient circuit while pressure is still developing in the pressure chamber, somewhere between 0.5 and 0.6 of the allotted inspiratory time, or between time markers $t_6$ and $t_{7.2}$. At the three-quarter point in the piston stroke, a valve in the piston opens to release cylinder pressure and prevent further generation of pressure, and the piston completes its forward travel. Two interesting features should be noted. First, the tidal volume (*patient* inspiration) has been delivered to the patient before *machine* inspiration is finished and while the power unit is still exerting pressure in the chamber containing the breathing bag. Second, expiration begins while the piston is still in forward motion. Obviously, the remainder of exhalation occurs during the return of the piston to its starting position.

There is an advantage to the Engström's pressure-airflow relationship, and it revolves about the slight time lag between the emptying of the breathing bag into the patient's airway and the termination of mechanical inspiration. In the normal respiratory tract the continued pressure in the breathing bag chamber helps to effect the maximum distribution of the inspired gas among the alveoli. In a sense the tidal volume is rapidly delivered to the airways by the pressure of early inspiration and then evenly dispersed throughout the lung by the steady pressure of the few moments until the piston releases its force. In the event of a drop in compliance of the lung or an increase in resistance, this same interval is a reserve period during which the continued generated pressure can ensure maximum delivery of the tidal volume. The manufacturer of this ventilator refers to the initial part of inspiration as the *dynamic inspiratory period* and to the last part as the *static pressure period.*

As soon as the power cylinder pressure drops, at one third the cycle, exhalation begins even though the piston is still completing its stroke. This interval comprises what is called *passive exhalation,* and the time of reverse travel of the piston the *negative phase.* During the former, pressures in the circuits are falling toward atmospheric, and no extraordinary influences act upon exhalation, but while the piston is reversing its position, the negative pressure is available.

Like the Emerson ventilator, the Engström is a controller only. At certain times in the cycle the patient may be able to take a spontaneous breath from the reservoir bag, but this does not constitute any sustained effort toward independent breathing. Pressures are adjustable up to 70 cm $H_2O$, and there are nomograms available to assist in selecting the proper air volumes for both adults and children. The gas compression effect is taken into consideration in such calculations.

**Positive-pressure, volume-cycled, electric, assistor-controller.** There are two types of instruments that fit this category, but they differ so in their construction, operation, and indications that little can be said for their common features except they are volume ventilators and are able to assist as well as control ventilation. It is this latter function that differentiates them from the two described above.

*Piston, linear-drive, single-circuit (Bourns\*).* This ventilator is designed only for the premature or term infant and has a maximum stroke tidal volume of 150 ml. A single-circuit device, the instrument is powered by an electrically operated piston-cylinder unit, utilizing a mechanism very different from that of the other piston machines. The Bourns ventilator has a linear rather than a rotary drive, schematically illustrated in Fig. 9-7. The drive wheel *(1)* oscillates back and forth and moves the piston drive shaft *(2)* in a similar fashion through a transmission gear *(3)*. The travel of the drive wheel thus determines the delivered tidal volume. The actual operation of the mechanism is governed by elaborate electronic circuitry through an electromagnetic clutch that has almost instantaneous response. Supplied with the ventilator is a specially designed criblike holder to confine the infant and yet leave him accessible to general care and even permit him to be maintained in an incubator. The patient is most easily connected to the breathing tubes by means of a custom-molded nasal mask[246] or through nasotracheal intubation.

For controlled ventilation the respirator has adjustments for rate, flow per stroke (in milliliters per second), periodic sighing, and stroke volume. The inspiratory/expiratory ratio can be varied and is set by means of selection of the proper flow. The principle involves, first, determination of the tidal volume and minute breathing frequency desired and second, adjustment of the milliliter per second flow that will deliver the tidal volume in that fraction of the ventilatory cycle allotted to inspiration. The machine, in delivering the calculated flow, automatically conforms to the predetermined inspiratory time. For example, if it is desired to deliver a tidal volume of 25 ml at a frequency of 50 per minute and to limit inspiration to 30% of the ventilatory

---

\*Augmentor-respirator (infant), Bourns, Inc., Ames, Iowa.

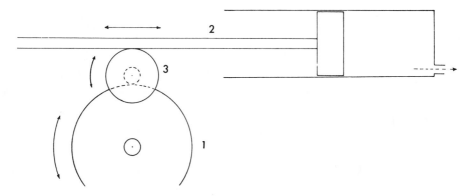

**Fig. 9-7.** Simplified sketch of the drive mechanism of the Bourns respirator, showing the linear travel of the piston. (See text for details.)

cycle, a flow of approximately 69 ml/sec is the only rate that can satisfy these conditions. To avoid the necessity of making this calculation every time the instrument is set up, the manufacturer provides a nomogram to give the required information quickly and accurately. At the same time, compensation must be made for the gas compression effect, since this is a critical value in the small tidal volumes used in infant ventilation.

For use as an assistor, the Bourns respirator has a variable resistance to activation of the machine. For the very weak patient only a small negative pressure at the start of inspiration will trigger the ventilator, and this can be increased whenever desired to aid the patient in his development of strong inspiratory effort in preparation for termination of assistance. The instrument will automatically take over ventilation if the rate falls below 60% of the established rate, for a period of 12 seconds, and an alarm will indicate this change in pattern.

*Compressor-bellows, double-circuit (Bennett\*).* One of the most comprehensive of ventilators, the MA-1 unit delivers a determined volume with pressure variable, but with pressure limits available as safety and warning devices. The instrument is compact with a large number of control dials, switches, and signals conveniently mounted on a panel. It is supplied with an adjustable heated humidifier, a monitoring spirometer, and an optional negative-pressure venturi. In addition to the usual controls governing tidal volume and minute breathing frequency, the MA-1 unit has adjustable maximal pressure limits up to 60 cm of water, maximum flows from 10 to 100 $\ell$/min, oxygen concentrations of five levels from 21% to 100%, artificial sigh with rate, pressure limit, and volume control, and expiratory resistance. There is also a mechanism to provide positive end-expiratory pressure (PEEP) controlled by a rate board that permits a ventilator frequency down to 1 cycle every 2½ minutes. Use of this appliance will be discussed under management of patients in ventilatory failure in Chapter 10. The ventilator is powered by the action of a compressor on a bellows, creating a double circuit.

There are other ventilators such as the Ohio Critical Care Ventilator,† similar in function to the MA-1, but differing in competitive details. This class of machine operates on the basic principle shown as simply as possible in Fig. 9-8. Power-circuit air, driven by a compressor or turbine *(A)* passes through a one-way valve *(B)* into an airtight chamber (usually a cylinder), which contains a bellows *(C)*. The bellows has valved ports *(D* and *E)* for inflow and outflow of the patient-circuit breathing gas. At the bottom of the bellows chamber is a balloon-type dump-valve *(F)*, which vents the chamber to atmosphere *(G)*. During inspiration, compressed air collapses the bellows upward, forcing air into the patient, and some of it inflates the balloon valve *F*. During exhalation, valve *E* closes; the bellows, which is weighted at its bottom, descends, and breathing gas flows into it. At the same time a valve, not shown, diverts the power gas to atmosphere, and the balloon valve *F* deflates, allowing the escape of cylinder gas as the bellows drops.

---

\*Respiration unit MA-1, Bennett Respiration Products, Inc., Santa Monica, Calif.
†Critical Care Ventilator, Ohio Medical Products, Division of Airco, Inc., Madison, Wisc.

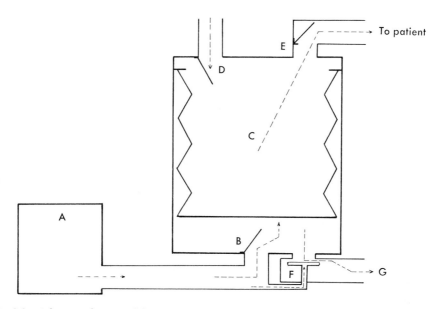

**Fig. 9-8.** Schematic drawing of the major elements of an electric, compressor-bellows, double-circuit, volume-cycled, assistor-controller ventilator. (See text for explanation of letter keys.)

When the MA-1 unit is used as a controller, inspiration is initiated by a timer and is volume limited at end-inspiration unless a preset pressure limit is reached first. Two techniques are available in the adjustment of pressure limits. In the first method, once the observed pressure in the system has been noted, the pressure limit may be set just above this value so that changes in the patient's respiratory system that might produce an increase in pressure will limit the delivered volume and indicate the change by activating a pressure limit signal. This is an effective means of monitoring ventilation. The second method involves setting the pressure limit to the highest range believed to be safe and then letting the ventilator deliver its volume unrestricted, according to changes in patient compliance and resistance. In a manner somewhat similar to the Bourns respirator, the flow of the MA-1 unit governs the inspiratory/expiratory ratio. With a predetermined volume to be delivered under conditions of a fixed frequency, the machine needs enough flow to accomplish its purpose. Guides are available from the manufacturer to initiate ventilation, but adjustments may be necessary as conditions change in the airways., Under any circumstance, should the time of inspiration exceed one half a controlled cycle, a warning light comes on and indicates the need to increase flow. This assures that an inspiratory/expiratory ratio will never be greater than 1.0. By adjusting the flow and carefully timing the ventilatory cycle, the operator can obtain a wide variety of ratios. In addition to negative pressure during exhalation, positive pressure is also available. Other ventilators often use a cap over the exhalation port, but the MA-1 ventilator introduces expiratory resistance by an adjustable control dial. The clinical use of the seeming paradox of resistance to exhalation will be detailed later.

This ventilator is easily used as an assistor. A patient-sensitivity control permits a wide range of inspiratory effort to initiate inspiration, but care must be taken to ensure an adequate flow for the needs of spontaneous breathing. For the patient with uncertain breathing patterns or who may be subject to fatigue and hypoventilation, the rate control of the instrument may be set to a limit lower than his own, and in the event of failure of spontaneous effort, the ventilator will support him.

***Positive-pressure, volume-cycled, pneumatic, assistor-controller ventilator.*** In their general delivery of breathing gas, ventilators of this group, exemplified by the Monaghan 225\* and the Ohio 550† ventilators, are similar to the machines just described. They operate with pressurized bellows, as illustrated in Fig. 9-8, and the only reason for noting them separately is to describe their internal gas control mechanism, which is so drastically different from any others. These instruments are often referred to as fluidic, or fluid-controlled ventilators, because they take advantage of some interesting and useful principles of gas flow that are part of the technology of fluidics. We will confine ourselves to the barest description of fluidics, and encourage those interested to follow with independent study.

Whereas most ventilators have numerous valves for the regulation of gas flow, the fluidic machine is noted for the paucity of its moving parts. The functional elements are known as fluidic devices, or fluid logic units, and operate only on pressurized gas, with no need for electrical power. The heart of the machine consists of channels with power jets through which gas flows, all comprising an integrated circuit. The inter-

---

\*Monaghan 225 respirator, Monaghan Co., Division of Sandoz, Inc., Littleton, Colo.
†Model 550 Ventilator, Ohio Medical Products, Division of Airco, Inc., Madison, Wisc.

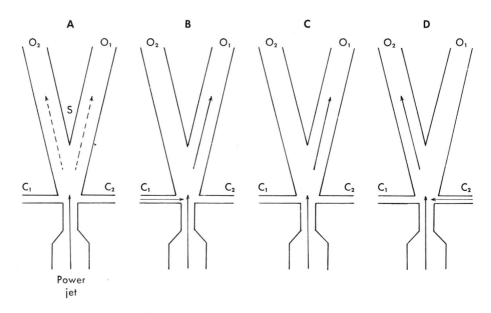

**Fig. 9-9.**   Bistable fluidic device, or a "flip-flop." (See text for description.)

actions among the streams of gas determine such factors as volumes delivered, timed increments of ventilation, pressures, entrainment, and many others. To avoid becoming more involved than is justified in technical and design details, we will describe two commonly used fluidic devices and let the student imagine how their seemingly simple functions might be expanded to perform many tasks.

Fig. 9-9 illustrates the principle of a bistable fluidic device, which is also known as a "flip-flop." The unit consists of a power jet nozzle that carries a stream of gas into a channel, which quickly bifurcates into output ports, $O_1$ and $O_2$. The ports are separated by a wedged partition, $S$, called a splitter. The exact configuration of the splitter and its distance from the nozzle are important engineering factors in determining the behavior of the gas flow. At the end of the nozzle, two control ports $C_1$ and $C_2$, enter the system, each smaller than the power supply channel or output tracts. Fig. 9-9, $A$, demonstrates the first important characteristic of a bistable device. Power gas entering the system can flow to *either* $O_1$ or $O_2$, as shown by the dashed arrows. Depending on the splitter design, some gas may go to both output ports. However, when a control port is activated, as in Fig. 9-9, $B$, by introducing through $C_1$ a flow of gas referred to as a signal, the power stream is diverted to $O_1$, if not already there. The second major characteristic of the device is shown in Fig. 9-9, $C$ and $D$. When the control $C_1$ signal stops, flow is continuous through $O_1$. It is considered stable in this pattern and will remain fixed until a signal from $C_2$ literally pushes the gas to $O_2$, where it will stay even after the signal ceases, until diverted again by $C_1$. The stream can thus be stable in either output port and thereby gains its designation of bistable. A third feature, although not limited to the flip-flop, is the mechanical work advantage realized when a small control signal gas flow can manipulate a larger main gas flow. Considerable power amplification is possible with several units in series, using the output of one as the control signal of another. Perhaps the student can also see how the bistable device can operate as a feedback unit, with downstream back pressures, for example, introduced as control signals to switch gas flow from one operation to another. In the ventilator the main valve is a flip-flop, with ventilation times, volume, patient triggering effort, and other functions modifying outflow through multiple integrated control signals.

In contrast, the monostable device of Fig. 9-10 is stable in only one position. Certain design features, shown in the illustration as a curvature in the lateral wall of the output port, $O_2$, but which might be a different location of the splitter or an angulation of the power nozzle, will cause the outflow always to follow one path unless diverted by a control signal. In Fig. 9-10, $A$, the gas stream automatically follows $O_2$ until a signal from the control port, $C_1$, diverts and holds it in $O_1$. When the control signal stops, the gas reverts to $O_2$. This simple design can be made more complex by the addition of other input controls, but it is very useful for on and off functions, such as the operation of an exhalation valve or of a breathing-phased nebulizer or the cycling of inspiratory positive-pressure breathing machines, which will be discussed later.

The student must understand that the use of fluidic mechanics in ventilators is a peripheral aspect of the technology. Fluidic devices can be integrated to function as computers, power amplifiers, and metering instruments, to name a few. About a

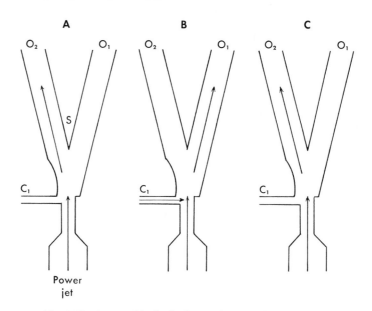

**Fig. 9-10.**  Monostable fluidic device. (See text for description.)

decade ago it was believed that fluidics would find a host of applications in industry and science, but the field was greatly overshadowed by the dominance of electronics. Yet fluidic units are comparatively easy and less expensive to make than electronic components; they have no intricate wiring and almost no moving parts. It would still seem as though this should be a productive area for continued research in respiratory therapy instrumentation.

*Positive-pressure, pressure-cycled pneumatic assistor-controller ventilator.* Ventilators in this classification, by virtue of their great versatility and wide usefulness, have become some of the most important instruments of the respiratory therapist. We will discuss suitable representatives of this group in greater detail than we have devoted to other types, not only because of their clinical importance but also because they so readily permit a review of certain critical ventilatory relationships and principles. This does not mean that they are the best ventilators for all patients, but they do have the most widespread applicability of all ventilating instruments in the general care of respiratory diseases. For our purposes in this section, we are interested in the use of these machines as true ventilators and will refer to them as *inspiratory positive-pressure ventilators* (IPPV); a little later we will cover other uses of these same units under the title of IPPB. With this specification, we will limit our discussion to only two ventilators as examples of the group, since both are very popular and in widespread use and there are significant and interesting differences in their functions.

There is no need to recapitulate the development of positive-pressure breathing, for there are some excellent reviews in the literature with extensive bibliographies, and the student is encouraged to study the background of this form of therapy in which he is expected to be an expert.[267] We have already described several ventilators, classified as positive pressure in nature, but as with many expressions in common use, the term *inspiratory positive pressure* connotes a certain type of mechanism. The IPPV and IPPB units are pneumatically powered, completely independent of any electrical current, and have a minimum of moving parts, most of which are valves. They are driven by gas pressure of 50 psig, the source of which can be a cylinder, central supply, or a compressor. In addition to a certain safety factor, the lack of need for electrical power affords considerable mobility, and the simpler mechanical structure facilitates maintenance and repair. Finally, the pneumatic positive-pressure ventilators are conveniently smaller and more compact than the electrically operated machines. These features are not necessarily determinants in themselves for the choice of a ventilator or for the evaluation of the performance of any of them, but they are practical considerations in the management and operation of a busy respiratory therapy department, especially when it is noted that the pneumatic machines are less costly than the other types.

The IPPV reduces the source pressure to a selected predetermined level, averaging between 10 and 30 cm of water, and delivers the breathing gas until equilibrium is established between the patient's lungs and the ventilator. End-inspiration and thus cycling of this ventilator are primarily dependent on a pressure buildup in the lung rather than on time or volume, although both time and volume exert influence under certain circumstances. The valving mechanism shuts off the gas flow when pressure balance is reached, and passive exhalation ensues. Whereas the volume-cycled machines deliver a volume at whatever pressure is needed to move it, the pressure-cycled instruments deliver a pressure that will produce a desired volume change. To express this in a somewhat oversimplified manner, we might say that, since every respiratory tract has characteristics that require a certain relationship between volume and pressure (compliance) to move air, theoretically it makes no difference which of the two factors determines end-inspiration; the other will follow accordingly. Based on this premise, the original pressure-cycled instruments were very simple, and pressure generation was directly dependent upon the flow of gas introduced into the apparatus from the source pressure. With his background in the physics of airflow, the student should now realize that such a direct relationship between flow and pressure cannot be satisfactory because of the pressure effect of increasing flow through a tubular conducting system—an effect that becomes increasingly important and influential in the presence of obstruction. Therefore the theoretical consideration mentioned above is not valid for real situations, and unrestrained flow-generated pressures cannot be depended upon to give us the resulting volume changes we wish. It is obvious that the factor of flow is an important one in the effective use of pressure-cycled ventilators, and to relate pressure and volume for the purpose of safe ventilation, flow control is a necessity. The IPPV units now suited for ventilation provide for this important factor but differ in the principle employed, a subject we will cover in our description of the two major machines.

Before pursuing the technical details further, we should make a point of practical importance. It is the nature of people to be impressed with size and apparent complexity of machinery and instruments, a characteristic that poses a frequent problem with the use of the IPPV. These units are relatively small, make little noise in operation, and to the uninitiated eye give the appearance of simplicity. As a result, many members of the hospital staff consider themselves qualified to operate the ventilators, with no more preparation than a brief orientation demonstration, perhaps supplemented by a review of the instrument's instructional brochure. Ignorance of the principles and mechanics of the IPPV has given many a distorted or downright erroneous impression of both its capabilities and its limitations, and in some hospitals such equipment is not used properly or for the correct indications, to the detriment of patient care. Far from being simple, except in physical design, the IPPV is a precision instrument based on some complex fluid-engineering principles, and the realization of its full clinical potential demands more operational skill and knowledge of physics and physiology than do most of the more impressive electrical machines. It is safe to say that, after a didactic introduction to IPPV, a full-time student therapist requires several months to develop the skill and confidence to use it safely and effectively, a fact that is not readily appreciated by many.

The IPPV is an assistor and a controller. To assist ventilation, it is supplied with a demand valve that responds to very slight patient inspiratory effort to activate gas flow. Demand valves differ in structure, but their general functions are the same. Both sides of the valve are atmospheric pressure just before inspiration, but when the patient makes a small effort to inspire, creating as little as 0.5 cm of water or less subatmospheric pressure, the valve opens to allow the flow of respiratory gas. Inspiration then continues until the preset pressure develops in the respiratory tract, and the absence of a pressure differential across the valve causes it to close. The amount of patient effort needed to start inspiratory flow is variable through a sensitivity control that makes it possible to assist the very weak effort or stimulate independent breathing by imposing a suitable work load on the patient. As a controller, the IPPV is able to cycle according to a rate determined by the operator, initiating inspiration through pneumatic timing devices. Expiration is triggered by pressure, but its length is subject to operator control. The patient control and automatic control abilities of the IPPV can be combined to give a backup assist to a patient with spontaneous but uncertain breathing. The apparatus is adjusted for controlled ventilation at a rate less than the patient's own, and should he become apneic or his rate fall off, the ventilator will take over. Negative pressure during exhalation is available to aid controlled ventilation if desired, activated by a simple venturi that uses source gas to introduce subatmospheric pressure in the patient line.

Although there is much good instructional material available from manufacturers describing and illustrating technical and operational aspects of their products, in conformance with our policy stated at the beginning of this chapter, we will consider some of the features of the two commonly used IPPVs. It is hoped that this will help the respiratory therapist to understand better those mechanisms of the ventilators that are critical to their safe and effective function.

*Flow-adjustable (Bird\*).* We will use the Mark 8 model as an example because it

---

\*Respirators, Mark 7, 8, Bird Corp., Richmond, Calif.

embodies the major characteristics in which we are interested. Working off a source gas pressure of no less than 50 psig, the Bird ventilator is a relatively small, two-chambered instrument whose basic operation is illustrated in the greatly simplified sketches of Fig. 9-11. Source gas *(A)* enters the partition between the chambers, called the *centerbody*, where its flow is controlled by an adjustable valve *(B)*, permitting rates from zero to approximately 80 $\ell$/min. Calibrations on the external valve are for reference only and do not indicate delivered flow. The chamber on the left is called the *ambient chamber* because it is in constant equilibrium with the atmosphere through a filter-equipped aperture *(C)*. Its counterpart is a *pressure chamber*, since this is where therapeutic pressure is developed; it is in direct communication with the patient's respiratory tract through tubing attached to the outflow port *(D)*.

CYCLING MECHANISM. The heart of the cycling mechanism is a sliding valve located in a channel in the centerbody *(E)*. Basically, this consists of a *ceramic cylinder* ground

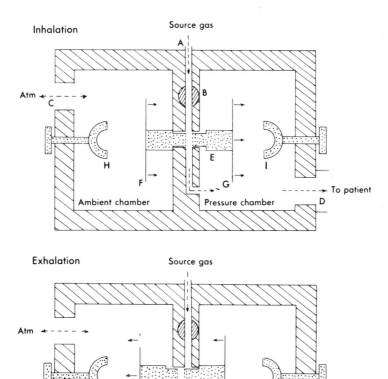

**Fig. 9-11.** Schematic illustrations of the inspiratory and expiratory mechanics of the Bird respirator. (See text for details.)

to close tolerance, with a vent through it (indicated by the dashed lines) and at each end of the cylinder an attached metal *clutch plate (F)* and *(G)*. The two illustrations show that the cylinder duct can align with the source gas inflow to allow its passage or can misalign to shut off the flow of gas; it should be noted that inspiratory gas enters the pressure chamber only. Each chamber has a permanent magnet *(H)* and *(I)*, whose positions in the chamber can be adjusted by outside threaded controls.

Magnet *(H)* in the ambient chamber constitutes the *sensitivity control*, so important to the function of the ventilator in the control mode because it determines the inspiratory effort required of the patient to trigger the start of inspiration. The patient is connected by airtight tubing to the pressure chamber, and if he creates a negative intrathoracic pressure through contraction of his inspiratory muscles, this negative pressure will be transmitted back to the pressure chamber of the ventilator. If such pressure is of sufficient force, the pressure gradient between the two chambers will move the ceramic valve toward the pressure chamber, opening up the source gas channel and initiating inspiration. The amount of inspiratory effort needed to open the valve depends on the proximity of magnet *H* to metal clutch plate *F*. Obviously, the closer together the magnet and the plate, the greater will be the negative pressure in the pressure chamber required to move the valve, and the greater will be the patient inspiratory effort. Conversely, if the magnet is withdrawn farther from the plate, its weaker hold on the plate is more easily overcome, and less work by the patient will start gas flow. This control is so sensitive that it can be adjusted to respond to but a fraction of a centimeter of water negative pressure to begin the respiratory cycle.

Once the sliding valve opens, gas flows into the pressure chamber until a preset pressure is reached in the chamber and the communicating respiratory tract; this constitutes the pressure-cycling characteristic of the ventilator. The amount of pressure required to stop inhalation is determined by the *pressure-control magnet (I)*, and again, operation depends on the relationship between magnet *I* and clutch plate *G*. The closer the magnet and plate, the greater will be the pressure needed to separate them as the rising pressure in the chamber acts on the sliding valve. As the adjustable magnet is advanced, higher pressures will build up in the chamber and in the patient's lungs; as it is withdrawn, lower pressures will activate the valve. On the outside of the instrument there is an aneroid manometer that records the pressure in the chamber, and this is referred to as the *system pressure*, the pressure delivered by the machine. It must be clearly understood that this pressure is not the *intrapulmonary pressure*, although the two are obviously related. Because of the nature of the bronchopulmonary tree, there is a pressure drop from ventilator to alveoli, and whereas the pressure in the instrument can be easily measured, that in the alveoli cannot, except indirectly. We can assume that as system pressure is increased, pulmonary pressure will follow accordingly; but from our earlier consideration of factors influencing gas flow, we know that increments of increasing pulmonary pressure may get progressively smaller as delivery pressure rises. It is possible to generate pressures up to about 60 cm of water, although such a level is used only in extraordinary circumstances. Calibrations on the pressure-control mechanism are helpful in setting a desired pressure, but final adjustment is made by observing the actual pressure recorded on the manometer. In Fig. 9-11 the exhalation sketch depicts the movement of the ceramic valve toward the ambient chamber, with interruption of gas flow; exhalation then proceeds passively, as air escapes from the patient through a special valve located at his end of the gas tubing in the breathing head assembly.

EXHALATION VALVE. The breathing head assembly, at the patient end of the gas delivery tubing, consists of several components. Here, the *mouthpiece,* or an adapter

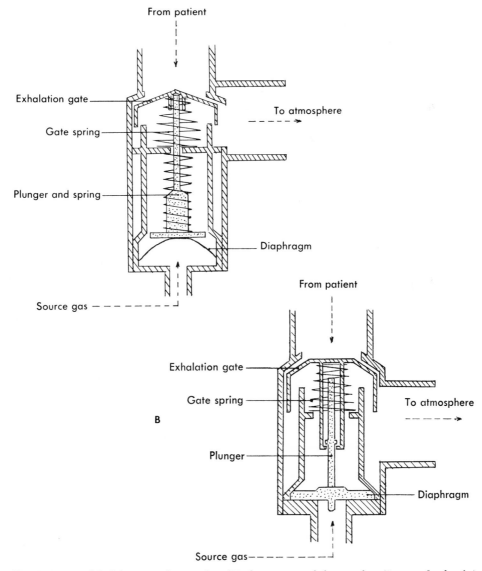

**Fig. 9-12.** Simplified diagrams of two styles of Bird respirator exhalation valve. (See text for details.)

to fit an intratracheal tube, delivers the breathing gas to the patient. In the unit also are the *exhalation valve,* a *nebulizer,* and the *negative-pressure venturi,* when used. Source gas is tapped from the main channel, below the cycling valve and carried by small-bore tubing to both the exhalation valve and the nebulizer. Fig. 9-12, *A,* diagrams the features of an older style exhalation valve, many of which may still be in use. The port is fitted with a spring-loaded plunger that acts against a caplike "gate," supplied with its own fine, weak spring. During inspiration the source gas pressure against the plunger forces the gate into the valve seat and closes the port. As soon as end-inspiration is reached and source gas flow ceases, the plunger retracts by its spring tension, allowing the port to open for instant exhalation. The gate spring, through its gentle action, offers very slight resistance to the outflow of gas, permitting the gate to open smoothly in response to the expiratory flow and pressure. It should be pointed out here that one of the most common causes of air trapping, especially in patients on controlled ventilation, is a failure of the gate spring. After considerable use, with frequent disassembling and handling for cleaning purposes, this fine spring often becomes stretched. Its tension and resistance to exhalation increase, impeding the passage of the terminal portion of exhaled air and retaining it in the airways. This event will be manifest by failure of the pressure manometer needle to return to atmospheric zero, leaving it "hung up" in the pressure zone of the gauge. Although there are other causes for this phenomenon, as soon as the therapist notes it, he should check the exhalation valve by inserting a pencil tip into the outflow port to see whether the trapped pressure can be released by freeing the gate. Should this be the problem, the gate must be replaced at once by one equipped with a good spring.

The current style of exhalation valve is shown in Fig. 9-12, *B.* It is slightly smaller than its predecessor, and much lighter, but its general operation is much the same. The plunger spring has been eliminated, and the exhalation gate provided with a hollow stem to accommodate the plunger. The new valve has fewer parts to disassemble and is designed for easier cleaning.

NEBULIZER. The same source of pressure supplying the exhalation valve is used to power the medication nebulizer, another component of the breathing head assembly. Either sidearm or mainstream nebulization can be used, and because the power gas flows only during inspiration, there is no nebulization during exhalation. In addition to supplying medication, the nebulizer plays an important role in determining the composition of inhaled gas and will be considered later.

NEGATIVE PRESSURE. If negative pressure during exhalation is desired, an adapter allows a venturi to be added to the breathing head assembly directly opposite the gate of the exhalation valve, in the passage designated *From patient* in Fig. 9-12. The power for the venturi is derived from a tap line of the source gas above the cycling valve, diagrammed in Fig. 9-13, the flow through which is controlled by a needle valve, adjustable from the outside of the instrument. The force of negative pressure generated by the venturi depends on the flow permitted by this control valve. Inside the ventilator there is a pressure cartridge with a spring-loaded *interrupter valve* in the venturi tap line, distal to the needle control valve. The small pressure chamber of the cartridge, however, is powered by a tap from the source gas after the cycling

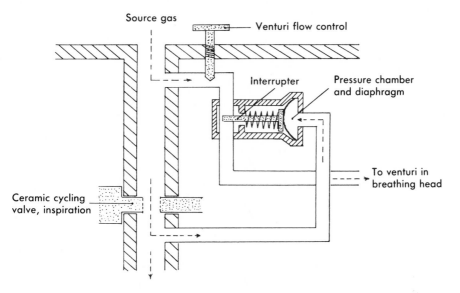

**Fig. 9-13.** Diagram of the control mechanism for the negative-pressure venturi of the Bird respirator. (See text for details.)

valve. During inspiration, as gas flows through the ceramic valve, it exerts pressure in the cartridge, forcing the spring-loaded interrupter to block the passage of gas from the needle valve to the venturi; but as soon as exhalation begins, the cessation of gas flow to the cartridge releases the pressure on the interrupter, and the latter springs back, allowing source gas to activate the venturi. Employing the usual principle of air entrainment, the fast flow of power gas through the venturi jet pulls into its stream air from the respiratory tract, creating an intrapulmonary subatmospheric pressure of −1 to −5 cm of water. The mixed gas escapes through the exhalation port with a distinctive sound.

EXPIRATORY TIMER. When the Bird respirator is used as a controller, the length of exhalation can be varied within a wide range through the action of an *expiratory timer*, housed in a cartridge in the instrument. Like the exhalation and interrupter valves just described, the expiratory timer employs a pressure chamber to activate a spring-loaded plunger. Fig. 9-14 diagrams the parts of the expiratory timer and shows their interrelated functions. For the sake of simplicity, the events of the in-spiratory phase are illustrated, despite the fact that the unit influences exhalation, but it is easier to depict the mechanics of preparation graphically and describe the final action. The pressure chamber, separated from the spring-loaded plunger by a diaphragm, is supplied by a tap line of the source gas below the ceramic cycling valve so that flow to the timer is limited to the inspiratory phase. During inspira-tion, then, the diaphragm compresses the plunger spring, extending the plunger into the ambient chamber of the ventilator. The pressure chamber has an outlet, the flow through which is controlled by a needle valve adjusted from the outside of the instrument and which terminates in a restricted ostium functioning as a bleed-off. If the timer control valve is closed, the unit is nonoperational, and the

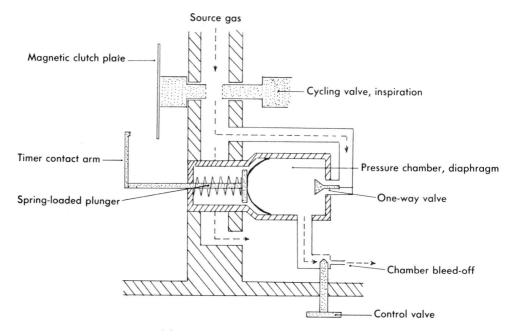

**Fig. 9-14.**   Diagram of the expiratory timer of the Bird respirator. (See text for details.)

pressure chamber is, in a sense, a dead-end street. For the expiratory timer to be activated, the control valve must be opened to allow gas to escape from the bleed-off, and the degree to which the valve is opened will determine the speed with which pressure is released from the chamber. When expiratory time control is started by opening the control valve, gas escapes from the bleed-off continuously, even while the pressure chamber is filling during inhalation, but its loss is small compared with the higher flow filling the chamber and does not interfere with diaphragmatic activation of the plunger. At end-inspiration, source gas is abruptly shut off to the pressure capsule, and a one-way valve in the capsule closes to prevent a retrograde loss of pressure through the source gas tap lines that supply the nebulizer and the air-mix venturi (to be described below). The bleed-off reduces chamber pressure at a rate determined by the control valve and allows a gradual return of the plunger. The distal end of the plunger is supplied with a right-angle extension, and as the plunger returns to its starting position, the extension contacts the magnetic clutch plate in the ambient chamber, pulls it away from its magnet, and initiates the next inspiratory cycle.

Thus, in summary, the duration of exhalation depends on the speed with which the control valve allows retraction of the spring-loaded plunger and its contact arm, tripping the cycling valve to start the next inhalation. Because the mechanism in no way interferes with the operation of the cycling valve, a patient may spontaneously initiate inhalation with his own effort. Fig. 9-14 makes it clear how readily the ventilator will adjust to the new cycle.

**AIR-MIX VENTURI.** The last of the major mechanical features of the Bird respirator to be discussed is the *air-mix* and the *main venturi* of the instrument, and anyone operating the ventilator must understand the workings of this system. In the preceding paragraphs we have referred frequently to the source gas of the ventilator without further specification as to its composition. As long as there is an adequate pressure available, any gas can be used to power the machine, but the ready accessibility of oxygen makes this the most commonly used of gases; and in everyday hospital practice it is usual to connect the ventilator to the nearest oxygen outlet. We have already been exposed to the risks of prolonged use of pure oxygen, so it is reasonable that provisions be made for reducing the concentration of source gas oxygen to safe levels for final delivery to the patient. This is the function of the air-mix control and the main venturi, and it is this function with which we will now concern ourselves.

In principle, the operation of the air-mix is very simple, as inflowing source oxygen is directed through a venturi, where it entrains air from the ambient chamber of the ventilator. The resulting mixture of less than 100% oxygen passes into the pressure chamber and on to the patient. Before considering the actual operation of the air-mix and the concentrations of oxygen it produces, let us look at the mechanism involved. Fig. 9-15 schematically shows the relationships between the components, sketch *A*, with the air-mix control in the "in" position, and *B*, with the control in the "out" position. The source gas is channeled into a narrow chamber with two outlets misaligned with one another, and in the chamber is the plunger of the air-mix control. We can see that, depending on the position of the plunger, its two baffles will direct the flow of source gas to one or the other outlet. With the plunger pushed in, source gas escapes undiluted into the pressure chamber of the ventilator for direct administration to the patient. Obviously, with oxygen as the power gas, the patient will receive 100% oxygen with the control in this position. When pulled out, the air-mix control shunts the source gas to the lower tap line, where it passes through a jet orifice in the venturi. Here, as shown in Fig. 9-15, *B*, air from the ambient chamber of the ventilator is entrained by the source gas jet stream and enters the pressure chamber subject to the influence of the spring-loaded venturi gate. As a result of this action, the breathing gas is a mixture of the source gas and room air. To avoid cluttering the illustrations, two items have been omitted from the air-mix control. One is a small metal flap over the source gas ostium to the pressure chamber, which acts as a one-way valve to prevent backflow of gas or loss of pressure through the tap lines, as described for the expiratory timer. The second is a small opening from the distal end of the plunger chamber into the pressure side of the ventilator. This acts as a pressure equalizer to prevent a cushion of gas from being trapped in the blind end of the plunger chamber to interfere with advancing the plunger and to prevent a vacuum in the same area from hindering withdrawal of the piston to the "out" position.

The function of the air-mix venturi mechanism is a dual one, for not only does it influence the oxygen concentration of the breathing gas but, equally important, it also determines the characteristics of the ventilator's airflow pattern. The two roles are interrelated and together constitute one of the main mechanical features of this ventilator. We will consider this aspect in detail because of its great importance. The structure of the venturi comprises what is termed a *pneumatic clutch*, and

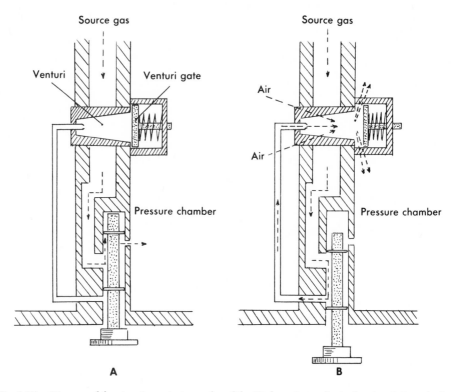

**Fig. 9-15.** Diagram of the air-mix venturi complex of the Bird respirator. In **A**, the air-mix is in the "in" position, delivering pure source gas to the pressure chamber, bypassing the venturi. In **B**, the air-mix is in the "out" position, diverting source gas through the venturi, where it is diluted with entrained air. A further description of this mechanism, along with the important pneumatic clutch action of the venturi, is found in the text.

according to the manufacturer, it permits the volume of gas going to the lung, and its flow, to vary independently throughout the inspiratory cycle, mimicking the accelerations and decelerations of gas flow characteristic of normal spontaneous breathing.[268] In essence, the clutch action is designed to modify the flow characteristics of inhaled gas according to the resistance and compliance status of the respiratory tract. The actual clutch action is the result of the combined operation of the venturi and its gate. As pulmonary resistance and compliance change in the expanding lung, these changes are reflected backward into the pressure chamber of the ventilator. Here they act on the venturi gate held in the outflow of the venturi by a sensitive spring, and the gate responds to increasing resistance in the ventilator's outflow tract by reducing the venturi output. By referring to Fig. 9-15, one can visualize pressure in the pressure chamber gradually building up during the inspiratory phase, slowly closing the gate to retard the flow of gas entering the chamber and, consequently, the flow of gas ventilating the lung. Thus, as inspiration proceeds and the resistance of end-inspiration increases, the impedance to airflow produces a back pressure that closes the venturi gate slowly and facilitates the maximum terminal flow of gas to the lung.

The student may recognize that the principle of the pneumatic clutch in this version of the pressure-cycled ventilator is designed to achieve the same objective as the sine curve we discussed in relation to the wheel and piston volume-cycled ventilator. We pointed out there that some importance was attached to a slow initial, as well as terminal, flow, best afforded by the rotary drive mechanism. The pressure-cycled ventilator starts inhalation with a substantial flow but slows down the flow as distal pressure develops. Some degree of the effectiveness of the pneumatic clutch may be demonstrated by comparing the relationships between gas flow and distal pressure of the Bird ventilator operating off 100% oxygen as source gas, both without and with the air-mix in use.

To understand better the difference between these two conditions, the student should be aware of an entirely different classification of ventilators, based on flow and pressure qualities.[264] Two basic types of ventilators are recognized—*flow generators* and *pressure generators*, differentiated as follows: Since the purpose of a mechanical ventilator is to inflate a flexible lung through a fairly rigid conducting system of constantly changing proportions, the ventilator must force air under pressure against the back pressure of airway and elastic resistance. The two factors involved that are determined by the ventilator are the flow and the delivery pressure (pressure at the mouth as opposed to alveolar pressure), and any given machine controls only one of these. In the presence of such changing lung characteristics as increased resistance and decreased compliance, if a ventilator at a given pressure maintains a constant flow of delivered gas, not influenced by the status of the lung and not hampered by increasing back pressure, the instrument is called a *flow generator*. On the other hand, if the machine holds the delivery pressure at the mouth constant while the flow responds to the lung characteristics by gradually diminishing in the face of back pressure, the ventilator is called a *pressure generator*. Knowing the relationship between flow and obstruction to gas flow, we know that to reach anything close to a pressure equilibrium on both sides of an obstruction (or, back pressure, generally), we must have a reduction in flow. We can visualize a flow of gas building up a pressure proximal to an obstruction in an airway much faster than in the airway distal to the obstruction; such a condition can cause a pressure-cycled ventilator to terminate inspiration before enough gas has reached the partially blocked alveoli to satisfy respiratory needs. The advantage of a pressure generator over a flow generator in ventilating a diseased respiratory tract is evident.

The basic original IPPB instrument was a flow generator with the delivered flow dependent on the source pressure applied; but as its use increased and its greater potential was recognized, as noted earlier in this section, the need for flow control became clear. The introduction of a manually variable flow adjustment, as in the Bird ventilator under discussion, represented a significant development in IPPV and materially increased both its effectiveness and its safety. Although it remained fundamentally a flow generator, because flow was still constant at any given combination of pressure and flow, the ventilator could be manually set, by trial and error and clinical observation, to accommodate a much wider variety of bronchopulmonary abnormalities. A further refinement of the pressure-cycled ventilator was the addition of the venturi apparatus, and we shall see shortly that this feature imparts to the instrument some of the characteristics of a pressure generator.

Let us first consider the operation of the Bird respirator with its air-mix control "in," eliminating the venturi. Now the instrument functions as an adjustable flow generator with independent pressure and flow settings. Source gas passes unmodified through the instrument inflow tract into the pressure chamber, where it develops the preset delivery pressure regardless of either static or changing conditions in the respiratory system that it is ventilating. Not only is the ventilator unable to vary its flow in response to developing impediments, such as accumulations of bronchial secretions, but also its flow remains linear and unchanged in the face of the normal resistances characteristic of the inspiratory phase. In other words, when once set for a given pressure-flow pattern, the instrument is inflexible in its operation. An excellent mechanical study of the performance of this ventilator emphasizes this facet of its performance, and Fig. 9-16 is diagrammatically adapted from one of the recorded pressure-flow relationships of that study.[269] At the outset of inhalation, gas flow rapidly reaches its maximum (as opposed to a sine curve flow) and maintains an unwavering rate throughout inhalation, despite the steadily rising pressure. It must be borne in mind that the amount of pressure recorded reflects airway back pressure against which the machine is working, and yet the flow of gas makes no adjustment to this resistance. It can well be imagined that with such a constant gas flow, the pressure drop along airways may so increase that alveolar ventilation, dependent upon pressure delivered to the alveoli, may be quite inadequate. Cer-

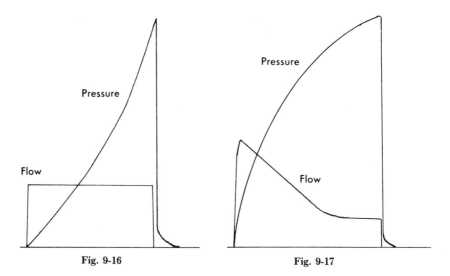

Fig. 9-16          Fig. 9-17

**Fig. 9-16.** Relationship between ventilator flow and pressure when these two factors are independently adjusted. At any given setting the flow remains constant even though resistance increases. (Modified from Edwards, W. L., and Sappenfield, R. S.: Anesth. Analg. **47:**77, 1968.)

**Fig. 9-17.** Relationship between ventilator flow and pressure when pneumatic clutching is active. With rising pressure, flow initially decreases, then levels as cycling pressure is reached. (Modified from Edwards, W. L., and Sappenfield, R. S.: Anesth. Analg. **47:**77, 1968.)

tainly, skillful operation of such a ventilator depends upon the ability to drop the constant flow to a level that will make possible the maximum alveolar ventilation consistent with the estimated resistance or compliance, but every such change must be manual and in response to airway conditions gross enough to be observed.

Activation of the venturi gives to the ventilator considerable versatility in coping with the characteristics of the airways. Source gas no longer enters the pressure chamber directly but is first used to power the venturi where it pulls in and mixes with air from the ambient chamber as described and illustrated in Fig. 9-15. Let us understand that the venturi does not make of the ventilator something it is not, for it is still basically a flow generator with the need to employ adjustable flow control, but the additional service of the venturi enhances the performance of the machine and supplements the action of the flow control. We have just seen that without the use of the air-mix, the instrument is an adjustable flow generator with a *rigid* flow, whereas the function of the venturi modifies it to what might be termed an adjustable flow generator with a *flexible* flow. For a given manual pressure-flow setting, the ventilator behaves somewhat like a pressure generator. The key to the successful function of the venturi lies in the performance of its gate, separating the mixed gases from the pressure chamber. The spring-loaded gate, acted on by the outflowing gas on one side and the developing pressure of the pressure chamber on the other, adjusts the venturi outlet to permit that flow of gases which will best compensate for the growing pressure. The sensitivity of the gate's responsiveness can be clearly seen if the outlet of the breathing head is alternately blocked and unblocked by the hand during gas flow. The gate is seen to open and shut in proportion to the applied obstruction and can be made to oscillate back and forth with rapid pressure changes. When the ventilator is cycling, the venturi gate can be seen to open abruptly with the start of inhalation, then gradually close as the cycle progresses.

Fig. 9-17 is another adaptation from the same study of ventilators referred to above and shows the effect of the pneumatic clutch on airflow. Graphically evident is the immediate drop in flow accompanying the rise in pressure for the first half of inspiration, after which the flow levels off until cycling pressure is reached. This response by flow to mounting pressure is called *flow sensitivity* and is the primary characteristic of a pressure generator. Because the Bird respirator is not a pressure generator, the flow sensitivity is not complete and it does not continue to the termination of flow, but for each manually set combination of pressure and flow, there is a significant degree of such sensitivity. We will describe more effective flow sensitivity when we discuss the next ventilator.

We cannot separate the pneumatic clutching action of the venturi from its oxygen-diluting function, for the two are interdependent. With the air-mix "in," the breathing gas is 100% oxygen if that is the source gas; and with the control retracted, the concentration is something less than 100%; but the question is how much less. When the venturi principle came into popular use, there was an unfortunate lack of clear understanding of its operation, and assumptions about its diluting action were accepted that have since been proved false. Although corrective action has been taken, manufacturer's specifications originally gave the impression, still persistent in some minds, that the air-mix venturi automatically produced a breathing gas with an oxygen concentration of 40%. Analyses of delivered gas, on the contrary, have frequently demonstrated oxygen concentrations over 90%, and in clinical use one rarely if at all finds the concentration less than 50%. Thus, although the venturi may be designed to produce a 40% air-oxygen mixture during unrestricted flow, when it functions against a resistance, its performance is completely changed. The major influence on the venturi is the factor of pressure, mediated through the venturi gate, and itself subject to the influence of flow. With the venturi output dependent upon so many variables, which themselves are interrelated, it is no wonder that we encounter a bizarre fluctuation of delivered oxygen concentrations that seem to have no rhyme or reason. However, we can get a clue to the relationships of these influences if we conduct the simple experiment of measuring the delivered oxygen concentration of a base line pressure-flow setting and then determine the concentration as pressure and flow are each individually increased and decreased. This will show us that if the original pressure-flow setting is changed so that pressure increases relative to flow, the resulting $F_{O_2}$ will rise. This change in the ratio may be either an actual increase in pressure or a decrease in flow. Obviously, a converse effect on the ratio will decrease the subsequent $F_{O_2}$, but the clinical situations to which we will be most frequently exposed usually involve pressure increases, so we will use this orientation for our discussion. Finally, a proportionate increase or decrease in pressure and flow will not significantly alter the oxygen concentration, since no ratio change will result.

Let us see how pressure can be so influential in determining the delivered oxygen content and how it uses the venturi gate. In our earlier description of the gate, we were concerned only with the general manner in which it acted as a clutch to compromise gas flow with opposing pressure and did not intimate that it might not be active throughout the entire respiratory phase. Actually, the gate does not necessarily remain open until end-inspiration and indeed can do so only under a given circumstance. Regardless of the time interval of inspiration, the venturi gate closes when the system pressure reaches somewhere between 10 and 15 cm of water pressure. This is felt to be a reasonably accurate range because the actual closing pressure of a given gate depends upon its physical state. Should it be worn or contaminated with foreign matter of adhesive nature, its closing point can be altered. Especially important in this regard is the condition of the gate spring, normally under a tension of 2 cm of water but which may be weakened by use or handling during maintenance or may be under increased tension after replacement. As we have done frequently throughout these pages, we will make a recommendation to the alert respiratory therapist and urge him to check the function of this important part, if through no other way than observing the gross action of the gate to see whether it is responsive or sluggish or, indeed, whether it is functioning at all and to take corrective action. This limitation on the activity of the gate was designed to permit it to exert its most effective clutching function when confronted with the usual flows and pressures encountered in clinical medicine. Now that we have established that increasing the ventilator pressure in relation to its flow will elevate the delivered oxygen concentration and have described the pressure point at which the venturi gate will close, let us see how these two mechanisms cooperate to influence the percentage of oxygen. There are two reasons why oxygen concentrations are unstable.

First, after the venturi gate closes, the *only* gas flow to the patient to complete his ventilation is *pure oxygen* through the medication nebulizer by way of the nebulizer tap line from the ventilator oxygen inflow tract. This gas, which has been activating the nebulizer since the beginning of inspiration, continues to flow into the patient until the preset system pressure is reached in the patient's airways, equilibrating with the ventilator to terminate inspiration by the cycling mechanism described earlier. Thus the longer inhalation lasts after closure of the venturi gate the more oxygen will flow undiluted through the nebulizer line and the higher will be the concentration of oxygen in the inspired mixture. This is why any change in the pressure-flow relationship that favors pressure, as noted above, will increase $F_{O_2}$. If pressure is increased while flow is kept constant, longer time will be required to reach the preset pressure, the postclosure time of the venturi gate will be lengthened, and nebulizer oxygen will raise the inspired oxygen concentration. If flow is reduced while pressure remains constant, the same circumstances will prevail and the actual flow time of nebulizer oxygen will be lengthened. If the cycling pressure set for the ventilator is less than the gate closure pressure, the gate will remain open throughout inspiration, and not only will the oxygen concentration be at its lowest but variations in the pressure/flow ratio (below the closure point) will effect little significant change in concentration.

Second, in addition to the nebulizer flow, another source of oxygen has been found that significantly increases its concentration in the inspired gas.[270] After the venturi gate closes, oxygen still flows into the venturi through its jet and, denied egress through the gate, backflows from the venturi into the ambient chamber of the ventilator. Here, the oxygen concentration may rise as high as 60%, and during inspiration the oxygen flow to the venturi is diluted, not with supposed atmospheric air but with air already highly enriched with oxygen.

We can summarize the action of the air-mix and the venturi in controlling delivered oxygen by comparing the sources of gas available during the initial and terminal portions of inhalation, with 100% oxygen as the source gas. With no dilution (air-mix control closed) both early inspiration and late inspiration are supplied by source oxygen and nebulizer oxygen; with dilution (air-mix control open) early inspiration is supplied by source oxygen, ambient chamber gas, and nebulizer oxygen, and late inspiration by nebulizer oxygen only.

There are many modifications of the flow-adjustable, positive-pressure pneumatic ventilator embodied in various accessories and models of the basic instrument, designed for such special purposes as minimizing dead space, adding a supplementary source of oxygen, correlating machine cycling with chest expansion, and accommodating the needs of the infant. Since it is not the purpose of this text to serve as a technical manual, we have limited our discussion to the fundamental principles that will be found in all variations of the ventilator, and it is felt that the student, through his clinical experience and personal investigation of equipment, should be able to apply his understanding of these principles to any specific instance.

*Flow-sensitive (Bennett\*).* We will describe the PR-2 respiration unit for it is the most sophisticated and complex, not only of all the Bennett models but of all pneumatic positive-pressure ventilators, and if the therapist understands its functions, he will have little difficulty with the others. Like the Bird respirator the PR-2 operates from a gas source pressure of 50 psig and exerts a pressure to inflate the lungs, but here the similarity ends. The physical design and the principles upon which the Bennett works are radically different from those of the Bird, and for this reason we will not follow the same descriptive format of the past few pages, since the two instruments cannot be compared item for item. Although we have included the PR-2 in the class of pressure-cycled assistor-controllers, we will have to expand this a bit to accommodate all its functions. To be all inclusive, we should describe the machine as a positive pressure-cycled, time-cycled, flow-sensitive, assistor-controller, a cumbersone designation but accurate. When used as an assistor, the PR-2 is pressure cycled and patient triggered by subatmospheric pressure. When it is used as a controller, end-inspiration is cycled either by preset pressure or by time, depending on which factor is activated first. Because the manufacturer has made available an adequate operating manual and some excellent teaching aids, we will not go into a minute description of the ventilator, but we will discuss some of the details that are unique to its function and with which all operators should be familiar.

**GENERAL FEATURES.** Unlike the Bird respirator, the PR-2 is not a chambered instrument but basically consists of a system of very complex pneumatic circuitry that intermittently feeds the breathing mixture to the patient under rigid control. Gas flow is regulated by one central valve, aided by several other automatic and manually operated controls, and three ingenious cylindrical pneumatic timing devices that integrate the functions of the components into the total output of the instrument. As source gas enters the machine, that which is to ventilate the patient passes directly to a unit which may be called a regulator-diluter. Here the gas is reduced from its source pressure to the working range of 0 to 45 cm of water by the adjustable manual pressure control, the exact level being determined by the ventilatory needs of the patient. This mechanism, unlike that in the Bird, which uses a movable magnet, is similar in its action to the adjustable cylinder gas–reducing valve, described in an earlier chapter, in that it employs a control attached to a spring-loaded diaphragm to oppose the incoming gas and limit its pressure. The regulator also contains a balloon that, when inflated, shuts off the outflow of gas from the regulator; and we shall see later that this works in conjunction with the timing mechanism to help establish ventilatory patterns. Pure source gas may be delivered to the patient, or a manually operated venturi may be activated to dilute the gas with atmospheric air. This venturi functions only as a diluter and plays no part in modifying the airflow pattern. As in the Bird respirator, the Bennett venturi is designed to dilute source oxygen to a 40% con-

---

\*Respiration Units PR-1, 2, Bennett Respiration Products, Inc., Santa Monica, Calif.

centration when operating with an unrestricted flow. However, during inspiration as obstruction to flow is encountered, the efficiency of the venturi decreases and the concentration of oxygen in the delivered gas increases above 40%. Additional oxygen mixes with the breathing gas through the nebulizer, described below. The instrument also contains another pressure regulator, called the unit regulator, that reduces source pressure to about 60 cm of water. Its function is to distribute gas to power several of the automatic components and has no direct communication with the patient.

Still other components work directly off source pressure without reduction. The adjustable pressure delivered by the patient regulator (regulator-diluter) is recorded on the face of the ventilator by a gauge calibrated in centimeters of water and labeled "control pressure." Adjacent to this is another similar gauge designated "system pressure," and the two must be differentiated. The control pressure is the pressure delivered by the patient regulator to the flow-control valve and is the pressure that will be reached in the outflow tubing and that will terminate inspiration if the ventilator is pressure cycled. The system pressure (often called mask pressure) records the actual pressure reached distal to the flow-control valve, or at the patient's mouth. For reasons already known, it does not indicate patient alveolar pressure. Under most circumstances the two gauges will record the same peak, but perhaps the student can already see that in the control mode in the face of significant airway resistance, because of the optional time-cycling capability of the PR-2, inspiration may end before the mask pressure has had time to reach the set control-pressure value. The careful observation of these two gauges is an important function of the respiratory therapist in the management of his patients.

Before describing the interesting details of the flow-control and cycling mechanisms, we shall enumerate the additional manual controls available on the PR-2 so that we will be familiar with them when we refer to them later in the discussion. Nebulization can be individually adjusted for either inspiration or expiration, or it can be activated continuously. Nebulization during exhalation enables the maximal amount of medication to be delivered to the patient, since aerosol fills the breathing tubes during this phase and is immediately available in quantity as soon as inspiration starts. The nebulization unit is powered by direct source gas pressure, but its phasing with respiration depends on an inflatable valve activated by gas at control pressure, tapped after the cycling mechanism. Respiratory rate can be adjusted from 1 to 45 breaths per minute, obviously only applicable when the machine is functioning as a controller. The regulating mechanism assures that expiration will never be less than 1.5 times the duration of inspiration, the physiologic reason for which will be learned later in this chapter, although circumstances may reduce the 1:1.5 ratio. Expiratory time can be prolonged, changing the I/E ratio, always favoring a lowered ratio such as 1:2, 1:3, etc. As with all patient-activated assistors, the sensitivity of the start of inhalation is adjustable over a wide range. Negative pressure during exhalation can be applied to the patient's airways by opening a venturi that works through the nebulizer control unit directly from source pressure. Peak and terminal flows are adjustable, and their functions will be discussed below. The student should note that we have not mentioned a manually operated flow control, which was so important in the Bird respirator. One of the major features of the PR-2 is the automatic regulation of flow, at any control-pressure setting; and we will now describe the mechanism responsible for this quality of flow sensitivity.

FLOW-SENSITIVE VALVE. Described by the manufacturer as the "valve that breathes with the patient," the Bennett valve is further affirmed to open with slight inspiratory pressure to permit a flow of gas that varies according to the balance between the delivered control pressure and the total resistance of the patient airways and to close automatically when the flow of gas through the valve reaches a low terminal point.[271] The Bennett valve is housed in the respirator in a horizontal position, front to rear, and is pictured in Fig. 9-18. It is a metal cylindrical drum, approximately 36 mm long by 26 mm in diameter, penetrated by two large and one small apertures, called windows. Eccentrically placed near the cylinder's wall, a rod runs lengthwise of the drum to function as a counterbalance. Projecting from the front end of the valve is a small lever that allows manual operation from outside the housing. Finally, attached to the outer surface of the valve are two rectangular vanes. The valve and its housing are precision made, and the cylinder is suspended with very close tolerance by jeweled bearings, front and rear.

We shall use four illustrations to show the basic function of the valve, of necessity simplifying both graphic and verbal descriptions. The sketches show a longitudinal section through the drum and its housing, exposing the major gas channels and showing the relative positions of the vanes, windows, and the counterbalance rod. In Fig. 9-19 the valve is in the resting state, as during the exhalation phase. Attention is drawn to the configuration of the drum housing with its three ports, *1*, *2*, and *3*. Port *1* is the entry for the main gas flow, which may be either pure source gas or an air mixture, coming directly from the regulator-diluter through the main inflow tract *(4)*. Port *2* is a vestibule leading into the outflow tract *(5)*, to which is connected the patient tubing, and port *3* is the site of action of the inspiratory sensitivity control. The drum housing, more detailed than indicated in the illustration, is provided with many small-caliber channels that receive gas from the various controls noted above or allow the escape of gas to them, all as part of the functioning of this critical center of providing just the correct character of flow, breath by breath. This view of the drum shows a cross section of the counterbalance rod and the position of the two large windows and the vanes in the resting state. Neither window approximates a major gas channel, and vane 2 (in port *2*) is against the upper wall of its port, as is vane 3. At this moment no gas is moving in the valve mechanism. The outflow tract *(5)* is provided with an adjustable restriction *(6)*, called the peak flow control, that obstructs the gas flow to the tubing. Its operation will be described with a subsequent illustration, as will the purposes of the three small channels connected to ports 2 and 3 and the outflow tract.

Fig. 9-20 depicts the events of immediate preinspiration, just before inspiratory gas starts to flow in assisted ventilation. The negative sign in port 2, with the airflow arrow directed toward the tubing, represents the negative inspiratory pressure exerted by the patient in an effort to trigger the cycle. This negative pressure draws down vane 2, giving the drum a counterclockwise rotation. The instrument has a

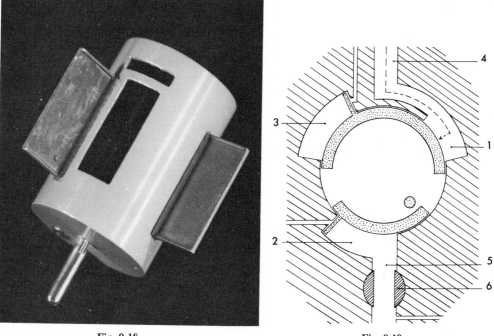

**Fig. 9-18**          **Fig. 9-19**

**Fig. 9-18.** Bennett valve drum, showing two of its windows, the vanes, and the projecting lever for manual operation.

**Fig. 9-19.** Bennett valve in resting position. (See text for description.)

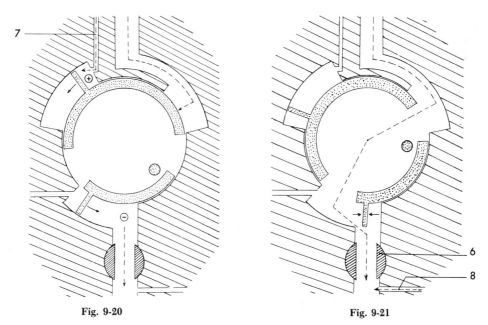

**Fig. 9-20**          **Fig. 9-21**

**Fig. 9-20.** Bennett valve just before inspiratory gas flow. (See text for description.)
**Fig. 9-21.** Bennett valve in midinspiration. (See text for description.)

sensitivity control to aid the patient in this effort, and its action is evident in port 3, where a flow of gas is seen moving down channel 7 into the port. Such a flow exerts a positive pressure on the upper side of vane 3, forcing it downward, again urging the drum in counterclockwise motion. The dual action of the negative and positive pressures on the two vanes rotates the drum with a minimum of work on its jeweled bearings, and by varying the gas flow to the upper vane, the cylinder can be rendered responsive to the weakest inspiratory effort. During controlled ventilation, without spontaneous patient effort, gas is supplied to vane 3 by the rate-control mechanism through the pneumatic timers mentioned above but yet to be described. Thus, whether assisted or controlled, inspiration is initiated, either in part or in total, by nudging the upper vane with a flow of gas to set the drum in motion. Care must be taken in assisting ventilation not to set the sensitivity flow too high, or cycling may be initiated without the patient's help and disturb the breathing pattern.

As the drum continues to rotate to allow inspiratory gas flow, we can illustrate an imaginary moment in midinspiration with Fig. 9-21. Movement of the cylinder has brought one window opposite port 1 and the other opposite port 2, effectively opening direct communication between the main inflow and outflow channels so that gas flows to the patient. It is at this time that the flow sensitivity of the valve is manifested. The exact position of the valve is determined by the resistance-compliance characteristics of the airways and lungs downstream, and in the illustration ports 1 and 2 are not fully opened. The two small arrows on each side of vane 2 indicate opposing forces responsible for the delicate balance of the drum. The arrow on the right represents the back pressure of downstream resistance, whereas that on the left reflects the force of the flowing gas. As resistance to flow develops, back pressure on the vane rotates the drum, reducing flow through the valve to a level that still permits a flow adequate to ventilate alveoli. This mechanism prevents a rapid buildup of pressure that could otherwise cycle the ventilator into exhalation before sufficient volume reached the lung and, by slowing the flow, allows the maximum volume of gas to navigate restricted airways. Such a flow-sensitive response achieves automatically that which requires manual operation on flow-controlled ventilators. To compare the flow sensitivity of the PR-2 with the Mark 8, Fig. 9-22 is adapted from the same source as Figs. 9-16 and 9-17.[269] Fig. 9-22, *A*, shows the very clear response of flow to steadily rising pressure, continuously to the end of inspiration, and demonstrates the gradual closure of the vaned drum as airway resistance increases. In Fig. 9-22, *B*, the real virtue of flow sensitivity is evident as flow through an obstructed passage meets an increase in resistance, with an ensuing sudden rise in pressure. At this point the Bennett valve abruptly retards flow to allow gas to ventilate the distal passage.

**TERMINAL FLOW.** Earlier it was stated that in the assist mode end-inspiration is cycled by pressure; although this assertion is essentially true, it must be slightly modified. The instrument is basically a pressure-cycled machine, but the actual closure of the valve depends on a *terminal flow point* of 1 $\ell$/min, which means that the valve will not close until the flow through it drops to 1 $\ell$/min, when with the aid of the weight of the counterbalance rod, the drum rotates fully clockwise and all flow stops. The terminal flow characteristic of the valve does not mean that it is

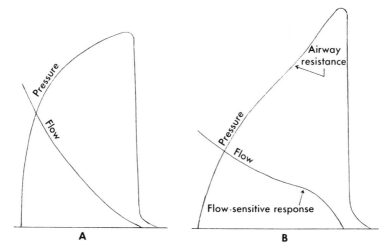

**Fig. 9-22.** Relationship between ventilatory flow and pressure in response to automatic flow-sensitivity control. (See text for details.) (Modified from Edwards, W. L., and Sappenfield, R. S.: Anesth. Analg. **47**:77, 1968.)

not pressure cycled because terminal flow, control pressure, and resistance are all related; it does mean that the valve is so constructed and mounted that the driving pressure of gas will keep flow active until the developing back pressure has retarded the flow to 1 $\ell$/min. To put it another way, as long as gas flow is in excess of 1 $\ell$/min, inspiration will not cycle off. It is apprent that when the machine is pressure cycling, the presence of a leak in the delivery system will let gas flow continuously without subsiding to the terminal flow point and inspiratory flow will not stop. Under certain circumstances leaks are difficult to avoid, especially if the respirator is used with a face mask or an intratracheal tube, but the instrument provides a means to compensate for such a loss of gas. The terminal flow control is a manually operated adjustment that introduces a flow of source gas at source pressure into the outflow tube below the peak flow control (8), as shown in Fig. 9-21. When the control is activated, gas is introduced through the same mechanism that regulates the inspiratory nebulizer so that it flows only during inspiration. The gas added to the Bennett valve's output by the terminal flow control in a sense "feeds" the system leak and allows the flow through the valve to drop to the terminal shutoff level of 1 $\ell$/min, even though the total output of the ventilator is greater than this. The same procedure for managing a leak can also be used during controlled ventilation, although in this situation compensation for gas loss can be achieved by varying the rate to give a longer time for lung inflation; often the latter is used as a backup for the terminal control technique, as a safety measure.

PEAK FLOW. In Fig. 9-21 the peak flow control (6) is a manually adjustable variable restriction in the gas outflow passage that merely reduces the diameter of the lumen. Its name derives from its ability to regulate the maximum flow that is available to the patient, reducing it from a high of 80 $\ell$/min when fully opened to approximately

10 ℓ/min when completely turned. The restriction, when activated, creates a back pressure on the Bennett valve, preventing the drum from opening widely. It serves two purposes. First, it reduces the initial blast of air striking the patient's airways as inspiration starts, sometimes a matter of discomfort about which the therapist should always inquire of the conscious patient. Second, if there is significant downstream obstruction, it prevents the development of sudden back pressure, which will result from the force of high-velocity gas. Thus the more restriction applied to the gas flow the more gradual will be the rise to the peak of the control pressure. To a considerable degree the Bennett peak flow control resembles, in its end result, the manual flow control of the Bird ventilator, but it is applied after the cycling mechanism instead of before and functions cooperatively with the flow-sensitive valve.

NEGATIVE PRESSURE. The final sketch of the Bennett valve (Fig. 9-23) shows the valve closed during exhalation, since it has rotated back to its starting position. However, instead of this exhalation phase being passive, it is subjected to a negative pressure for the therapeutic effects of that pressure, a function we have noted in connection with other ventilators previously. A control knob on the instrument regulates a flow of source gas at source pressure from the expiratory nebulization mechanism to a venturi located beneath the body of the machine. From the venturi two lines extend to the circuitry. One goes to a special exhalation valve manifold at the patient end of the gas flow tubing. The Bennett exhalation valve consists of a small balloon that inflates by gas flow from the cycling valve during inspiration to

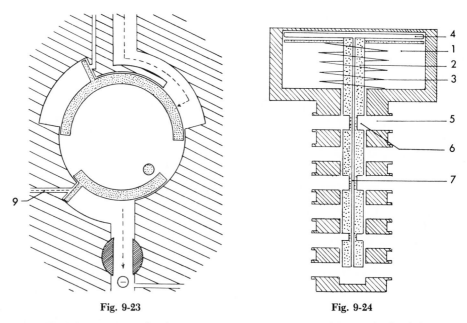

**Fig. 9-23**                **Fig. 9-24**

**Fig. 9-23.** Bennett valve during expiratory negative pressure. (See text for details.)
**Fig. 9-24.** Diagrammatic sketch of a Bennett timing accumulator. (See text for details.)

close an aperture to the atmosphere and collapses during exhalation to allow the escape of exhaled air. The negative-pressure venturi line enters the manifold between the balloon and the patient, and when the venturi is activated, negative pressure is generated in the entire conducting system, from the cycling valve to the patient's alveoli. Subatmospheric pressures down to −6 cm of water are available, depending on the extent to which the control is opened, and the negative force ceases as soon as inspiration begins. In Fig. 9-23 the system negative pressure is indicated by the negative sign in the outflow tract at the tip of the dashed arrow. The second line (9) from the negative-pressure venturi is connected to the blind end of port 2. We know that patient cycling of inhalation is achieved by creating a small negative pressure in port 2, so we can understand that an uncontrolled negative pressure of the degree generated by the venturi would rotate the drum wide open as soon as end-inspiration had been reached and the venturi set into action. To prevent this serious interference with cycling, the same amount of negative pressure applied to the exhalation manifold is applied to the upper surface of the vane in port 2. This perfect balance of forces across the vane keeps the drum closed during the negative-pressure phase, and because of this balance, the same small inspiratory negative-pressure effort will trigger inhalation and shut off the venturi.

TIMING ACCUMULATORS. The timing mechanism of the PR-2 respirator is composed of three interconnected and interrelated piston-in-cylinder devices known as *timing accumulators*, plainly visible protruding from the top of the instrument, one or all three of which are in motion whenever the ventilator is operating. It would be unnecessarily time consuming and needless to diagram in its entirety the circuitry joining these units with one another and with other components of the machine. Such information is available through instructional material; yet we should not pass over these interesting and vital mechanisms without at least describing their general structure and functions.[272] The three timing accumulators are identical in design and consist of spring-loaded grooved pistons, topped by inflatable balloons, and they ride in vertical cylinders supplied with a number of gas inlets and outlets. Fig. 9-24 is a schematic representation of one of the units, not to scale and not showing the exact relative positions of the gas connections, since it is a two-dimensional projection of a three-dimensional object with radially placed outlets; but it does show the functioning parts that are responsible for the smooth operation of the respirator. The upper, visible portion of the cylinder (1) is transparent, and through its wall can be seen the upper end of the piston (2) with its recoil spring (3), surmounted by a collapsed balloon that is supported by a metal disc (4). The lower part of the cylinder is narrow, pierced by six pairs of small gas conduits (5), and that part of the piston in the narrowed cylinder has three circular grooves cut into it (6). Finally, a narrow channel runs the length of the piston, open at its lower end and communicating with the balloon at its upper end (7). The paired openings in the cylinder are connected in an intricate fashion among the three accumulators—the sensitivity, rate, and expiratory time controls, the Bennett valve, and the gas outflow tract.

Each accumulator functions as a multiple-action valve, dispatching gas flow according to the position of its piston. When the piston grooves are aligned with gas channels in the cylinder, gas flows across the unit; when they are misaligned, flow is blocked. The changing patterns of valvular action result from gas moving up the narrow channel at the core of the piston, inflating the balloon. As the balloon swells, the piston is forced downward, changing the lineup between its grooves and the gas passages, and it is returned to its resting position by the action of its spring when freed of the driving gas pressure.

If we orient the three accumulators from a front view of the respirator and designate them as left, middle, and right, we can briefly describe the principal role played by each. During ventilatory assistance, only the *middle timing accumulator* is operating, and it functions in this circumstance as a regulator of the inspiratory sensitivity mechanism. Opening the sensitivity control allows gas to pass from the unit regulator through an open channel across the cylinder of the middle timer to port 3 of the Bennett valve housing by way of gas line 7 (Fig. 9-20). Here it helps the patient to initiate inspiration, but once flow starts, a gas line from the outflow tract back to the bottom of the middle accumulator inflates the middle accumulator's balloon, depressing the piston and terminating flow to the Bennett valve. During exhalation, the accumulator's balloon deflates and the groove realignment readies flow to the drum vane for the next cycle. When the instrument is used for respiratory control, all three timing accumulators function, and although to the casual observer their action may appear to be random in nature, they are actually performing with split-second precision. The *middle timer* now acts to coordinate the action of the other two by blocking and releasing gas flow to their balloons in the proper timing sequence, correlating this with the flow leaving the vaned drum through its communication with the outflow tract. Thus it senses the start and stop of airflow and prepares the circuitry of the other accumulators for suitable response. The *left timing accumulator* is activated by the rate control and starts inspiration by sending gas to the same vane on the Bennett valve as does the sensitivity control. The breathing rate is determined by the length of time devoted to exhalation, and the more gas sent to the left accumulator balloon by the rate control the shorter will be exhalation and the faster this timer will open gas flow to the vaned drum from the unit regulator. The left accumulator acts in concert with the right timer to maintain an I/E ratio of 1 : 1.5 at any rate by taking proportionately more time to line up its channels than does the right. In addition, gas to the left accumulator balloon from the rate control can be retarded by the expiratory time control, prolonging the time it takes to align its flow passage and thus extending the expiratory time. When this occurs, the I/E ratio is reduced to 1 : 2, 1 : 3, etc. The *right accumulator* starts exhalation by terminating inhalation. During inhalation the middle timer directs gas to the balloon of the right timer, and this opens a circuit through the right timer from the unit regulator to the balloon in the patient regulator, which inflates and shuts off inspiratory flow. The hazard of describing individually several concomitant functions is to give a picture of intermittent action. In reality, all the interrelated movements of the timing accumulators noted above are smoothly integrated into a continuously repetitive cycle but one that can be modified at will by the trained operator and that will also respond to spontaneous patient effort.

In summary, the Bennett PR-2 ventilator is a versatile instrument that can deliver either assisted or controlled mechanical ventilation, or a combination of both, to allow the patient spontaneous assisted breathing with backup control in the event of recurrent failure. It is a pressure generator, since it delivers gas at a preset pressure, and its flow varies according to resistance in distal airways through the operation of an automatic flow-sensitive outflow valve. Because of this mechanism, manual adjustment of gas flow into the ventilator is unnecessary for most circumstances, but to overcome severe obstruction, the gas leaving the valve for the outflow tract can be retarded so as to delay the point of time in inspiration that peak gas flow will be reached. In the assist mode the instrument is pressure cycled, but inspiration will not terminate until flow through the valve drops below 1 $\ell$/min. When used as a controller, the PR-2 is time cycled through the action of the timing accumulators, which allows the determination of total ventilatory rate and the inspiratory/expiratory ratio, not to exceed 1:1.5. However, should conditions permit the buildup of control pressure in the airways before the end of the preset inspiratory time interval, the machine will pressure cycle. Because of the ease with which the drum valve operates, a controlled patient can take a spontaneous breath at any time, and the accumulators immediately rephase themselves to continue control as soon as spontaneous effort ceases.

## PHYSIOLOGIC EFFECT OF MECHANICAL VENTILATION

Mechanical ventilation cannot be used either safely or effectively until those responsible for it are knowledgeable in its effect upon the physiology as well as proficient in its mechanics. When artificially ventilating a patient, we deliberately attempt to change a physiologic condition, hopefully from a poor to an improved status; but we are nonetheless interfering with a level of function, even if that function is pathologic. It is vital that we know what effect our therapy is likely to have on the patient, not only in terms of the objectives we are trying to achieve but also, equally as important, in terms of the effect upon organs or systems not directly related to the primary disease and in terms of unwanted adverse sequelae. It is a safe generalization to state that a form of treatment potent enough to alter or correct the progress of a disease is most apt to have some accompanying side effects that may be undesirable. We have already noted with emphasis the caution needed in the administration of oxygen and will now consider the physiologic responses, good and bad, to mechanical ventilation. The comments that follow will apply primarily to positive-pressure breathing, except where otherwise noted. For convenience, we will discuss separately the effects on *ventilation*, *circulation*, and *metabolism*.

### Effect on ventilation

With assisted mechanical ventilation we can generally expect an improvement in total ventilation, manifested by an increased minute breathing volume, improved alveolar ventilation, a better distribution of inspired gas, a normalization of blood gases, and a reduction in the patient's work of breathing. It should be apparent to the student that these responses are interrelated and depend on one another but that the degree to which any given one is favorably affected will be determined by the underlying disease and the effectiveness of the ventilator. It is most usual to expect an increase in minute volume and tidal volume, which are dynamic compartments of the total lung volumes, whereas changes in static volumes, the functional residual capacity and the residual volume, are more variable, depending on the bronchopulmonary condition.[273] Theoretically, all five of the functions noted above should be improved or stimulated by mechanical assistance, and if they are not, the cause will be one of the following: (1) The respiratory tract may present a severity of obstruction or a reduction in compliance beyond the ability of the ventilator to surmount. We have described enough of the principles and characteristics of ventilators for the student to accept the fact that such instruments are too severely limited in both scope and flexibility to compensate for all types of failure. (2) Most instances of inadequate mechanical ventilation in daily hospital practice are the result of the wrong choice of instrument for a given circumstance or improper technique in its administration. Both of these responsibilities require in-depth experience in assisted ventilation but are critical to successful therapy. It can be assumed as obvious now that the beneficial effects of mechanical ventilation can be realized only when consideration is given to the establishment of breathing rates and the use of flows consistent with the conducting potential of the airways, coordinated with just the proper delivery pressure. If the student looks into the growth history of positive-pressure breathing, he will encounter strong opposing views of its efficacy and safety, especially reported during its early years of use. There is little doubt, in retrospect, that many of the unfavorable opinions originated from failure to achieve satisfactory ventilation because the disease was untreatable with available equipment, the equipment was ill chosen, or especially because the equipment was not effectively used.

The relationship between the distribution of inspired gas in the lung, alveolar ventilation, and the correction of abnormal blood gases and pH is apparent, and in these areas positive-pressure breathing performs some of its most important functions. For the overall stabilization of ventilation, it is not enough merely to increase the gas flow to alveoli already ventilated if there are alveoli persistently nonventilated. A major contribution of PPB is its ability to effect a more normal and uniform distribution of inspired gas to all lung areas by opening up to gas exchange lobules and other pulmonary units that have been nonparticipating. This claim for PPB is made notwithstanding some opinions to the contrary. A study was made of voluntary hyperventilation and IPPB in normal subjects and patients with emphysema.[273] In the normals essentially equal increases in tidal volume were recorded during both hyperventilation and PPB assist, but in the patient group the increase in tidal volume was significantly greater with mechanical aid. In all subjects experiencing an increase in tidal volume, alveolar distribution of air was improved as measured by the nitrogen-washout test, and it is interesting to note that this distribution was improved in patients who could not hyperventilate spontaneously but needed the PPB assistance. In more precise physiologic terms there was an implied improvement in the ventilation/perfusion ratio. On the other hand, another group of patients was reported to show increases in alveolar-arterial oxygen tension differences during positive-pressure breathing.[274] This suggested that the inspired air was not normally distributed among the alveoli in relation to the alveolar perfusion. It was concluded that, since emphysema is characterized by an abnormal $\dot{V}/\dot{Q}$, PPB might not be expected to improve this relationship in lungs so diseased. However, in comparing divergent results, it is often difficult, if not impossible, to determine how uniform were the techniques employed; unless comparable equipment is used and close attention given to rates, flows, and pressures, comparison is on shaky ground. Many years of clinical observation substantiate the view that an improved $\dot{V}/\dot{Q}$ ratio incidental to better alveolar distribution of inspired gas is a significant result of properly applied PPB.

Thus improvement in alveolar ventilation, the major objective of the therapy of respiratory failure, coincides with bettering the $\dot{V}/\dot{Q}$ ratio. More effective alveolar ventilation is evidenced by a decrease in arterial blood carbon dioxide tension and an elevation of arterial blood pH. It must be noted that the effect of PPB on carbon dioxide and pH, well documented and universally accepted, does not necessarily depend upon its ability to expand the general distribution of inspired gas, discussed above. Such changes may be accomplished by the hyperventilation of existing functioning alveoli, taking advantage of the easy diffusibility of carbon dioxide. However, it has been aptly demonstrated that not only does PPB decrease the carbon dioxide but it also elevates the arterial blood oxygen tension of hypoxia, even when ambient air is the source gas without added oxygen.[275, 276] This was taken as evidence of an increased uniformity of alveolar ventilation and an improved $\dot{V}/\dot{Q}$ ratio.

Last, but by no means least, an important physiologic service of positive-pressure breathing is a significant reduction in the work energy expended by the patient in labored breathing. The respiratory therapist will frequently see the gratifying physical relaxation enjoyed by a patient as a mechanical ventilator assumes a major portion of his work. This response to assisted ventilation not rarely is sought to prevent a patient, still compensating, from slipping into failure from the cumulative effect of respiratory fatigue. Again, it must be strongly emphasized that merely subjecting a patient to mechanical ventilation does not assure him relief from his struggle to breathe, since unless properly administered, ventilatory "assistance" may seriously handicap him further. Obviously, to aid the patient and lessen his work, ventilation must be adequate for his needs. Although this may appear to be so basic as to be redundant, it is an aspect that must be carefully considered to prevent the spontaneously breathing patient from "fighting" the machine. Unless the ventilator can deliver inspired air rapidly enough, the patient will work harder to augment the gas from the instrument, and if flows are too rapid or forceful, the patient may oppose the gas with expiratory efforts. It has been noted that with pressures in excess of 25 cm of water, and with unadjusted flows, alveolar hypoventilation may persist, and the resulting struggle of the patient to get air can increase the work of breathing 250% without benefit.[267] An excellent investigation into the work of breathing explains how effective ventilation helps the patient.[274] It will be recalled that carbon dioxide is metabolically produced by contraction of muscles, including the muscles of ventilation. Indeed, in severe respiratory disability, the energy of all the muscles brought into use to move tidal air may account for a major portion of the carbon dioxide production as well as the oxygen utilization. In short, most of the patient's work may go into driving the machinery that supplies the body's energy fuel, leaving little for other activities. Also relevant to the discussion is the note that the more efficient a muscle is the less carbon dioxide it produces per unit of work performed compared with a less efficient muscle.

The level of arterial carbon dioxide tension is dependent upon both the production of $CO_2$ by the body and the effectiveness of alveolar ventilation and can be expressed in the following proportionality:

$$P_{a_{CO_2}} \cong \frac{\dot{V}_{CO_2}}{\dot{V}_A}$$

Reduction in the carbon dioxide tension is thus the result of increasing the alveolar ventilation or limiting the $CO_2$ production. In severe airway obstructive disease voluntary hyperventilation is not apt to decrease the arterial $CO_2$ tension significantly because the uneven alveolar ventilation accompanying obstruction prevents the deep breathing from improving the alveolar ventilation. If, by a strenuous effort, the patient is able to effect a better alveolar ventilation, the work involved will increase the $CO_2$ production simultaneously to maintain the same general proportion in the above equation. It has been determined that the muscles of respiration use one third less oxygen when passively moved; and thus positive-pressure ventilation increases the alveolar gas exchange, with less patient work, and without raising the $CO_2$ production.

### Effect on circulation

With the close functional and anatomic relationship between the respiratory and circulatory systems, it is not surprising that interference with the performance of one of them will affect the other. The great potential hazard of circulatory response to mechanical ventilation makes it mandatory for the therapist to understand fully what does and can happen to cardiovascular function when a patient is artificially ventilated.

In our study of the physiology of ventilation, we learned that ventilatory muscle contraction expands the diameters of the thorax, lowering the intrathoracic pressure so that ambient air flows into the lung. The pressure within the thoracic cavity is never above atmospheric with quiet breathing but, rather is slightly below even at the resting level, and it exceeds atmospheric only during forced exhalation as the expiratory reserve volume is moved. This is illustrated in the balloon-in-box sketches of Fig. 3-5, which depict the fluctuations of intrathoracic pressure from its average resting value of about $-5$ cm of water, with ventilatory excursions. The cardiovascular system is designed to function with its central power source, the heart, in a subatmospheric pressure, and as noted in Chapter 5, the "thoracic pump" is necessary for venous return to the heart and for an adequate cardiac output. Thus airflow into and out of the lungs and the circulation of blood to and from the heart are both accomplished most efficiently when the ventilatory cycle starts with a subatmospheric pressure that increases in negativity during inhalation and decreases during exhalation but never exceeds atmospheric except under conditions of stress. Obviously, this normal intrathoracic pressure environment is reversed when positive-pressure ventilation is employed, as inspiratory gas under pressure inflates the lung, raising the intrapulmonary pressure, which is then transmitted through the lung into the pleural "space" to elevate the intrathoracic pressure during inhalation. Passive exhalation returns the pressure to its resting subatmospheric level, as the patient exhales into the ambient atmosphere, and in a functional sense is temporarily disassociated from the machine. Fig. 9-25 is a schematic example of two sets of tidal volume curves, comparing the pressure relationships between normal spontaneous breathing and pressure ventilation. Here the resting level of voluntary ventilation is shown as $-2$ cm of water, and as air enters the lung, the pressure drops to $-7$ cm of water, a net pressure change of 5 cm of water; but the pressure at all points is below atmospheric. In contrast, the pressure-ventilated lung starts its cycle from the same resting level of $-2$ cm of water intrathoracic pressure, but as air is forced into the lung a driving pressure of 5 cm of water is transmitted through the alveoli to the pleural space, raising the intrathoracic pressure to 3 cm of water at end-inspiration. Here several points along the pressure curve are above atmospheric.

For completeness a differentiation should be made here between intra-alveolar and intrathoracic pressure fluctuations. As long as the airways are open in unassisted breathing, alveolar pressure immediately equilibrates with atmospheric whenever airflow stops. Thus at the two points of no flow, resting end-expiration (pre-inspiration) and end-inspiration, intra-alveolar pressure is zero gauge. With pressure breathing, positive pressure is maintained in the alveoli from the start of inspiration until the end-expiratory level is again reached. Fig. 9-26 compares alveolar pressures in these two circumstances.

The significance of intrathoracic pressure deviations in their effect on cardiovascular function is one of the most important clinical aspects of mechanical ventilation. During all phases of normal or abnormal pulmonary airflow, those elements of the circulatory system that are located in the thorax, especially the heart and large veins,

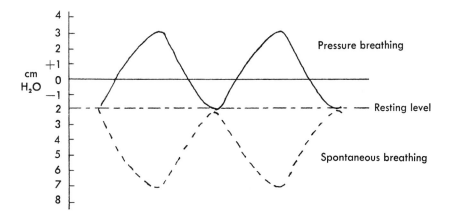

**Fig. 9-25.** Comparison of *intrathoracic pressure* in positive pressure and spontaneous tidal ventilation with driving pressures of 5 cm $H_2O$.

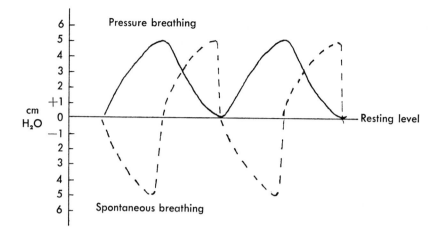

**Fig. 9-26.** Comparison of *intra-alveolar pressure* in positive pressure and spontaneous tidal ventilation with driving pressures of 5 cm $H_2O$.

are subjected to the ambient pressure generated in the thorax, so let us describe details of the circulatory response to both normal and pressure ventilation. The fall in intrathoracic pressure that accompanies a normal spontaneous inspiration enhances the flow of venous blood to the thoracic vessels and hence into the right atrium, increasing the right ventricular output and flow to the lungs. Temporarily, less blood moves from the lungs to the left atrium as the intrathoracic negative pressure fills up the pulmonary vessels, and left ventricular output falls. During passive exhalation, the events are reversed as the increasing (although still subatmospheric) intrathoracic pressure dampens venous return and right atrial filling and output but, at the same time, in a sense, squeezing blood from the pulmonary vessels to increase left atrial filling and left ventricular output. When the lung is ventilated under positive pressure, venous return, right atrial filling, and pulmonary blood flow are impaired; but the pressure squeezing the lung, now during inspiration, increases left heart filling and output. However, this lasts for but a few heart strokes, and if the pressure is continued, flow to and from the left heart falls. Exhalation lets the intrathoracic pressure return to normal, encouraging venous return and an increase in pulmonary flow but retarding left ventricular output. Let us compare these sequences in natural and pressure breathing. During normal spontaneous ventilation, the fluctuations in intrathoracic blood flow are rhythmically synchronized with the breathing pattern, a decrease in one component during inhalation increasing during exhalation, and so on. Thus, whereas venous return accelerates in inhalation and left ventricular output falls, both are reversed in exhalation; the net result, cycle after cycle, is a smooth-flowing circulation. The same description can be given of pressure breathing, with the time sequences of the kinetics turned about, but the efficiency of the net result is markedly modified by one significant factor—supra-atmospheric pressure. Several excellent studies have clarified the effect of positive pressure on circulation to explain why such pressure interferes with cardiac function, and we will consider the relevant data.[277-282]

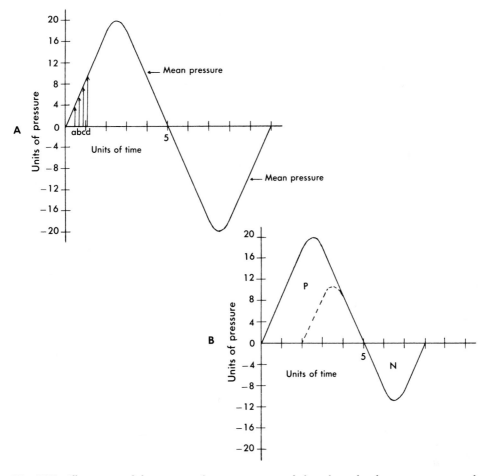

**Fig. 9-27.** Illustrations of the concept of mean pressure and the relationship between pressure and time. **A,** Sketch of a sine curve, **B,** Asymmetric biphasic curve. (See text for description.)

It is necessary to understand the concepts of *mean pressure* and the *pressure-time relationship,* since they are the keys to the problem. Fig. 9-27, *A,* is a biphasic sinelike curve, plotting positive and negative pressures against arbitrary units of time, first traveling from its starting point to a peak pressure of 20 and back to zero pressure in 5 time units then dropping to −20 units of pressure and back in another 5 time units. For the first 5 time units, positive pressure is being exerted, and for the last 5, negative pressure of the same magnitude. As we look at the curve, our common sense tells us that the net or final result of these two opposing pressures will be to negate one another, since they will average out to zero. The *mean* pressure of the entire cycle then will be zero, since means is an arithmetical average. Each half of the curve has its own mean pressure, which is easy to visualize because of the regularity of the curve, but this is not so in curves with changing contours. The mean value of any curve is the average of an infinite number of points along the curve (*a, b, c, d,* etc., in Fig. 9-27, *A*), and although we cannot measure an infinite number of values, the more that are measured, the more accurate will be the calculation. In practice, the calculation of the mean of an irregular curve is done by methods of mathematical calculus or with accurate and rapid electronic calculators, necessary instruments in the modern laboratory. It is obvious in our illustration that the mean pressure of the terminal half of the curve is the same as that of the first but with the opposite sign. If we refer back to Fig. 9-25, we can see that the mean pressure of the upper, positive ventilatory pattern is 0.5 cm of water, whereas that of natural breathing is $-4.5$ cm of water (the resting level is already at $-2$ cm $H_2O$). The *pressure-time relationship* is the length of time that a pressure is active and refers to the duration of a mean pressure. For example, in the first half of Fig. 9-27, *A*, the pressure continuously changes from time 0 to time 5, but it represents a mean pressure of 10, for 5 time units; and the second half of the curve represents a mean of $-10$ units of pressure for another 5 units of time. The same interpretations can be derived for the tidal excursions of Fig. 9-25.

It may be evident at this stage that whatever effect pressure will have on circulation will be directly related to the mean pressure to which the circulation is exposed and to the time of this exposure or, in other words, the pressure-time effect. In ventilation the time interval is the duration of the respiratory cycle, or its components, and the pressure is the intrathoracic, which in clinical practice must be measured indirectly. It was noted in the earlier discussion of the lung-thorax relation and compliance that to avoid the risks of a direct measurement of intrathoracic pressure, esophageal pressure is often used, since it reflects changes within the chest, but the student will frequently see reference to *mask pressure* and *mouth pressure* in relation to the kinetics of mechanical ventilation. They refer to the pressure of the ventilating gas as measured at the subject's mouth or administering appliance or the pressure in the trachea of patients who have been intubated. Although the mask pressure is not quantitatively the same as the intrathoracic pressure, the mean values of both are linearly related and thus can be used interchangeably to monitor qualitative changes. When using mask or mouth pressures, the student should remember that the end-expiratory level will be at zero gauge, not subatmospheric.

In Fig. 9-27, *B*, let us consider the positive segment to represent the pressure-time curve of a positive-pressure ventilator generating an arbitrary maximum mask pressure over a 5-unit time period. Regardless of what the mean pressure might be, in a general way the area under the curve *(P)* can be thought of as proportional to the pressure-time effect of the ventilatory pattern, since it represents the total pressure for the total time. The larger the area under a given pressure curve the greater potential effect it will have on circulation. Let us now imagine a subatmospheric pressure applied to the patient's airway during exhalation that lowers the mask pressure as indicated by the last part of the curve, enclosing pressure-time area *(N)*. The net circulatory effect of the pressure over the entire cycle will be proportional to the difference between the areas *P* and *N*, graphically depicted by superimposing *N* on *P*, with the dotted outline. The mean mask pressure for the whole ventilatory cycle has been lowered by the addition of terminal negative pressure, proportionately reducing the effect on circulation that would be expected from the original pressure.

At this point we might pause and summarize our information on the circulatory response to positive intrathoracic pressure. We can say that the determining factor is the relation between the height of the mean intrathoracic (or mask) pressure and the duration of pressure, and we know that the total mean cycle pressure can be kept low by the addition of negative mask pressure during exhalation. In the above description of the circulatory sequences through the natural or pressure-generated ventilatory cycle, we noted the different effects on right and left hearts, depending upon the respiratory phase.

However, the picture can be simplified and the "meat" of the matter illustrated in its crudest form as shown in Fig. 9-28, which demonstrates the basic relationship between intrathoracic pressure and the circulation. The thorax is represented by a box with a gas inlet, containing the heart and major vessels. To avoid clutter in the illustration, the lungs are not included although this does not imply that they play no role. It is assumed, however, that whatever pressure is delivered to the lungs is readily and fully transmitted to the thoracic cavity. Exceptions to this assumption will be noted later. Both diagrams depict inhalation *(A)* during natural spontaneous breathing and *(B)* during positive-pressure ventilation. Despite the circulatory fluctuations during each ventilatory cycle, the mean intrathoracic pressure of natural breathing is sub-atmospheric; thus the net presure effect on blood flow is that of low pressure. This is indicated by the negative sign within the chest cavity and the effect of this *mean negativity* on circulation. Venous return is enhanced, and the negative pressure is shown as

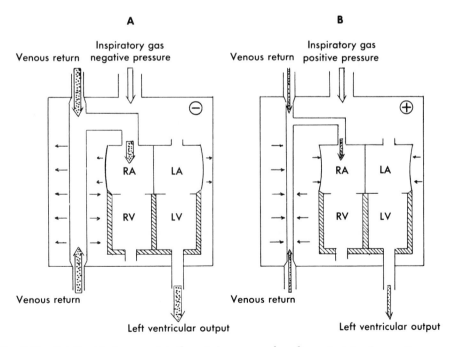

**Fig. 9-28.** Relationship between intrathoracic pressure and cardiac output in, **A,** negative-pressure and, **B,** positive-pressure breathing. (Details are explained in the text.)

dilating the intrathoracic veins and encouraging filling of the atria. In contrast, positive-pressure inhalation produces a higher, or relatively positive, mean intrathoracic pressure, the net circulatory effect of which is just the opposite of natural breathing. The *mean positivity* in the chest depresses venous return by blocking its flow into the thoracic veins. The student is encouraged to consider the conditions demonstrated in Fig. 9-28, *A*, as the normal status, the natural environment in which the heart and supporting vessels developed and grew. In this environment the circulatory dynamics of both inspiration and expiration are such that the body's needs are most efficiently met. It is not so much that the mean negative pressure of spontaneous breathing excessively encourages venous return and a subsequent increase above normal of left ventricular output as it is that *deviations* from the normal mean intrathoracic pressure adversely affect the circulatory efficiency. Therefore, in the positive–pressure breathing of Fig. 9-28, *B*, regardless of whether the left heart filling and output may be temporarily increased by the rising pressure in the thorax, the net effect of subjecting the heart and its tributary veins to an abnormally high mean pressure is to impede venous return and to reduce the arterial blood supplied to the systemic circulation.

When venous blood flows toward the heart from the peripheral areas of the body and encounters an abnormally high pressure as it attempts to enter the thoracic vessels, portions of it will pool in vascular reservoirs, mostly in the huge network of veins and capillaries of the abdominal organs.[283] This can effectively remove from circulation a volume of blood large enough to reduce the left ventricular output, as noted above, and constitute a serious potential danger to the hypoxic patient by reducing his cerebral blood flow and further compromising the oxygen supply to his brain. Lesser degrees of the effect of excessively high intrathoracic pressure on cerebral blood flow can be demonstrated in the normal subject by voluntary breath holding at end-inspiration while exerting a strong expiratory effort against the closed glottis. Impaired venous return is manifested by distended neck veins, suffusion of the facial skin, and eventual loss of consciousness or at least faintness. In the mechanically ventilated patient, continued interference with venous return and left ventricular output can lead to a full-blown state of clinical shock, with all the signs and symptoms described for this condition earlier. When precipitated by mechanical ventilation, such vascular collapse is termed *respirator shock*.

So far we have been concerned only with the mechanisms responsible for the physiologic influence of intrathoracic pressure on the circulation, but let us now see how important all of this is in clinical medicine to which the respiratory therapist is exposed. Data from the references cited at the beginning of this discussion, as well as from the observations of those who have managed patients under mechanical ventilation, attest to the reality of this phenomenon. When the mean mask delivery pressure exceeds 7 cm of water, there is a measurable decrease in the left ventricular output, although it need not be clinically evident.[277] In relaxed patients without specific bronchopulmonary disease who were ventilated at a fixed tidal volume and rate, measurement of the mean intrathoracic pressure showed an elevation above normal, ranging from 3.5 to 6 cm of water.[278] The degree to which circulation is impaired and the risk there is in store for the patient are dependent upon three modifying factors in addition to the level of pressure.

*Cardiac status.* The integrity of the heart and circulatory system is an important influence on the effect of an increased intrathoracic pressure. As noted above, even small pressures interfere with cardiac output, and it can be anticipated that anyone subjected to pressure will be so affected. However, the normal healthy heart has a great functional reserve and can tolerate considerable resistance to its action. There is no rule to follow to estimate the risk of circulatory depression from pressure breathing, and the large majority of patients so treated suffer no apparent ill effects. Some have been supported on positive-pressure ventilation for several consecutive weeks without evidence of a compromised circulation. There is no doubt that the patient with overt or potential cardiac disease is a high-risk candidate for trouble. Part of the management of the ventilated patient is a close surveillance of his cardiac condition, with appropriate measures taken to support a failing heart so that the needed ventilation can be carried out. Certainly, a circulatory complication might be considered a more likely possibility in an elderly patient than in a young one or in a patient with long-standing pulmonary disease than in one with a new, acute disease. It is this varying response of each individual and the uncertainty of his reaction to the pressure of mechanical ventilation that make skillful and intelligent management the keys to successful therapy.

*Pulmonary status.* Positive pressure generated in a ventilator flows into the alveoli and from there is transmitted across alveolar walls to the thoracic cavity. The ease and the degree to which such transpulmonary transmission of pressure occurs are a function of the physical state of the lung. The more compliant the lung, the more readily will intrapulmonary pressure carry into the thorax, since the flexible lung easily responds to pressure applied to it. The patient with normal bronchi and lungs who needs mechanical ventilatory for nonpulmonary hypoventilation is the most likely to demonstrate circulatory interference, a risk greatly enhanced, of course, by concomitant heart disease. In contrast, the patient whose disease has left his lung relatively stiff, with significant loss of compliance, is least likely to transmit intrapulmonary pressure to the thoracic cavity. His lungs can tolerate high positive pressures and need such force to move an adequate tidal volume of air. However, such a patient is not free of hazard, since the pressure needed to distend the alveoli also compresses the pulmonary capillaries embedded in alveolar walls, impedes blood flow, and stresses the right ventricle with increased resistance. On the other hand, should the compliance of the chest wall rather than the lung be reduced, there will be a rapid transmission of pressure to the thorax as expansion of the latter is limited. Perhaps the therapist can visualize the difficulty in ventilating a patient with basically normal lungs but whose chest wall is partially immobilized by pain or injury or even extensive postoperative dressings. The compliant lungs and noncompliant rib cage will combine to generate the maximum intrathoracic pressure for any given mask pressure. Finally, allied to the reduced chest wall compliance just described is the resistance to ventilation of the agitated or unrelaxed patient who may have no intrinsic thoracic disability. The patient who "fights" the instrument because poor technique denies him an adequate flow or who is wittingly or otherwise uncooperative will have increased transmission of intrapulmonary pressure. His muscular activity prevents the necessary chest wall (and diaphragmatic) flexibility for compliant submission to a developing intrathoracic pressure.

*Ventilatory pattern.* The pattern by which positive-pressured air is delivered to a patient incorporates the concept of the pressure-time effect, recently discussed, but applies it to the practical use of mechanical ventilation. Attention was drawn to the importance of pattern when it was observed that a rise in intrathoracic pressure during positive-pressure breathing could be kept minimal if the inspiratory phase was limited to no more than one third the total cycle time. When we now relate pressure and time to the physiologic process of ventilation, the matter is not as simple as our definition and graphic representation of peak and mean pressures, and it becomes evident that an effective ventilatory pressure-time pattern must be more complex than those used in Fig. 9-27.

The immediate effect of elevated intrathoracic pressure is to interfere with right atrial filling and subsequently to reduce left ventricular output. Thus each atrial diastole is a point of time during which pressure may exert its influence on venous return, and there is another important relationship to consider, that between cardiac rate and the pressure-time curve. Fig. 9-29 is designed to demonstrate the potential differences in cardiac response to various combinations of the cardiac rhythm and pressure. The vertical bars at the top of the sketches indicate the times of atrial diastole in a heart with a rate of 60 beats per minute, the small arrows showing where each atrial diastole falls in the ventilatory cycle. For the sake of comparative uniformity the oblique first arrow represents the last atrial diastole of the previous ventilatory cycle; thus each cycle is correlated with four diastoles. Generation and degeneration of pressure follow linear paths in the three triangular ventilatory patterns of *A*, *B*, and *C*, and the mean pressure of each is necessarily 10 units, since the range is from 0 to 20 units. In curve *A* the final mean pressure affecting the four diastoles is the same as that of the total cycle, that is, 10 units, and even though inspiratory time is reduced in *B*, the pressure mean of the points of diastole is unchanged. Because of the relationship between the

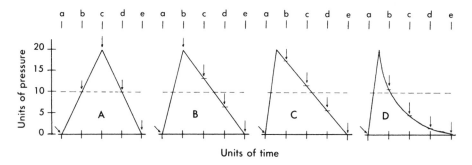

**Fig. 9-29.** Diagrams illustrating the effect of the relationship between cardiac diastoles and the intrathoracic pressure curve of positive-pressure breathing upon the resulting mean pressures affecting cardiac output. (See text for details.)

heart rhythm and ventilatory time intervals, the student who remembers geometry can see that the diastolic pressure means in both these sketches must be identical. A further, sharp reduction in the inspiratory time of *C*, however, changes the diastole-pressure relation, and the mean of the pressures coinciding with the diastoles has here dropped to 8 units. Careful examination of these illustrations should make it apparent that when diastole occurs with the peak pressure, the mean will be the same as the mean of the cycle. This clear-cut relationship is easy to see in the examples used, the data for which were chosen for simplicity, but with any combination of cardiac rate and ventilatory cycle, it can be demonstrated that the average of diastole-associated pressures will be lower if a diastole does not coincide with peak pressure and if a maximum number of diastoles fall in low-pressure areas of the cycle. This view of the relation of positive intrathoracic pressure and heart action is more of academic interest than anything else, since it is not practical to attempt to correlate the two clinically; but it does give emphasis to the fact that mechanical ventilation has a significant effect on circulation.

The next step in our discussion is of great clinical importance, however. Fortunately, passive exhalation does not follow the simple linear deceleration of the sketches used so far but has a configuration more like that of Fig. 9-29, *D*, somewhat exaggerated.[17] The curved contour of exhalation makes for an early drop in pressure and a reduction of mean pressure during exhalation. Although the mean *inspiratory* pressure of *D* is 10 units, as in the other patterns, more of the *exhalation* curve lies below the 10 units pressure line, showing that mean exhalation pressure is something less than 10 units. It is not necessary mathematically to try to calculate the mean of the curved pressure-drop line, as long as the ventilatory and circulatory advantages of this configuration are appreciated by the student. The projections of diastoles *c* and *d* fall well below the 10 units pressure level so that mean intrathoracic pressure affecting atrial diastolic filling is the least in *D* of the four patterns illustrated. The student should note that the time relationships of *C* and *D* are the same and that the projections of the atrial diastoles of *D* onto the lower pressure levels are entirely due to the curved shape of the exhalation line. Apart from changing the diastole-pressure relation, the transformation from a straight to curved exhalation line decreases the important pressure-time relation, since the area under sketch *D* is less than the area of the others, and for all practical purposes this is the major contribution of such a ventilation pattern. Modern mechanical ventilators allow the operator great flexibility in determining the most advantageous pressure-time curves for each patient's ventilatory and cardiac status, which is a critical consideration in treating the patient in failure.

The curves in Fig. 9-30 illustrate three clinical points. The patient ventilated by curve *a* experiences a rapid buildup in his intrathoracic pressure, which is held as a plateau for a major portion of his cycle before falling precipitiously. The area under this curve is extensive, implying the prolonged exposure of the intrathoracic circulatory system to the steady effects of a high mean pressure. Maximum interference with venous return and consequent left ventricular output can be anticipated from such a pattern. Later we will describe a clinical condition for which such a pressure-time curve is highly therapeutic, but for our present purposes we can consider it a

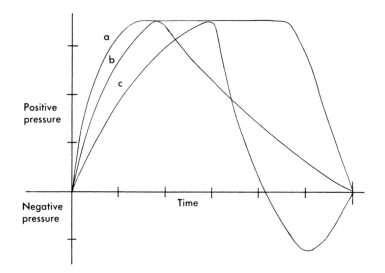

**Fig. 9-30.** Three pressure-time ventilatory patterns with the same range of positive pressure. Curve *a*, with its sustained peak pressure, has the greatest total pressure effect on circulation. Curve *b* reduces pressure-time by a slower rise and immediate descent. Curve *c* uses terminal negative pressure to offset some of the positive-pressure effect.

serious hazard. Pattern *b* demonstrates a marked modification of pattern *a*. The inspiratory time is slightly prolonged but is still less than one third the cycle, and it delays somewhat the initial exposure of the circulation to high pressure. The key difference in these two patterns is the immediate drop in pressure as soon as peak has been reached and the rapid falloff to the end of exhalation. The effect on the circulation of curve *b* would be less than that of curve *a* to the same degree that the area under *b* is smaller than the area under *a*. There are occasions when inspiratory needs cannot be fulfilled in the early one third of the cycle because factors of obstruction and low compliance necessitate longer inflationary periods. If possible, duration of exhalation is increased accordingly to maintain a favorable inspiratory/expiratory ratio of 1:1.5 or 1:2 to keep the mean pressure down, but sometimes in assisted ventilation the patient will not tolerate the resulting reduction in ventilatory rate. In such a case, should the prolonged inspiration pose a threat of reduced cardiac output, terminal expiratory negative pressure can be introduced into the system, as in curve *c*. Such a precaution is also applicable to any situation in which, even with a well-balanced ventilatory ratio, cardiac action is embarrassed from other causes. The rapid drop in pressure to below atmospheric increases the venous return during exhalation to make up for a deficit incurred during inspiration. Employing the concept of net pressure referred to earlier, it can be seen that the final effective mean intrathoracic pressure of this type of curve is proportional to the difference between the areas under the curve, above and below the zero line.

Let us summarize the physiologic effect of positive-pressure ventilation on the circulatory system from a clinical viewpoint. Although the primary objective of mechanical ventilation is to ensure an adequate tidal alveolar air exchange, the therapist must always be aware of the side effects of such treatment, especially on cardiac function. When considered over cycle after cycle, the supra-atmospheric pressure generated in the patient's chest retards the return of venous blood to the right atrium. The important consequence of this is a drop in the cardiac output, with eventual reduced circulating systemic flow that may develop into a full-blown circulatory collapse or shock. The normal heart can tolerate the restrictive action of high mean intrathoracic pressure for prolonged periods of time, but a heart actually or potentially weakened from disease or one subjected to excessively high pressure may be seriously affected. The degree to which venous return is impeded is proportional to the height of the mean pressure developed in the thorax and the length of time such pressure continues. This gives rise to the concept of the pressure-time relationship, which in a given circumstance with available data on instant-to-instant pressure and time, can be graphically expressed as a curve by plotting pressure against ventilatory cycle time.

The inspiratory-to-expiratory time ratio is an important factor in assuring adequate ventilation while minimizing the adverse circulatory effects of positive pressure. In general, if an I/E ratio is established so that expiration is longer than inspiration, the mean intrathoracic pressure will be lowered to a level of relative safety. The setting of an I/E ratio requires skill, understanding, and patience of the operator, for the final ventilatory pattern must be able to satisfy inspiratory needs while keeping inspiratory pressure time to a minimum. In our discussion of ventilators, we described the mechanisms for adjusting inspiratory and expiratory times in some of them and found that others had fixed I/E ratios.

*Negative pressure* during exhalation is available to produce the maximum reduction of mean intrathoracic pressure. Generated by a venturi, 3 to 5 cm of water subatmospheric pressure applied to the airways, when used with a favorable I/E ratio, can reduce the mean pressure in the chest almost to atmospheric. For reasons to be noted below, negative pressure in exhalation should not be used on a routine basis but reserved for those patients in whom peripheral cardiovascular collapse is an immediate or actual threat. Its use is monitored by close observation of heart rate and blood pressure, and elevation of the first with depression of the second in a patient maintained on positive-pressure ventilation is a most probable indication for instituting negative pressure, regardless of the cause of cardiac dysfunction. Although all other appropriate measures to combat shock are also used, it is not uncommon to observe how easily the stability of the blood pressure can be manipulated by varying the combination of positive and negative pressures.

Artificially induced subatmospheric airway pressure is not without its own inherent hazards, and because it entails a calculated risk its use is restricted to the support of failing circulation only. The two potential dangers of negative expiratory pressure are *air trapping* and *pulmonary edema*. Fig. 6-2 can be used to illustrate the risk of air trapping if we visualize the ventilatory pressures as intraluminal, with positive pressure inflating the alveolus and negative pressure deflating it. The illustrated bronchiolar collapse due to extraluminal positive pressure would then be caused by intra-luminal negative pressure. This hazard is especially great in patients with chronic bronchopulmonary disease, in whom diseased airways are a major characteristic and many of the smaller passages lack enough connective tissue support to maintain their integrity in the face of subatmospheric pressure. The therapist can understand the seriousness of further restricting the alveolar gas exchange in a patient already in ventilatory failure by cutting short his exhalation with airway collapse, retaining air in his lungs and significantly elevating his functional residual capacity. This is why it is necessary to reject the temptation to use negative pressure as a means of aspirating secretions or overcoming airway obstruction, for the suction needed to accomplish these objectives is just as apt to have the opposite effect. The risk of air trapping can be minimized by introducing subatmospheric pressure gradually and limiting it to the least that will achieve the desired purpose.

Negative intrapulmonary pressure also subjects the patient to the danger of pul-monary edema. Like the effect of positive pressure on venous return, the probability of circulatory harm from negative pressure depends on the general health and stability of the pulmonary circulation. Venous return is greatly enhanced during the negative-pressure phase of exhalation as the mean intrathoracic pressure precipitously drops and the pulmonary vasculature fills with blood, creating at least a temporary state of pulmonary congestion. Should some defective function of the left heart make it slow to accept the pulmonary venous outflow, pulmonary vascular hydrostatic pressure will rise and the gradient between the high intravascular pressure and the subatmospheric intra-alveolar pressure will force blood water into the alveoli. The same condition can prevail without an undue rise in hydrostatic pressure if there is an abnormal increase in the permeability of the pulmonary capillaries so that the usually well-tolerated cap-illary to alveolar–pressure gradient is enough to move fluid from circulation to alveoli. The therapist working in a hospital with a busy pulmonary service will occasionally encounter one of the most difficult patients to ventilate because of a serious physio-logic paradox. This is the patient with severe obstruction or impaired compliance who needs relatively high pressure for alveolar ventilation but who has concurrent heart disease, often with myocardial damage from an inadequate coronary artery circulation. Because of the unstable cardiovascular system, not only do high ventilatory pressures easily embarrass venous return and precipitate respirator shock but the corrective measure of expiratory negative pressure induces pulmonary edema. In an extreme example of such a patient, the adjustment of the negative pressure within the range of only a few centimeters of water may find a dropping blood pressure and dry lungs re-placed by a rising pressure but accompanied by the wet lungs of edema. The careful and delicate titration of positive and negative pressures against alveolar ventilation and circulatory stability requires the ultimate in physiologic understanding and technical proficiency.

Our discussion of the effect of mechanical ventilation on circulation would not be complete unless we commented on this relationship in *negative-pressure* breathing for comparison. After the above discussion of the action of positive-pressure ventilation, the student may be surprised to be told that the same deleterious effect can be found in the patient treated by a tank respirator. In our description of this instrument, we noted that chest expansion and subsequent pulmonary inflation result from the action of subatmospheric pressure on the external surface of the thorax, and the comment was made that this principle is more nearly like that of natural breathing than is positive-pressure breathing. This was a valid observation, since with this technique, intrathoracic pressure never exceeds atmospheric, but there is another factor. If we refer to Fig. 3-15, we will see that in the body respirator negative pressure is applied not only to the thorax but to the rest of the body as well, with the exception of the head and neck. However, because of the relative flexibility of the abdomen compared with the chest, the pressure is readily transmitted into the former, and this is not physiologically similar to natural breathing when inspiration generates positive intra-abdominal pressure. The drop in abdominal pressure destroys the normal gradient from abdomen to thorax that aids the return of venous blood to the heart. In consequence there is a dilatation of the vast network of abdominal capillaries, as described above in reference to positive-pressure breathing, and pooling of venous blood. Just as with positive-pressure ventilation, the pooled blood is effectively removed from circulation, reducing right atrial filling and ventricular output. Thus the same hazard of circulatory failure is encountered in both types of ventilation. During the years of the poliomyelitis epidemics, when body respirators were extensively used, the circulatory depression caused by distal venous pooling was called "tank shock." With the large number of patients so treated, this complication undoubtedly would have been more prevalent than it was except that most of the patients were young, with good cardiovascular function. The student can now see an advantage of the chest cuirass other than convenience, since with subatmospheric pressure applied only to the thorax, the circulatory insufficiency produced by both intrapulmonary positive and body surface negative pressures is circumvented.

### Effect on metabolism

In this context, *metabolism* is used to include the function of systems other than the cardiorespiratory system and responses of that system other than those included in the above discussion. An acute and progressively deteriorating state similar to the respiratory distress syndrome in infants has been described in some patients supported by continuous positive-pressure ventilation.[284] Affected patients demonstrate severe dyspnea, tachypnea, hypoxemia refractory to oxygen administration, a large alveolar-arterial oxygen tension gradient, a loss of pulmonary compliance, and a chest x-ray film identical to that seen in acute pulmonary edema. We have considered the damage sustained by the lung after exposure to high oxygen tensions, but in the patients under discussion, unusually high concentrations of oxygen were not used and oxygen toxicity was not considered the cause. With a variety of underlying diseases necessitating mechanical ventilation, it was postulated that damage to pulmonary surface-active material might be responsible for the precipitous loss of lung function. A comprehensive study was made of this condition, reviewing the pulmonary and metabolic status of 100 patients undergoing prolonged mechanical ventilation.[285] In addition to the signs and symptoms noted above, nineteen of these patients exhibited a significant retention of body water and either a weight gain or failure to lose weight as anticipated. Also, they showed a drop in concentration of serum sodium (hyponatremia) and a reduction in hematocrit, both consistent with an increase in blood volume (hypervolemia) due to retained water (hydremia). This clinical state is called the *adult respiratory distress syndrome (ARDS)*, and being a syndrome, may have a score of etiologies. We are noting it here because two of its outstanding characteristics, progressive hypoxemia and decreasing compliance, may make a patient who is so affected the most difficult to manage. Mechanical ventilation itself does not cause ARDS, but associated water retention can.

An association between pressure breathing, both positive and negative, and kidney function has long been recognized. A normal subject under continuous positive-pressure breathing may experience a reduction in urinary flow as much as 50%, attributed to a reduced renal blood flow, whereas negative-pressure breathing induces an increased in these functions.[286, 287] It was suggested that renal circulation is at least temporarily compromised to compensate for circulatory deficiencies during the stress of positive-pressure ventilation and that one of the mechanisms involved may be an alteration in the so-called *antidiuretic hormone* (ADH). This is a substance secreted by the pituitary gland that is instrumental in regulating body fluid content and concentration by appropriate adjustment of urinary output. By virtue of its name, one can see that the more hormone present the less excretion of urine and the greater retention of water there will be. The relation of the action of ADH to the patient undergoing mechanical ventilation may lie in the experimental observation that vagal reflexes from the cardiac atria seem to influence ADH activity in response to pressure changes in the atria, and we now know that positive-pressure ventilation markedly alters right heart blood flow and pressure.[288]

Thus, as pointed out in the study noted above,[285] a potentially serious physiologic effect of mechanical ventilation may be the disturbance of the usual body fluid–ADH balance and the selective accumulation of abnormal amounts of water in the lungs, since peripheral edema is not noticeable in the absence of frank cardiac failure. The latter cannot always be ruled out, but the degree of pulmonary fluid appears out of proportion to the sparse indications for heart failure. Certainly the interference with pulmonary function in these patients can reasonably be attributed to pulmonary congestion and edema, an interpretation confirmed by the often rapid and dramatic improvement in the clinical condition and the x-ray picture of the lungs after the administration of a diuretic. It is obvious that management of the ventilated patient must include close attention to maintaining a safe balance between fluid intake and output, since although dehydration must be avoided, so must the risk of overhydration in the event of an increase in ADH activity.

The therapist may feel confused by the apparent paradox of positive-pressure breathing acting to limit the blood volume of the lung as described under its circulatory effects and also precipitating pulmonary edema as just noted. In our first consideration of the physiologic action of positive-pressure breathing, we described the usual, or expected, effect of pressure, whereas the hazardous metabolic disturbances accompany long-term ventilation, during which many of the body's reserve functions and compensations become depleted. This underscores the lability of physiologic response, especially under the stress of severe disease, and emphasizes the need for intelligent observation of the patient, with an awareness of the possible complications that may develop.

# Chapter 10

# RESPIRATORY THERAPY MANAGEMENT OF VENTILATORY FAILURE

Ventilatory failure is a multisystem derangement even though it focuses so dramatically on the function of the lung, and its successful management involves several facets of therapy. In patients with inadequate ventilation, good nursing is a critical factor, nutrition and fluid needs must be met, the control of infection may determine the eventual prognosis, and special care must often be given to cardiac function. Our interest is limited to those aspects of treatment that directly relate to the responsibility of the respiratory therapist. However, he must be aware of and understand the purpose of the efforts and the concern of other medical disciplines involved. Cooperation among members of the medical team is essential, and the rapport among themselves is as important as that between them and the patient. We will discuss such aspects of the management of failure as *airway patency, selection of ventilators, ventilatory patterns, monitoring ventilation,* and *positive-pressure breathing.* Unavoidably, there will be repetition and many references to material previously discussed in other chapters as well as cross-references among the subtopics themselves. However, we will use this to good advantage and summarize and correlate many principles of physiology and therapy and showing their practical application to patient care.

## IMPORTANCE OF PATENT AIRWAYS

By now we have been well oriented toward the great hazard of airway obstruction and its pathologic origins and can justifiably relate it to the problems of assisting the patient in ventilatory failure by the following dictum: *The effectiveness of mechanical ventilation is directly proportional to the patency of the airways.* The importance of the health of the bronchial tree gives it priority in our discussion. Airway obstruction is a major obstacle to ventilation and an almost constant challenge to the skill of the respiratory therapist—obvious in the patient suffering from chronic bronchopulmonary disease or insidiously developing in a patient otherwise afflicted. Not only is the attempt to administer artificial ventilation against severe obstruction usually futile but the efforts may be demonstrably harmful. Such an attempt may cause a serious increase in dead space ventilation and reduce effective alveolar tidal exchange, since the mechanically driven air rapidly generates back pressure to shorten inspiratory time. It may also encourage air trapping, with a subsequent increase in functional residual capacity and an elevation in the resting level, further burdening a lung that may already be abnormally distended.

Before instituting ventilation, the therapist should make an estimate of the status of the patient's airways. This in no way conflicts with the role of the attending physician, nor does it usurp any of his function; since if the therapist is to carry the burden of supervising therapy, it is the therapist's right and obligation to become acquainted with the problem he faces. The therapist should learn something of the patient's background, either from the physician directly or through a study of the clinical chart, to determine whether airway obstruction has been a clinical feature. A significant smoking history may be a valuable warning clue in the patient with no apparent current obstruction; it should caution the therapist to be on the alert for a later complication. At the bedside the experienced therapist can listen for telltale gross wheezes or rhonchi and, if in doubt, he can use the stethoscope for better evaluation. Once therapy is under way, indications of obstruction should always be sought. Periodic observation of the assisted patient's ventilation should reveal if exhalation is unduly prolonged or effortful, if the pattern is irregular, or if the rate significantly increases. In the assisted or controlled patient, obstruction may be evidenced by marked shortening of inspiratory time, noted by listening to the cycling of the machine. Air trapping can often be detected by slowing of a tidal volume–metering device to reach its end-expiratory base line or by an elevation of this base line.

The pharmacologic agents most frequently used in the treatment of airway obstruction were covered in earlier pages, and we will now consider the mechanical techniques available that may be used before the start of ventilation or introduced into the program at any time needed. The three important procedures with which we must be familiar are *bronchoscopy, intubation,* and *tracheobronchial aspiration.*

## Bronchoscopy

Two types of bronchoscopy are now in widespread use—rigid, and flexible, or fiberoptic, bronchoscopy. There are similarities and differences in the instruments used, their indications, and techniques. We will first describe the older procedure, the introduction of the rigid scope into the airways.

*Rigid bronchoscopy.* Bronchoscopy is a procedure that is both therapeutic and diagnostic, requiring the services of a skilled and experienced physician, usually a specialist in the fields of either otorhinolaryngology (diseases of the ear, nose, and throat) or thoracic surgery. It is extensively used for direct visual examination of a suspected lesion in the bronchial tree or of one previously noted by x-ray examination. If the lesion is available, the bronchoscopist can often remove a small specimen (biopsy) for histologic examination. The instrument is a long, lighted telescopic tube, with a tip that can be rotated through several degrees by remote control, and provided with lenses for looking into bronchial orifices. The procedure is usually performed in a room provided for it, although in extraordinary emergency situations it can be done at the bedside. The pharynx and larynx are locally anesthetized and, with the patient supine and head hyperextended, the operator introduces the tube through the mouth into the airway. Each side is examined in turn, and as the instrument is advanced deep into the main bronchi, the orifices of the branches are visualized. A long metal aspirator is inserted down the tube and secretions are sucked out; often large plugs that may have obstructed large bronchi are removed.

The value of bronchoscopy in treating and preventing serious atelectasis is obvious. Because the procedure is carried out under sterile precautions, the secretions obtained can be cultured to determine the extent of any infectious process that may be active. In many patients suffering acute obstruction from secretions, a single drainage by this technique is often adequate, but if the disease is extensive enough to require repeated suctioning, other methods to be described below are preferred. Certainly, bronchoscopy is the most direct approach to the problem of excessive secretions, but it has little if any value in diffuse bronchospastic obstruction. Indeed, the mechanical irritation of the procedure itself may precipitate or worsen bronchial spasm. There are varying degrees of patient discomfort, both during and after the procedure; many patients complain of soreness of the throat for several hours. The introduction of the instrument into the respiratory tract constitutes an obstruction to breathing, and this can be a serious hazard to the patient already severely hypoxic. Finally, when rapid relief of acute obstruction is needed, the responsible personnel may not be immediately available for the most opportune use of bronchoscopy, and delay may not be justified. Major problems with the rigid bronchoscope include its instability to reach all bronchi easily, its potential risk for inflicting patient injury, and the need for a special room for its use. Of the two types of bronchoscopies, however, the rigid procedure is the more useful in recovering biopsy material or foreign bodies and for controlling intrabronchial bleeding.

***Flexible (fiberoptic) bronchoscopy.*** Endobronchial examinations and therapy enjoyed giant steps forward with the application of fiberoptic technology to medicine. Fiberoptic instruments basically consist of bundles of large numbers of fine glass fibers, each fiber capable of transmitting light. When connected to an electrical light source, the bundles of fibers provide a bright spot of light distally, even though the bundles are twisted on themselves into loops and knots. The importance of such flexibility is immediately evident, permitting the construction of a snakelike cable of light, able to reach into the depths of the respiratory tract. The flexible scope, like the rigid one, can be used for collecting biopsies and for aspiration of secretions, and it allows simultaneous administration of oxygen. Its great virtue lies in the wide range of circumstances in which it can be used. Local anesthesia is needed, but bronchoscopy can be performed at the bedside or while the patient is seated in a chair. Whereas the rigid scope is seldom used by any except specialists in otorhinolaryngology and thoracic surgery, the fiberoptic scope is being increasingly used by the internist specializing in pulmonary disease.

## Intubation

We will explore intubation in considerable detail because it is almost a standard procedure in the patient with severe ventilatory failure, and the therapist will work extensively with patients so treated. In contrast to bronchoscopy, which is a short-term technique, intubation is the placing of a rigid or semirigid tube in the respiratory tract and leaving it for varying periods of time, from a few hours to permanently, to assure patency of the upper airway.

The following points should be noted about intubation: First, the tube itself is space occupying in the airway, and its use constitutes somewhat of a compromise in that the tube reduces the caliber of the natural lumen, although it ensures that the narrower passage is clear. Second, intubation is indicated for the access it provides to the bronchial tree for the aspiration of secretions (to be described in detail below). Third, it is a means of administering mechanical ventilation. Under certain limited circumstances, pressured air may be given to a patient by means of a face mask, but a moment's reflection will bring to mind several practical inadequacies of such a measure.

1. Because of the great variations in contours of the human face, a secure fit between mask and face is difficult to achieve, and if delivered pressure is to be responsible for ventilation, a leak in the system is hazardous.
2. With the best-designed face mask, considerable pressure must be applied to hold it in place to prevent slippage as well as leaks. The dependability of head straps or a harness is highly questionable, and with the force required, the risk of pressure necrosis of the skin is very real. The alternative method of the therapist manually holding the mask in place can be effective sometimes for short periods but is obviously impractical for prolonged supportive therapy.
3. There is a great risk of oropharyngeal obstruction by the lax tongue in the unconscious patient, a complication that is often precipitated by the supine position and the pressure of a mask. In such circumstances a mouth airway must always be used to hold the tongue out of the way and to provide a good channel for the delivered air.
4. In the presence of significant airway resistance, the flaccid cheeks may absorb enough of the ventilating pressure that pulmonary ventilation is compromised. Thus, except for short-term emergency treatment, the use of face masks is not suitable for positive-pressure ventilation, and a substantial airway must be provided.

For this last indication the tubes are almost always "cuffed." The cuff is a rubber, balloonlike item that fits over the lower end of the airway tube and has a narrow rubber tube extending outside the body by which the cuff can be inflated with air. The simple illustration in Fig. 10-1 shows the general relationships of the parts involved. As the cuff distends with air, it seals the airway to prevent the retrograde flow of gas cephalad under pressure. Thus all gas movement is through the indwelling tube. The outer end of the inflating tube has a small pilot balloon that distends with the cuff and serves as a monitor because should the cuff develop a leak, the pilot balloon will also deflate. The cuff is usually filled with air by a syringe, and a clamp is placed proximal to the pilot balloon. More details of cuffs and their management will be described later under the subject of tracheostomy.

There are three types of intubating tubes in general clinical use—the *oral endotracheal tube*, the *nasotracheal tube*, and the *tracheostomy tube*. The individual features of each will be described, but characteristics common to all and the general

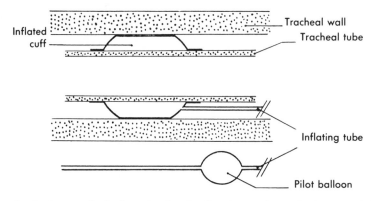

**Fig. 10-1.** Sketch of intratracheal tube with inflated cuff in place, in longitudinal section of the trachea. Air is introduced into the cuff through an inflating tube, which extends through the surgical incision to the outside. A pilot balloon warns of accidental deflation of the cuff after a clamp is placed distal to it on the inflating tube.

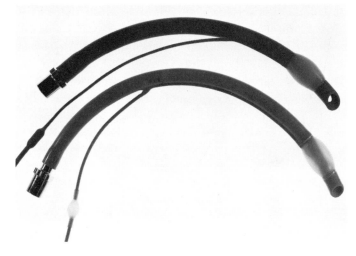

**Fig. 10-2.** Endotracheal tubes with inflated cuffs and pilot balloons.

principles of intubation and patient care will be discussed with the tracheostomy as the model.

*Oral endotracheal intubation.* Endotracheal tubes are of rubber or plastic and come in a variety of sizes from 12 cm long with an inside diameter of 2.5 mm to about 38 cm long and 11 mm inside diameter. They are curved to facilitate introduction into the respiratory track and are available with attached cuffs, as shown in Fig. 10-2. Oral endotracheal intubation has long been used to maintain an open airway during surgery, usually instituted after induction of the anesthesia, but with the increasing incidence of pulmonary diseases, it has become an important part of medical management of the conscious or unconscious patient in ventilatory failure.

The base of the tongue, the pharynx, and the larynx are rendered insensitive with local anesthetic nebulized or directly applied to the area and sometimes infiltrated into the larynx by injection. With the patient in the supine position, the way is readied for intubation by introducing a laryngoscope into the pharynx. This is an instrument consisting of a handle containing batteries and a small bulb, at approximately right angles to which is a blade that may be straight or curved. Thus, under direct lighted vision, the tip of the laryngoscope blade displaces the epiglottis and exposes the larynx. The endotracheal tube can then be inserted between the vocal cords through the larynx into the trachea just far enough that the cuff clears the larynx. A small oral airway or some other effective "bite block" is fastened between the patient's teeth to prevent accidental compression of the tube by closure of the jaws.

Endotracheal intubation, for the most part, is fairly simple, but it carries serious potential risks. At the outset, there is the possibility of an adverse reaction to the local anesthetic, a great hazard to any patient but more so in one with defective ventilation. The larynx is a sensitive organ and often responds to irritation or trauma by becoming spastic, completely occluding the airway, and attempts to force the tube may seriously damage the vocal cords. It is important that every effort be made to pass the cords on the first attempt, since repeated probing will stimulate an almost immediate edema of the cords, greatly hampering the procedure and risking the life of the patient. Intubation should still be considered a medical procedure, not a technical one, and its responsibilities entail such legal and ethical considerations that its use should be reserved for the professionally trained physician. There is no doubt that a good therapist could be trained to perform intubation, but the skill and finesse with which it is done are directly proportional to the frequency of its performance. Even though it is widely used in patients receiving respiratory therapy, the actual number of times per week or per month that the average therapist would have occasion to intubate is negligible when compared with its frequency in the daily work of the anesthesiologist. It is recognized that there may be circumstances in which trained professional personnel are not readily available, and emergency or routine intubation must depend on the therapist. In this situation then, if competent respiratory therapists are available, they definitely should be given the responsibility. However, to maintain their expertise they should practice intubation regularly and frequently in the surgery. In summary, each hospital must work out its own solution to providing emergency intubation, but, whenever possible, a trained physician, especially an anesthesiologist, should be on first call. It should be remembered that even the most skillful operator is at a serious disadvantage when faced with the task of intubating a larynx already spastic and edematous from a bungled earlier unsuccessful attempt.

The advantages of oral endotracheal intubation are summarized in a study of this technique.[289] As noted above, a good airway can be obtained by an expert operator in a short time without the risk and inconvenience of a surgical procedure, as is necessary for tracheotomy. There is no tissue destruction or scarring and no anatomic distortion so that a repeat intubation can be done whenever necessary. Extubation (removal of the tube) time was found to be shorter than with a tracheostomy because there seemed to be less patient and physician dependence on nonsurgical than on surgical intubation. Of great significance was the observation that the return of an effective cough was almost immediate after extubation, whereas there is always some delay after surgical violation of the trachea. Finally, the prior oral intubation of the trachea makes much safer and easier a subsequent tracheotomy, a point that will be emphasized below in the discussion of the latter procedure.

In comparison, the disadvantages of oral intubation are of less significance. The most important is some degree of patient intolerance to the awkwardness and inconvenience of the large tube through the mouth. Frequently, much continuous assurance must be given the patient, supported by sedation to allay his apprehension and reduce discomfort, obviously not a problem in the unconscious or mentally obtunded patient. Occasionally an agitated patient may pull out the tube, but after replacement, proper restraint will prevent recurrence. Laryngeal edema may be troublesome in the postintubation period, but this has not proved to be a serious hazard, and reintubation can always be done if needed. Until fairly recently it was almost a dictum that oral endotracheal intubation be terminated at 48 hours and that if further therapy were necessary, tracheotomy be done. With increasing experience in its use, the duration of intubation has been greatly expanded, and in the study referred to above, tubes were left in place for periods ranging from 21 to 171 hours with no ill effects.

*Nasotracheal intubation.* The objectives of nasotracheal intubation, as well as the tube employed, are similar to those of oral intubation. In this case, however, the tube is introduced first through the nose rather than the mouth and then into the trachea. Although "blind" passage of the tube through the larynx can be attempted, it is much safer to use the same direct visual approach as with oral intubation once the tube has passed the nasal cavity. Nasotracheal intubation has been most extensively used in children but is now finding increasing favor in the treatment of adults, and a study compares its effectiveness with that of tracheostomy in the latter group.[290] With a variety of underlying conditions necessitating intubation, nasotracheal tubes were used for periods ranging from 12 hours to 14 days. The advantages of this procedure are the same as those described for oral intubation with the additional feature of better patient tolerance and less discomfort, since the mouth is free of the large tube. Similarly, the disadvantages are basically those noted above, with the possible additional risk of some kinking of the tube as it navigates the tortuous nasal passages.

The opinion is frequently heard that a nasotracheal tube must be smaller than an oral or tracheostomy tube and that resistance to airflow will be accordingly increased. The report cited above disputes this, implying that there need be no difference between the oral and nasal tubes, although it would seem reasonable that unfavorable nasal conditions might limit the size of tube that could be effectively used. It further states that despite its greater length, the nasotracheal tube may be less resistant than a loosely fitted tracheostomy tube. It is interesting to note that the survey of the oral endotracheal technique referred to earlier found the use of naso-tracheal tubes in adults much less satisfactory than the use of oral tubes and was accompanied by a sharp difference in patient survival. In all probability the differences in opinion reflect the results of personal experiences and interest in one technique over the other rather than any significant inherent difference in these two similar procedures. The therapist will perhaps note that just as we were unable to describe one best mechanical ventilator, endowed with all virtues and no vices, so there is no single intubation technique to satisfy all needs.

**Tracheostomy intubation.** The greatest portion of our discussion on airway patency and intubation will be devoted to the intubation of the tracheotomized airway, for this is the standard against which all other techniques are evaluated. Let us first define two terms widely used, often erroneously interchangeably. *Tracheotomy* is a surgical procedure that produces an opening in the trachea (the suffix *-tomy* means "a cutting or incision"), and a *tracheostomy* is the opening so made in the trachea (the suffix *-stomy* coming from the Greek *stoma,* "mouth"). A *tracheostomy tube* is therefore a tube designed to be placed in the trachea through a tracheostomy. This technique has been a lifesaving procedure for some three centuries, to and including the present, and is the most precise and definitive way to establish and maintain a free upper airway. Many of the comments to be made will apply to both oral and nasal tracheal intubation as well, and to avoid unnecessary repetition, the reader will be left to relate them in his own mind.

The indications for a tracheostomy can be enumerated as follows: (1) to establish and/or maintain a patent and accessible airway after endotracheal intubation or when the latter is not considered desirable; (2) with a cuffed tube, to prevent aspiration of regurgitated gastric contents or blood from facial or oral trauma, as in a comatose patient or one with obtunded reflexes; (3) to permit the aspiration of bronchopulmonary secretions, a maneuver easier through a tracheostomy tube than through the longer endotracheal tube; (4) with a cuffed tube, to permit long-term, positive-pressure mechanical ventilation; and (5) to reduce the anatomic dead space and relieve the work of breathing. By short-circuiting the nasal, oral, and pharyngeal passages, the tracheostomy tube affords the spontaneously breathing patient less distance to move air from atmosphere to alveoli. Reference will be made to this again later, but it should be observed that the cost of reducing the dead space is a reduction in the lumen of the upper airway, since the tracheostomy tube itself is an obstruction. It has been shown that resistance to breathing does not drop significantly below normal in the adult patient until the internal diameter of the tube exceeds 9.5 mm, and this is larger than the three most commonly used tubes.[291]

*Tracheotomy.* Tracheotomy itself is not to be taken lightly, since it is a surgical procedure carried out on a patient with a severely compromised major system. Emergency tracheotomies have been performed under a variety of circumstances, and many will be, of necessity, in the future. However, every attempt should be made to see that conditions for it are as ideal as possible, and in the modern hospital the bedside tracheotomy is denounced. Even in the most critical situations, tracheotomy should be an elective procedure, done in the operating room with due regard for preparation and careful technique. With the recognition of airway obstruction severe enough to warrant mechanical interference, the patient should immediately be intubated endotracheally to assure his survival; supportive therapy should be given, and surgery performed, when both the patient's condition and the operating facilities are at their best. The techniques of tracheotomy may vary, but in general the incision into and through the skin and subcutaneous tissue is made high enough so that the trachea can be entered at the level of either the second or third cartilage. This site is essential so that the tip of the tube will not impinge on the carina. Selection of a tube of proper size and shape is critically important, for the tube must be neither too tight nor too loose if the complications that will be described later are to be avoided. Once firmly in place, the tracheostomy tube is secured by a fabric tape around the patient's neck. Tracheotomy carries with it definite surgical risks; the mortality directly attributed to the procedure, as opposed to the underlying disease, is estimated at 3% and serious complications at nearly 50% in some series.[290] The three most important immediate surgical complications can be classified as follows.

BLEEDING. Bleeding is an exceptionally potential hazard, for not only is the involved anatomic area naturally very vascular but congestion in the vessels is often increased as a result of the hemodynamic changes incidental to both pulmonary disease and supportive ventilation. Every bleeding source must be meticulously attended because these patients can ill afford the stress of excessive blood loss.

TISSUE EMPHYSEMA. The great variety of neck contours seriously challenge the surgeons, and the probing and dissection in some patients hold the risk of invading the apices of the lungs with subsequent pneumothorax. Not rarely, air escapes from the opened trachea and works its way through exposed tissues to accumulate under the skin of the face, neck, and thorax, a condition known as *subcutaneous emphysema*. More serious is the movement of air along the paths of the major airways into the mediastinum, *mediastinal emphysema*, where it builds up in response to the negative pressure of the patient's inspiratory efforts and may embarrass the intrathoracic cardiorespiratory mechanics. Fortunately, most of the time such events are correctable or tolerated by the body, but since they can occur even when tracheotomy is done with operating room care, the therapist can understand the risk of operating in haste.

CARDIOVASCULAR COLLAPSE. There are two types of adverse cardiovascular reactions to the tracheotomy procedure itself, similar in their end results but differing markedly in their mechanisms. First, one of the immediate hazards is acute cardiac arrest, most often encountered during a hurried tracheotomy but fortunately becoming less frequent with adherence to currently accepted practices. At one time believed to be due to some vagal reflex accompanying the trauma of surgery, arrest is now attributed to a severe and sudden hypoxia superimposed on the hypoxia of the underlying disease, as ventilation is impaired during the manipulations of the procedure. This is the major reason for prior intubation and efforts to improve oxygenation before surgery and for maintaining good mechanical or manual ventilation until the new airway is adequately functioning. Second, cardiovascular and sometimes respiratory collapse may be the paradoxical result of rapidly achieving a good airway during tracheotomy.[292] Shortly after the airway is secured and secretions cleaned out, the patient may become acutely hypotensive and pulseless and go into complete apnea. This reaction is believed to be due to the sudden washout of accumulated carbon dioxide from the body as alveolar ventilation is precipitously increased and the respiratory acidosis reversed. Such a rapid swing in acid-base balance is known to produce arrhythmias and hypotension. The accompanying apnea is the sequela of cerebral blood flow reduction from both the circulatory failure and vascular dilatation of sudden hypocapnia. Before, during, and immediately after tracheotomy, the patient's blood pressure should be checked frequently and vasopressors kept close at hand to prevent the shock from becoming irreversible.

It might be of interest to note that a secondary, but definitely helpful, benefit of preoperative intubation is the increased ease of locating, mobilizing, and handling a trachea already identified and supported by an indwelling tube. In summary, we can say that the incidence and seriousness of tracheotomy complications are inversely related to the degree that the procedure is performed under elective, controlled conditions.

*Tubes and cuffs.* There are many types of tracheostomy tubes now available. For many years only silver tubes were used, but disposable plastic tubes have become popular and for the most part have replaced the metal. We will, however, first describe the traditional silver tube (Fig. 10-3) because it is occasionally used, and its parts can be disassembled for descriptive purposes. Then we will consider the features of plastic tubes that have given them their position of prominence.

SILVER TUBES. The tubes are curved to accommodate the anatomy of the trachea and to facilitate introduction and removal, varying from an outside diameter of 3 mm and a length along the outside of the curve of 1.75 inches to an outside diameter of 14 mm and a length of over 4 inches. Unfortunately, sizing of tubes involves at least two scales and mixes metric with English units of measurement. It is not critical that the respiratory therapist be familiar with the details of such data, for he will have available for his purposes a large enough variety of adapters that he will be able to service any tracheotomized patients under his jurisdiction, but if he is interested, equipment catalogues are available with specifications of the many types. The tracheostomy tube is basically a cannula within a cannula (Fig. 10-3). The outer cannula maintains the patency of the airway, whereas the inner cannula is removable for cleaning to prevent secretions from obstructing the tip. If there were but a single tube and it became plugged with secretions, it would have to be removed, thereby disrupting the entire surgical area. This is avoided by the removable inner cannula. The styluslike accessory is called an obturator, and it is used only for the initial introduction of the outer cannula to prevent scraping of the tracheal wall. Once the outer cannula is in place, the obturator is withdrawn and the inner cannula inserted. The two cannulae are held snugly together by a locking mechanism on the metal units or by friction on the plastic. The head of the inner cannula is designed to accept adapters that permit the attachment of ventilators to the system.

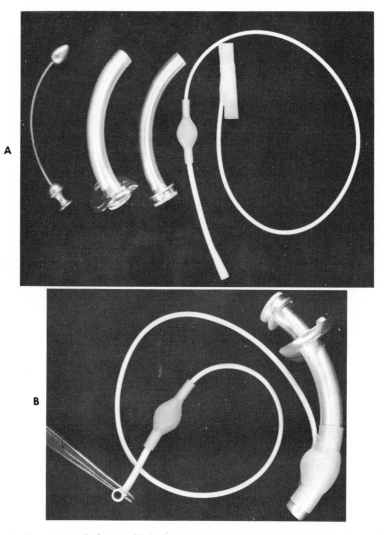

**Fig. 10-3.   A,** Components of a disassembled silver tracheostomy tube. On the left is a stylus, or obturator, used only during insertion of the outer cannula, followed by the outer and inner cannulae, and a cuff. **B,** Cuff is in place and inflated, and the inner cannula is seen protruding slightly from the outer tube.

We have made frequent references to the cuffs used on intubation tubes, and because of their importance in making effective ventilation available to patients, we shall describe them in a bit more detail. A typical cuff for a metal tracheostomy tube is an elastic sleeve whose central segment is thinner-walled than its ends and which is slipped over the distal portion of the outer cannula. A small-caliber elastic tube runs from the center of the cuff, along the outer cannula, and through the tracheostomy incision to the outside. A syringe is used to instill air through this filling tube to inflate the distensible center of the cuff, effectively sealing off the trachea around the outer cannula and preventing retrograde air leaks from ventilator positive pressure. The inflating tube is closed by a plug or a clamp. Between its outer end and the patient, the tube is provided with a pilot balloon, which inflates with the distal cuff. This allows the therapist to monitor the integrity of the inflated cuff for if the cuff should collapse from a leak, the pilot balloon would also deflate. Separate cuffs vary in size from 4 mm to about 13 mm, and success of subsequent ventilation may depend on the proper application of the proper size cuff. As shown in Fig. 10-3, the ends of the cuff are narrower and less elastic than the easily distensible midportion. The tight fit of the ends of the cuff holds it in place on the outer cannula of the tube to prevent both leakage and slippage; a special cement is often used for additional support.

A very informative and practical study of tracheostomy cuffs describes two basic types, the single-lumen and the double-lumen.[293] The single-lumen cuff is a simple tube of thin rubber with snug ends and a distensible body supplied with an inflating tube. It distends evenly in all directions, exerting pressure equally on all mucosal contact points, and it holds the tracheostomy tube in the center of the trachea. However, it tends to leak air and to ride up and down on the outer cannula as it is subjected to the motion of the patient and manipulation of attached equipment. The double-lumen cuff is double walled. As it is inflated, the inner wall is compressed against the outer cannula, securely holding the cuff in place while the outer wall distends to occlude the airway between the tube and trachea. A disadvantage of the double-lumen cuff is its tendency to bulge mostly in one direction, opposite the attachment of its inflating tube. Not only does this create unequal pressure on the inner tracheal wall but it also displaces the cannula from the center of the airway to an eccentric location. In spite of these undesirable characteristics, because of its stability, the double-lumen cuff is probably the more desirable of the two.

PLASTIC TUBES. Plastic tracheostomy tubes generally follow the pattern described for silver tubes, but they have some decided advantages of their own. There are many brands on the market, each with special features supposedly making it superior to its competitors. It would be time wasting to attempt to cover the details of all, and again the student is encouraged to study advertising literature and inspect several tubes for a broad view of the field. A major advantage of the plastic trach tube is its disposability. Each tube is packaged sterile and after use is thrown away, to be replaced by another new one as needed. Additionally, the tubes are light in weight with no sharp edges—features that reduce the risk of tracheal injury during movement of patient or tube. Plastic tends to soften slightly at body temperature, allowing the tube to conform to the tracheal contour for a maximum fit. An important asset is the bonded cuff already sealed onto the cannula, eliminating a sometimes difficult task and assuring that the cuff will not slip off the end of the tube.

Fig. 10-4 shows a common and popular plastic tracheostomy tube. Like many others it has no inner cannula, making frequent suctioning of secretions necessary to prevent obstruction. A feature of great value, found with most tubes now used, is the low-pressure cuff. Designed to occlude the airway with a minimum of intra-cuff air pressure, thereby reducing the hazard of pressure damage to the tracheal mucosa, low-pressure cuffs are generally of two basic types. The cuff shown in Fig. 10-4 is constructed with a large surface for mucosal contact, thus distributing its

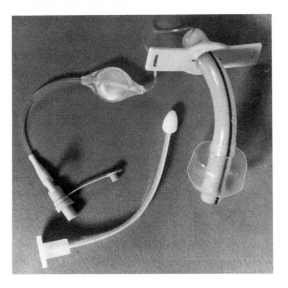

**Fig. 10-4.** Plastic, low-pressure cuff tracheostomy tube.

pressure over a broad area of mucosa. Lower total pressure is needed for a good seal than if the cuff-tracheal interface were smaller. The second type of low-pressure cuff contains a spongy, air-cell substance, which can be deflated by syringe aspiration for insertion into the airway and which needs little inflation for sealing because of the self-expansion of its air-foam.

We have been emphasizing the primary function of an inflated trach tube cuff, sealing the trachea between the tube cannula and the tracheal wall for use with a positive-pressure ventilator. Usually, whenever the patient is not being ventilated, the cuff need not be inflated, but there may be an exception. A secondary use of the inflated cuff is prevention of aspiration into the airways of vomitus, secretions pooling in the hypopharynx, or food in patients who are obtunded or with dulled epiglottal reflexes. The length of time a cuff should remain inflated for these reasons alone is a matter of clinical judgment, but in selected patients such protection of the airways may be lifesaving. Always, before the cuff is deflated for any reason, the hypopharynx must be suctioned of any material to prevent its aspiration past the collapsed cuff into the bronchial tree.

Proper cuff inflation requires skill but is somewhat easier if the patient is on a ventilator. In general, the older practice of instilling a fixed volume of air, such as 5 or 10 ml, into the cuff is no longer advised. With the tip of a 5 or 10 ml syringe inserted into the end of the inflating tube, air is slowly introduced while the ventilator is attached and operating. Inspiratory air leakage is noted, and cuff inflation is stopped as soon as the leak ceases. Air is then slowly withdrawn from the cuff until a slight leak is once again heard. At this point just enough air can be reintroduced into the cuff to stop the leak, with assurance that occlusion of the cuff is achieved with minimal pressure. As an alternative, the "minimal leak" technique can be used by plugging the filling tube while a slight leak persists. This utilizes the small inspiratory leak to blow cephalad for easier removal, secretions tending to pool around the cuff.

*Management of the intubated patient.* The management of the tracheotomized patient mechanically ventilated through a cuffed tube constitutes one of the respiratory therapist's greatest responsibilities. It can be flatly stated that no member of the hospital team is as qualified or as able as a trained and mature respiratory therapist to supervise the ventilatory care of such a patient. There is not yet universal agreement on this point, and some conflict is evident between nursing and respiratory therapy services. For the most part this is understandable, stemming from the facts that respiratory therapy is new, it involves patient care to a degree formerly reserved for nursing, and there is a shortage of therapists to meet hospitals' needs. Because of the intense care required for these patients, there is need for both nursing and respiratory therapy working cooperatively, and in those hospitals where respiratory therapy functions at its highest level, conflicts dissolve as each service concentrates on its contribution to overall care.

There are several factors that the therapist must bear in mind in addition to the attention he directs toward the efficient functioning of his ventilator. He must remember that the patient is entirely dependent upon all medical and nursing attendants and can do little for himself. If the patient is alert, he will initially be apprehensive and justifiably may be greatly frightened. Reassurance by the therapist through words and action is a *critical* part of therapy, for the patient's emotional status may markedly influence his breathing pattern or his acceptance of mechanical ventilation. The therapist must create an atmosphere of calmness and confidence for the patient, aware that the patient watches every move and listens to every word. It must be remembered that the cuffed patient cannot talk because his vocal cords are bypassed by the tracheostomy tube. He can speak only after disconnection from the ventilator, deflation of the cuff, and obstruction of the outer opening of the tube so that exhaled air can leak around the tube through the larynx. This may be tiring and should be reserved for those instances when the patient desires to communicate, or when it is necessary to get information from him essential to therapy.

It was noted above that adapters are used to attach the ventilator to the end of the inner cannula. For the most part, these are plastic and come in sets to accommodate all sizes of tubes. They are generally held into the inner cannula (a further reduction in the caliber of the airway) by friction, connecting the airway to the machine by a flex tube. It is important to adjust this joint in such a manner that there is a minimum of strain on the connector to reduce the risk of accidental dislodgement, which would completely separate the patient from his major, if not only, source of ventilation. There is available a swivel connector that permits patient mobility without loosening.

The inflated cuff is a potential danger to the respiratory tract because of its constant pressure on the tracheal mucosa, which may cause areas of mucosal necrosis. To avoid this possibility, the cuff should be deflated for approximately 5 minutes every hour, but if the patient's ventilatory status is so critical that he cannot tolerate this length of time, then deflation should be done more frequently for shorter periods. Whenever the ventilator is not in operation, the cuff should be deflated, except as noted above, where aspiration is a risk. Because some cuffs are defective and may break, the therapist must be on the watch for evidence of a leak, the first instance of which may be the failure of end-inspiratory cycling of a pressure-cycled ventilator or the prolongation of inspiration if the leak is relatively small. The ear of an alert and experienced therapist will pick up changes in the cycling patterns of his equipment, but these warnings will be absent in time-cycled ventilators. The pilot balloon is usually a reliable indication of the inflation of the cuff, but on occasion the inflation tube may become pinched at the tracheal stoma so that the pilot balloon remains filled even after collapse of the cuff. In the event that a defective cuff is detected or suspected, the therapist should notify the responsible physician at once.

The constant potential hazard to the intubated patient, as noted frequently, is obstruction, especially from accumulated secretions. One of the safeguards against this is effective aspiration, the technique of which will be described separately below. In addition, if an inner cannula is present, it should be removed and cleaned every 4 hours, or more frequently if needed; for long-term care the entire tube should be removed and changed weekly, even in the absence of malfunction, a responsibility of the physician who did the original surgery or a skilled therapist.[294] The final protection against secretion buildup is adequate humidification, and we do not exaggerate when we say that not only will intubation fail to achieve its purpose but it may be positively harmful to the patient if humidity is lacking. While the patient's dead space has been reduced by tracheotomy, so has his natural humidification mechanism been bypassed, and little can be more detrimental to his respiratory hygiene than a flow of dry air or gas (even room air) directly into his trachea. While the patient is being ventilated, humidification will be provided by the many effective devices available as attachments, especially heated units such as the Cascade humidifier, which delivers water vapor, not aerosolized water, with the latter's capability of carrying bacteria into equipment or the patient's respiratory tract. However, humidification must not be overlooked when the patient is removed from the machine for significant periods of time. A tracheostomy mask or collar that conveniently fits over the opening of the cannula, or a T-tube are satisfactory if used with a good humidifier. It is felt by many that secretions will seldom be a serious problem if the patient is supplied with adequate vapor and water aerosol, since most secretions will be wet enough to be easily aspirated. Water in the inspired gas serves another purpose than maintaining general health of the respiratory tract. No matter how good is the fit of a tracheostomy tube, there is always some motion of it in response to respiration, patient activity, and handling of the attachments; and a bit of excess water in and about the tube acts as a lubricant to minimize frictional damage to the local mucosa.

Many of the patients who are intubated need supplemental oxygen therapy. Our concern here is not with the indications for or the hazards of oxygen per se, for we have already considered these factors earlier and will discuss them again later on; our concern, rather, is with the method of administration. As in the case of humidity mentioned above, during mechanical ventilation oxygen will be provided as needed through the instrument, but a word is in order concerning its use when the patient is not being ventilated. The safest technique is the use of a tracheostomy mask, which can combine both oxygen and humidification. Unfortunately, there is an old technique still in use that is to be condemned. This is the insertion of an oxygen catheter directly into the tracheostomy tube. Although arterial oxygen levels can be increased, such a procedure offers a significant resistance to exhalation with a potential danger that outweighs any benefit. This subject was studied with convincing results of the ventilatory burden it imposes.[295] We have already indicated that the tube itself increases the airflow resistance in the respiratory tract, and it is reasonable that the introduction of a catheter, no matter how small, will further increase such resistance. When to this is added the resistance of an oxygen flow directly opposing the passive outflow of air, we can only wonder that such a procedure was ever considered safe. The study logically concluded, but with quantitative proof, that peak expiratory resistance increased as the size of the tracheostomy tube decreased, as the size of the oxygen catheter increased, and as the oxygen flow increased. Should a therapist encounter this procedure in use or being contemplated, it is hoped that he will use his greatest diplomacy and tact in suggesting an alternate technique.

*Complications of tracheostomy.* In addition to the hazards of the surgical procedure of tracheotomy and the clinical precautions to be considered in the management of a tracheotomized patient, there are complications that can be attributed to the presence of the tracheostomy tube itself. Although the medical care of such complications is a responsibility of the attending physician, the respiratory therapist should be acquainted with them, for he may be the first to note their onset and so stimulate immediate corrective action. Some latitude may be expected in determining what phenomena constitute complications due to a tracheostomy, but we will include the most important in the following classification.

### OBSTRUCTION

FROM SECRETIONS. This has already been discussed and is repeated only for emphasis of its importance, but it most certainly is a direct result of the aggravation of pre-existing secretions by intubation.

FROM THE CUFF. A loosely fitted, single-lumen cuff may partially or completely slip off the end of the cannula, obstructing the airway locally or in either main stem bronchus. This is most apt to occur following rupture of the cuff after it has been in operation, during manipulation of the cannula with the cuff deflated, or during removal of the tube. Clinical and mechanical signs and symptoms of airway obstruction accompanied by inability to inflate the cuff should bring this probability immediately to mind. Because of its better grip on the cannula, a double-lumen cuff is unlikely to become completely dislodged, even when deflated, but it may herniate or hang over the end of the cannula. When it is then inflated, it will occlude both the trachea and the tracheostomy tube as it distends freely across the opening of the cannula. The resulting severe dyspnea in the spontaneously breathing patient will be relieved by deflation of the cuff, and the obstructive response of an attached ventilator will be replaced by evidence of a leak. In such a condition a probing suction catheter will encounter the obstructing inflated cuff but will pass freely when the cuff is emptied of air.

FROM THE CANNULA. Should the tracheotomy incision be placed too low or too long a tube be installed, the tip of the cannula may impinge on the carina, with resulting severe obstruction. When intubation has been completed and mechanical ventilation started, the attending physician or the responsible therapist should always check to be sure that the cannula is not directed down one or the other main stem bronchi. Should this occur, all the ventilation will go to one lung, whereas the other will become severely atelectatic from complete deprivation of its air supply. Suspicion of this complication should be aroused by the inability to achieve satisfactory ventilation with the respirator (because of the reduced volume of only one functioning lung) and is confirmed by the lack of breath sounds in the bypassed lung as the chest is examined by stethoscope. Immediate correction is mandatory, since this is life threatening.

FROM ABRADED MUCOSA. It has been suggested that many of the instances of obstruction following tracheal intubation may be the result of what has been termed the "snowplow effect" of the tracheal cannula.[296] While the rigid tube remains fairly stable, the respiratory tract moves with the breathing cycle, riding upward during exhalation and downward during inhalation. As a result, if the tube is not centered in the airway and its tip is allowed to rest on the inner tracheal wall, the cephalad expiratory movement scrapes the tracheal mucosa against the unyielding edge of the cannular opening. Debrided epithelium, mixed with secretions, has been demonstrated to form a mass of significant size to obstruct a bronchus and require bronchoscopic removal. Selection of tubes of the proper length and, if necessary, supporting them by packing about the tracheotomy opening will minimize this traumatic risk.

FROM TRACHEAL STENOSIS. Obstruction from tracheal stenosis is a serious complication that becomes evident during the weeks following extubation or removal of the tracheostomy tube. As the trachea heals from the double trauma of tracheostomy and intubation, its passage may narrow from fibrous scarring or from the growth of granulation, tissue which is a soft, easy-bleeding mass of proliferating blood vessels, often replacing destroyed tissue. Stenosis usually occurs at the stoma, or incisional opening of the tracheostomy, or at the site of the trach tube pressure. The stoma probably heals by the joining of severed tracheal cartilage ends, and if the rings are surgically shortened, stenosis results. On the other hand, cuff site tracheal stenosis is often preceded by severe pressure necrosis damage, as the distended cuff impairs local blood supply, causing tissue death and ulceration. Not only is the mucosa injured but the tracheal wall as well, with exposure and destruction of cartilaginous rings. This stage is referred to as *tracheomalacia*, which means a weakness of the tracheal wall usually causing the trachea to dilate. Postmortem studies suggest that some degree of necrosis is probably present in all intubated tracheas.[297] The lesion is circumferential, extending around the trachea, and as destroyed tissue is replaced by granulation and scar, a gradually contracting ring constricts the trachea.[298] Regardless of the cause, if stenosis is symptomatic, interfering with airflow, surgical repair is needed.

There are many informative articles in the pulmonary literature describing stenosis of the trachea after intubation, and the student is advised to make use of them. A recent survey of forty patients, electively tracheotomized for ventilatory assistance, revealed the following: (1) 10% had complicating bleeding; (2) 17.5% had some problem with tracheostomy management; (3) 16% had asymptomatic narrowing of the stoma site; (4) 16% had asymptomatic defects at the cuff site; and (5) 8% required tracheal resection for stomal stenosis. This study strongly suggests postextubation evaluation of the trachea by fiberoptic bronchoscopy or x-ray examination.[299]

### HEMORRHAGE

FROM THE INCISIONAL SITE. Inadequate hemostasis (control of bleeding) during surgery may allow a recurrence of bleeding from the operative site after therapy has been started. The danger of brisk bleeding is obvious, but even a hidden slow oozing of blood is hazardous, since blood may accumulate about the upper part of the cannula in the trachea and be aspirated into the bronchi when the cuff is deflated during routine care.

FROM TRACHEAL TRAUMA. Erosion of the tracheal mucosa as described above with "snowplowing" can produce surface bleeding, with subsequent aspiration. Less common, but far more serious, is a frank perforation of the tracheal wall by the indwelling cannula, with damage to a neighboring artery. This may lead to rapid and fatal exsanguination.

TISSUE EMPHYSEMA. The escape of air into body tissues during surgery has already been noted when intrathoracic negative pressure can draw air through the planes of exposed cut tissues, letting it migrate to the mediastinum and subcutaneous areas. During positive-pressure ventilation this is unlikely unless the patient is "fighting" the machine because it is not meeting his needs, in which case his inspiratory efforts may suck air into the tissues around the incision. However, should there be damage to the airway below the level of the tracheal cuff (as from the end of the cannula), positive-pressure ventilation may force air into the tissues, producing extensive subcutaneous emphysema.

INFECTION. Some physicians believe that infection is the most troublesome, if not the most significant, of tracheostomy complications.[300] It may range from a relatively minor wound sepsis to an overwhelming pneumonia. A frequent major problem is differentiating the infection due to invasion of the respiratory tract through a tracheotomy from that of the underlying pulmonary disease, and at times this is not possible to do with certainty. Many patients have preexisting bronchopulmonary infection at the time of their tracheotomies, and, indeed, such infections may be prominent etiologic factors in the obstructions for which the tracheotomies are performed. There can be little doubt that intubating the trachea increases the possibility of infection, with the deliberate perpetuation of an open wound into the air passages, bypassing the natural filtering mechanism of the upper tract. Handling the cannula, frequent introduction of a catheter into the trachea, attaching ventilators to the tube, and serous seepage about the incision all contribute to the risk of infection. However, even positive bacterial cultures of aspirates or wound discharges are not conclusive evidence of a clinical infection; they may be from local contaminants. For the diagnosis of a significant infection, there must be signs and symptoms other than just bacteriologic. Despite the increased chances for sepsis through a tracheostomy, it is not rare to note rapid clearing of a pulmonary infection after the establishment of good bronchial drainage and the aspiration of obstructing secretions.

Especially troublesome is the bacterium *Pseudomonas aeruginosa*, about which the therapist will hear many references. Its frequent culture from tracheotomized patients and their equipment is a constant cause for concern. Because it thrives in dampness, it is a frequent contaminant of equipment and utensils, but an unusual overgrowth of the organism in a patient weakened by disease can be pathogenic in its own right—a serious hazard to the already handicapped patient. Meticulous care is necessary for the tracheotomized patient, and attention to his wound or his tube should be only under conditions of surgically sterile technique. The incision should be treated as any surgical site, with cleaning and asepsis as indicated, and it should be kept dressed as sterile as is consistent with its use. An awareness of the risk of infection in the patient in ventilatory failure will help all attending personnel to exercise caution and avoid carelessness.

*Summary.* The importance of tracheostomy therapy justifies a summation of its place in the management of ventilatory failure. If at all avoidable, tracheotomy should never be done as a hurried emergency procedure, since such a circumstance carries with it high mortality and morbidity. Prior intubation should be performed to secure a good airway, for not only does it give technical assistance to the operating surgeon but it also prevents the serious hypoxia that is so likely to damage the patient, even to the point of triggering cardiac arrest. At the same time, overventilation must be avoided or the patient is subjected to the risk of acute alkalosis with cardiovascular collapse and cerebral hypoxia. These two seemingly paradoxical precautions point up the great skill needed to safeguard the patient during the procedure. During follow-up management, medical attendants must watch especially carefully for cuff failure and take all necessary care to prevent tracheal damage. In general, to minimize bleeding and infection the tracheostomy must be treated like the surgical site it is.

Tracheotomy is surgery performed on a physiologically unstable patient in critical condition, and in a real sense it is chosen as the lesser of two evils. The fatality rate among tracheotomized patients has been reported as high as 38% in one group of 300.[301] This is not an indictment against the therapy but, rather, reflects the gravity of the diseases making it necessary. On the other hand, after a careful review it was estimated that a similar 38% of over 400 patients survived their illnesses because they did undergo tracheotomy.[300] In addition to the advantages of airway suctioning and the ability to assist ventilation, tracheotomy carries a physiologic benefit of its own, as shown by a study of the character of spontaneous breathing in a group of emphysematous patients.[302] The subjects experienced a reduction in total ventilation, attributed to a reduction in the volume of the dead space, which was more than enough to offset the increased resistance afforded by the tracheostomy tube, compared with the resistance of mouth breathing. That this was true was indicated in the lowered oxygen consumption, showing a significant reduction in the physical work of breathing. Because less oxygen was needed for ventilatory efforts, arterial oxygen saturation rose, probably aided by a concomitant improvement in the alveolar ventilation-perfusion relationship.

### Tracheobronchial aspiration

Aspiration is such an important part of tracheostomy care that it warrants special discussion, for upon its effectiveness may rest the success of the tracheotomy and all other associated therapy. Unfortunately, aspiration, or as it is sometimes called, "bronchial toilet," is a facet of patient care that is frequently done ineffectually and harmfully. Except for other specially trained personnel, such as those employed in intensive care units, aspiration of the respiratory tract is best done by the experienced respiratory therapist, for he is able to correlate the procedure with the operation of a ventilator or oxygen therapy equipment. Even more significant, his training has impressed upon him the importance of maintaining a free airway, on which the successful performance of his work depends. Aspiration is not satisfactorily left to the general ward nursing staff, who, shorthanded and pressed for time, may delegate it to nonprofessional nursing personnel. At best, the instruction and experience in bronchial suctioning vary greatly among nursing school curricula. It is not a difficult task, but it does require understanding of its objectives and hazards and great care. We will discuss it in terms of the equipment used, the preparation, and the details of the aspirating technique.

**Equipment.** A special catheter with a perforated tip through which secretions may be drawn is used to pass into the respiratory tract. It may be of rubber, but many hospitals have found disposable plastic to be more practical and convenient. No matter which type is used, the catheter must be smooth along its length and at its tip; one that has been cut to leave a rough or sharp distal end should never be used. The catheter must be fully sterilized according to standard procedures, and because the ventilated patient will probably need frequent attention, many should be immediately available. For this reason the individually packed, sterile, disposable units have become popular. If rubber is preferred, several can be stacked in layers, separated by toweling, and made up in a sterile pack to be left at the bedside where they can be uncovered individually as needed. For each patient the diameter of the intrabronchial catheter should be no greater than one half the diameter of the tracheostomy tube so that aspiration will not generate dangerous intrapulmonary negative pressure.[303] This is especially important to protect the easily compressed airways of children and the diseased bronchioles of emphysematous patients.

As shown in Fig. 10-5, a collecting bottle for the bronchial secretions is attached to the suction source by suitable tubing and the bottle in turn connected to the stem of a glass Y-tube connector. The catheter is attached to one arm of the Y-tube, the other arm left free. After each episode of suctioning the airways, the catheter is discarded, either in the trash if disposable or in a container to be cleaned and sterilized if of rubber. Gone are the days of the single catheter used repeatedly time and again, often left lying on the bedsheet, even dangling to the floor, or futilely immersed in a "germicidal" solution. Examination of such solutions has demonstrated that they very soon become cesspools of bacteria. Once common practice, such mishandling of catheters is inexcusable in the modern hospital.

**Preparation.** The therapist must carefully open the wrapping of a catheter, making sure he does not touch it with the bare hand, letting it rest on its sterile covering or some other sterile surface. He must then thoroughly wash his hands, preferably

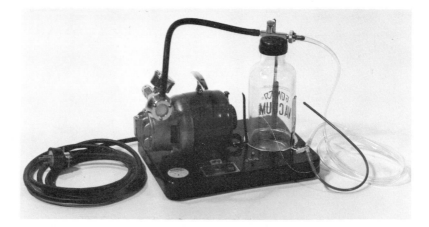

**Fig. 10-5.** Tracheobronchial aspiration setup using a suction pump. The aspirating catheter is connected to one arm of a Y-connector, the other arm is left free for thumb-controlled suction. Aspirate is collected in a jar located between the Y-connector and the pump.

scrubbing them with a brush and antiseptic soap, dry them with a sterile towel, and put a sterile glove on his dominant hand. With the unsterile hand the therapist holds the Y-connector and, with the gloved hand, attaches the catheter to one arm of the Y-tube. The ventilator can be disconnected from the tracheostomy tube by an associate, or if the therapist is alone, he can do it with his uncovered hand. He will take this opportunity to aspirate the mouth and pharynx of secretions, and then deflate the cuff, both to relieve tracheal pressure and to provide the spontaneously breathing patient with some additional airway during the aspiration. If advisable, according to the schedule established for the individual patient, he or his helper can remove the inner cannula for replacement by a fresh sterile one following suctioning. Removal of the ventilator, deflation of the cuff, and removal of the inner cannula can be done by the unaided therapist before scrubbing if the patient is able to tolerate the time off assisted ventilation. Finally, the suction is turned on, and the procedure is ready to begin with a fresh sterile catheter.

We have described the classical aseptic technique, proper performance of which is universally accepted. However, it is time-consuming and awkward without assistance, and often the clinical situation demands faster, more efficient action. An alternative technique that has proved to be safe and effective omits the hand scrubbing and sterile glove. Instead, the operator manipulates the catheter into and out of the airways with a surgical clamp. When not in use, the clamp is kept in a cylindrical container of an effective chemical sterilizer and its tip rinsed in sterile water before the catheter is picked up.

**Aspiration.** No one without a clear understanding of the anatomic structures of the respiratory tract and a responsible appreciation of the vital role played by the bronchial mucosa in protecting the body from infection should be permitted to aspirate the airways. All instrumentation of the tract is traumatic to its delicate lining, and the utmost gentleness is required to keep injury to a minimum. During the preparation of the patient and equipment, the patient's airway should be flooded with 100% oxygen for 1 to 2 minutes. During each interruption in aspiration and at the conclusion of the procedure, oxygenation should be repeated. Cardiac arrhythmias have been noted in many patients being aspirated, believed to be due to accompanying hypoxia.

The operator's sterile hand holds the catheter, and the unsterile hand holds the glass Y-tube connector; with the free end of the Y-tube left open so that *no suction* is applied, the operator gently introduces the catheter into the trachea and one of the main stem bronchi as far as it will easily go. Since both lungs will be aspirated, it generally makes no difference which is treated first, but the catheter will readily enter either bronchus if the patient's head is turned to the opposite side. As soon as the catheter's progress has stopped, the therapist occludes the open end of the Y-connector and applies suction for 2 to 3 seconds. Aspiration is stopped by releasing the Y-connector, the catheter is withdrawn a short distance, and aspiration is again activated. This procedure is repeated in two to four steps until the catheter is in the trachea, at which time it is then withdrawn. The following must be remembered: *The catheter is never moved along the axis of the airway while suction is being applied.* While it is stationary and aspirating, the catheter may safely be gently rotated by an easy twirling motion to allow maximum exposure to secretions. It must *not* be plunged up and down in the bronchial tree, since it will then ream the respiratory mucosa and denude the airways of much of the all-important cilia. Following vigorous and injurious ramrodding of the bronchi, histologic examination of sediment from the collecting jar has often revealed large sheets of respiratory epithelium with cilia that have been stripped from and sucked out of the airways. Should additional aspiration be needed, the catheter is reintroduced and the sequence repeated, but once withdrawal has started, it should be completed with intermittent suctioning along the way. The opposite lung is then attended, preferably with a new sterile catheter.

The intervals between aspirating sessions will necessarily vary from patient to patient according to need, but aspiration should be carried out routinely at least every 30 to 60 minutes. The duration of each aspiration will depend on the patient's tolerance but should not be prolonged beyond 15 seconds even though the patient does not appear adversely affected. Many patients suffer severe apprehension over the procedure, viewing it with great dread and fear, and in some it precipitates distressing coughing and choking. The patient must be closely observed during suctioning because cardiac arrest can occur, especially if the procedure is prolonged. It is felt that arrest is the result of severe hypoxia resulting from the loss of oxygen and lung volume through the catheter.[297] The therapist must remember that he is suctioning not only secretions from the lungs but also lung air, reducing the oxygen available to the patient and shrinking the volume of the lungs.

To make the most of bronchial aspiration the therapist should mobilize the secretions as much as possible by humidification. We have adequately emphasized the importance of aerosolized moisture in the breathing gas, but if the secretions are still excessively viscid, they may be rendered more fluid by using a steady intratracheal saline drip in the patient not on a ventilator. When this is not feasible, the instillation of 10 to 15 ml of saline directly into the tracheostomy tube prior to suctioning may increase the aspirate yield. If secretions are predominantly purulent, preaspiration injection into the airways of either N-acetylcysteine or pancreatic dornase is a helpful preparation for suctioning.

As noted above, the introduction of an aspirating catheter may reveal an obstruction above the carina. Difficulty in passing the catheter may be the result of its impingement against the tracheal wall, a dislodged or herniated cuff, or dried secretions occluding the distal end of the cannula. If the cuff is at fault, the entire tube must be removed and completely replaced. The therapist should be alert to these possibilities, for he may note their presence during routine aspiration before they have had a deleterious effect on the patient.

Finally, aspiration through an endotracheal or nasotracheal tube follows the same basic principles described for a tracheotomy. The added distance of the indwelling tube through which the catheter must be passed makes the procedure more awkward and probably a bit less effective. Generally, smaller catheters must be used because of the reduced lumen of the tube and the need to avoid serious additional obstruction by the catheter. For the maintenance of clear airways in the intubated patient whose major problem is not obstructive, aspiration through the tube will usually be satisfactory. If secretions are an important pathologic factor and need frequent attention, the patient should be tracheotomized for the assurance of maximum airway clearance.

## MANAGEMENT OF THE VENTILATED PATIENT

Because he is among the most critically ill in the hospital, the patient being supported for ventilatory failure must be treated in an area specifically devoted to intensive care. Attempts to manage such a patient on general medical or surgical floors is inconsistent with good medical practice. Some hospitals have respiratory care units, intensive care areas limited to the acute pulmonary patient. This is theoretically the ideal because it permits maximum concentration of personnel and equipment for each patient. A major drawback is the inevitable duplication of services required to care for patients in the general intensive care unit, or other special care areas, who cannot be moved because of pressing nonpulmonary needs. Probably, in most average general hospitals, the mechanically ventilated patient is best managed in the intensive care unit.

The patient on a mechanical ventilator requires constant close attention and observation by both nurses and respiratory therapists who are knowledgeable in the clinical aspects of inadequate ventilation. As has been pointed out before, the ventilated patient is dependent for every breath on his respirator and the skill of his attendants. The possibility of mechanical failure and the sudden changes that may develop in the patient's physiology make it mandatory that he not be left alone for an instant. It is not enough to have people around; they must be people who know how to respond to the patient's needs and to any emergency that may arise. This obviously leads to the conclusion that the management of the ventilated patient must be delegated only to those with special training in respiratory care at medical, nursing, and technical levels.

The physician ultimately responsible for the therapeutic details must be experienced in clinical chest medicine and versed in basic cardiopulmonary physiology and pulmonary function evaluation. This extent of preparedness often requires the combined efforts of the patient's attending physician and a specialized consultant. An insight of the interacting physiologic and biochemical forces active in respiratory failure comes only with prolonged exposure, and even the most competent general physician seldom has enough constant experience with this condition to be fully confident in its management, at least during the most acute phases. Certainly, a new house staff should not be given responsibility for the care of respiratory failure without close supervision, for at the present time undergraduate medical education does not give these people adequate preparation. From a teaching point of view the consolidation of respiratory patients in a special care unit provides an unparalleled opportunity to train young physicians in this field and give them the basic knowledge and experience in the minimum time to make them proficient in respiratory care.

General nursing education usually includes pulmonary physiology and respiratory diseases only as segments of overall comprehensive courses, and the nurse who will care for ventilatory failure patients must have additional training. In hospitals with effective respiratory therapy departments, this should be easily accomplished, and it is the responsibility of such departments to make available to all nurses who are interested a course of instruction in the principles and practices of respiratory therapy, with emphasis on acute care.

Let us now consider some of the practical aspects of supporting the patient with a failed ventilatory system.

## Choice of a ventilator

*General factors in selection.* We have established that there is no single best ventilator, that there are several machines which are good, with qualifications, yet each has its champions; and we are accustomed to hearing debates extolling the virtues of one over another. The personal preferences among physicians and therapists alike are based on many factors, among which are experience with one type of ventilator, confidence in one over the others, admiration for a particular mechanical principle, and economy. All of these are important considerations but are dependent more upon whim than upon the specific objectives sought in each individual patient being ventilated. It can be emphasized again that generally the skill and experience of the operating therapist are more important than the specific type of respirator used; but in our discussion of the principles of the various units in common use, we indicated features both favorable and unfavorable. Some of the desirable characteristics that we would like to see in a ventilator would certainly include at least the following:

1. The machine should be able to operate for long periods with a minimum of servicing and maximum freedom from the risk of mechanical breakdown.
2. There should be provisions for operating the instrument on room air, pure oxygen, a variable mixture of both, and any other gas desired.

3. Whether the ventilator is basically pressure cycled or volume cycled, there should be dependable control over, or a safe limit to, the generated pressure.
4. Especially important and strongly emphasized earlier, there should be a variable flow control, either manual or automatic.
5. Desirable, but not always essential, is a combination of both control and assist capabilities or greater versatility in handling the changing patterns of breathing so commonly encountered.
6. Negative pressure during exhalation should be available for the patient undergoing prolonged controlled ventilation.
7. There must be provisions for adequate humidification of inspired gas, a need upon which the patient's survival may depend.
8. For the patient under controlled breathing, there should be a means of adjusting the inspiratory-to-expiratory time ratio or at least a provision to assure that inspiration does not exceed expiration.
9. There should be available some means to monitor the delivered tidal volume.
10. The ventilator should have built-in mechanisms, or attachments, to provide positive end-expiratory pressure and intermittent mandatory ventilation maneuvers, which will be described later in the chapter.

This is not an exhaustive list, and the therapist can probably add several more criteria he would like to see met before he would have full confidence in any machine. In summary, we may state that the choice of a ventilator will often depend upon which one of all those available in a given hospital is felt to be the safest and most effective for a given patient with due regard for the number, skill, and experience of the therapists who will be responsible for its operation. This choice will be made from among the groups described in the classification of Chapter 9, negative-pressure versus positive-pressure, assistor versus controller, and electric versus pneumatic.

As a recapitulation of some of the features of the major ventilators, Table 10-1 compares their adjustable, variable, and fixed characteristics while operating as controllers.

**Table 10-1.** *Adjustable, variable, and fixed functions of controllers**

| Ventilator | Tidal volume | Pressure | Flow | Minute rate | I/E |
|---|---|---|---|---|---|
| Tank | V | A (neg) | V | A | V |
| Chest | V | A (neg) | V | V | A |
| Engström | A | V | V | A | F |
| Emerson | A | V | V | V | A |
| Bourns | A | V | A | A | V |
| Bennett MA-1 | A | V | A | A | V |
| Monaghan 225 | A | V | A | A | V |
| Bird M-7, 8 | V | A | A | V | A |
| Bennett PR-2 | V | A | A† | A | F‡ |

*A = adjustable; V = variable, depending on A, other variables, and condition of machine-patient circuit; F = fixed by machine.
†Flow self-adjusting, with additional modification by rate control.
‡Fixed at a maximum but may be lowered by expiratory timer.

*Clinical guides to selection.* Let us now consider the possible clinical indications that might favor one type of ventilator over another, grouping patients according to normal lungs, restrictive disease, and obstruction, with the understanding that in actual practice individual circumstances are often complicated by a combination of these factors.

*Patients with normal lungs and thorax.* This group usually includes those with neurologic or muscular pathology interfering with ventilation. The generalization may be made that a patient in ventilatory failure who has a normal lung-thorax and clear airways can be adequately ventilated with any of the standard respirators, since the only problem is the simple transportation of air into the alveoli against no abnormal barriers. If the removal of bronchial secretions or the risk of aspiration of oral or regurgitated gastric contents is not a clinical consideration, intubation may be avoided and the patient ventilated by the negative-pressure body respirator. The elective use of the tank implies the need for minimal medical and nursing attention and the ability to control rather than assist the patient's breathing. It is in this group of patients also that the chest respirator has its greatest application, especially in those being weaned from the large tank or who need support of their own spontaneous breathing, such as during the sleeping hours. However, the cumbersome tank ventilator, and the difficult-to-fit-and-adjust chest ventilator, are being used less and less frequently, since increased skills in the management of the intubated patient almost exclusively employ positive-pressure ventilation. The choice of respirator is therefore based on convenience and comfort rather than on the need to combat a physiologic limitation to gas exchange. Although the management of ventilation is fairly easy, it is not without its hazard, for as will be emphasized below, the risk of serious over-ventilation is great.

*Patients with restrictive lung disease.* Restriction that limits ventilation may be due to involvement of the thorax, as with trauma, and of the pulmonary parenchyma. The primary ventilatory problem in this case is the markedly reduced lung-thorax compliance, which necessitates high driving pressures to deliver adequate tidal and minute volumes. In this circumstance many physicians and therapists favor the use of a volume positive-pressure ventilator that can deliver the necessary tidal volume at whatever pressure is required. The obvious disadvantage of the pressure-cycled respirator is premature end-inspiratory cycling before delivery of the tidal volume if the pressure needs of air delivery exceed the capability of the machine. The factors that will determine whether a volume or pressure ventilator will be necessary are the degree of restriction and the skill of the respiratory therapist. Pressure-cycled ventilators can be successfully used against a considerable loss of compliance and in many patients with chest injury, but success depends on close attention to the pressure-time relationships of the mechanical adjustments by an experienced therapist.

Two observations may help to clarify this problem for the student. First, regardless of the instrument used, the patient with severe restrictive disease is faced with the hazard of the deleterious effects of high intrathoracic pressures that we have already considered in detail. Because of this and progressive loss of compliance, some patients just cannot be sustained with any equipment or techniques now available. In such patients it is more academic than realistic to debate the virtues of delivering air at almost unlimited pressure if the therapy itself puts the patients under increasing risk. Second, in patients with "pure" restriction, the volume-cycled ventilators can support all but those noted above and are probably preferred, especially when there is anything less than ideal technical supervision. However, except in such diseases as the respiratory distress syndrome of the newborn and adults, and a few fibrotic or granulomatous conditions, restriction is frequently associated with obstructive disease, to be described next, and in this case the ventilator preference may be reversed.

*Patients with obstructive disease.* By and large, most patients with obstructive disease present the dual problems of increased airway resistance and reduced compliance and may confront the therapist with his greatest technical challenge. The chief prerequisite of a respirator to manage the obstructed patient is variable flow control, reasons for which have been adequately covered earlier. There is widespread disagreement on the efficacy of pressure versus volume ventilators, but it is futile to engage in debate. With a mechanically dependable instrument that has flow control, the clinical results obtained depend entirely upon the skill and experience of the operator. Theoretically, it makes little difference whether a ventilator is volume cycled or pressure cycled if it possesses flow control, but practically, this reduces the selection to the IPPV type. It is true that the Engström respirator has a sort of "automatic" flow control, in a sense, active during its so-called "static pressure period" to allow the gas flow to accommodate to resistance. However, at the usual ventilatory rates this time interval is less than 0.75 second. In contrast, the IPPVs have direct or indirect control over flow. Reference to Table 10-1 shows that four respirators have manually adjustable flows, one of which is also self-adjusting and another modified by manipulation of its I/E ratio. With pressure and flow critical factors in the kinetics of ventilating obstructed airways, only two have the distinct advantage of independent control over these two parameters. We should point out here that for the respiratory therapist who understands basic pulmonary physiology and mechanics as well as the detailed functions of his equipment, it makes little difference whether a volume is delivered to a patient at a required pressure or a pressure is delivered to achieve a desired volume, as long as the flow of the gas can be adjusted to ensure its delivery. It is the responsibility of the therapist to determine, in his own mind, what variables will respond to changes in adjustable controls for each ventilator he is expected to use. The opinion is expressed here that in the face of the unstable and interacting forces of obstruction and loss of compliance, the patient whose ventilation fails because of chronic obstructive disease can best be managed by a ventilator which gives independent control over pressure, flow, and I/E ratio. Both skill and patience are needed, since frequent resetting of controls assures the maintenance of ventilation through the shifting course of the disease, but maximum flexibility is thereby available to the therapist who is able to give tailor-made treatment to his patient.

***Summary.*** There are no hard-and-fast criteria for respirator selection, and whatever guidelines one may have are becoming harder to follow because new makes and models of equipment continue to flood the market. With the exception of fluidic control, there has been no innovation in operating principle for a number of years, only more elaborate styling and increasing costs. The following personal observations and opinions are offered to help the therapist formulate his own views.

1. Respiratory therapy literature of ventilatory care contains few references to economy, as if the grave nature of respiratory failure precludes such a consideration. The student is urged to note the cost differential between most pressure-cycled and volume-cycled ventilators. It is suggested that most patients can be successfully supported on flow-adjustable, pressure-cycled machines (Bird Mark 7 or 8, Bennett PR class) and that these are practical for general use because of their portability, adaptability to emergencies, versatility in ventilating normal and obstructed lungs, and economy of cost and space.

2. More skill is required to use the full potential of pressure-cycled ventilators than volume-cycled. Thus availability of personnel trained and experienced in the operation of pressure-cycled units may be an important factor in choosing a machine.

3. Significantly reduced compliance is a strong indication for ventilation by volume cycling.

4. Negative pressure ventilators should be limited to the uncommon patient whose ventilatory failure is due to neuromuscular disease rather than obstruction or loss of compliance, whose physical condition requires little medical or nursing attention, and where the equipment is compatible with available space and the comfort of other patients. There is actually little need for the large tank ventilator and only rare indications for the chest cuirass.

5. Assistor-controllers have always had distinct advantage over assistors, although current techniques in mechanical ventilation, to be described soon, have made this difference less important.

## Instituting and maintaining ventilation

Most of this section will refer to the patient who is apneic or whose breathing is weak and ineffective and who thus needs complete ventilatory control. It will usually be obvious where comments also apply to the assisted patient, but where necessary, this will be stipulated.

*Initiating tidal volume and rate.* The first problem to be faced by the respiratory care team is the determination of a suitable tidal volume and rate. For the adult patient with no spontaneous breathing, a rate is generally established somewhere between 15 and 20 breaths per minute, although this decision may have to be modified by tidal volume needs. Because of the great variations in body mass among the many patients being mechanically ventilated, the choice of tidal volume can be a difficult one. Obviously, an attempt is made to establish a pattern of breathing that will give the patient the best alveolar gas exchange, and the *only* way this can be determined is to measure arterial oxygen and carbon dioxide tensions and pH. We will emphasize a little later the necessity of this technique throughout the entire management period, but it should be stressed here that in many instances ventilation cannot be delayed while waiting for laboratory data. Often the initiation of artificial ventilation must rely upon clinical evaluation, and especially upon a background of extensive experience in treating respiratory failure. The highly skilled therapist will base his judgment on the size of the patient, the depth and ease of chest movements during ventilation, and the many combinations of pressures and volumes that he has had occasion to use in the past. It is quite remarkable how effective this clinical approach can be when later confirmed by blood gas determinations.

The therapist is not without some assistance in setting combined tidal volumes and rates, since there are available nomograms to use as initial guidelines to get ventilation under way. Two such are provided for use with the Engström respirator, one each for children and adults.[304, 305] These are complex charts based on a series of mathematical equations that consider such factors as estimated basal alveolar ventilation, body surface area, sex, age, breathing frequency, and tubing size. More applicable for general use is the Radford nomogram, a reproduction of which will be found in Appendix 13.[306] It should be clearly understood that no nomogram or formula for determining tidal or minute volumes is precise. The nomogram is used only to suggest a reasonable starting point with a minimum of delay, with necessary modifications as indicated by clinical observation or physiologic data. However, the Radford nomogram is useful because of the ease and speed with which it can be used, factors of great importance in the often hurried atmosphere of the failing patient.

The Radford nomogram bases its values on the three parameters of weight, respiratory rate, and sex, but it is vitally important to understand that the data refer to *basal* requirements in *healthy* subjects. This means that the chart is composed of information obtained from large numbers of healthy individuals, of a variety of sizes and ages, of both sexes, at complete rest, with all bodily functions at a minimal level of activity. Obviously, then, the direct information provided by the nomogram does not apply to the patient whose physiologic disturbance of his disease may raise his metabolic activity far above the basal level. To compensate for such effects of illness, provisions are made to adjust the nomogram values by specific percentages, according to the clinical situation. The effect of a tracheostomy on ventilatory needs is illustrated in the chart of nomogram corrections, permitting the reduction of basal tidal volume by a significant amount. Also, the adjustment referred to as the dead space of "anesthesia apparatus" reflects the anesthesia orientation of the nomogram but can equally be applied to a ventilator. When the nomogram is used for the apneic patient, respiratory frequency must be established that is consistent with the age as well as the tidal volume. If the patient has spontaneous breathing, the tidal volume actually moved by him is measured and compared with that predicted by the graph to see whether air movement is adequate or intervention is indicated. If the limitations of this nomogram are kept in mind and the therapist has good clinical understanding and judgment, he will find the chart useful. It should not be used by inexperienced personnel as a substitute for a clear understanding of the principles of mechanical ventilation.

On the basis of information from many sources as well as personal experience, the average basal tidal volumes by age, weight, and sex, from birth through adulthood are summarized in Table 10-2.[306-312]

**Table 10-2.** *Estimated basal tidal volume by age, weight, and sex*

| Age (yr) | Normal frequency | Average weight (lb) | Tidal volume (ml) | |
|---|---|---|---|---|
| | | | Male | Female |
| Newborn | 30-40 | 8 | 18- 22 | 18- 22 |
| 1 | 25-35 | 22 | 55- 70 | 55- 70 |
| 2 | ±28 | 27 | 80 | 80 |
| 3 | ±25 | 32 | 100 | 100 |
| 4- 6 | 20-25 | 36- 44 | 125-150 | 125-145 |
| 7- 9 | 20-25 | 50- 65 | 160-180 | 155-175 |
| 10-14 | 20-25 | 65-100 | 200-265 | 185-245 |
| 15-16 | 16-18 | 100-115 | 300-330 | 280-300 |
| Adult | 12-18 | 120 | 350 | 320 |
| | | 130 | 370 | 340 |
| | | 150 | 400 | 360 |
| | | 175 | 450 | 400 |
| | | 200 | 500 | 440 |
| | | 225 | 540 | 460 |

It might be added that the tidal volumes of premature infants can be as low as 6 ml, making necessary the use of respirator exhalation heads that have as close to no dead space as possible. There is no need for the student to memorize Table 10-2, for it is intended only to emphasize the tremendous variation in tidal volumes with which he must contend, and with continued experience he will become familiar with a few key values that will enable him to start safe therapy while awaiting more specific guides.

***Establishing a ventilatory pattern.*** We will be concerned not with theoretical pressure of flow curves but, rather, with those factors that contribute to establishing a pattern of breathing most helpful to the patient, emphasizing the clinical problems faced by the therapist.

*Relation of pressure, rate, and volume.* Once the desired frequency and tidal volume have been determined, volume-cycled ventilators are preset and activated and the actual delivered volume measured by a suitable meter. Slight adjustments are often necessary, since the volume controls are not perfectly precise. If a pressure-cycled ventilator is used, a moderate to low starting pressure is chosen to initiate ventilation and is gradually increased to deliver the desired volume. Whatever instrument is used, an attempt is generally made to keep the pressure below 40 cm of water to minimize interference with the circulation, although this may be difficult in the presence of a significant reduction in compliance. To illustrate this with an oversimplified example, let us assume that we wish to deliver a tidal volume of 400 ml at a frequency of 16 per minute but find that a pressure of 50 cm of water is needed. Because we know from our earlier studies of physiology that compliance tends to vary inversely with respiratory frequency, we will slow down the controlled rate and see whether ventilation can be accomplished with less force. Perhaps we will find that at a rate of 12 breaths per minute, the ventilator can deliver 533 ml of air at a pressure of but 40 cm of water, in which case we will provide the same total minute ventilation. Whether this increase in tidal volume is to the patient's advantage will be a matter of medical judgment to determine, but this fictitious example is presented to demonstrate the need for versatility by both therapist and ventilator in accommodating the requirements of respiratory failure.

Frequently patients will have spontaneous breathing but of a character too weak, rapid, or irregular to effect adequate alveolar gas exchange, and it is often possible to "override" such spontaneous breathing with a volume ventilator. If complete control cannot be achieved at once over a rapid rate, the volume ventilator is adjusted to the patient's frequency, and then attempts are made to reduce the rate of the instrument gradually, allowing the patient to accommodate to the slowing pace, which relieves him of much of the effort of breathing. The power of the volume-cycled respirators tends to discourage patient competition unless the spontaneous drive is strong, and in such instances safe ventilation may not be possible without modifying the patient's pattern, to be described below, or switching to a different type of ventilator. Semi-controlled ventilation may be achieved with a pressure-cycled machine in a patient with rapid but weak spontaneous breathing. This technique assists the patient's breathing rather than taking complete control over it but at the same time modifies its pattern. The instrument is adjusted for automatic controlled breathing at a rate less than the patient's own, and he is allowed to override the ventilator. If the patient is rationally responsive as he benefits from the assist to his breathing, he sometimes can be encouraged to relax his efforts and give in to the control of the respirator, letting his rate subside to a more efficient level. Even when the patient cannot be brought under full control, continued reassuring support by the therapist will often help the rapid breather to slow his efforts so that satisfactory, restful, assisted ventilation will assure good tidal air exchange. No matter what the technique, the object is to relieve the patient of excessive work, to reduce frequency to the normal range for his age and size, and to deliver to him an adequate tidal and minute volume.

*Inspiratory/expiratory ratio.* There are no shortcuts to setting up a safe and effective respirator. Although the pressure-cycled machines are the most versatile and sensitive with the potential for fine control if properly used, they require the most skill and experience. It must be repeated here for emphasis that in the hands of the untrained, such ventilators may constitute in themselves a serious hazard to the welfare of the patient. During fully controlled ventilation, attention must be given to the inspiratory-to-expiratory time ratio, the rationale for which has been sufficiently covered earlier. Inspiratory time must never exceed expiratory time, and in most instances a ratio of 1:1.5 or 1:2 will be safe. The surest way to establish the ratio is to use a stopwatch, but many experienced therapists have so trained their ears that they are remarkably accurate in balancing the respiratory phases merely by listening as they adjust the controls. This important step is not always easily or quickly accomplished, and the manner in which it is done depends on the instrument used. With some, the matter is simply the adjustment of control switches (Emerson); with others, it depends on regulating the flow control (Bourns, Bennett MA-1); and with yet others, the ratio is machine fixed (Engström, Bennett PR-2). However, we know that even

**Table 10-3.**  *Relationship between P, V, inspiratory time, and frequency*

|  | P ↑ | | | P ↓ | | | V̇ ↑ | | | V̇ ↓ | | |
|---|---|---|---|---|---|---|---|---|---|---|---|---|
| P | ⧅ | ⧅ | ⧅ | ⧅ | ⧅ | ⧅ | → | ↓ | ↑ | → | ↓ | ↑ |
| V̇ | → | ↓ | ↑ | → | ↓ | ↑ | ⧅ | ⧅ | ⧅ | ⧅ | ⧅ | ⧅ |
| Inspiratory time | ↑ | ↑↑ | → | ↓ | → | ↓↓ | ↓ | ↓↓ | → | ↑ | → | ↑↑ |
| Frequency | ↓ | ↓↓ | → | ↑ | → | ↑↑ | ↑ | ↑↑ | → | ↓ | → | ↓↓ |

with the PR-2 the ratio can be modified so that it is not entirely nonadjustable. On the other hand, the Bird respirator, because it is so amenable to custom setting, offers a good example to use for reviewing the intricacies of the I/E ratio.

Fundamentally, controlled inspiratory time depends on the flow at a given pressure setting, whereas expiration is regulated by its own mechanism, and the student must remember the interrelationships among flow, pressure, time, and frequency. For convenience, these are summarized in Table 10-3, which does nothing more than compact in columns what already we have described in some detail. The table compares the effects of various combinations of pressure and flow on inspiratory time and frequency. Horizontal arrows mean no change; double arrows imply a greater response than a single arrow. For example, increasing the pressure while decreasing flow increases (prolongs) inspiratory time more than if flow were kept stable. Once the desired combination of mask pressure and tidal volume has been established, the I/E ratio is adjusted by individually timing inspiration and expiration, while still maintaining a constant frequency. Let us suppose that we have set a Bird-type ventilator so that a delivery pressure of 30 cm of water provides the tidal volume we feel the patient needs and we wish the breathing pattern to be one of 20 breaths per minute with an I/E ratio of 1:2. This means that each breath will be of 3 seconds' duration, of which inspiration will comprise 1 second and exhalation 2 seconds. We will first adjust the control that regulates the time interval between inspirations to get our expiratory time. This will remain independent of other controls, since it is activated by end-inspiration, and its duration is determined by the speed of its bleed-off. The 1-second inspiratory phase will be set by appropriately changing the flow, increasing it to reduce inspiration and decreasing to prolong it. In the absence of any variable factors that might change the dynamics of ventilation we should now have set the respirator to deliver our predetermined tidal volume at a safe pressure, at a frequency consistent with the size and age of the patient, and with a phase ratio that we feel will protect the patient from harmful pressure effects.

However, if our patient has chronic bronchopulmonary obstructive disease, we must be prepared to make frequent readjustments because the compliance-obstruction status of his airways changes frequently. In addition to bronchospasm, which may well be present, the shifting of secretions in the respiratory tract and their periodic removal by therapeutic aspiration will keep the status of the airways in a state of continual flux. This is why the obstructed patient must be kept under constant observation and the controls of his respirator frequently changed to maintain as constant ventilation as possible in the face of an unstable tract. Such a patient may put the respiratory therapist's skill to a severe test and often requires his full-time services. Let us now imagine that the compliance drops in the patient we attended in the preceding paragraph. We will find that our machine can no longer deliver the required tidal volume at the initial pressure of 30 cm of water; to restore this volume we must increase the system pressure. As soon as we do this, we note that the inspiratory time increases, since more time is required to transmit the higher pressure to the patient's lungs at the original flow. With a prolongation of inspiration, not only is the I/E ratio disturbed, but the total frequency drops because the expiratory time is unaffected and remains unchanged. Obviously, to restore the initial ventilatory pattern, we will have to increase the flow accordingly and bring the inspiratory time back to its original value. If our patient's problem is primarily one of loss of compliance, we can continue to increase both pressure and flow to deliver a constant tidal volume, up to the limits of the ventilator or to the limit of physiologic safety for the patient. On the other hand, if varying degrees of airway obstruction complicate the condition, our task will be much more difficult.

*Ventilating obstructed airways.* We are well aware of the problems of ventilating an obstructed passage with pressure-driven air and the great need to be able to vary the flow to compensate for such obstruction. If our patient suddenly reduces the effective caliber of his bronchi by spasm or an outpouring of secretions, the back pressure so generated will match the system pressure and cycle end-inspiration before delivery of the full tidal volume and, in this instance, inspiratory time will be markedly shortened. We have a choice of two maneuvers to try to restore tidal ventilation. First, we can increase the system pressure as we did with the compliance defect above, which will prolong the inspiratory time; but our knowledge of gas kinetics tells us that overcoming the pressure drop due to obstruction by this method will probably elevate the intrathoracic pressure to dangerously high levels. Second, we can make use of the variable flow control of our ventilator and drop the flow, which will significantly reduce the pressure gradient across the obstruction and deliver a larger pressure (and gas volume) distally with a minimum system pressure and prolong inspiratory time. The response of inspiratory time to both these combinations of pressure and flow are indicated in Table 10-3. However, merely slowing the delivered flow will not necessarily be satisfactory, since overcoming the obstruction may require an inspiratory time so long that the reduced minute rate will prevent an adequate minute alveolar ventilation despite the desired pressure and tidal volume. Also, if the inspiratory time is too prolonged, it can seriously upset the optimum I/E ratio. When faced with this problem, the therapist must be prepared to spend a considerable period of time trying to achieve a compromise balance among the many factors involved because there is no standard procedural guide to follow. He will probably find that a combination of lowering the flow and elevating the pressure in gradual steps will give him the best control over the ventilation. In addition, he may find that he will have to settle for a reduced frequency to accommodate a necessarily prolonged inspiratory time and then will try to increase the tidal volume enough to assure a safe minute volume. At any rate he will be aware that a change in either pressure or flow will change the entire balance between pressure, flow, inspiratory time, and frequency; and he will soon develop the patience required to reset controls as he finds it necessary to keep up with ventilation needs. His goal will be the lowest system pressure at the lowest flow that will deliver the desired tidal volume at a normal frequency and with a safe I/E ratio.

Reference should be made here to the automatic flow adjustability of the Bennett PR respirator. The sensitivity of the main valve slows down gas flow in the presence of distal obstruction but allows flow to continue to the patient as long as it is in excess of $1 \ell$/min. The pneumatic timers prevent the I/E ratio from exceeding $1:1.5$. In this instrument some manual influence over flow can be achieved by reducing machine output through use of the peak flow control, and, of course, the delivered pressure can also be adjusted. The automatic responsiveness of the Bennett respirator does not mean that it is a simple instrument to operate, since its safe and effective use requires a full understanding of the mechanical relationships of its parts. It is again emphasized that the choice between these two major positive-pressure ventilators is a matter of the operator's preference for either partial automatic function or freer control over each variable setting.

*Periodic hyperventilation.* If the student will observe his own quiet breathing during a prolonged period of bodily relaxation, as during a reading session, he will note a phenomenon so natural that he is usually unaware of it. Every now and then he will unconsciously sigh, often rather deeply. The significance of this act and its importance to mechanical ventilation became clear with the rapid increase in use of ventilators. During periods of physical inaction, as metabolic needs approach basal levels, depth of ventilation decreases and the distribution of intrapulmonary inspired air becomes irregular. Some pulmonary units are poorly expanded by the low level of ventilation and get less-than-adequate air exchange. This sets up localized areas of decreased ventilation-perfusion ratios, which actually constitute small physiologic shunts. In the normal subject, with active respiratory control mechanisms, this presents no hazard because the natural periodic sigh hyperinflates the lung, expanding and aerating all segments. It had been frequently noted, however, that patients who were maintained on supposedly adequate mechanically ventilated patterns often suffered deterioration of their pulmonary status and became progressively more difficult to ventilate. A detailed study on anesthetized patients demonstrated the cause for this unfavorable response.[313] Ventilatory and physiologic studies showed that prolonged artificial ventilation at an unvarying tidal volume level leads to a gradual and progressive atelectasis. As increasing respiratory units become airless, significant arteriovenous shunting, or venous admixture, develops, and the pulmonary compliance steadily drops. Further, it was found that this phenomenon could be both prevented and corrected by periodic hyperinflation of the lungs, the introduction into the breathing pattern of an artificial sigh.

Part of the management of the ventilated patient on complete control is the use of the periodic sigh, and most volume respirators have a mechanism to accomplish this automatically. Controls allow one or more deep breaths to be delivered at preset intervals. With other instruments it is advisable to hyperinflate the lungs with two deep breaths at least every half hour. Manual sighing can be done with the Bird respirator by holding open the cycling valve, for which purpose a rod is provided that extends to the outside of the instrument from the ambient end of the valve. The Bennett PR ventilators can be used to sigh the patient by holding open the rotating valve with a finger on its small projecting rod and increasing the terminal flow. Clinical judgment dictates the hyperinflating volume to be so used, but the short duration of the maneuver holds little risk for the patient.

*Sustained hyperventilation.* In general, hyperventilation is as physiologically unsound as is hypoventilation, and because it is our responsibility to understand the effects of what we do to our patients, we will review in some detail the basic hazards of mechanical hyperventilation. We will then consider how hyperventilation *may* be used with benefit under close control in selected circumstances.

In earlier chapters we discussed response of the acid-base balance of the body to ventilation and the hazards of respiratory alkalosis accompanying hyperventilation. It should be readily appreciated that the patient in respiratory failure is already severely ill and there is no justification for subjecting him to additional physiologic trauma, since the consequences of ventilator-induced alkalosis are potentially grave. The patient may suffer tetany—-convulsive spasms due to marked increased reactivity of muscles. A warning of this impending condition may be jumpiness of the patient in response to ordinary stimuli or may be elicited by tapping the patient's cheek and noting a spasmodic contraction of the facial muscles of the tested side. Especially hazardous is an interference with cerebral blood flow, about which more will be said in detail below. A fall in the concentration of serum potassium has been frequently noted in respiratory alkalosis, believed to be due to movement of potassium ions from the serum into the cells to replace hydrogen ions that are depleted because of the alkalosis. The hypokalemia (low serum potassium concentration) renders the myocardium susceptible to arrhythmias, especially if the heart is already hypoxic or if it is under digitalis treatment. In the latter instance, digitalis toxicity may be precipitated. Finally, alkalosis produces an unfavorable shift in the oxygen dissociation curve, impairing the cellular uptake of oxygen.

The greatest caution must be exercised in ventilating the patient with normal lungs, for he is the easiest to ventilate. It was noted above that in the absence of obstruction or loss of compliance, almost any standard respirator can be used effectively. With such a patient, however, there is the ever-present risk of overzealous therapy, especially true if the therapist is simultaneously supervising the management of a patient who is hard to ventilate.

Let us consider the patient with chronic bronchopulmonary disease who is in respiratory acidosis with characteristically elevated arterial carbon dioxide tension and low pH. It is natural that all members of the medical team are anxious to restore the blood values to normal as soon as possible, since this gives reassurance of effective treatment and subsiding danger; but it is unnecessary to bring down the carbon dioxide level precipitously. This is especially true if the hypercarbia is of significant duration and less important if it is acutely elevated. Thus, if the hypercarbia has suddenly risen, it can be more safely corrected rapidly than if it gradually rose over a long time. There are two physiologic reasons for this differentiation—one somewhat speculative, the other positive. First, with vascular dilatation of the cerebral circulation as a major response to high levels of carbon dioxide, any increase in cerebral blood flow due to sudden hypercarbia in all probability is somewhat "extra," being superimposed on whatever has been the usual perfusion of the brain in the given subject, and the removal of this additional flow by rapid excretion of carbon dioxide returns the cerebral blood flow to its own normal. In contrast, prolonged hypercarbia may condition the cerebral circulation to an increased level of perfusion and, when suddenly reduced, will produce an ischemia of the brain by deprivation of its usual blood supply. This reaction may manifest itself as a period of mental sluggishness or confusion or may produce the signs and symptoms of an acute stroke, with characteristic speech difficulties or muscular weakness, depending on the location of the brain area affected and the severity of the condition. By and large, chronic hypercarbia is more likely to be found in advanced-age patients, since respiratory failure may develop only after many years, whereas sudden, acute uncompensated hypercarbia is more prevalent in the younger patients subject to chest and head trauma, narcosis and anesthesia, and central nervous system infectious diseases. Thus the patient with acute failure superimposed on chronic hypercarbia often has a preexisting compromised cerebral circulation due to degenerative vascular disease, and his brain is more sensitive to alterations in its circulation than is the one with normal circulation.

We are most commonly concerned with the second reason, which is related to the acid-base status of the body. The more acute the hypercarbia, the more uncompensated is the acidosis, simply because there has not been time for the body to meet the challenge by increasing its available supply of buffering bicarbonate. Basically, the problem in this instance is one of a suddenly high carbon dioxide tension and low pH, and if the excess carbon dioxide can be excreted by the ventilatory route, the acid-base balance will readily return to normal. Much more treacherous to manage is the patient with a chronic but low-grade hypercarbia due to long-standing disease in whom a respiratory infection, for example, has acutely depressed ventilation, pushing him into overt failure. This patient may have as high a carbon dioxide tension in his blood as the one cited above, but his pH will not be as low because he already has an increased bicarbonate accompanying his chronic hypercarbia and is thereby in partial compensated respiratory acidosis. If the excess carbon dioxide should be rapidly depleted, and it need not even reach a normal level, large quantities of extra bicarbonate will be left circulating, and the pH can easily jump from a severe acidemia to an iatrogenic alkalemia of serious proportions. As an example of the tremendous acid-base swing that can result from overly aggressive treatment, there is the recorded instance of an arterial pH that leaped from 7.10 to 7.80 in 10 minutes.[314] One can only speculate what effect this must have had on the cerebral circulation and the conductivity of the myocardium. The therapist must keep in mind that in many, if not most patients, intensive therapy can lower the carbon dioxide tension fairly readily, but hyperbasemia can be removed only by renal excretion, and it may take a normally functioning kidney 2 to 3 days to rid the body of an excess load of the antacid. Since many patients in respiratory failure have imperfect renal function, the result of either hypoxia or other accompanying disease, it is easy to see how they may be driven from the frying pan into the fire in terms of their acid-base balance if they are not treated prudently.

The use of buffers poses another ventilation problem with which the therapist should be familiar because it may compound the effect of the elevated bicarbonate of metabolic compensation in respiratory acidosis. There has been a great deal of disagreement over the use of buffers in respiratory acidosis, stemming mostly from a failure to appreciate the physiologic differences between respiratory and metabolic acidosis. For years, part of the standard treatment of metabolic acidosis has been the intravenous administration of sodium bicarbonate (or sodium lactate, which is metabolized in the body to produce bicarbonate) to neutralize excess acid according to the following nonspecific reaction:

$$NaHCO_3 + HA \rightleftharpoons NaA + H_2CO_3$$
$$H_2CO_3 \rightleftharpoons H_2O + CO_2 \uparrow$$

Success of this reaction depends on the ability of the body to remove, by blowing off through the lungs, the carbon dioxide formed. The patient with metabolic acidosis, as from the accumulation of organic acids accompanying diabetes or renal failure, can readily remove large volumes of carbon dioxide if he has no associated pulmonary disease. Indeed, one of the clinical characteristics of such a patient is severe hyperventilation. However, the student will recall that metabolic acidosis disturbs the Henderson-Hasselbalch equation by decreasing the numerator as the normal body bicarbonate is depleted by the abnormal circulating acids. In such a circumstance it is logical to replace bicarbonate therapeutically and so restore normal balance. The biochemical situation is different in respiratory acidosis, especially if it is chronic. In the first place, if we substitute for acid *HA* in the above reaction the characteristic acid of respiratory failure, $H_2CO_3$, the added $NaHCO_3$ merely builds up to high levels because the inherent disability of respiratory acidosis is the inability of the body to blow off even normal amounts of carbon dioxide. Second, when we view respiratory acidosis in terms of acid-base balance, we find it is the result of an increase in the denominator of the H-H equation, not fundamentally a deficiency in bicarbonate. In short, we return to the basic principle of therapy of respiratory acidosis—acid-base balance can be restored only by actively ridding the body of excess carbon dioxide, not by adding increasing amounts of bicarbonate. Suppose a patient has the extreme physiologic values we used earlier in Table 4-6 to illustrate acid-base balance, with a bicarbonate-to-carbon dioxide ratio of 24/2.4 mM/$\ell$ and a pH of 7.10. Even if we add enough bicarbonate to the patient's blood to raise its level to 48 mM/$\ell$, restore a 20/1 ratio, and bring the pH up to 7.40, we still will not correct his basic defect. As long as his $CO_2$ remains elevated, he will be in severe failure although temporarily compensated.

Since it is established that mechanically ventilating the patient in ventilatory failure is the fundamental treatment, let us return to our subject of hyperventilation and see just what are its risks. We will use as examples two fictitious treatment situations as shown in Fig. 10-6, making certain assumptions for the sake of clarity.

Let us imagine a patient before respiratory failure with the blood findings of box *A*, the acid-base ratio expressed in millimoles per liter with the equivalent carbon dioxide tension and the pH consistent with the ratio. Let us now assume our patient develops ventilatory failure (box *B*) with no evident compensation at this stage and a subsequent marked drop in his pH. At this point we can permit normal renal compensation to do what it can to minimize the acidemia (box *C*), or we can actively assist this function with the parenteral administration of bicarbonate (box *E*). If we follow the first course, we may find that the physiologic conservation of bicarbonate will elevate the numerator of the H-H equation, let us say for example, to 36 mM/ℓ and partially relieve the acidemia by raising the pH to 7.28. Because the carbon dioxide tension is still high and thus the underlying hypoventilation uncorrected, we place the patient on a mechanical ventilator and, in our enthusiasm to restore his carbon dioxide to normal, overventilate him. After a few hours of therapy we may find that we have completely corrected his hypercarbia, but because renal bicarbonate excretion lags behind carbon dioxide removal, perhaps the patient's bicarbonate has dropped only to 30 mM/ℓ and we have now pushed the patient from a severe respira-

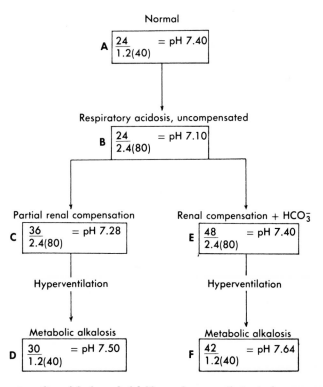

**Fig. 10-6.** Schematic outline of the hazard of deliberate hyperventilation in the treatment of respiratory acidosis. The mechanisms by which metabolic alkalosis can be induced are described in detail in the text.

tory acidemia to a moderate metabolic alkalemia. Although a metabolic swing of this magnitude may not be of any great significance in most patients, it may be in some, and it indicates the ease with which therapy can overcompensate.

Let us now consider the possibilities if we follow the second course and give the patient bicarbonate because it seems reasonable to treat acidity with an antacid. The combination of renal compensation plus administered bicarbonate (box *E*) may effect rapid and complete ratio balance and quickly restore the pH to normal. Assisted ventilation will still be necessary, of course, and the student should realize that starting with a higher bicarbonate level in this instance, with effective ventilation, will make it difficult, if not impossible, to avoid leaving the patient with a significant bicarbonate excess. Box *F* assumes a response similar to that described in the first course, namely a rapid removal of carbon dioxide but with a concomitant reduction in bicarbonate of only 6 mM/$\ell$, giving the patient a severe metabolic alkalemia.

The therapist who thoroughly understands these concepts is now ready to consider exceptions. We often see a patient on a mechanical ventilator who needs a depth of ventilation, to maintain adequate blood oxygenation, in excess of that required for a normal carbon dioxide tension. This is the result of uneven patency of airways to various lung units, preventing uniform distribution of inspired air at tidal volumes judged to be adequate by carbon dioxide blood levels. In other words, easily diffusable carbon dioxide can be sufficiently excreted by ventilation that is unable to correct hypoxemia. In the absence of serious pathology such as surfactant deficiency or massive atelectasis, the problem can frequently be solved by delivering to the patient large tidal volumes, sometimes double or triple that considered normal. Even though the ventilatory rate of a controlled patient can be reduced in an attempt to keep minute ventilation to a minimum, hyperventilation often results, with the rising arterial pH of alkalemia. Unless we can protect the patient from the potential harm of our induced alkalosis, we are not justified in adding another risk to his survival.

For the patient on controlled ventilation there are two general procedures that can be used to maintain his acid-base balance in the face of deliberate hyperventilation. First, rebreathed volume or dead space ($V_{Drb}$)[32] can be added to the patient tubing, between the patient and the exhalation valve, generally a piece of flex tubing of known volume. At the beginning of each inhalation the patient breathes this volume of carbon dioxide–rich air trapped in the tubing from the previous exhalation, thus supporting the desired arterial carbon dioxide level despite hyperventilation. It is convenient to have available for this purpose precut lengths of tubing of 50 and 100 ml capacities, measured by water filling. In general, rebreathed volumes of 50 to 300 ml satisfy most needs, but the final determinant is the arterial carbon dioxide tension and pH. Some hospitals routinely include 50 to 100 ml $V_{Drb}$ in adult ventilatory circuits and hyperventilate all patients, but it is advisable to use this technique selectively and only when needed. Second, the same objective of elevating inhaled carbon dioxide concentrations can be achieved by adding carbon dioxide to the air-oxygen inspired gas mixture through a special mixing valve, which limits the maximum concentration of carbon dioxide to 3%.* The $CO_2$ mixer is accurate with usual gas flows

*$CO_2$ Ratio Controller, Veriflow Corporation, Richmond, Calif.

as long as supply pressure from the oxygen-air mixer to the $CO_2$ mixer is 40 psi, and the $CO_2$ pressure to the $CO_2$ mixer is between 50 and 70 psi. One study found the $CO_2$ mixer more convenient to use than the addition of dead space tubing in controlling $P_{a_{CO_2}}$, and demonstrated that carbon dioxide concentrations greater than 3% were neither well tolerated nor necessary.[315]

For the ventilated patient with spontaneous but inadequate breathing, deliberate hyperventilation is probably best and easiest carried out in conjunction with intermittent mandatory ventilation, to be discussed next.

With the above discussion as a background to impress upon the student the need for caution in establishing the depth of mechanical ventilation, let us now consider what role, if any, buffers can play in managing respiratory failure. To begin with, the student may wonder why there should be a controversy over a procedure that apparently holds so much risk. Until the tremendous development of interest over the past two decades in pulmonary diseases and their physiologic effects, the training of most physicians oriented their views of acid-base disturbances as being metabolically generated. The physician was well versed in recognizing acidosis and alkalosis resulting from metabolic, gastrointestinal, and renal diseases and the surgical and postoperative states, to mention a few of the common conditions. He was thus used to treating acidosis, generally, with bicarbonate replacement, and it has been difficult for him to accept the concept of "acidosis" where this was not an immediate need. Naturally, as chest medicine has become an increasingly important specialty, there has been a growing understanding of the influence of pulmonary physiology on the acid-base status, and successive groups of young physicians are becoming more skilled in respiratory management.

Perhaps the student can see for himself where the judicious use of bicarbonate may contribute to the overall treatment of ventilatory failure. It is indicated in those patients who have severe acidosis, with a reduction in pH to levels that are a hazard to cellular survival, in whom there has been a negligible metabolic compensatory response. This is exemplified by the patient who does not have chronic hypercarbia due to long-standing bronchopulmonary disease and in whom there is no chronically elevated bicarbonate but who, for one reason or other, develops sudden carbon dioxide retention. To avoid the damage to this patient's enzyme systems and other cellular functions by subjecting them to a severely acidotic environment, *partial* neutralization of the patient's acidosis by increasing his store of bicarbonate is justifiable. Partial neutralization is further indicated in patients with a combination of metabolic and respiratory acidosis, for in them the ventilator therapy will not correct the underlying metabolic disorder, and the careful use of both modalities will maintain the smoothest acid-base balance. However, such therapy is acceptable only if the physician recognizes it as a stopgap measure to be employed until results can be obtained from definitive assisted ventilation and if he is fully aware of the potential risk of overcompensation. As a general rule of thumb, bicarbonate therapy can be recommended, even in obvious respiratory acidemia, when the pH is less than 7.20 if it is discontinued above this level. The patient will be spared the harmful effects of a high hydrogen ion concentration, but his risk of therapeutically induced alkalosis will be minimal. In contrast, the use of supplemental bicarbonate in the patient with an already elevated bicarbonate level from renal compensation is extremely hazardous, and the development of a metabolic alkalosis is almost inevitable. It is a wise precaution for the therapist asked to set up mechanical ventilation to inquire of the medical attendant whether the patient has been given bicarbonate.

We can summarize our comments on the risks of hyperventilation by stating that although the primary need of the patient in ventilatory failure is a mechanically increased alveolar ventilation, such ventilation must be done cautiously and carefully. Especially must judgment be used in treating the patient with chronic hypercarbia and superimposed acute failure, for too great enthusiasm can easily precipitate a potentially harmful metabolic alkalosis to replace his acidosis. Supplemental systemic buffers must be used with great reservation, if at all, and every member of the therapeutic team must be aware of the risk involved. The final objective of mechanical ventilation is to return carbon dioxide tension and pH to as close to normal as possible, not to overcompensate. There are times when the so-called normals for a given patient may not be identical with the normals associated with a healthy subject. In some patients with chronic hypercarbia and with adequate compensation prior to acute failure, it may be satisfactory to return carbon dioxide levels to those with which they have become adjusted. The therapist can be assured that his treatment is safe and effective if he first stops the rise in carbon dioxide tension and drop in pH and then notes that both are beginning to return to normal. From then on, as long as the progress is steady, it makes little difference how long the treatment takes, and it is safer to bring down a high carbon dioxide over a period of 2 to 3 days than in a matter of hours.

*Intermittent mandatory ventilation (IMV).* This ventilatory technique has two applications in the management of the mechanically ventilated patient. We will describe here the principle of IMV and its role in the support of the patient in ventilatory failure, and later, its use in discontinuing mechanical ventilation. *Intermittent mandatory ventilation* describes a method of operating a ventilator which enables the patient to breathe spontaneously at his choice, bypassing the ventilator, while still delivering to him at variable and predetermined volumes and frequencies, machine-powered breaths.[316, 317] The adjective *mandatory* refers to the ventilator cycle, over which the patient has no control.

The most important concept that the student must grasp at this time is the nature of the patient's spontaneous breathing. All ventilators in common use provide for the patient to cycle the machine spontaneously on demand. The breath so generated is then delivered by the ventilator like any other controlled breath at the preset volume and time. It is an *assisted* rather than a true spontaneous breath, since unless the patient "fights the machine" and prematurely terminates inhalation or otherwise disturbs the inspiratory/expiratory ratio, he has no control over the breath. Also, malfunction or inept operation of the ventilator may make its activation by patient effort difficult or impossible. In contrast, a spontaneous breath of the IMV technique is completely *unassisted*, since patient-generated inspiration *does not cycle the ventilator* but bypasses it through a valved circuit, to bring in gas from another source. Not only is initiation of the breath an option of the patient but also full control over its force, duration, and depth.

Fig. 10-7, *A*, is a schematic diagram of a basic volume ventilator setup to which an IMV bypass circuit can be added. Source gas, *A*, supplies ventilator, *B*, and from outflow port, *C*, it passes through humidifier, *D*, patient tubing, *E*, and into exhalation manifold, *F*. During inhalation, pressurized gas from the ventilator inflates balloon-valve, *G*, and gas is directed into intubated patient at *H*. At end-inspiration, the drop in ventilator pressure deflates the balloon-valve and the patient exhales to atmosphere through port *I*.

An IMV system consists of combined ventilator and spontaneous breathing circuits. Fig. 10-7, *B*, demonstrates the relationship of a spontaneous circuit to a ventilator circuit with which it is joined. Source gas, *A*, is carried through

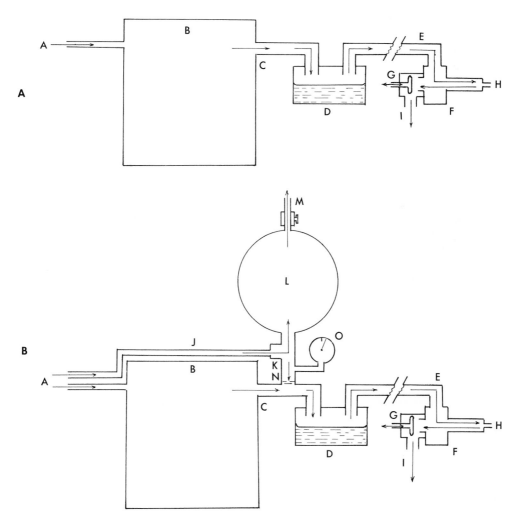

**Fig. 10-7.  A,** Simple ventilation setup. **B,** With an added IMV circuit. (See text for description.)

the bypass line, *J*, to the wide bore tubing, *K*, of the spontaneous circuit. At the distal end of the circuit, a 3-liter anesthesia-type bag, *L*, functions as a reservoir for the continuously flowing breathing gas. The bag bleed-off port may be fitted with an adjustable screw clamp, *M*. The proximal end of the spontaneous circuit is teed or wyed into the ventilator circuit between ventilator and humidifier, where a one-way valve, *N*, permits flow only from the spontaneous circuit into the ventilator circuit. We will describe the purpose of the manometer, *O*, tied into the spontaneous breathing circuit when we consider the mechanical ventilatory technique of positive end-expiratory pressure (PEEP) in another dozen or so pages.

During ventilator delivery, high pressure in the machine circuit closes the one-way valve, preventing gas entering the spontaneous circuit. Breathing gas flows steadily into the reservoir bag, and its rate, or the loss of gas through the escape port orifice, should be so adjusted that the reservoir bag does not collapse whenever the patient takes a spontaneous breath. Theoretically, overdistention of the bag by flows greatly in excess of patient needs should not present a serious problem. The increased pressure in the circuit as gas gathers between breaths will allow gas to escape through the one-way valve and vent through the exhalation valve to atmosphere. Only during ventilator delivery, when the balloon-valve blocks egress, will outflow be interrupted. However, in the interests of conservation of gas and maximum precision of technique, seepage of gas through the one-way valve can be prevented by permitting only moderate distention of the reservoir bag. When the patient starts a spontaneous breath, inspiratory subatmospheric pressure in the ventilator circuit opens the one-way valve, and the patient inhales a tidal volume from the reservoir and through the humidifier at a rate and depth of his choice. Exhalation pressure closes the valve, and gas flows out to atmosphere.

There is no single routine method of using IMV, and the following general guides may be of help to the inexperienced reader. In some hospitals an IMV system is incorporated in all initial ventilator setups. More experience will be necessary to advise us if it should be immediately available for all patients on ventilators or if it should be used with more selectivity, although there is little doubt that IMV has made mechanical ventilation safer and more effective in many circumstances. It is obviously of no use in the apneic patient but can or should be available when spontaneous breathing returns.

The basic purpose of IMV is to permit the mechanically ventilated patient to breathe on his own when he desires so that he may maintain or regain function of his ventilatory system and avoid developing dependence on the machine. In general, the ventilator is initially set to provide fully for the patient's needs, using tidal volumes in the 12 to 15 ml/kg body weight range. Triggering sensitivity of the ventilator must be reduced (resistance to patient triggering increased) so that the patient's inspiratory efforts will open the valve to the IMV bypass circuit rather than initiate a machine cycle. The sensitivity control may be completely inactivated, or as a safety measure only partially so, and thus in the event of gas supply failure to the bypass, a strong patient inspiratory effort will produce a ventilator breath. As spontaneous breathing becomes significant, ventilator breathing (this is the IMV) is gradually reduced in frequency, allowing the patient to assume more responsibility for his ventilation. At any given time the IMV rate should be the lowest that is able to maintain normal arterial blood gases and pH, provided the spontaneous rate does not exceed 30 breaths per minute. The speed with which IMV is reduced must be highly individualized and based on close observation of the patient. Not uncommonly it is necessary to retreat to higher ventilator rates, allowing the patient more time to adjust to independent breathing. The point at which IMV is discontinued depends entirely on the patient. Ventilator timing mechanisms now provide for IMV rates as low as one breath every 1 to 2 minutes. Thus the transition from controlled, through assisted, to independent breathing can be as gradual as needed.

In the interest of classification and definition, IMV can be designated as a modification of controlled rather than assisted ventilation. Ventilator breaths cannot be initiated by the patient because patient-generated inspiratory efforts open the bypass circuit instead of triggering the machine. Thus, with an IMV circuit in operation, machine assist is not possible. On the other hand, regardless of their frequency, because the ventilator breaths are preset and not influenced by the patient, they are control breaths. IMV therefore is a decreasing mechanically controlled breathing that permits the gradual, simultaneous return of spontaneous, unassisted breathing.

We noted above that IMV provides activity for ventilatory muscles and helps to prevent ventilator dependence. There are two additional physiological benefits of great significance. *First*, in contrast to machine breathing, the parameters of which are arbitrarily selected to a considerable degree, the true spontaneous breathing of IMV can be the patient's respiratory center response to real gas exchange needs. In other words, as spontaneous breathing gradually becomes a larger segment of total breathing, the patient's own drive can set a ventilatory pattern, and especially a blood carbon dioxide level, more suitable for his needs than we can deliver by machine, based on clinical evaluation and blood gas analysis. A frequently encountered problem is a sequel to ventilator hyperventilation, described a few pages back. Efforts to establish a spontaneous pattern may be frustrated if the dominant ventilator breaths are so large that they produce a hypocarbic alkalosis. The lowered hydrogen ion concentration may be inadequate to stimulate the respiratory center to independent action, and until corrected, will necessitate continuation of machine ventilation. *Second*, under the influence of positive-pressure ventilation, intrathoracic pressure rises abnormally during each tidal volume, elevating the mean pleural pressure, as we have seen. The major risk of such pressure is its retarding effect on venous return and cardiac output. The spontaneous breaths of IMV, on the other hand, are accompanied by subatmospheric intrathoracic pressure, as illustrated in Fig. 9-25. Over a time period, the net intrathoracic pressure is a function of the ratio of machine-to-spontaneous breaths, decreasing as the patient takes over more of his own breathing. For patients in overt or potential cardiac failure this may be the most important benefit of IMV.

Intermittent mandatory ventilation has certainly contributed to patient safety and comfort in many instances, but it must not be viewed as an indispensable ingredient in all ventilator management or as a solution to all management problems. For example, we must be careful not to burden some patients too early or too frequently with their own breathing. They may have an adequate central drive to breathe spontaneously, but because of their disease, may not possess adequate musculoskeletal power to convert the drive into significant tidal volumes. For such patients, triggered assisted machine breathing may be safer and more effective than IMV until resolution of the underlying disease. Thus the timing of introducing IMV may be a critical factor, requiring keen clinical judgment. Again, although many users advise IMV for all ventilated patients, experience continues to show that the tachypneic, shallow spontaneous breather is not always a good subject for it. At times, hyperventilating with the machine will dull the patient's spontaneous drive through alkalosis and slow his rate. Mindful of the hazards of alkalosis, the student can appreciate that such deliberate manipulation of breathing and acid-base balance must be undertaken with great caution. In such circumstances the techniques of spontaneous breathing suppression, to be described next, may be of considerable short-term use before attempting to institute IMV.

We will again consider IMV in conjunction with positive end-expiratory pressure breathing and as part of the process of weaning a patient from his ventilator.

***Suppressing ventilation.*** It may be impossible to ventilate adequately a patient with strong spontaneous breathing no matter what instrument is used. Although machine override is often possible, a pattern of breathing that is rapid and shallow or grossly irregular may be forceful enough not to submit to the drive of a preset ventilator. In addition, the patient may "fight the machine," consciously or otherwise, because he is severely hypoxic, is fearful or apprehensive, or is mentally unable to cooperate. In such a patient, to continue to assist him is only to perpetuate his pattern, leading to a steady deterioration of his respiratory status. Most often the patient will be breathing very rapidly with shallow tidal volumes and is subjected to the following two hazards: First, the tremendous amount of physical work expended in rapid breathing will gradually deplete his energy. Second, rapid shallow breathing is essentially dead space breathing, and although at great energy cost the patient may move large minute air volumes, all that he accomplishes is ventilation of his dead space, leaving his alveoli relatively unventilated. If he is responsive to metabolic oxygen needs, the resulting hypoxia will continue the ineffective, tiring respiratory pattern. As a general rule, this risk is not great in adults until the frequency exceeds 25, and then, depending upon the conductance (opposite of resistance) and compliance of the lung-thorax, rate increases are apt to be accompanied by reduced tidal volumes.

The condition of the patient with strong, ineffective spontaneous respirations who cannot be brought under at least partial control is a grave one, and his very survival may depend on the ability of the medical team to correct the deficiency. As soon as it becomes evident that effective assistance or conformance to control is not possible, there is nothing to gain and much to lose by further delay. The decision must be made to abolish the patient's own breathing and place him under complete ventilator control. This is a responsibility of the patient's attending physician, although the technical management will fall on the assigned therapist. The responsibility that this technique entails cannot be emphasized too strongly, for when we decide to interfere with natural processes as vital as breathing, thus asserting that we can do better for the patient than he can do himself, we are assuming a great burden. The therapist should appreciate that this is not exactly the same as attempting to restore to a patient a function that he has lost completely through injury or disease. Instead, it is the use of our judgment as to the quality and performance of the patient's ability to provide his basic physiologic need, deciding that he is inadequate in this function, destroying it, and supplanting it with an artificial substitute of our choosing. This statement is not intended to overdramatize a procedure for which there is no alternative if the patient is to survive, but it is important that the therapist realize the full depth of his commitment to the patient who is completely helpless and totally dependent on his medical attendants. Respiratory suppression should be undertaken only where facilities are adequate for complete care and in the physical presence of a responsible physician and respiratory therapist. We will describe the three common techniques currently used—suppression by oxygen, by morphine, and by neuromuscular blocking agents.

*Oxygen suppression of breathing.* This procedure is especially effective for the patient with long-standing chronic hypercapnia, whose ventilation has been dependent to a considerable degree upon the hypoxic drive that has replaced the damaged function of his respiratory center. It is of interest that in this instance we employ, as therapy, a technique we strongly condemn otherwise. Earlier we discussed in detail the role played by chemoreceptors in the event of respiratory center failure accompanying progressive and chronic pulmonary disease. We stressed the great hazard in administering oxygen promiscuously to such a patient for fear of satisfying hypoxia, thus inactivating the hypoxic chemoreceptor drive and rendering the patient apneic. Now we do exactly that—inactivate the hypoxic chemoreceptor drive—so that we can eliminate the patient's own breathing and ventilate him artificially. The patient is given 100% oxygen through the assisting ventilator or by means of a tracheotomy mask, if he is so intubated, for a period not to exceed 10 minutes; results should be realized in that length of time if at all. As he becomes hypopneic and his respiratory energy decreases, he is put on ventilator control and the oxygen concentration is reduced to a safe level. Close observation must be maintained to ensure that the patient remains under adequate control and does not return to his previous pattern. If this procedure is unsuccessful, one of the following procedures must be employed.

*Morphine suppression of breathing.* Morphine sulfate is a potent addicting narcotic with the ability to relieve pain, produce lethargy, and induce a deep-to-stuporous sleep. One of its most specific activities, however, is its depression of respiration by directly suppressing the activity of the medullary respiratory center. Like high concentrations of oxygen, morphine is contraindicated in general medical use in any patient with compromised breathing, and many deaths have been attributed to it in patients with asthma, chronic bronchopulmonary disease, and cerebral injury. The respiratory depressant effect of morphine is directly related to dose and is evident to slight degrees even with small doses given, for example, for pain relief. The respiratory response is a decrease in both frequency and tidal volume.

When used to stop spontaneous breathing, morphine can be best controlled if given by intravenous injection. By this route, maximum respiratory depression for a given dose occurs within 10 minutes, compared with 1 hour or more if given intramuscularly. There are no hard-and-fast rules for its administration, but a good basic program is 5 mg intravenously, repeated every 10 minutes until the desired effect is realized, to a maximum of 20 mg for the series. In most patients, if morphine is to be effective, it will be before this amount of the drug has been used. For maintenance 2 to 3 mg can be given as needed to keep the patient well relaxed. The duration of morphine therapy is usually too short to warrant concern over addiction, but there are occasional side effects that can prove troublesome. Among the most common are nausea and vomiting, which sometimes preclude further use of the drug. Occasionally morphine causes hypotension and must be used cautiously, if at all, in the patient in incipient or overt shock. The automatic movements of the intestine, or peristalsis, are retarded or stopped by morphine, and this can lead to gaseous distention of the bowel severe enough to impair diaphragmatic motion and interfere with ventilation. The patient's face and neck may appear flushed, and he may complain of itching of the skin or nose as the effects of the drug subside. Generally speaking, the intravenous administration of morphine is a safe and effective method of suppressing unwanted spontaneous ventilation and relaxing the patient so that he may be ventilated effectively. It has often been lifesaving.

*Neuromuscular blocking agents to suppress breathing.* A neuromuscular blocking agent is a drug that blocks the transmission of motor nerve impulses to skeletal muscles, effectively paralyzing those muscles. They are widely used in surgery to gain maximum muscular relaxation along with anesthesia, making manipulation of muscular tissues much easier by eliminating their normal tonal contraction. In respiratory therapy there are two indications for neuromuscular blocking—momentary paralysis for ease of endotracheal intubation of a tense or agitated patient, and prolonged action to override unwanted spontaneous breathing in a patient on a mechanical ventilator. In neither instance is total body paralysis desired, but only enough muscular relaxation to achieve the desired results.

These drugs must be used under the closest supervision, and a patient under their influence must *never* be left unattended. If the patient is alert prior to the administration of blocking agents, he should first be tranquilized or sedated, since the completely helpless feeling of paralysis to a patient aware of his condition can be one of the most frightening of experiences.

We will not take the time to examine pharmacologic differences of the several blocking drugs available to the anesthesiologist, but will note the major characteristics of three of them often used in the control of ventilation—*d*-tubocurarine, succinylcholine, and pancuronium bromide.

*d*-TUBOCURARINE. *d*-Tubocurarine is a plant alkaloid whose paralyzing action has been known for centuries and which has been widely used in anesthesiology for many years. When given intravenously, the route of choice, its action is evident in 3 to 5 minutes, lasting about 40 minutes; doses of 15 mg may be used almost as needed until the desired effect is reached. In case of a mishap or overdosage, neostigmine methylsulfate should be available as an antidote. *d*-Tubocurarine has potential side effects. Large doses may precipitate hypotension, already a threat to a mechanically ventilated patient. Perhaps even more relevant to patients in respiratory failure is the severe bronchospasm that may follow curarine's use. The bronchospasm is attributed to the release, by the drug, of histamine from its cellular stores into the plasma, and one of the major physiologic effects of histamine is broncho-constriction.[318]

SUCCINYLCHOLINE (ANECTINE). Although a neuromuscular blocking agent like *d*-tubo-curarine, succinylcholine differs chemically and in its mode of action. Also given intra-venously, it starts acting in less than 1 minute, reaches its maximum in 2 minutes, and disappears within 5 minutes. It has been used in general surgery to provide rapid relaxation for short procedures such as instrumentation. For respiratory suppression a single dose of 20 mg may be given to test the patient's response or to initiate ventila-tion and may be repeated as needed until a good ventilatory pattern is established. A smoother response will accompany its prolonged administration in an intravenous infusion, as a 0.1% solution, run at a rate of 2 to 3 mg/min. By this method, because the action is so short, very close control over the depth of paralysis can be maintained merely by adjusting the infusion flow. Acute cardiovascular collapse may follow intra-venous succinylcholine administration. It is believed this is due to a sudden rise in serum potassium concentration (hyperkalemia) with resulting myocardial depression and ventricular arrhythmias.[319]

PANCURONIUM BROMIDE (PAVULON). Pancuronium bromide is one of the newer para-lyzing drugs recently made available, and although the total experience with it so far is meager compared with the two just described, it appears to have been well re-ceived.[320] Major advantages of pancuronium bromide include its nearly complete freedom from unwanted cardiovascular effects and its failure to stimulate histamine release. Its potency is some five times that of *d*-tubocurarine, and it has no effect on consciousness, pain awareness, or mental activity. Nevertheless, because it is a neuromuscular blocking agent, it is as potentially dangerous as *d*-tubocurarine and succinylcholine. Dosage varies with the duration of effect intended. By intra-venous injection 2 to 4 mg are usually adequate for intubation, with effects evident in 2 to 3 minutes and a duration of action of up to 90 minutes. For maintenance of paralysis during control of ventilation, 4 to 5 mg of pancuronium bromide can be given at intervals of 1 to 3 hours, depending on response. Some prefer to use succinylcho-line for intubation and pancuronium bromide for long-term control.

**Correcting hypoxia.** The general subject of oxygen therapy was described in Chapter 8, and we will only attempt to correlate certain aspects of it with mechanical ventilation and some specific needs of respiratory failure. Most of the emphasis in our discussion of ventilators centered about the importance of alveolar ventilation and the removal of carbon dioxide, but we must not forget that the most pressing need of the patient in failure is the correction of hypoxia. Unless ventilation can assure him a viable level of arterial oxygen, our efforts will be of no avail. In all in-stances of significant ventilatory failure we will have to contend with hypoventilation hypoxia or physiological shunt hypoxia, along with the management problems already discussed. Correction of these two types of hypoxia will be discussed separately.

*Hypoventilation hypoxia.* We have been almost dogmatic in our insistence that oxygen administration for failure due to hypoventilation be accompanied by assisted ventilation to avoid the potential hazard of worsening the patient's ventilatory drive, but now that the fundamental precautions of such therapy are well understood, let us examine the state of failure to see if any modifications are justified. Obviously, we are not concerned with the risk of apnea in all hypoxic patients, and if we feel that a given patient has an adequate alveolar ventilation, we do not hesitate to give him oxygen as needed. Perhaps there are patients with some degree of hypoventilation who also can be treated with oxygen unsupported by mechanical ventilation. There are many who feel that a trial of oxygen therapy may safely be given when hypercarbia and acidemia appear to be less a risk to the patient than his hypoxemia, thereby hopefully avoiding the need for unnecessary intubation and the additional risks inherent in artificial ventilation.

This has been studied by several investigators, and the following program has proved successful in many patient when combined with vigorous therapy to establish or maintain airway patency.[257, 321, 322] Arterial blood gas values are obtained as soon as possible while the patient is breathing room air. If the oxygen tension is less than 60 mm Hg (some use 50 mm Hg as the limit) and the pH is above 7.30, the patient is started on a very low oxygen flow, usually by catheter. Since the method employs trial and error, follow-up blood studies are essential, and if a given level of oxygen flow maintains the blood values within the limits specified above, it is continued. If hypoxia is still not corrected, the oxygen flow is increased by very small increments until an arterial oxygen tension of at least 60 mm Hg is reached, provided the pH does not fall at the same time. Should it not be possible to oxygenate the patient without the development of progressive acidemia, he is intubated and given supported mechanical ventilation. This is a conservative approach and, if followed under careful observation, may be expected to be successful in many patients whose ventilatory defects are due to readily reversible conditions. If oxygen is given by nasal cannula, 2 to 3 $\ell$/min often suffices for moderate hypoxia and is unlikely to cause alarming elevations in arterial carbon dioxide tension unless the ventilation-perfusion balance is seriously disturbed.[323] The venturi mask lends itself well to this type of therapy, since it will deliver a prefixed and relatively stable oxygen concentration at high enough flows to satisfy almost any ventilatory demand; but, of course, it does not guarantee any specific blood oxygen level.[249, 259, 324]

If mechanical ventilation is necessary to prevent progressive hypercarbia and respiratory acidemia, the therapist will have to use the ventilator as a medium to supply oxygen. In Chapter 9 he learned how unreliable is the oxygen diluter on the pressure-cycled machine, and yet he is aware of the need to avoid the delivery of high oxygen concentrations because of the risk of fatal lung damage with prolonged administration. He also has learned that the ventilatory problem he is trying to solve may make it difficult to avoid high inspired oxygen concentrations if he is using a pressure-cycled ventilator in the face of reduced pulmonary compliance. The relationship between the prolonged inspiration often necessary to ventilate stiff lungs and the subsequent rise in oxygen in the inspired air makes control of the oxygen delivered to such a patient very difficult.

There are steps to take to control the delivered oxygen concentration, depending on the type of ventilator used. It is fairly simple in the volume ventilator by adding oxygen to the air that is the basic gas used by the machine. The structure of the volume machine makes available a chamber in which the gases can readily be mixed, and for each instrument there is provided by the manufacturer either a guide table or a mechanical control by which to adjust the oxygen flow to obtain a given concentration under specific operating conditions. It is still necessary to analyze samples of delivered gas to determine the exact concentrations in case of malfunction or maladjustment of the diluting mechanism. The problem is a bit more complicated in the pressure-cycled ventilator, and there are three general ways it can be met. First, it is often satisfactory to operate the ventilator off a source of compressed air, a compressor, central supply, or a cylinder and to add oxygen to the patient-supply circuit. A large humidifier is a good place to accomplish this. Such a method is strictly trial and error, and the mixed gas must be measured for its oxygen content. Changes in the breathing pattern, especially in the assist mode, can change the balance between source and added gases, necessitating frequent examination of the delivered gas to maintain any stability in oxygen delivery. When such supplementary oxygen is added to the patient breathing circuit and is allowed to flow throughout the ventilatory cycle, it will render inaccurate the exhaled gas measurements often used to monitor tidal or minute volumes. Second, a tank of a prepared known concentration of oxygen can be used as the power source gas, a popular mixture being 40% oxygen in 60% nitrogen, since this concentration of oxygen is generally safe and effective. There are some practical disadvantages to this technique, however. Prepared cylinder gases are expensive, and they are cumbersome to move and store in the patient's room, especially where the respiratory care service is adjusted to a central oxygen supply. More important is the need to operate the respirator on the so-called "100% oxygen setting," since dilution of the source cylinder gas by entrained room air will defeat the purpose of its use. For the Bird respirator this means the loss of one of its most valuable characteristics, pneumatic clutching, which depends on activation of the venturi by an open air-mix control, as explained in Chapter 9. Third, mixing valves are available that can mix source oxygen with air to deliver predetermined oxygen concentrations.[325] They are designed to maintain constant concentrations at all available flows as long as the mixed gases have similar densities, as do oxygen and air. These appliances are useful for volume ventilators as well as for the therapeutic administration of unassisted oxygen but present the same difficulty for the Bird respirator as does the cylinder gas.

The use of helium oxygen mixtures will be noted only in passing because of its detailed coverage in Chapter 8. Helium-oxygen should always be considered when oxygenation of a mechanically ventilated patient is unsuccessful because of severe diffuse bronchial obstruction. A pressure-cycled ventilator is a good vehicle for the administration of the mixture if the patient has a well-cuffed airway tube, but it must be operated with its air-mix closed.

*Physiological shunt hypoxia.* Most of the discussion so far has centered about patients whose greatest needs are the correction of hypercarbia and acidemia, with oxygen support until spontaneous breathing is again normal. However, there are many whose major problem is a hypoxia that persists in the face of normal total alveolar ventilation, as judged by arterial carbon dioxide tensions and pH, or despite satisfactory support of an associated hypoventilation. We will review the principles of management of this condition, based on several good studies and increasing experience.[326-330]

As defined in the last chapter, the basic functional defect in shunt hypoxia is a reduction in ventilation/perfusion ratios in scattered areas of the lung. This may derive from the following: (1) small airway or alveolar inspiratory obstruction, producing so-called microatelectasis, resulting from accumulated secretions, edema, or alveolar exudates; and (2) a lack of surfactant, often replaced by a glassy appearing film described as a hyaline membrane, with its associated increase in alveolar surface tension, and which may be caused by (a) congenital absence due to prematurity (respiratory distress syndrome of the newborn) or (b) destruction by systemic shock, oxygen toxicity, infection, and probably other unknown factors (respiratory distress syndrome of the adult). It is important to emphasize again that ventilation/perfusion hypoxia often occurs with hypoventilation failure, complicating its management, but the principle of its therapy is the same no matter what the etiology.

Both alveolar inspiratory obstruction and increased alveolar surface tension (reduced lung compliance) elevate the pressure necessary to initiate inflation, and the latter requires yet additional force to maintain alveolar distention adequate for gas exchange. Thus the two basic principles of correction of shunt hypoxia are (1) adjustment of inspiration to permit time for the distribution of gas into the slowly ventilating obstructed lobules; and (2) maintenance of sufficient intra-alveolar pressure to resist abnormally high collapsing force and to limit expiratory alveolar deflation. Two techniques in current use are referred to as *inflation hold* and *positive end-expiratory pressure*.

**INFLATION HOLD** (FIG. 10-8). A frequent problem in the management of ventilator patients is the ventilation of lung units that are partially blocked by bronchial disease. These areas are referred to as "slow spaces" because of the reduced flow of air into them. Inflation hold is a technique used with IPPV to prolong distention of the lung so that more time is available to ventilate the slow spaces. It is of two general types, depending on the control mechanism provided by the manufacturer—peak inflation hold and plateau inflation hold.

**PEAK INFLATION HOLD.** Fig. 10-8, *B*, shows the increasing pressure of inhalation

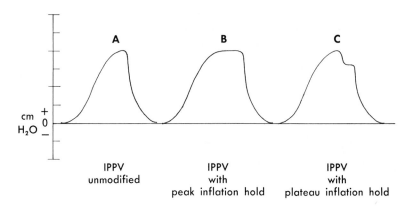

**Fig. 10-8.** Inflation hold. Pressure wave forms of two types are compared with unmodified pressure inhalation. (See text for description.)

reaching its maximum, or *peak pressure*, at end-inspiration. At this point the driving force of the ventilator, such as the bellows of a volume machine, holds the lung at its predetermined distended volume for a variable and preset time, before cycling out of the inspiratory phase. Holding inflation gives time for better inspired air distribution than if end-inspiration were only a momentary pause. The peak pressure generated to deliver the desired volume represents so-called mouth or airway pressure, not intra-alveolar pressure. When the hold is released, exhalation follows the natural passive recoil mechanism to zero gauge resting level. The student should recall that the longer the positive pressure of end-inspiratory inflation is held the greater will be its possible circulatory effects.

PLATEAU INFLATION HOLD. Although it is true that peak inflation hold creates an end-inspiratory plateau, as demonstrated in the sketch, the term *plateau* as we use it here refers to a variation of this pattern. In Fig. 10-8, *C*, inflating pressure is seen to reach the same peak as in *A*, but inspiration cycles off as scheduled. Manual activation of a control delays the opening of the exhalation valve, and thus for a moment neither gas flow nor pressure moves into or out of the lung. In this brief interval, pressure equalization between airways and alveoli takes place as air that is already in the airways moves further into the harder-to-ventilate alveoli, expanding its volume and dropping its pressure below that at the mouth. The pressure drop is seen in Fig. 10-8, *C*, as a small plateau in the expiratory downslope of the pressure curve, shortly below the peak level. In reality, the plateau causes a hesitation in the descent of the ventilator manometer needle, which may be from 1 to 10 cm of water below peak pressure.

During these moments of no gas flow, between peak and plateau pressures, if we assume that there is complete pressure equilibration throughout the respiratory tract, the mouth pressure as recorded by the ventilator manometer also represents alveolar pressure at the distal end of the tract. The plateau pressure is thus considered to be at least a close approximation of pressure in the alveoli. Measurement of plateau alveolar pressure is both therapeutically and diagnostically useful. Therapeutically, it performs a service similar to that of the peak inflation hold, providing time for ventilation of poorly communicating lung units. Diagnostically, plateau pressure supplies valuable information about the state of a mechanically ventilated lung.

Mouth pressure reflects the force required to inflate the lung against the resistance both of the airways and the elastic recoil of the combined lung and chest wall. One of our concerns in the mechanically ventilated patient is evaluating his lung-thorax compliance, the amount of lung inflation that can be achieved per unit of ventilating pressure applied. To measure this compliance we must eliminate the factor of airway resistance and consider only the pressure relating to the lung-thorax system. This can be done with the plateau hold maneuver, since during the interval between the end of inhalation and the opening of the exhalation valve, once pressure has equilibrated, there is no gas flow in the airways. With cessation of gas flow the contribution of airway resistance to ventilating pressure is removed, and the pressure at the plateau represents the recoil force of the lung-thorax, or conversely, the force needed to inflate the lung-thorax. The therapist can closely estimate what is referred to as the *static compliance* of lung and thorax by dividing the patient's tidal volume by his plateau pressure, a calculation that should be done frequently during acute stages of mechanical ventilation. It should be emphasized that a true static compliance value depends on an accurate volume measurement, for which adequate meters are available, and a static state of no gas flow in the airways, which cannot always be guaranteed with certainty. The time interval for the completion of inspired air distribution among all the lung units depends on the extent of airway patency. In some patients, airway obstruction may be so severe that distribution takes several seconds, and in the presence of severe airway disease, it is possible that a plateau might not be reached before the start of the next ventilator cycle. Thus, to be sure the pressure reading is truly static, expiration should be blocked until it is certain that a real plateau is reached. Although this can be done much more easily with special tools in the laboratory than by the gross method of observing movements of a manometer needle, bedside measurements are fortunately accurate enough for our clinical needs. It would probably be better, however, if we referred to the compliance as *effective static compliance*, a term that acknowledges the possible presence of slight airflow within or between the lungs, even though upper airways may be completely static.

*Positive end-expiratory pressure (PEEP).* One of the most difficult management problems is the patient with persistent hypoxemia, and often hyperventilation, despite the administration of oxygen concentrations of up to 100%. Such a patient may have no significant carbon dioxide retention and may be frankly hypocarbic from hypoxia-induced overbreathing. Obviously, associated airway obstruction further compounds the problem.

The primary functional defect in this situation is widespread physiological arteriovenous shunting, or venous admixture. Although shunting occurs in a number of diseases, one of its most serious manifestations is as a component of the infant and adult respiratory distress syndromes, where it is the product of accumulated intrabronchial, intra-alveolar, and interstitial pulmonary fluid. The fluid interferes with ventilation by (1) physically excluding air; and (2) interfering with action of bronchiolar and alveolar surfactant, causing collapse of bronchioles and alveoli, which in turn (a) decreases pulmonary compliance and (b) reduces functional residual capacity (FRC). The clinical problem therefore is correction of a progressive shunt hypoxia, resulting from airway and alveolar collapse and decreased compliance and FRC.

PEEP is a maneuver that maintains pressure above atmospheric in the patient's lungs at the end of expiration. This combats the collapsing tendency of small airways and alveoli, deprived of effective surfactant, by increasing the FRC. Alveolar inflating force against the resistance of surface tension is inversely proportional to alveolar size. Thus, if more air than normal can be left in the alveoli at end-exhalation (increased FRC), less air pressure will be needed to inflate them (increased compliance). At the same time, because the bronchioles and alveoli are kept in a hyperinflated state at end-exhalation, distribution of inspired gas is greatly enhanced. More effective than inflation hold, the increased FRC improves ventilation of slow spaces and permits air entry into bronchioles and alveoli that otherwise would be partially or completely collapsed. The reversal of severe hypoxemia is sometimes dramatic, but it cannot be stressed too strongly that for this technique to succeed, patency of large and medium airways must be assured, since significant obstruction at these levels can render PEEP quite useless.

To summarize, positive end-expiratory pressure (PEEP) is a procedure that purposely increases functional residual capacity (FRC) when disease has neutralized effective action of pulmonary surfactant. The increased FRC improves compliance, reduces bronchiolar and alveolar occlusion from collapse, and improves pulmonary air entry and distribution.

The mechanics of increasing FRC by retaining gas pressure in alveoli at end-expiration is fundamentally simple, but safe clinical application requires sound understanding of the desired objective. Unfortunately, it is not enough that the student learn the principles and use of PEEP; he must also cope with the confusion of nonuniform terminology relating to the subject. A problem of definition stems from differences in the use of PEEP on patients who are (1) on controlled or assisted mechanical ventilation or (2) breathing spontaneously without mechanical assistance. These differences will be described, but it can be noted at this time that there is one universal need for effective PEEP—an airtight breathing system. With one exception, which will be explained, this means fitting the patient with a cuffed endotracheal or tracheostomy tube.

Terminology of the use of end-expiratory pressure thus depends on whether the patient is on a ventilator or is breathing spontaneously. The matter is not this easily settled, however. For example, note the definitions suggested by the ACCP-ATS Joint Committee on Nomenclature, and by an editorial in *Respiratory Care*.[32, 331]

1. ACCP-ATS Joint Committee
   a. Positive End-Expiratory Pressure (PEEP): A residual pressure above atmospheric maintained at the airway opening at the end of expiration. This may be used *during spontaneous or mechanical ventilation.** 
   b. Constant Positive Pressure Breathing (CPPB) (Constant Positive Airway Pressure—CPAP): A pressure above atmospheric maintained at the airway opening throughout the respiratory cycle during spontaneous breathing.
2. Editorial, *Respiratory Care*
   a. Positive End-Expiratory Pressure (PEEP) is *mechanical ventilation** against a threshold resistance.
   b. Continuous Positive Pressure Breathing (CPPB) is nonventilator breathing against a threshold resistance.
   c. CPAP is the same as CPPB.

There is a major difference between the two definitions of PEEP, relating to its application during spontaneous breathing. We will see soon, also, that there is a situation where neither of the definitions limited to spontaneous breathing applies. Finally, to add more confusion, there is popular use of the expression, *continuous positive pressure ventilation* (CPPV), as a counterpart to the previously discussed inspiratory positive-pressure ventilation (IPPV) indicating the presence of positive pressure during both phases of ventilation.

---

*Italics added.

We will discuss PEEP under the three categories of (1) *PEEP with controlled mechanical ventilation;* (2) *PEEP with assisted mechanical ventilation;* and (3) *PEEP with unassisted spontaneous ventilation.* It is used most frequently on patients with controlled mechanical ventilation, so under this heading we will review most of the details of the technique, describing the other two in terms of how they differ.

PEEP WITH CONTROLLED MECHANICAL VENTILATION. In the interest of conciseness and brevity, we will refer to this category as *controlled-PEEP,* understanding that the control status implies the use of a mechanical ventilator.

1. *Mechanics of controlled-PEEP.* The reader's attention is drawn to Fig. 10-9, a modification of Fig. 10-7, *B,* illustrating the addition of PEEP capability to IMV circuitry on a volume ventilator system. Breathing gas *A* is delivered by ventilator *B* through humidifier *D* to the patient at *H*. Expired air passes through the ventilator-regulated exhalation valve, *F,* and by tubing of suitable length, *P,* into the resistance of a column of water, *Q*. In the closed, airtight circuit, high-pressure exhaled air bubbles out into the atmosphere, but back pressure of the water column prevents intra-alveolar and airway pressures from dropping to atmosphere at the end of exhalation. The amount of pressure, in centimeters of water, remaining in the system at the lung-thorax resting level, keeping alveoli partially inflated and the FRC enlarged, is a function of the distance in centimeters from the end of the exhalation tube to the top of the water column, *R*. When PEEP was first introduced into respiratory therapy, the water-sealed exhalation tube was the usual method of increasing FRC. Now, however, most ventilators have a built-in, manually operated variable control, which produces a plateau of end-expiratory positive pressure by limiting deflation of the exhalation valve diaphragm, *G,* retaining pressurized air in the alveoli. Although water column and mechanical back-pressure devices are calibrated, tubing resistance to airflow may influence the actual PEEP produced. For accurate monitoring, it is recommended that a manometer, *S,* be integrated into the system as close as possible to the patient.

PEEP and IMV are frequently used together, and special attention must be given to the balance of pressure across one-way valve, *N,* Fig. 10-9. PEEP exerts a continuous positive pressure on the ventilator circuit, holding the valve closed, and since the spontaneous circuit is at atmosphere, the patient must make an inspiratory effort of a force exceeding that of the PEEP to open the valve for a spontaneous breath. Two similar techniques will eliminate the problem. First, adjustment of source gas flow, or of controlled reservoir bag bleed-off, can allow sufficient pressure to develop in the spontaneous circuit to create a slight leak through the one-way valve. The leak may be detected at the exhalation valve port and indicates an erasure of the high to low pressure gradient across the valve from ventilatory circuit to spontaneous circuit. Second, better flow control can be realized by incorporating a manometer, *O,* into the spontaneous circuit and carefully adjusting gas release from the reservoir bag until the spontaneous circuit manometer approximates the patient circuit manometer, *S*. Slight negative inspiratory pressure by the patient will then open the valve for easy spontaneous breathing.

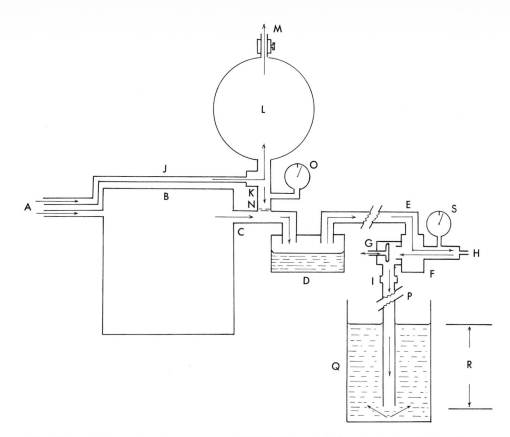

**Fig. 10-9.** Positive end-expiratory pressure (PEEP) with controlled mechanical ventilation. (See text for description.)

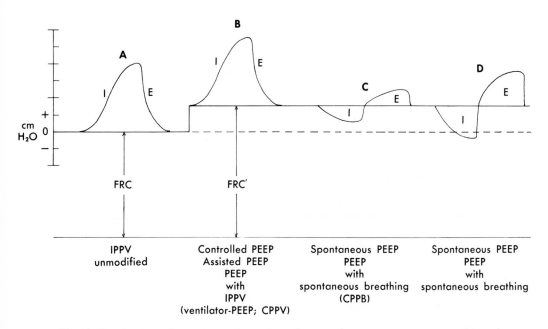

**Fig. 10-10.** Positive end-expiratory pressure (PEEP). Intrapulmonary pressure curves and lung-thorax resting levels in three applications of PEEP. (See text for description.)

Let us consider intrapulmonary pressure curves *A* and *B* in Fig. 10-10. The graph is dimensionless and combines pressure with volumes, as the polarity of intrapulmonary pressures is shown with accompanying imaginary FRCs. Curve *A* is a normal curve, for comparison, showing inspiratory and end-expiratory pulmonary pressures of zero gauge and a "normal" FRC volume. Curve *B* uses the same pressure pattern as *A* but differs from *A* in the position of its resting level. The level is elevated because end-expiratory pressure, equal to the difference between the old and new resting levels, has prevented the alveoli from deflating to their volumes in *A*, and consequently FRC has increased to FRC'. The student should note that to maintain a tidal volume after setting a PEEP level, peak inspiratory pressure must also be raised. In time, however, as PEEP activates more alveolar units, improved compliance may allow reductions in peak pressure without sacrifice of tidal volumes.

2. *Hazards of PEEP.* The use of high pulmonary pressure to hyperinflate the lungs is not without hazards, and some series report complications in as many as 50% of patients so treated. The major adverse effects of PEEP are:

a. *High-pressure physical lung damage (barotrauma).* A common manifestation is *subcutaneous emphysema,* the leakage of air from alveoli and its migration along vascular and bronchial paths to the lung roots, expanding out beneath the skin of the upper body. *Pneumothorax,* air leakage into the thorax from alveolar rupture, with varying degrees of lung collapse, while more serious is less frequent and usually results from end-expiratory pressures in excess of 20 cm of water.

b. *Reduced cardiovascular function.* If high PEEP can be transmitted to the intrathoracic space, it can retard venous return and reduce cardiac output. Fortunately, in most patients needing the benefits of PEEP, disease has so reduced compliance that the lungs are too "stiff" to carry intrapulmonary pressure to intrathoracic structures, and depressed circulation is avoided. Also, despite high pressure, in some instances myocardial function improves with increased oxygenation.

c. *Reduced urinary output.* We learned earlier that positive pressure ventilation, by elevating intrathoracic pressure, can reduce urinary flow. The addition of PEEP may aggravate this response and require the use of diuretics for correction and control.

The incidence and severity of these complications of PEEP are "dose related," that is, the higher the pressure and the greater the length of time it is applied the greater the chance of side effects. Incorporation of intermittent mandatory ventilation in the management plan will help minimize complications. Each patient-generated breath, if allowed to exhale to atmosphere, will lower the long-term mean effective intrathoracic pressure, relieving strain on other systems.

3. *Indications for, and contraindications of, PEEP.* The general indication for PEEP was described in the opening paragraph of this discussion, but there were no guidelines for its use in specific circumstances. It should be apparent to the reader that there can be no hard-and-fast rules for using PEEP, any more than for starting a patient on mechanical ventilation. The two dangers against which we try to protect

these patients are progressive hypoxia and oxygen toxicity as a consequence of treating the hypoxia. When our efforts are inadequate, then we use PEEP. As a rule of thumb, we should at least be prepared to initiate PEEP, when arterial oxygen tension continues to drop below 50 mm Hg, in a patient on IPPV, who is ventilated with an oxygen concentration greater than 50%. Not all patients with hypoxemia are suitable candidates for PEEP. A relative contraindication is, of course, significant hypotension. This is not absolute, because in a given circumstance it may be evident that risk to survival from hypoxia is greater than from hypotension. Also, pharmacologic agents can be used to support circulation, and improved myocardial oxygenation from better gas exchange may protect the cardiovascular system from pressure effects, despite continuation of PEEP.

Perhaps more important contraindications to PEEP are known pulmonary hyperinflation prior to onset of critical hypoxia and a normal or high compliance. The direct effect of PEEP increases both FRC and compliance, and if they are already elevated, little benefit can be expected. In a general way, we can say that PEEP is probably inadvisable for a patient with pulmonary emphysema. Areas of the lung already hyperinflated will be further distended, and excessive intra-alveolar pressure may divert pulmonary capillary flow to low-pressurized, poorly ventilated alveoli, increasing venous admixture and worsening hypoxia. The decision to use or withhold PEEP requires careful scrutiny of clinical and laboratory data, establishing priorities of risk to the patient. It should never be employed as a routine procedure, but only when it is judged that the hazards of an increased FRC and elevated intrathoracic pressure are less than the risks of continued hypoxia or oxygen toxicity.

4. *Initiating and discontinuing PEEP.* So far we have been concerned mostly with the principles of PEEP, and now it is time to consider such practical matters as levels of pressure used and how to start and discontinue it. Although there is no formula available to help us determine what PEEP should be, it is probably safe to say that end-expiratory pressures of 5 to 15 cm of water will accommodate most needs, but often pressures of 20 to 30 cm of water are needed, and rarely pressures more than 50 cm of water. There is no accepted "safe" level of PEEP. For many patients who have maintained fair cardiopulmonary stability, careful clinical observation, with blood gas determinations as needed, can safely guide the use of low PEEP levels. In the very acute patient, when end-expiratory pressures of more than 20 cm of water are needed, more specific cardiovascular monitoring is necessary. Currently popular for this purpose is the Swan-Ganz catheter, described earlier, which allows the titration of PEEP against cardiac output and degrees of arteriovenous shunt. With this information so-called "optimal PEEP" can be determined as the highest pressure that maximally decreases shunt without impeding cardiac output.[317, 332] A modification, described as "best PEEP" can be calculated at the bedside, without using the Swan-Ganz catheter.[333] Too much pressure decreases compliance, since overdistention of alveoli exceeds the number of lung units opened up to ventilation. Thus optimum lung function should accompany a level of PEEP that produces maximum compliance. In clinical use the effective static compliance is measured by dividing the tidal volume by the difference between plateau pressure and positive end-expiratory pressure

(*not* atmospheric zero gauge). This value is calculated for increasing PEEP levels until additional increments of pressure do not increase compliance. The final end-expiratory pressure is the "best PEEP." Such a relatively simple maneuver is not intended to replace invasive monitoring techniques, where the latter are indicated, and in patients with crushed chests, for example, where compliance is disrupted, it is inapplicable. Nevertheless, many patients can be safely managed by the "best PEEP" technique, coupled with knowledgeable clinical observation, and the hazard of intracardiac and intrapulmonary arterial catheterization avoided.

When PEEP is successful, we then have the task of reducing both PEEP and the high concentration of inspired oxygen. Assuming no complications from PEEP, it is advisable to maintain the elevated pressure while dropping inspired oxygen by increments of 10% to 15%, keeping arterial oxygen tension between 60 and 100 mm Hg. When the $F_{I_{O_2}}$ is 40% or less, the PEEP should then be lowered in steps of 5 cm of water until abolished. All patients require tailored schedules, of course, and many can be weaned from PEEP abruptly, whereas others may need a long and gradual withdrawal.

PEEP WITH ASSISTED MECHANICAL VENTILATION. Enabling a patient to trigger a ventilator, provided with PEEP, into a demand cycle for an assisted breath, requires the same attention to inspiratory effort as does the use of PEEP with IMV discussed a few pages back. Without IMV, spontaneous inspiratory effort should trigger an assisted ventilator breath. Thus machine sensitivity must be increased (as opposed to the use of IMV) so the patient will not have to overcome the PEEP to activate the ventilator. On modern volume ventilators the sensitivity mechanism can be readjusted, changing the triggering level from slightly subatmospheric to just below any desired PEEP; then initiating a machine-assisted breath calls for no more patient effort with PEEP than without it.[334]

In general, the airway pressure curves of machine-assist, patient-triggered breaths are the same as control breaths under static conditions. Thus curve *B* in Fig. 10-10 represents both controlleed-PEEP and assisted-PEEP. It would be more accurate, however, to include a small downward deflection at the start of inspiration of an assist curve, representing patient triggering effort.

Now that assisted-PEEP is technically possible, we should evaluate its role in acute respiratory care.[335] It would appear that the technique of intermittent mandatory ventilation (IMV) has replaced mechanically assisted ventilation to a considerable degree, but the student must remember that the sudden popularity of a new procedure does not mean that all its predecessors are automatically invalid. Despite the many welcome virtues of IMV, there are still occasional instances when it is advisable to encourage simply an inspiratory effort, even if the patient is unable to effect an adequate follow-up tidal volume. Here, true assisted ventilation is very helpful, and if PEEP is indicated, it can and should be used. It has been suggested that assisted-PEEP might occasionally be useful, in selected patients, when administered by face mask in an attempt to avoid tracheal intubation.[336] Even though perhaps limited in its scope, assisted-PEEP does put at our disposal another valuable tool in the management of ventilatory support.

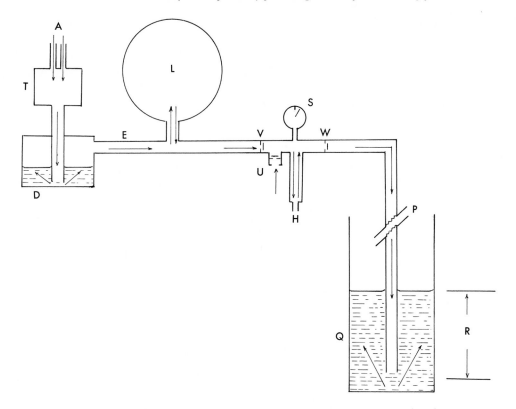

**Fig. 10-11.** Positive end-expiratory pressure (PEEP) with unassisted spontaneous breathing in an intubated patient. (See text for description.)

**PEEP WITH UNASSISTED SPONTANEOUS VENTILATION.** Positive end-expiratory pressure may be indicated in an intubated patient recently weaned from a ventilator or in one whose own breathing has not needed mechanical support but who can be intubated for PEEP. In some circumstances, PEEP can be used for short periods with a tightly fitted face mask. The simplest circuit for *spontaneous-PEEP* is shown in Fig. 10-11. Modifications can be added to this basic design, but it demonstrates the key elements. Breathing gas mixture from blender, *T*, flows through humidifier, *D*, into patient inspiratory tubing, *E*. Reservoir bag, *L*, makes available adequate gas for any size of tidal volume required by an intubated or tightly masked patient at *H*. As depicted in Fig. 10-9, an extended exhalation tube is immersed in a water column or attached to an adjustable mechanical resistor to create PEEP, the magnitude of which is accurately measured by manometer, *S*. The airways and lungs of a relaxed patient equilibrate with the supra-atmospheric pressure in the gas-conducting system, which to the lungs, in a sense, is now "ambient pressure." Spontaneous inhalation and exhalation therefore starts and terminates, respectively, at an elevated lung-thorax resting level, and FRC is enlarged.

Valving in such a system is unnecessary as long as breathing gas supply is adequate and is adjusted to flow steadily through the PEEP generator. It is wise, however, to anticipate the potential disaster of supply failure and include protective safety mechanisms. In the event of a loss of source gas, atmospheric air is immediately available to the patient through emergency one-way valve, *U*. Under the same circumstances, one-way valve, *V*, prevents exhaled air from taking the retrograde path of least resistance into the inspiratory arm of the patient tubing, creating a large dead space. One-way valve, *W*, similarly prevents rebreathing of gas in the exhalation tubing, in the absence of the rinsing effect of a steady source gas flow.

The technique just described is commonly referred to as CPAP (constant or continuous positive airway pressure) and as CPPB (constant or continuous positive pressure breathing) in accord with the two sets of definitions given earlier by the ACCP-ATS Joint Committee and the editorial office of *Respiratory Care*. CPAP (CPPB) implies spontaneous breathing without mechanical assistance against resistance to exhalation for the purpose of increasing FRC. The student's attention is directed to Fig. 10–9, where it can be observed that the circuit through the ventilator is a typical PEEP system, with an end-exhalation resistance to machine-assisted breathing. In contrast, the bypass circuit for spontaneous breathing is essentially the same as the system we have just described for CPAP. In other words, when we add PEEP and IMV capabilities to a ventilator circuit, we are providing both PEEP and CPAP (or CPPB). The battle of semantics over terminology and definitions does seem a bit ridiculous in this light because whether the patient is treated with PEEP or CPAP (CPPB) can depend on how he breathes—it may be his decision, not ours.[337-341]

Early in the description of the PEEP principle, reference was made to one exception to the need for airtight intubation. The respiratory distress syndrome of infants is

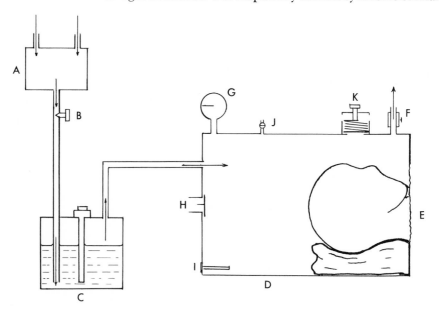

**Fig. 10-12.** Positive end-expiratory pressure (PEEP) with unassisted spontaneous breathing in a non-intubated infant. (See text for description.)

an extremely grave condition, most often afflicting the prematurely born. The disease is characterized by progressively falling compliance due to a surfactant lack of prematurity. Many infants need full ventilator support with intubation, but others with spontaneous breathing may need only assistance in maintaining alveolar patency and can benefit from PEEP. Intubation in these small patients is difficult, and a PEEP technique has been developed for them that is noninvasive.[342]

Fig. 10-12 schematically diagrams the major elements of a spontaneous-PEEP system that is, in reality, a miniature hyperbaric chamber. It surrounds the infant's head with a supra-atmospheric pressure, which elevates the lung-thorax resting level, and increases the FRC. Air-oxygen mixture from a blender and flowmeter, *A*, passes through a flow control valve, *B*, a heated humidifier, *C*, and into a rigid transparent plastic cylinder enclosing the patient's head, *D*. An adjustable soft plastic diaphragm, called an iris, which opens and closes like a camera shutter, forms a partial seal about the infant's neck, *E;* complete airtightness is unnecessary. A balance between entry gas flow and flow out of an adjustable escape port, *F*, maintains desired chamber pressure, which is recorded on an aneroid manometer, *G*. The unit is also supplied with a fitting for emergency manual bag ventilation or sighing, *H*, a thermometer for monitoring chamber temperature, *I*, a sampling port for analysis of chamber gas, *J*, and an adjustable safety pressure relief valve to limit chamber pressure, especially during manual ventilation, *K*. This can also be an underwater seal instead of a mechanical valve. Not shown is a hinged lid on top for easy access to the patient.

Attention is directed to Fig. 10-10, curve *C*, which has the biphasic intrapulmonary pressure contour of a spontaneous breath. Inspiration generates airflow by lowering intrapulmonary pressure, *I*, and at end-inspiration, as flow stops momentarily, pressure equilibrates with ambient and returns to baseline. Exhalation, *E*, elevates intrapulmonary pressure to force air out, then at end-exhalation pressure again returns to baseline. Two important facts should be noted. First, despite the intrapulmonary pressure oscillations about the baseline during the ventilatory phases, breaths start and stop (end-expiration) at the elevated resting level. Second, and again despite the pressure variation of the breathing curve, all that matters is that end-expiration is at a higher than atmospheric pressure. This is what increases the FRC.

Curve *D* amplifies these points. Assume the patient takes an occasional extra large breath or that his regular pattern is large enough that he creates a slight negative pressure in his lungs at peak exhalation. The fact that inspiratory pulmonary pressure dips into the negative range in no way interferes with or negates the function or purpose of PEEP. End-expiration still falls at the desired positive pressure of an elevated resting level, and the FRC is correspondingly enlarged. Also, if the patient has the power to create large pressure swings and big tidal volumes, this reflects favorably on his functional status. The student is asked to note, however, that in a curve *D* situation, the expressions *constant* or *continuous positive airway pressure* or *positive-pressure breathing* are technically incorrect because of the possibility of inspiratory negative peak pressures. For this reason a term such as *spontaneous-PEEP*, or some other that emphasizes the terminal pressure, is more appropriate than are *CPAP* or *CPPB*, as defined earlier.

*Monitoring mechanical ventilation.* The need for close observation of the mechanically ventilated patient has been amply emphasized, as has the value of a respiratory care unit for this purpose. No matter what the physical circumstances are under which treatment is being given, there are certain things for which the therapist looks and which he checks, and procedures which he follows that experience has shown to be necessary for the patient's safety. We will describe three types of monitoring—clinical, physiological, and mechanical—although there are overlapping areas among them.

*Clinical monitoring.* Clinical monitoring involves observing the patient and evaluating his condition and the effectiveness of his ventilation based on signs and symptoms and the therapist's critical knowledge of the physiology of the disease and the expectations of therapy. No sophisticated diagnostic equipment is used. The therapist is interested in the physical and mental comfort of the patient because the patient's attitude is vital to his recovery. Since the intubated patient cannot speak, the therapist must be on the watch for signs of pain, restlessness, and apprehension. Often communication can be established through the use of pencil and paper, and although too-frequent annoying questions are to be avoided, the therapist should inquire periodically of the feelings of the patient. The alert and observant therapist soon learns the characteristics of his patient and how best to manage him. The patient's color should be watched and both cyanosis and pallor noted. We know that cyanosis is a crude quantitative gauge of hypoxemia, but it is a good determinant of changes in oxygenation. Excessive pallor, especially if accompanied by cold moist skin, may indicate developing cardiovascular collapse.

Much valuable information concerning the work of breathing and the effectiveness of therapy can be obtained by noting the muscular components of ventilation. This is especially true before the start of treatment in the patient being assisted rather than controlled in his breathing and during breaks in controlled ventilation, as when the patient is being aspirated or equipment is being serviced. Increasing or decreasing use of the accessory ventilatory muscles is noted and is an excellent indication of the energy used by the patient. The therapist should frequently observe the mobility of the upper abdomen, or epigastrium, both when the patient is on and when he is off the ventilator. To do this properly he should expose the upper half of the patient's abdomen and kneel by the side of the bed so that he can sight across the patient at the abdominal level. Retraction of the epigastrium during the inspiratory phase and protrusion during exhalation constitute paradoxical breathing, described in Chapter 6, and indicate a severe disturbance in the efficiency of ventilation. If present while the patient is being mechanically assisted, they mean that he is completely uncoordinated with the instrument, that he is working against it, and that therapy is worsening rather than helping him. The degree to which the epigastrium rises during inhalation is a function of the descent of the diaphragm and a rough indication of the tidal volume. Like the evaluation of cyanosis, the volumetric implication of epigastric movement is valuable as a monitor of changes rather than a quantitative measurement. To appreciate the abdominal motion, the therapist should lay his hand gently on the patient, between the xiphoid cartilage and the umbilicus, and observe as well as feel the movement of his hand. In the obstructed patient with spontaneous breathing, assisted or unassisted, the therapist may be able to feel the expiratory contraction of the abdominal wall as the patient works to express air against heavy resistance. Finally, in addition to judging the muscular aspect of ventilation, the therapist will be able to ascertain by inspection and palpation of the abdomen whether there is abdominal distention. The accumulation of intestinal gas postoperatively and the swallowing of air by a dyspneic patient given short-term ventilatory assistance through a face mask or mouthpiece can produce serious distention of the abdomen. Not infrequently distention builds up an intra-abdominal pressure so great that it seriously interferes with the inspirational descent of the diaphragm. In such an instance the therapist will observe the abdomen to be rounded, its skin stretched smooth, and the wall tense to the touch. A gentle but sharp slap will elicit a tympanic, or drumlike, response. If the therapist notes such distention, he should bring it to the attention of the attending physician or nurse, for unless it can be relieved, it may make effective ventilation impossible.

Auscultation of the chest is an examination of the breath sounds through a stethoscope and is a technique with which the therapist should become familiar. It should be clear to him that his use of a stethoscope is limited, for diagnostic auscultation is a fine art employed by a physician and takes many years to develop to a point of proficiency. However, the use of a stethoscope will enable the therapist to evaluate the distribution of air in the patient's chest and to evaluate the degree of obstruction. When the ventilator has been set up to the therapist's satisfaction, he should listen to the chest with the scope—anteriorly, posteriorly, and in the axillae—comparing the sounds in related areas of both lungs from the apices to the bases. Closing his eyes for maximum concentration, he listens for the intensity of airflow to determine whether there are areas that are not being adequately ventilated.

Since many of his patients suffer severe obstruction and have mobile secretions, it is not uncommon to find areas of lung poorly aerated and patterns of air distribution that change from hour to hour. In this regard, special mention should be made of a hazard of intubation referred to earlier in this chapter and illustrated in Fig. 10-13. This is the placement of a tracheal tube too low so that its tip passes the carina into one

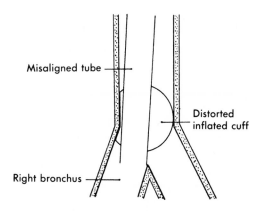

**Fig. 10-13.** Low position of tracheal tube so that its tip enters one main bronchus. The inflated cuff effectively occludes the other air passage, limiting ventilation to only one lung.

or the other main bronchi. This is generally the result of a hasty insertion of an endotracheal or nasotracheal tube, intubation by unskilled personnel, or the use of too long a tracheostomy tube. With most if not all the delivered gas directed into only one lung, the serious disturbance to the ventilation-perfusion balance is obvious. Severe physiologic shunting can increase the venous admixture to the point that hypoxia may be fatal, and in the obstructed patient the resistance to the total airflow's diversion to one lung will prevent compensation for the hypoventilation of the blocked lung, and hypercapnia is probable. Usually the clinical appearance of the patient will warn of this complication, but if the occlusion is not complete, the ineffective ventilation may be attributed to underlying disease and correction attempted by such irrelevant measures as increasing airflow, the use of bronchodilators, etc. Thus, in an intubated patient, signs of sudden disruption of ventilatory pattern, accompanied by auscultatory signs of reduced airflow to one lung, should raise the immediate suspicion of a misplaced or slipped tube or a displaced cuff, and the responsible physician should be alerted at once. With experience the therapist will be able to differentiate the breath sounds encountered in obstructive disease and described in Chapter 6. This will help him in evaluating the status of the airways by recognizing obstruction as primarily due to bronchospasm rather than to secretions; and the better his understanding of the patient, the better will be his services.

With his knowledge of the effect of mechanical ventilation on circulation, the therapist will want to keep himself informed on his patient's cardiovascular status by frequent checking of heart rate and blood pressure. Although these parameters are traditionally the responsibility of the nursing service, there need be no conflict. Indeed, this is a function whereby cooperation between the nurse and the therapist will be to the advantage of the patient. In a special-care unit, rates and pressures are recorded frequently, and the therapist may not need to do the measurements routinely. However, the therapist is aware of the speed with which the ventilated patient's condition may change, and he should monitor these values as often as he feels necessary, and especially if he finds it necessary to increase inspiratory pressure to a high level in an unstable patient or one receiving prolonged therapy.

There is no rule to follow, but in the patient whose cardiac condition is in doubt or who has known cardiac weakness, heart rate and pressure may have to be recorded as often as every 15 minutes until stability is assured and then at least hourly thereafter. At any time the therapist feels there is a progressive or significant rise in heart rate or a drop in pressure, the attending nurse or physician or the medical director of the respiratory therapy department should be immediately notified. If the responsible physician decides that cardiac output is falling and shock developing, he will start corrective measures, and although the therapist knows the role played by expiratory negative pressure in this situation, the physician is the one to order it. However, the tactful therapist may offer his services to adjust the ventilator for negative pressure, thus reminding the physician of the availability of this effective measure. If the physician gives approval, it is then the responsibility of the therapist to reevaluate the ventilatory pattern in terms of the I/E ratio and extend the expiratory time as long as possible, while reducing inspiratory pressure as much as is consistent with ventilatory needs. If cardiac rate, dropping blood pressure, and other signs of shock, as described in Chapter 5, are unrelieved, negative pressure during exhalation may be introduced. The physiologic rationale for this maneuver as well as its own risks were detailed in Chapter 9. Let us only repeat here that negative expiratory pressure should never be used indiscriminately and only for correction of reduced cardiac output resulting from positive-pressure ventilation. The hazards of air trapping and pulmonary edema must be watched for closely. Negative pressure should be started gradually, balancing its effect against the blood pressure, and usually 3 to 5 cm of water are adequate. To maintain the same alveolar ventilation as before the introduction of subatmospheric pressure, the therapist may have to increase the tidal volume to make up for additional air removed by expiratory suction at the expense of the functional residual capacity,[343] since in a sense this amounts to increasing the physiologic dead space. Skill is needed to use expiratory pressure safely and effectively, since the procedure entails balancing the negative pressure necessary to protect the cardiac output against a possible increase in positive pressure (if a pressure-cycled machine is being used), to maintain ventilation in the face of the negative-pressure effect on lung volume, and still realize a net drop in intrathoracic pressure.

*Physiologic monitoring.* In contrast to clinical observation, physiologic monitoring refers to the laboratory measurements of the physiologic responses to disease and treatment. One does not supplant the other, for laboratory findings are of only limited value unless interpreted in the light of what is actually happening to the patient as a whole; but at the same time clinical examinations cannot give us the precise information we need of what is happening inside the patient. The current therapy of ventilatory failure is predicated on the availability of facilities to give us this physiologic insight, and the use of modern respirators in controlled treatment is dangerous guesswork without such information. Thus the hospital that is to treat failure must have not only good respiratory therapists but also a pulmonary function laboratory. The organization of such a facility and its relationship to the respiratory therapy service will be noted in the final chapter, but let us say here that whatever the structure needed to meet the needs of an individual hospital, the pulmonary function laboratory must work closely with respiratory therapy and its findings made readily available to the therapists. Although the services of such a laboratory may be diverse, in our concern with management of ventilatory failure, physiologic monitoring, for the most part, means measurement of arterial oxygen and carbon dioxide tensions and pH, and the calculation of bicarbonate level. By this time the therapist's orientation toward his work should be firmly fixed on the importance of these values.

In all probability, before the therapist is called to attend a patient, the diagnostic workup will have included blood gas studies on the basis of which, with clinical findings, the decision to institute therapy was made. Frequently the therapist will see a patient admitted as an emergency, obviously in need of ventilatory assistance, and earlier in this chapter we commented on the therapeutic approach while awaiting physiologic data. Whatever the situation, arterial gas values constitute the basis for definitive therapy and should be obtained as soon as possible. The question is frequently raised concerning the frequency of blood gas examinations during therapy, and for this there can be only one answer—as often as is necessary to assure the most effective and safest ventilation. Not rarely is it needed every 15 minutes until the medical team feels confident that management is proper. When the response to therapy is satisfactory, clinical and physiologic signs of stability become evident, and the frequency of blood gas determinations can be gradually reduced. For the sake of safety, once the acute phase has passed and the patient can be considered at a maintenance plateau or recovering, gas tensions and pH determinations should be done at least twice daily. Often this can be modified, however, if hypoxia is felt to be permanently corrected, and monitoring is reduced to carbon dioxide tension and pH measurements. The therapist must keep in mind that, despite his skill or the sophistication of his equipment, the adequacy of his patient's alveolar ventilation can be ascertained only by these last two values.

Until the past 3 to 4 years, arterial sampling was a procedure limited to physicians, reminiscent of a similar limitation on venoclysis up to about two decades ago. Fortunately, there is increasing recognition that such restrictions, based on habit more than reason, are uneconomical and not in the best interests of patient care. Arterial blood sampling not only can but should be done by respiratory therapists, pulmonary laboratory technicians, and nurses participating in pulmonary care. Obviously, not every therapist and nurse needs to be skilled in the procedure, and assigning this responsibility so that all shifts are covered is a simple administrative task. We should have learned several years ago, when special "intravenous teams" of nurses were organized, that the skill of performance is directly proportional to the frequency of performance. Therapists and technicians who draw arterial blood samples several times daily not only inflict minimal trauma on patients but they are excellent tutors for the medical house staff and students. We will not go into details of technique because there are many good teaching aids available, but it is important to emphasize that while arterial sampling is generally safe and easy, there is always the potential for injury. Those performing it must be careful, responsible people.

The therapist might wonder why venous blood cannot be used for monitoring, since it is considered more readily attainable. The basic objection to venous blood is that, because it is usually drawn from an extremity, it reflects the local metabolic activity of the area drained by the vein chosen and in a sense indicates what is left over after perfusion of local tissues. Arterial blood, on the other hand, shows directly the ability of the lungs to effect gas exchange before any extraction of oxygen or addition of carbon dioxide by the tissues. If venous blood is withdrawn after a needle has been left in the vein without a tourniquet about the extremity for 1 minute, there will be some correlation between venous and arterial carbon dioxide tension and pH but little for oxygen tension.

Arterial blood sampling in infants can be a very difficult procedure, and in some adults repeated "arterial sticks" are hampered by poorly accessible vessels and occasionally threaten vessel integrity. As an alternative to direct arterial sampling, a technique utilizing "arterialized" capillary blood has become popular and practical. Commonly known as a "finger stick," this procedure consists of puncturing the end of the finger (or toe or heel of an infant) with a sharp blade to obtain a free flow of capillary blood. Prior to puncture the hand is immersed in hot water for 10 minutes, a technique that has been demonstrated to render blood in the capillaries similar in its characteristics to arterial blood. The blood is collected in a glass capillary or a properly prepared small syringe and analyzed in the same manner as arterial blood. For some time this technique has been considered satisfactory for carbon dioxide tension and pH, but many questioned its reliability for oxygen tension. More comparative experience with it, however, has indicated that all three capillary parameters correlate well enough with arterial blood to be clinically accurate.[344,345] Acceptance of this technique has made physiologic data readily available because this is a procedure that can be done as often as necessary to monitor mechanical ventilation while at the same time sparing the patient repeated arterial punctures. The reliable respiratory therapist may be given freedom to obtain and examine arterialized capillary blood according to his own judgment to fulfill his responsibility for maintaining ventilation. He is thus aware of the condition and needs of his patient at all times.

In Chapter 5 and again in the discussion of "optimal PEEP," reference was made to the Swan-Ganz catheter. It and the central venous catheter are primarily tools for cardiac monitoring, but they sometimes are valuable in following patients in ventilatory failure, especially if on ventilator support. The data from such intracardiac and intravascular monitoring were described earlier, and we will only note here that prevention or rapid correction of cardiovascular complications of mechanical ventilation may be a critical factor in patient survival. Not all patients in ventilatory failure need these invasive measures, but their availability is one more option in management.

Of more immediate urgency for the mechanically ventilated patient is an electronic monitor to count cardiac rate, to signal deviations above and below preset ranges, and to display electrical cardiac complexes on a small oscilloscope. There have been unfortunate instances of unnoticed heart stoppage in mechanically ventilated patients. Many efficient commercial models are available, and one of them should be part of all standard ventilator setups.

*Mechanical monitoring.* For the most part, mechanical monitoring resolves into the use of spirometers to measure tidal and minute volumes. Some ventilators are equipped with such meters, but they often give only an approximation of the amount of air delivered. Extremely useful is a portable meter, the Wright respirometer.* With a face the size of a small clock, the instrument is a flowmeter constructed as a small air turbine with one dial calibrated in liters up to 100 liters and a second dial calibrated in 10 ml increments up to 1 liter. Its minimum flow response is less than 2 lpm, but it should not be subjected to flows exceeding 300 lpm. It is easily adapted to the exhalation port of any ventilator to measure the exhaled air as a gauge of tidal volume, a practical but not always accurate assumption. Obviously, it cannot be so used with expiratory negative pressure. The meter can give rough but usable information about three characteristics of ventilation. First, severe airway obstruction will cause the small needle to "hang up" in response to interference with exhaled flow. Second, in controlled ventilation, if the needle finishes its rotation before the next inspiration begins, it indicates terminal air trapping. Third, if the ventilator pressure and metered tidal volume are noted simultaneously, a working compliance can be calculated. Although not of diagnostic accuracy, this compliance is of importance in monitoring changes in the lung during prolonged ventilation.

---

*Wright respirometer, Anesthesia Associates, Inc., Hudson, N.Y.

Electronic monitors are available that will emit visible and audible signals if preset ranges of rate or phase are not met or are exceeded and if the ventilator fails or disconnects from the patient.*† Such instruments have a definite value, and with the current interest in instrumentation in so many fields of medicine, there will doubtless be other developments in monitoring respiratory function as there have been for cardiac function. Any assistance that gives support to the patient is desirable, but mechanical or electronic monitors must not be relied on as a substitute for the personal attention of a skilled therapist. A monitor will not correct a deficiency, and its value depends entirely on the capability of the personnel responding to its call.

### Weaning from the ventilator

As with all the other aspects of ventilator care, the process of weaning, or gradual removal of the patient from his respirator, must be tailored to the needs of each patient, and only general suggestions can be offered. The therapist must accept the fact that supported ventilation, and especially controlled ventilation, is a harrowing and frightening experience for anyone, accompanied by much psychic trauma. During the course of therapy, the patient develops an understandable dependence upon the machine that was responsible for his survival. No sooner has the successfully treated patient survived the terror of breathlessness, able to relax with the support of his ventilator, than he hears his medical team discussing the possibility of taking it away from him. The thought may panic him because he is far from sure that, since he needed mechanical help so recently, he is able to do without it now. Two dicta of weaning may be stated together. Remove the patient from his ventilator as soon as possible, but prepare him for it carefully. There are two general weaning techniques, each with many possible variations—*weaning with unattached ventilator* and *weaning with attached ventilator*. Both systems have advantages, but the student should view them as craftsmen's tools. There are many ways in which they can be used, and they are used according to the need of the work, the work is not fitted to the tool. Despite the aura of scientific precision created by rhythmical ventilators, bedside monitors, and laboratory data slips, separation of a patient from his ventilator is very nearly pure art. The two approaches to weaning will be discussed separately and will reflect both personal experience and the reported experience of others.[346-350]

*Weaning with unattached ventilator.* Weaning with an unattached ventilator is the older of the two techniques and consists of removal of the ventilator from the patient according to a time schedule. Generally, the longer a patient is ventilated the more difficult and the longer is the weaning period. In addition, the state of intubation with power-induced ventilation is both unnatural and unphysiologic and carries the risk of secondary infection and injury to the lung the longer it persists. The objective of mechanical ventilation therefore is to support the patient through acute respiratory failure, control or improve the etiology of the failure, and restore the patient to spontaneous unassisted breathing as soon as possible. Conditioning of the patient for this move should start well in advance, not by telling him that he will be taken off the

---

*Monitaire, ventilation monitor, Monitor Instrument Co., Inc., Hamden, Conn.
†D. H. Taylor solid state IPPV monitor, Respiratory Function Labs, Inc., Syracuse, N.Y.

ventilator on a given day so that he will anticipate it fearfully, but by giving him encouraging reports of his progress while he is still supported. From the earliest moment in therapy he should be told repeatedly that mechanical ventilation is a temporary measure, designed to give him rest from the stress of breathing until he is better. Many factors will influence the decision to wean. Arterial blood gases and pH should be normal or acceptable for the patient's condition, with a $P_{a_{O_2}}$ of at least 70 mm Hg on 40% $F_{I_{O_2}}$. It is felt that, off the ventilator, the patient should have (1) a peak inspiratory pressure numerically no less than −20 cm of water, as measured by an aneroid manometer attached to a piece of breathing tubing with a suitable tracheal adaptor; (2) vital capacity of 15 ml/kg body weight; (3) the ability to double minute ventilation voluntarily; (4) a dead space/tidal volume ratio ($V_D/V_T$) of less than 0.6; and (5) an alveolar-arterial $P_{O_2}$ difference, breathing 100% oxygen (A-a $D_{O_2}$ on 100% oxygen) of less than 350 mm Hg.

Infection should be controlled and the patient's mental attitude one of cooperation. It is very helpful to watch carefully the patient's behavior when he is removed from the ventilator for the short periods required for aspiration or servicing his tracheostomy tube or ventilator, and if spontaneous breathing is evident at these times, some estimate of its adequacy can be noted. Certainly, such spontaneous breathing must return before weaning can even be considered, and it is often helpful to ask the patient to take an occasional breath while still on control to see if he can override the machine. He may have to be urged to this effort, since it is so easy for him to conform to the ventilator that he may not exert himself to see whether he can breathe unless encouraged to do so. For short periods of time the patient can be put on assisted ventilation, with take-over control at a lower rate, and the explanation can be given that he must exercise his ventilatory muscles, which have become weak from disuse. Most patients accept as reasonable this need to try breathing on their own, and such periods can be extended to as long as is acceptable to them. The therapist should keep reassuring the patient that, should he tire or even fall asleep, the ventilator will automatically start to function.

Once a patient's spontaneous breathing has been demonstrated to him, he is ready for the next step. While disconnected from the ventilator for tracheostomy care, the patient can be asked if he would like to breathe on his own for a few minutes with the therapist in attendance, and he should be provided with a tracheostomy mask for the delivery of humidified oxygen or air. Supported ventilation should be resumed before the patient tires, but these intervals of spontaneous breathing *with the cuff deflated* are gradually increased until he is breathing on his own most of the time, with occasional periods of restful support. It may be necessary to provide assisted ventilation during the sleeping hours for a little longer.

The student will find that some authors speak deprecatingly of this so-called "trial-and-error" method of removing patients from ventilator support for periods of time and at intervals that are quite arbitrary. Still, this is a time-tested method that has been successful when supervised by conscientious and knowledgeable medical personnel. It does not take an experienced therapist long to evaluate his patient's ventilatory stamina and to set up a gradual program of ventilator withdrawal that is safe and effective. Some experts advocate removing the patient from his ventilator for a fixed short period of time and gradually shorten the intervals between. As an example, this might mean letting the patient breathe unassisted for 2 minutes of an hour, then 2 minutes each half-hour, quarter-hour, and so on, until mechanical aid is discontinued. When weaning has started in earnest, oxygenation and humidification in the free-breathing intervals are important. A T-tube blow-by attached to the end of the tracheal tube provides a flow of inspired gas from which the patient breathes. It is advised that inspired oxygen concentration be 10% higher than had been delivered by the ventilator.[350] Humidification should be as close to 100% as possible because the prevention of respiratory mucosal drying is critical at this stage. When the patient can breathe unassisted around the clock, is moving a reasonable amount of air without undue effort, and can walk for short distances consistent with his general physical condition, and when ventilation is satisfactory and stable by blood gas values, it is time to consider removal of the intratracheal tube.

*Extubation.* If the weaning schedule has been gradual, removal of the tube will present little difficulty, whether it is nasotracheal, orotracheal, or tracheostomy. Cleaning of mouth and hypopharynx by suction should precede removal of supralaryngeal tubes, but once they are out, no special care is needed unless there has been local tissue tube damage. Humidified oxygen in the same concentration that had been used is continued by face mask, then with further improvement it is reduced or eliminated as indicated.

Removal of a tracheostomy tube is not difficult, but the residual stoma must be covered with one or two gauze pads held loosely with tape. It is treated as any open wound until healed, a matter of a few days in the absence of complications. Many patients are apprehensive about the tracheostomy, but they can be reassured with some simple instructions. Most ventilated patients have excessive sputum production and a cough. A patient newly extubated should be taught to support the tracheal stoma during cough by applying a firm squeezing pressure to the throat over the dressing with the full palm of one hand. With encouragement he soon learns to cough past the tracheostomy and bring secretions into the mouth for expectoration. Depending on the flow of secretions, annoying ostial leakage can be expected for 2 to 3 days, and dressings should be changed frequently. Pressurized aerosol therapy can be used with a mouthpiece, shortly after extubation, with little loss of inspired air through the tracheal defect, because the patient uses manual support and is soon able to breathe past it.

Sometimes it is desirable to prevent immediate closure of the stoma, especially when profuse secretions make continued aspiration necessary while a weak patient is regaining his own cough power. The use of Kistner tracheostomy tubes or Moore buttons can be very helpful. These are basically short tubes that can be inserted through the tracheostomy and are held in place by flanges on their inner ends. Caps are available for occlusion, some have one-way valves for air intake only, and their small sizes offer little intratracheal airflow resistance.

We will consider two modifications of tracheostomy tube removal that involve special preparation for the actual extubation.

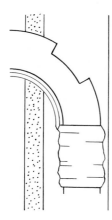

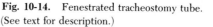

**Fig. 10-14.** Fenestrated tracheostomy tube. (See text for description.)

**USING A FENESTRATED TRACHEOSTOMY TUBE.** For the tracheostomized patient who was difficult to wean, who perhaps is borderline hypoxic, and who may need occasional ventilator support or pressure breathing therapy, the cuffed fenestrated tube can be substituted for the regular style. As illustrated in Fig. 10-14, this tube has an opening (fenestration) cut into its convex surface, and it is supplied with an inner cannula. With the cannula removed and the cuff deflated, the patient can move air through the tube in the usual manner, and by mouth through the fenestration and around the tube. This allows maximum airflow against minimal resistance, supposedly expedites easier coughing and oral removal of secretions, and facilitates phonation, if the tube is plugged. With the cuff inflated and the inner cannula in place occluding the fenestration, pressure-breathing aerosols or assisted mechanical ventilation can be used in a closed system.

The fenestrated tube therefore is a kind of half-step between ventilator weaning and extubation. It allows the patient a little longer to establish ventilatory and gas-exchange stability before becoming fully independent. At the proper time the fenestrated tube is removed, and the patient is managed as described above.

**PLUGGING THE TRACHEOSTOMY TUBE.** This consists of deflating the cuff, then occluding the tube with a stopper that blocks about half the orifice, and after a variable period of time, replacing it with a fully occluding plug. The purpose is to acclimate the patient gradually to breathing through a narrower airway than that provided by the patent tube and to prepare him for the restrictions of his own nasal and laryngeal passages. However, there is an important point here that should be clearly understood. Trach tube plugging had its origin when tracheostomies were performed mostly for conditions such as laryngeal croup, diphtheria, and the like, or to prevent aspiration of oral secretions in patients with bulbar poliomyelitis who were supported in tank respirators. These patients usually had normal lungs and normal conductance distal to their tracheal tubes. It was reasonable to test their ability to breathe against improving proximal obstruction or to evaluate the degree of return of neuromuscular ventilatory function before extubation. This may still be useful for patients with non-pulmonary ventilatory failure. The many patients we see who are intubated and ventilated for airway obstructive disease present a different problem. Any type of intratracheal tube is space occupying and an impedance to airflow, even when fully patent, and its presence is justified only as long as it is used to support ventilation or remove secretions. There is little rationale in plugging tracheostomy tubes in such patients, adding more obstruction to their already existing difficulties, for which they were intensively treated in the first place. In general, when an intubated patient with obstructive disease shows signs of improving spontaneous breathing, he will breathe considerably better when the tube is removed.

***Weaning with attached ventilator.*** This specifically refers to the use of intermittent mandatory ventilation (IMV) as a means of removing a patient from mechanical ventilation. In our earlier discussion we considered it as a part of general ventilatory management, but of necessity touched upon its role in weaning. IMV was originally intended as a weaning device, to be activated in the ventilator circuit as the patient improved. We have already learned, however, that IMV can be available, if felt advantageous, from the beginning of mechanical ventilation.

There are two major advantages to IMV weaning. First, with a spontaneous breathing circuit present, the patient himself may determine the onset of his weaning by generating breaths on his own. Thus his own ventilatory drive may set the pattern for further management. In the absence of patient breaths, perhaps because mechanical breathing is not permitting his respiratory center to express itself, the ventilator rate can be gradually reduced until spontaneous breathing begins. Clinical judgment is responsible for setting the pattern, but as the machine breaths lessen and the patient breaths increase in frequency, the transition from controlled to free breathing can be smooth and effortless. With some patients, discontinuance of the ventilator is possible when IMV breaths are 2 to 4 a minute, while in others machine rates as low as 1 breath per minute may be needed before full reliance can be put on the patient.

The second advantage of IMV is that it allows the patient to benefit from the same gas mixture and PEEP in both machine and spontaneous breathing. There is no change of equipment, no adjusting of oxygen mixtures, no supplementary end-expiratory pressure equipment needed.

No technique is foolproof, and IMV is not an exception. Some patients still require trials off the ventilator, on a T-piece, even though they have been on an IMV system. This does not negate the value of IMV, since perhaps without it, weaning would have been even more difficult. There is no uniform agreement that IMV is the best weaning procedure to follow, and advocates of unattached ventilator weaning strongly support their method. There is little doubt, however, that IMV has given us a tremendous option in our choice of managing the weaning patient. Principles of extubation are the same as those already discussed.

## INSPIRATORY POSITIVE-PRESSURE BREATHING

So far, we have discussed the use of inspiratory positive pressure in the delivery of assisted or controlled ventilation for the patient with inadequate breathing, and now we will consider IPPB as a treatment entity for less acute conditions. IPPB has come rapidly onto the medical scene, enjoying both widespread use and acclamation and considerable condemnation. As with many innovations, pressure breathing suffered from initial overuse without due regard for proper indications or technique, and when expectations that were never claimed for it did not materialize, many users became disenchanted with it. Much, if not all, of the controversy over the value or harm of IPPB was the result of lack of clear understanding of its capabilities and what can be expected of it. In addition, the advent of IPPB preceded the development of respiratory therapy as a skilled technical specialty, and pressure breathing was used by many people with little concept of its objectives or knowledge of the mechanics of the instruments or their physiologic effects. It is little wonder that results were less than spectacular and the treatment blamed rather than those treating.

### Equipment

Most IPPB instruments function according to the principles described for IPPVs, and although the ventilators themselves can be used for intermittent therapy, there are units much simpler in structure designed just for this purpose. Without the need for the many critical controls of ventilators, treatment instruments are generally smaller in size, and many are portable, independent of gas cylinders or centrally supplied air with their own built-in compressors. Advertising brochures and operating manuals from manufacturers will give the student an overview of the specifications of the many competitive units on the market, and we will not pursue the topic further.

### Indications for IPPB

Pressure breathing is generally used for its following physiologic effects: (1) to increase alveolar and total ventilation, (2) to elevate arterial oxygen saturation, (3) to reduce arterial carbon dioxide tension, and (4) to reduce cardiac output. The special use of the last effect will be discussed separately below. Its indications include many clinical entities, such as acute and chronic bronchitis, pulmonary emphysema, bronchiectasis, lung abscess, postpneumonia, and preoperative and postoperative states, to list the most common.

IPPB is indicated for two broad clinical objectives. First, it is used to improve the general intrapulmonary distribution of inspired air, thereby restoring a disturbed ventilation-perfusion balance to as nearly normal as possible, eliminating venous admixture and lowering carbon dioxide tension. Pressure breathing is especially valuable in preventing postoperative atelectasis by assuring adequate lung expansion during the recovery period. Its judicious and energetic use may prevent potential hypercarbia and subsequent respiratory failure in a susceptible patient, such as one with emphysema who is the victim of trauma or a respiratory infection. Second, IPPB is widely used as a vehicle for deep pulmonary aerosol therapy because it will effect maximum aerosol distribution. It is valuable in the treatment of bronchospasm and as an aid to the removal of secretions, and it can be used to deliver any of the aerosols discussed in an earlier chapter. In this regard, surgeons have found it valuable preoperatively to assure maximum airway clearance for the prevention of postsurgical atelectasis and infection, especially in those with known bronchial disease or who are heavy cigarette smokers.

Frequently, IPPB with an aerosolized bronchodilator is followed by chest physiotherapy, as described in the next chapter, to facilitate maximum clearance of secretions from the airways. The use of ultrasonically nebulized saline, or saline/propylene glycol may be given after the IPPB to water down secretions for later removal by physical therapy. There are many treatment programs that include IPPB, and it is imperative that *IPPB never be used on a dogmatically routine basis.* This is one fault that has exposed the procedure to criticism as noted in the preface to this edition. There should be a specific objective that IPPB is expected to accomplish in every patient for whom it is prescribed. As yet there are no standard guidelines to judge the efficacy of IPPB therapy, but it is a responsibility of the attending physician to use whatever means are available to evaluate its effects and to indicate its discontinuance. Good clinical observation and examination and judicious use of simple pulmonary laboratory tests will be sufficient in most instances.

There are two cautions in the administration of IPPB that cannot be overstressed, and failure to consider them in the past has contributed to resistance to its use. First, probably most IPPB therapy is poorly done, and many patients would have been just as well, or perhaps better, without it. Unless a trained attendant such as a respiratory therapist or technician can remain with the patient throughout the treatment and actively participate in it, it is doubtful that the therapy will have any beneficial effects. This does not mean that the therapist should sit in a corner of the room reading the newspaper. The experienced therapist or technician may feel that IPPB treatments are unglamorous when compared with management of controlled ventilation; this is only because of his familiarity with it. It still remains one of his most valuable contributions to medicine, and as deserving of his best efforts as any other procedure. In a new patient, IPPB can cause disturbing apprehension, and he must be watched and advised continuously. We often consider that a veteran user of IPPB can take care of himself, and we tend to let such a patient treat himself. *This is a serious error.* A patient cannot be expected to be responsible for the proper performance on himself of a procedure that requires as much skill as does IPPB. That is our job, as professionals. When left alone for self-treatment, patients almost invariably forget small details of breathing techniques or slouch into positions more comfortable for them but which completely negate the function of the therapy. It is up to the therapist to watch each patient during the entire treatment, instructing and advising him, breath by breath if necessary, to help him meet the goals set for him.

In summary, this means that the minimum criteria for IPPB therapy are that it be given by someone skilled in its use, on a one-to-one therapist-patient relationship during each treatment. I am fully aware that this is an ideal still a long way from realization, but if we are to be honest with our patients and ourselves, we must recognize that correction of this basic deficiency should be one of our highest priorities, before we look around for new and seemingly greener fields to conquer.

Second, in our enthusiasm for aggressive action, we sometimes forget that a patient is not a disease but is a person with a disease, and by virtue of his illness he has less than his normal physical stamina. Subjecting him to a program that may promise to ease his problems, but that pushes him to the edge of exhaustion, will earn him disappointing, diminishing returns. Combining procedures for additive benefit is to be encouraged, as part of a specific therapeutic plan, but it must be done with care and a regard for the patient's well-being. To prescribe 15 minutes of IPPB, followed by 30 minutes of ultrasonic aerosol inhalation, then 15 minutes of chest physical therapy, on a 2-hour basis for a 100-pound, 70-year-old woman, may stress her to a dangerous point. We frequently must compromise what we would like to do for or to our patient, with concern for the patient's discomfort. Overtreatment is potentially dangerous, but it is preventable by establishing a treatment plan for each patient and prescribing only those procedures that contribute to the plan. Duration of, and intervals between, treatments must be tailored to the specific needs of each patient, progress followed closely, and the program adjusted on a daily basis. This is honest and rational respiratory therapy.

**Technique of IPPB administration**

Before initiating therapy on a new patient, if meaningful communication is possible, the therapist must be absolutely certain to explain to the patient what is going to be done. Without delivering an academic lecture, the therapist should tell the patient the nature of the treatment and in a general way what is expected of it. Resistance or hostility of a patient toward therapy is usually due to one or more of the following: (1) he is irrational from illness or age; (2) he is expressing fright through hostility; and (3) he does not understand what is expected of him. A few moments of reassuring explanation will make the treatment helpful for the patient and easy on the therapist.

For best results the patient should be seated upright in a relatively straight chair, although this is not always possible for the hospitalized patient. Nevertheless, every effort should be made to avoid a slouched position, which will hamper diaphragmatic mobility. Obesity is a serious hazard to good ventilatory mechanics, and in the supine position, especially if the head of the bed is elevated, abdominal pressure may prevent all but very small diaphragmatic descent. Ventilation can often be greatly helped by IPPB if the patient can be helped to stand by the bed during a treatment. Sitting in a chair usually worsens the problem. A mouthpiece is preferred to a mask, and at first a noseclip is best, although this can often be omitted shortly. The edentulous patient presents a problem in achieving necessary airtightness, but a trial of several mouthpieces of different shapes, especially with flanges, will generally locate one that is satisfactory. These appliances should be fitted so that the patient can become acclimated to them before the start of treatment. All initial control settings will be tentative, but sensitivity should be relatively free and pressure started somewhere between 10 and 15 cm of water. The control of flow-adjustable instruments can be set somewhere in the middle of the available range.

As treatment is begun, the patient is instructed to breathe slowly and easily and encouraged to allow the machine to do the work. There is a tendency for respiratory frequency to increase, and the patient often appears to be chased by the respirator so that the therapist may have to urge the patient to maintain a normal rate. Especially is the anxious patient or the patient trying hard to please likely to overbreathe, and this must be prevented because it is easy for him to become alkalotic. Not only is alkalosis itself a potential hazard but the hypocarbia reduces central ventilatory drive. On cessation of pressure-assisted breathing there may be a period of hypoventilation until eucarbia returns, during which time blood oxygen levels may drop dangerously low. This consequence of intermittent therapy must be kept in mind.

Pressure and flow may have to be adjusted often during an initial treatment until the patient's pattern stabilizes, but most patients do well quickly, reassured by the therapist's relaxed and confident manner. If overbreathing cannot be corrected by the patient's voluntary efforts, dangerous hypocarbia can be prevented by inserting between the patient and the exhalation valve a piece of breathing tubing, 50 to 150 ml in capacity, for rebreathing of carbon dioxide–rich exhaled air. This should be a temporary expedient, if possible, and efforts continued to help the patient establish a better breathing pattern. It is prudent to inquire after the patient's feelings to determine whether he is experiencing dizziness or getting tired. Water, or medication to be aerosolized, must be in the nebulizer at all times, and the treatment must never be given dry; if medication is used, the patient should be instructed to hold his breath momentarily at end-inspiration to permit maximum particle distribution.

Once the patient appears at ease with the procedure, if he is obstructed, he should be encouraged to prolong his exhalation within the limits of comfort. If he has difficulty doing this himself, the therapist can put a *retard cap* over the exhalation port of the instrument. This is a cap that has several holes of different diameters to provide varying degrees of back pressure for slowing down and prolonging exhalation. It is especially useful when air trapping due to bronchiolar collapse is a problem, since the back pressure developed at the port will help to maintain airway patency to end-expiration. Expiratory retard should not be confused with inspiratory hold, described earlier. Retard does not maintain a pressure plateau but merely delays alveolar-bronchiolar decompression by lengthening exhalation time; in contrast, exhalation following inspiratory hold is usually of normal duration and pattern. The therapist should also teach the patient to aid exhalation by abdominal contraction. This is often difficult for him to grasp, but it will be easier if the therapist will demonstrate on himself in front of the patient. Then, with his hand on the patient's epigastrium, the therapist can exert gentle but firm pressure during the terminal third of exhalation, pointing out to the patient how this increases the removal of air. Finally, the patient is allowed to try epigastric retraction himself, but he will need close supervision and must not be allowed to tire himself with this maneuver. For the patient with a severe obstructive problem, there is available an inflatable swathlike belt that can be fitted about his middle and upper abdomen. Coordinated with the ventilator, the belt inflates during exhalation, exerting a forceful squeeze on the abdomen. It does not take the place of active exercise of the abdominal muscles, but sometimes it is helpful in instructing the patient in the purpose of forced terminal expiration and demonstrating to him what can be accomplished.

Generally, an IPPB treatment of 20 to 30 minutes is sufficient at a frequency of three to four times daily, although it is obvious that the schedule must be fitted to each patient's needs. However, the indications for treatment are usually such that an intensity of this degree is necessary, at least at first. Care must be taken not to let IPPB become so routine that all patients are treated alike. On the other hand, both the patient's attending physician and the respiratory therapist need some sort of a working standard procedure to present to a patient for whom therapy is proposed. It is probably safe to answer a patient who inquires how long he will need treatments that he will need them every day while in the hospital and as an outpatient for up to 2 weeks, at which time his conditions will be reviewed. Thus outpatient services must be available, and in many hospitals they may carry the burden of IPPB therapy. An obvious problem arises in this case, since it is rarely possible for a patient to return to the outpatient service three to four times daily unless there are provisions for all-day care at the hospital. The desirable will have to be compromised for the feasible, and if only one treatment can be given, it is definitely better than none. For the patient previously treated more intensely as an inpatient, once a day is probably satisfactory; for the outpatient starting therapy it may be the only arrangement possible. Careful evaluation by both physician and therapist is needed to determine when therapy should be stopped, and to follow a tapering schedule is often better than to stop abruptly.

An increasingly popular solution to the outpatient problem is self-administered home therapy, with the patient borrowing, renting, or purchasing his own IPPB unit, and many instruments are manufactured just for this purpose. Home therapy may be satisfactory if it is subject to certain conditions. First, a series of treatments should be given by a trained therapist in either the inpatient or outpatient service until such time as the therapist is confident that the patient knows the procedure well. There are some patients who never can treat themselves safely or satisfactorily, and the therapist should frankly make this known to the responsible physician. Second, before the hospitalized patient takes his instrument home, the therapist should go over it carefully with him, reviewing the technique of its use, showing him how the components operate, and instructing him in its care and cleaning. The outpatient should bring his machine to the ambulatory service for the same purposes, and often arrangements can be made to have the patient's unit delivered to the hospital so that he can be instructed when he picks it up. It is a reponsibility of the patient's physician to follow the progress of home care and, if necessary, to send the patient back to the therapist for an occasional checkup on technique. Experience has shown that many patients on home-care programs are forgotten and tend to become negligent in their treatment.

### Treatment of acute pulmonary edema

The student is advised to review the causes and clinical picture of pulmonary edema as discussed in Chapter 5. Its treatment is included here because of the importance of IPPB, although the overall management will be described briefly to familiarize the therapist with this condition which he will be called on so frequently to treat. The following is modified from a previously published discussion of pulmonary edema.[48] In the management of full-blown acute edema, speed is essential, and treatment can be considered in four categories: (1) physical and mental relaxation,

(2) improvement of cardiovascular function, (3) relief of hypoxia, and (4) retardation of venous return.

*Physical and mental relaxation.* Physical and mental relaxation is a responsibility of the attending physician rather than the respiratory therapist. The patient is allowed to assume a position of comfort, which is usually sitting because of his severe dyspnea. Many patients are extremely apprehensive, and morphine sulfate is the drug of choice to relieve anxiety and promote muscular relaxation. Not only is the patient's mental state improved but morphine reduces peripheral vascular tone through suppression of vasomotor centers and thus directly affects an underlying mechanism responsible for the edema. If circulation is adequate to ensure absorption, the narcotic can be given subcutaneously in doses of 10 to 15 mg at 30-minute intervals to a total of four doses if necessary. Should shock be present, reducing tissue perfusion, intravenous administration will be necessary, if the drug is given at all. Ventilation must be observed closely, since a respiratory center already depressed by the hypoxia accompanying acute edema will be seriously aggravated by morphine. Also, since wheezes may be present in both acute pulmonary edema and obstructive bronchial diseases such as asthma and bronchitis, it is important that the latter diagnoses be excluded because the use of morphine could be catastrophic. Should serious hypoventilation or apnea follow the drug, morphine antagonists such as levallorphan tartrate (Lorfan) or nalorphine (Nalline) and respiratory stimulants such as ethamivan (Emivan) or nikethamide (Coramine) may be necessary, in addition to artificial ventilation.

*Improvement of cardiovascular function.* A critical part of the physician's evaluation of pulmonary edema is his determination of whether the condition is due to cardiac failure, for if it is, successful therapy will depend upon restoring compensation. Digitalis, or one of its analogues, is specifically indicated for cardiac failure, either causing or complicating pulmonary edema, but it has no value in the absence of such failure. The physiologic effects of digitalis, even when given intravenously, are not evident for at least 15 minutes, and thus it does not rank in priority over the use of morphine for the treatment of hypoxia. It should also be remembered that the initial response of digitalis may be an aggravation of symptoms as a result of the marked increase in pulmonary vascular pressure due to digitalis action. It is often better to withhold use of digitalis until the acute emergency has passed or is well under control. Aminophylline is useful in relieving the bronchospasm that is often present and in lessening pulmonary-capillary transudate. Diuretics are of value only when congestive heart failure is present and have little effect on pulmonary edema per se.

*Relief of hypoxia and retardation of venous return.* The relief of hypoxia and retardation of venous return will be discussed together because they are managed simultaneously. The treatment of hypoxemia is of the highest priority, and a significant increase in alveolar oxygen tension is necessary to increase diffusion across the fluid barrier of edema. The first move is to give the patient 100% oxygen while readying other measures, preferably by means of a nonrebreathing mask, and oxygen therapy will be continued during the next step of retarding venous return. For many years the reduction of pulmonary blood volume has been recognized as a prime objective in the relief of the acute phase of pulmonary edema, and there are three techniques that will reduce the volume of blood returning to the right atrium.

*Phlebotomy.* The physical removal of blood from circulation will certainly reduce the pulmonary blood volume, and it was customary in the past to withdraw up to 500 ml rapidly. This can be hazardous, however, since if acute edema has already precipitated circulatory collapse, blood loss will further aggravate shock. This technique has largely been abandoned.

*Tourniquets.* Applied to the extremities, tourniquets will effectively reduce venous return and are much safer than phlebotomy. Rubber straps or blood-pressure cuffs may be used and are applied with a force greater than that of the estimated venous pressure but less than the arterial diastolic pressure. Peripheral pulses must be palpable at all times to avoid the risk of ischemic necrosis. Only three extremities are occluded at a time, and the tourniquets are rotated so that each extremity is free, in sequence, for 20 minutes. When the acute phase is over, the restrictions are released, one at a time at 20-minute intervals, to avoid flooding the pulmonary circulation with a sudden return of flow. This technique is safe and effective and should be used while waiting for and during the next maneuver.

*Intrapulmonary pressure.* Pressure-controlled inflation of the lungs is more rapid and effective than either phlebotomy or tourniquets, and its administration by IPPB is an important function of the respiratory therapist. As noted earlier, this is an instance in which the usually undesirable generation of high intrathoracic pressures may be lifesaving rather than a hazard. Instead of regulating his ventilator to minimize its circulatory effect, the therapist does just the opposite. He uses pressures up to 40 cm of water or higher and flows high enough to reach peak pressure in the shortest possible time. This allows the maintenance of a plateau of high pressure at end-inspiration and blocks the return of venous blood into thoracic vessels. To a considerable degree the volume of blood so retarded can be regulated and controlled in a manner not possible with phlebotomy or tourniquets. In the acutely ill patient, almost a breath-by-breath adjustment of the IPPB unit will be required because of the rapid and difficult breathing; but the great assistance the patient receives from the ventilator gradually eases his work of breathing, reducing frequency and increasing tidal volume. Oxygen is now given through the ventilator so that hypoxia, pulmonary edema, and congestion are effectively treated together. It is common practice to nebulize 20% to 50% ethyl alcohol during treatment, taking advantage of its antifoaming properties to mobilize the edema froth as well as to benefit from the systemic effects after absorption into the circulation. The patient with combined shock and edema is difficult to treat, for positive pressure is a hazard to one, and negative pressure is a hazard to the other. Still, by progressing cautiously, the therapist can provide relief of hypoxia from oxygen administered by gentle pressure breathing and may reverse circulatory collapse and reduce edema. The combined judgment and talents of physician and therapist may determine the outcome.

In summary, it can be stated that acute pulmonary edema is one of the specific indications for IPPB and that IPPB has become an accepted part of its treatment.

Chapter 11

# CHRONIC CARE AND REHABILITATION OF RESPIRATORY FAILURE

The steadily improving care of patients with acute ventilatory failure is presenting its own problem. As more survive the acute phases of respiratory disease, there is an increasing population of people with chronic pulmonary insufficiency, displaying a wide spectrum of disability. It makes little difference whether they were originally diagnosed as having pulmonary emphysema, fibrotic tuberculosis, chronic asthma, or any of several other conditions, since in their chronic state they have one thing in common—the inability to move to and from their lungs sufficient air for physiologic needs, without being distressingly conscious of the physical effort required. The high incidence of repeated hospitalizations and the progressive disability of these patients make necessary all-out efforts to set up purposeful and supervised chronic-care programs for them, to include not only supportive measures but also vigorous efforts to rehabilitate those with significant cardiopulmonary reserve. This is long-term therapy, for which both trained personnel and physical facilities are in short demand. Many chronically handicapped patients require daily care, some of which can be provided in ambulatory centers, but desperately needed for pulmonary rehabilitation are hospitals primarily intended for the chronic respiratory patient. Only the barest beginning of chronic care can be given in the average general hospital, both the philosophy and cost of which prohibit significant follow-up.

The overall objectives of pulmonary rehabilitation are not different from those of other disabling diseases—to increase the patient's physical comfort and performance and help him to maintain or regain economic productivity or improved self-care. There is not yet a solidly based therapeutic pattern for such goals, but the following outline gives the needs that should be considered and provided for rehabilitation of chronic bronchopulmonary disease:

A. Medical therapy
1. Control of respiratory infection
2. Maintenance of clear airways
   a. Aerosol therapy
   b. Assisted ventilation
   c. Postural drainage exercises
3. Correction of inefficient ventilation—ventilatory exercises
4. Improvement in ambulation

    a. Graded walking exercises (with or without oxygen)
    b. Physical conditioning exercises
  5. Psychosomatic support
    a. Group therapy
    b. Individual therapy as indicated
  6. Evaluation of cardiopulmonary function
B. Economic and social adjustment
  1. Occupational retraining and placement
    a. Work classification
    b. Employer support
  2. Family counseling
    a. Education
    b. Home planning

We will not consider in detail all the items listed for some are self-evident and others already have been adequately covered. There is no need, for example, to comment further on the control of infection other than to say that its importance is reflected in the position it occupies in the total program and to emphasize that unless it can be achieved, none of the other measures will be of much avail. Aerosol therapy and assisted ventilation (IPPB) have been considered in depth relative to their uses in acute medicine, but they are just as important in chronic care, employing the same techniques already described. General physical conditioning is still mostly the responsibility of the physiotherapist, even though, as we shall soon see, other physical techniques are very much a part of the respiratory therapist's services. Comments will be made later on some of the other aspects of rehabilitation, but we will first discuss respiratory therapy procedures that are usually employed in the postacute state for either immediate recuperation or for prolonged care.

Although the role of the respiratory therapist may seem more dramatic in the care of the patient in acute respiratory failure, it is no less valuable after passage of the crisis. Many of the same therapeutic and diagnostic techniques will apply then as before, but there are some reserved mostly for the convalescent period. We tend to sigh with relief when respiratory compensation is restored to a patient in failure and perhaps congratulate ourselves for normal blood gas values. However, as far as the patient is concerned, this may mark only the start of a long period of disability, threatened with unpredictable relapses and characterized by frustrating physical disability. We are still responsible for the patient, but our aims are somewhat different now, and from here on we will try to accomplish two things simultaneously. First, we will attempt to restore as much function as possible to his ventilatory mechanism, and, second, we will try to keep him out of further episodes of failure. Both are large tasks.

To begin our discussion, let us define the respiratory therapy of chronic pulmonary care as those measures intended to improve respiratory performance rather than to save an acutely threatened life. The chronic state can develop gradually according to its own progression, or it may follow an acute illness, but the management will generally be the same. Chronic care may be started in the hospital as an outgrowth of acute care, or it may be initiated in the ambulatory patient who has never been hospitalized. We will discuss techniques that theoretically and traditionally belong to physiotherapy but that have become not only useful adjuncts to respiratory therapy but an integral part of it. These techniques apply specifically to the treatment of diseases of the chest and, in the United States at least, have been less emphasized by physiotherapists than have other aspects of their field. However, the respiratory therapist found these physically oriented procedures of great interest and use to him, and in the natural evolution of respiratory therapy, they have been incorporated into his general function. The encroachment of respiratory care upon the domain of physiotherapy therefore was not intentional but developed only as a means to give a full spectrum of care to the respiratory patient.

With the respiratory therapist responsible for administering the basic aids to ventilation and for maintaining the patient during acute illness, it is only reasonable that he also have at his disposal any procedures that may further aid his patient's breathing and that will permit him to continue caring for the patient during convalescence and rehabilitation. We will see that some physiotherapy is indicated as a part of pressure breathing treatments, for example, and it is not in the interest of efficiency or good medicine to make the simultaneous services of two technicians necessary when one can do the job or to send the patient back and forth between two departments when only one is needed. The greatest justification for allocating chest physiotherapy to the respiratory therapist, however, is his specialized knowledge of, as well as interest in, pulmonary physiology and mechanics. It is hoped that the future education of the respiratory therapist will involve him more deeply in the techniques of chronic care, but at this time his training should include the following physical procedures: postural drainage, chest percussion, chest vibration, cough control, acute chest compression, pursed-lip breathing, abdominal breathing, and other ventilatory exercises. These are the subjects we will discuss below, but to understand the objectives and techniques of postural drainage, the therapist must know the segmental anatomy of the lung and the spatial relationships of segments and bronchi.

## RESPIRATORY THERAPY OF CHRONIC CARE
### Postural drainage

The purpose of postural drainage is to increase the removal of bronchial secretions by so positioning the patient that gravity will aid their cephalad movement. As employed by the respiratory therapist, "tipping," to use the British expression, is often an important part of an IPPB treatment. He will have frequent occasion to stop therapy, tip the patient, percuss and vibrate his chest, and then resume pressure breathing. In theory, the therapist should have the prior consent of the patient's physician to perform these added services, but in hospitals where the medical staff is properly informed in chest therapy, a reliable therapist may be permitted to use his judgment. In the sophisticated respiratory therapy department, such physiotherapy is considered not as "added services" but as much a part of patient treatment as is the use of a respirator. Before initiating drainage, the therapist must consider such factors of the patient's general condition as related diseases, other infirmities, and age, but there are few who cannot benefit from some form of this therapy. This statement does not imply that all patients given IPPB must have postural drainage, for drainage is specifically reserved for those with significant secretions that cannot be readily removed by other means. It is true, however, that IPPB will often fail to achieve its purpose if stubborn secretions are permitted to obstruct the airways, and much time and effort can be wasted on fruitless therapy.

Patients for whom postural drainage is indicated will mostly fall in the following disease categories, listed in order of frequency: obstructive bronchitis-emphysema, bronchiectasis, resolving pneumonia, lung abscess, necrotizing pneumonia. Of the patients the therapist drains, by far the most will have bronchitis-emphysema, and their retained secretions will usually involve the basal segments of the lower lobes. Thus, in a general way, referring to the therapist's average daily work, postural drainage will mean positioning the patient to remove secretions from the lower lobe basal segments, and especially the posterior basal segment, either side or both. The other diseases listed may require treatment of different segments with localization by x-ray examination or bronchography. When a physician specifically orders postural drainage, he should indicate the area to be treated. This he probably will do if the disease is other than bronchitis-emphysema, but often with the latter, he will merely request "IPPB and postural drainage," which implies treatment to the posterior, lateral, and anterior basal segments bilaterally. Drainage undertaken on the therapist's initiative should be confined to these segments. There are several good manuals on postural drainage describing and illustrating in detail the many available positions and their relationship to the bronchial tree.[351-353] It would be a redundant use of time to reproduce them all on these pages, for the therapist can consult such sources and familiarize himself with all the techniques. Since our interest is in the common daily use of postural drainage, we will confine our discussion to basal segment drainage only but with some recommendations that will apply to all techniques.

Fig. 11-1 illustrates two methods of posterior basal segment drainage. Position *A* is the one preferred if the patient's condition will permit tipping him head down. There are three important points to assure effectiveness with maximum comfort. First, the angle of 45 degrees between the patient's trunk and the horizontal is relatively critical, since this puts the posterior basal segment bronchus in the most favorable position for gravity drainage. Second, the back should be kept as straight as possible, avoiding a tendency to sag, since this will impair effective drainage and strain the back muscles. Third, the patient's arms should be supported or he will be unable to maintain his position with any degree of comfort; a footstool, a pile of books, or any other suitable object on which the patient can rest his crossed arms may be used. It is not always easy to find a satisfactory surface across which the patient can lie at the desired angle. Many beds are too low or have too much give to them. If a bed is used, it should be adjustable to accommodate the patient's height and its mattress firm enough to be free of sagging. A tilt-table that will allow the entire body to be put at a 45-degree angle is ideal, and this should be part of the equipment of an ambulatory care service of the respiratory therapy department, to which many patients can be brought for therapy. Such a table must have shoulder supports to prevent the patient from sliding off its end. Position *B* shows an alternate technique

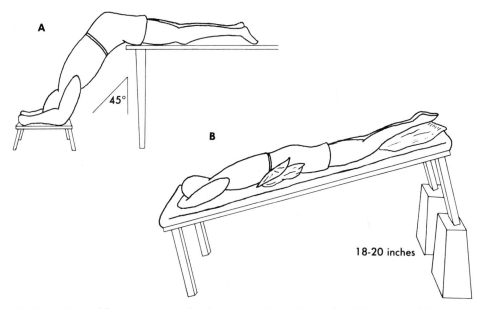

**Fig. 11-1.**   Postural drainage, posterior basal segments. Position **A** is preferred. **B** is reserved for patients for whom the head-down position is not indicated.

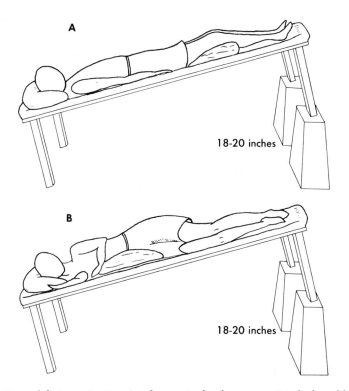

**Fig. 11-2.**   Postural drainage. Position **A** is for anterior basal segments. **B** is for lateral basal segments.

for those patients for whom the head-down position is contraindicated. Drainage will be aided if the patient is placed in the prone position with two pillows under the hips and the foot of the bed elevated about 18 to 20 inches. The bed may be raised by blocks of suitable size under the foot legs or by an automobile jack under the foot end to which an extension angle iron has been welded to prevent rocking. Strength of the head legs must be assured because elevation of the foot places a tremendous strain on the head of the bed. This method is not quite as effective as the head-down position because the body assumes an angle of no more than about 15 degrees, but it has the advantage that it can be maintained for long periods of time. Fig. 11-2, *A*, shows the position that will drain the anterior basal segment, with the foot of the bed raised 18 to 20 inches and a pillow under the knees for comfort. Fig. 11-2, *B*, demonstrates the position for lateral basal drainage, depending upon the side on which the patient is placed. A pillow or two is placed under the waist to keep the spine straight.

Judgment will determine whether all three positions should be used in sequence during any one treatment. From a practical point of view, considering the elements of time and patient fatigue, it is probably advisable to use the head-down technique whenever possible and as the first maneuver and, if therapeutic results are satisfactory, to do no more. On the other hand, if the patient presents a particularly difficult secretion problem, it may be necessary to rotate him through a series of all three positions. Initially, a patient may be able to tolerate the head-down technique for only a minute, but he will soon adjust to it for as long as is necessary. When the patient is in position, the therapist should warn him not to make a deliberate effort to cough vigorously, since this will markedly raise intracranial pressure. Rather, the patient should be instructed frequently to "clear his throat" with sharp grunting sounds but with only gentle effort. This maneuver will elevate intrathoracic pressure momentarily at intervals, transmitting short bursts of high-velocity air in the bronchi to loosen and move secretions. Both the patient and the therapist should understand that the value of postural drainage is not in the immediate production of a great flow of secretions, since very often the treatment will seemingly accomplish little. Its function is to mobilize secretions intrabronchially for easier removal with a less effortful cough long after the tipping. If drainage should be effective at once, so much the better, and if it precipitates hard coughing, the patient should sit up until the cough subsides.

## Chest percussion

Percussion, also known as tapping or clapping, is a technique of striking the patient's chest to loosen bronchial secretions as an aid to postural drainage. The striking force must be against the bare skin, delivered by the therapist's hand held slightly cupped with fingers and thumb closed so a cushion of air is trapped between the hand and chest wall. The therapist, holding his arm with the elbow partially flexed and wrist loose, whips his hand sharply down onto the patient's chest over the area being drained. Best results come from using both hands alternately in rapid sequence for several seconds at a time. It is a noisy procedure, but, far from being painful to the patient, it is stimulating and the coarse vibrations set up in the thorax literally shake loose secretions. Naturally, care must be exercised by the therapist to avoid tender areas or sites of trauma or surgery. It is not a difficult technique to master, but skill and experience are needed to determine the force to use for a given chest wall thickness and to maintain a uniform blow throughout the procedure.

### Chest vibration

Like percussion, chest vibration is an accompaniment to postural drainage and has the same objective as percussion but through a little different technique. In the classical maneuver the therapist lays one hand on the patient's chest over the involved area and places his other hand on top of the first. Then, while exerting slight to moderate pressure on the chest wall, he rapidly produces an even vibratory motion of his hands. In contrast to the more violent percussion, this procedure sets up fine vibrations that are transmitted to the secretions. More effective is the use of an electric hand vibrator. This instrument not only assures prolonged uniform vibrations to loosen secretions but is also relaxing to the patient.

The combination of IPPB, postural drainage, chest percussion, and vibration thus can be considered as a treatment unit, and the physical therapy elements have proved themselves very helpful in increasing the efficiency of pressure breathing and aerosol therapy. In practice, the therapist will often start IPPB in the usual manner and then, upon noting the apparent presence of resistant secretions that the patient raises with great difficulty, if at all, will stop and position the patient for drainage. He will apply percussion and vibration over the basal areas, giving the patient ample opportunity to cough as needed. Again he will resume IPPB and so continue to alternate between pneumatic, aerosol, and physical therapy according to the results he obtains. The ability and judgment of the respiratory therapist to use such combined therapy effectively rank equally with his skill at maintaining mechanical ventilation.

### Cough control

To the patient with a basically normal respiratory tract, a cough is usually a necessary nuisance that gives him relief from bronchial irritation. To the patient with chronic pulmonary disease, on the other hand, an effective cough may mean the difference between adequate and inadequate air exchange, and this he may not be able to accomplish. In general, patients who need some type of cough assistance will be found among those with (1) postoperative or posttraumatic pulmonary restriction (thoracic or abdominal), (2) postventilator weakness, or (3) air trapping. The patient with restriction, usually because of pain, has limited inspiration and is unable to generate enough propulsive power to remove secretions effectively. The therapist can help such a patient by supporting his lower thorax bilaterally with the hands. As the patient inhales, the therapist moves with the expanding chest but still maintains resistance against which the patient must work. At the limit of the patient's inspiration, the pressure exerted by the therapist gives impetus to the start of a cough, and continued compression increases the force and velocity of the exhaled air. The therapist can repeat this maneuver several times to mobilize secretions and may be able to teach some patients to do it themselves, although this is usually less effective.

The patient recently weaned from a mechanical ventilator and the patient with air trapping, as from emphysema, may have adequate inspiratory capacities but lack expulsive power for effective removal of secretions. The reasons for their problems differ, however. Prolonged assisted ventilation may allow one patient to lose tone and strength of his ventilatory muscles so that, although he can move tidal air satisfactorily, he cannot generate cough power. Also, irritation of his throat from intubation or actual laryngeal damage may limit cough. On the other hand, the patient with bronchiolar damage may have commendable vital and inspiratory capacities, but the buildup of intrathoracic pressure during cough compresses the weakened bronchiolar walls to stop the cough before it has had time to be effective. Both these patients can be taught to overcome their problems, a responsibility of the respiratory therapist. The therapist instructs the patients to start their coughs from a midinspiratory position rather than the usual full inspiration, which is more natural. This reduces the volume of air to be removed by the weak patient and lowers the intrathoracic pressure of the air-trapping patient. To compensate for resultant loss of expulsive force, the patients are then told to exhale in a rapid series of "machine gun" bursts of short, sharp coughs, repeated several times always from a midinspiratory position or even the end-expiratory resting level. This technique relieves the weak patient of the strain of a prolonged hard cough, and the staccato rhythm at a relatively low velocity minimizes airway collapse in the air-trapping patient.

### Acute chest compression

Acute chest compression is related to the procedure just described for cough control, but it has a specific and often acute indication, especially in the patient with severe emphysema and air trapping. Not only may the mechanism of air trapping interfere with effective cough, as already noted, but it may place the patient's life in jeopardy. The emphysematous patient with chronic bronchial secretions may suddenly be stimulated by the need to cough, take a deep breath, start his cough, and suddenly find his airflow shut off before end-expiration. At this point he may be unable either to exhale or inhale, and his chest becomes "frozen" and immobile. He continues to strain in an attempt to move air, his neck veins distend from the intrathoracic pressure, his face becomes cyanotic, and he is suddenly in acute danger of suffocation. Fortunately, most such episodes are self-limiting, as perhaps weakness causes enough relaxation of intrathoracic pressure to permit air to move, but the experience is frightening to patient and family alike, and it severely strains the heart and subjects the brain to acute hypoxia. The respiratory therapist should be prepared to manage this event, since overbreathing from IPPB and breathing exercises may precipitate an attack of acute air trapping. Should this happen or the patient give a history of its occurrence at home, family members should be taught how to treat it. The technique is simple but effective and is applied as soon as the patient's distress is seen because, of course, he will be unable to speak. If the patient is relatively slight in stature, the therapist, standing behind him, places both hands over the lateral costal margins and lower chest and exerts a series of strong short compressions, releasing completely between each. This develops bursts of enough intrapulmonary pressure to break through airway obstruction and allow completion of exhalation. If the patient is large, with a heavy chest wall, the therapist can exert greater expulsive force by standing to the patient's side and, grasping him in a bear hug around the lower thorax, sharply squeezing him laterally against his own body. The occurrence of acute air trapping whenever an attempt is made to cough indicates the need for intensive therapy to remove offending secretions but at the same time is a warning to use caution in treatment and to try to maintain the patient's ventilation at a level of low velocity.

Forceful compression of the costal margins, as described, is not without its hazards, since rib fracture, lung puncture, and injury to liver are possible. A newer, and perhaps more effective technique has received much publicity recently, and although primarily intended to rescue the victim of food choking, can just as well be used to break air trapping. To avoid unnecessary repetition the student is referred to an excellent published description of the so-called "Heimlich maneuver," or *external subdiaphragmatic compression.*[354] All therapists should be familiar with this procedure.

The principle behind it is similar to that of chest compression, but as its descriptive name indicates, pressure is generated below the diaphragm, in the abdomen, rather than in the chest. For the standing or seated patient the operator stands behind, encircling the patient's waist with the arms. A clenched fist, grasped by the other hand, is pressed into the patient's abdomen between the xiphoid and umbilicus, with sharp upward thrusts. For the supine patient the operator straddles the hips and, with one hand placed over the other, presses the upper abdomen inward and upward, quickly and forcefully, with the heel of the lower hand.

The repeated epigastric compressions force the diaphragm upward and squeeze the lung. Pressure so generated, transmitted to the airways can literally blow out obstructions from the hypopharynx, larynx, and trachea. Especially helpful for the patient choking from a bolus of food, a child who has aspirated a foreign body, or a near-drowning victim, subdiaphragmatic compression may well replace chest compression for relief to the air trapper.

Apparently, serious complications of the Heimlich maneuver are rare, but at least one instance of stomach rupture has been reported.[355] The procedure has been performed many times with success, but the accumulated body of experience is still small at this time. As a result, the American Medical Association Commission of Emergency Medical Services recommends that, ". . . the National Academy of Sciences-National Research Council, the American Heart Association . . . determine the place of the Heimlich maneuver in the instruction of the public in proper emergency care practices."[356]

### Pursed-lip breathing

Pursed-lip breathing is a simple maneuver that many patients learn for themselves without knowing why, but because it is so useful in breathing exercises and breath control, it should be taught to those unaware of it. Its purpose is to prevent the air trapping due to bronchiolar collapse, serving the same purpose as the retard cap on the exhalation port of the IPPB respirator, and it is almost exclusively used for emphysema. The patient is instructed to purse his lips as if whistling during exhalation, controlling the velocity of his exhaled air to the slowest that is consistent with his ventilation. A variation of this, which is not really pursed-lip, consists of placing the tongue on the roof of the mouth and releasing the air slowly as if saying the letter "s." This has no inherent gain over pursing the lips and is certainly noisier. In either case, resistance of the mouth transmits back pressure throughout the bronchial tree, and its gradual release during exhalation prevents intrathoracic pressure from compressing shut those bronchioles weakened by disease. When used with the forceful abdominal-breathing exercises to be described next, the pursed-lip retard of airflow is continued to the end of the prolonged exhalation. At other times, such as during the breath control of quiet breathing or moderate exercise, the pursed-lip retard may be released at midexhalation to allow a normal terminal flow, since the naturally slowing velocity of passive end-expiration carries little risk of air trapping.

## Abdominal breathing

Of the many available exercises directed toward improving the mechanics of ventilation, we will describe but four, for it is felt that these have the widest application in the general treatment of respiratory deficiencies. Many of the others are designed to improve skeletal muscle performance and posture, but we will let the therapist pursue their uses at his leisure. When we discussed the mechanics of ventilation, we learned how such pulmonary pathology as obstruction, destruction of alveoli, and air trapping upset the normal ventilatory pattern, lowering the diaphragm and effectively removing it from useful ventilation and throwing the burden of air movement on the thorax. We learned how inefficient is thoracic breathing, with its need to activate accessory ventilatory muscles, and how the subsequent distortion of a barrel chest aggravates the problem. In this section we will be interested in the patient with thoracic breathing, especially if paradoxical, for the thoracic breather is expending much more energy moving his chest wall than he would if he had only to move his more flexible abdominal wall. The additional oxygen need for the work of breathing seriously compounds the disability of his underlying disease. Abdominal-breathing exercises are designed to ease ventilatory work by gradually changing the pattern from thoracic to abdominal. This is a slow and difficult process and requires the utmost patience of the respiratory therapist. He should understand that it is often very difficult for a patient who has developed a thoracic breathing pattern to revert to abdominal, and many never do accomplish it. It is quite remarkable that what was once a natural function, when lost, is so difficult to relearn. There is no set method of teaching effective breathing, but we will present suggested techniques upon which the therapist can improve with experience and modify according to need. Before starting a breathing exercise, the therapist should have the patient take two or three inhalations of a bronchodilator aerosol and permit him to relax mentally and physically. Before teaching a new exercise, he should demonstrate it plainly to the patient, explaining the purpose of each move and how best the patient can accomplish it.

***Forced-exhalation abdominal breathing.*** The purpose of this exercise is to strengthen the contractile force of the abdominal wall muscles so that they can effectively elevate the diaphragm and empty the lungs. Although it can be done in almost any position, it is best taught in the supine with a pillow under the patient's head and his knees drawn up comfortably to relax the anterior abdominal wall. The principles of technique are illustrated in Fig. 11-3. The patient's hand is placed on his epigastrium, not to exert pressure but only to focus his attention to this area (*A*). Much of the success of therapy will depend on the degree to which the therapist can keep the patient's mind on epigastric movement. Exercise is always started in the same manner, by exhaling from the resting level through pursed lips. At the same time the patient is instructed to pull in his upper abdomen gradually, with conscious force, prolonging exhalation as long as he can (*B*). At end-exhalation he is told to inhale easily through his nose, letting his upper abdomen balloon out (*C*), and the cycle is repeated. From now on, however, exhalation will start from end-inspiration, and the patient is urged to let the air flow out slowly through pursed lips until near the end of normal expiration and then forcibly to contract the upper abdomen to extend expiration to its maximum. He is advised to think of all his breathing as taking place in his abdomen rather than in his chest; therefore, as he fills with air, his abdomen should swell, lifting up his hand, and as he expels air, his hand should fall with his receding abdomen.

During the maneuver the therapist must keep reminding the patient to concentrate on all respiratory movement as taking place in the area in contact with his hand and to disregard his chest completely. Many patients, trying hard to cooperate, will suddenly forget the sequence they were taught, contracting the epigastric wall during inhalation and attempting to relax it during exhalation, and may even stop

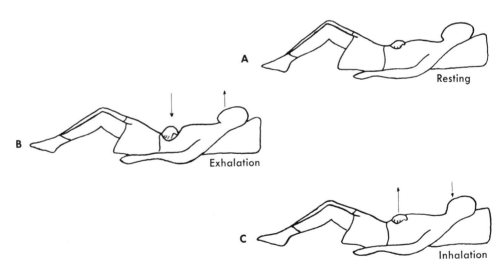

**Fig. 11-3.**   Forced-exhalation abdominal breathing. (See text for description.)

breathing in their confusion. The therapist will find two things of help. The first is the steady repetition over several breathing cycles of "breath in, abdomen out, breath out, abdomen in" to help fix the rhythm in the patient's mind. The second is the placement of a hand over the patient's hand on the abdominal wall to exert gentle but firm pressure, depressing the epigastrium during the prolongation of exhalation. Much practice may be required for this seemingly simple procedure, but as proficiency is acquired, the patient is encouraged to make a positive effort to keep the chest immobile while ventilating completely with the abdomen.

If the patient has exceptionally poor coordination and is unable to achieve adequate expiratory contraction of his abdomen, the surface on which he is lying may be tilted so that the body inclines cephalad about 20 degrees. A pillow may be used under the head, but care is taken that it does not extend beneath the shoulders. In this position the force of gravity shifts the abdominal contents against the diaphragm to assist in elevating it. This technique is useful only to get the procedure under way because success depends on developing sufficient abdominal strength to raise the diaphragm against gravity.

For the breathing exercise to be of value, it must be performed regularly and frequently, not just in the presence of the therapist. A regular schedule of exercise must be set up, perhaps as much as 5 to 10 minutes every hour until clinical results justify reducing it.

To vary the forced exhalation exercise, the patient may be taught to do it in the seated position, employing the added techniques of forward bending as shown in Fig. 11-4. The patient relaxes in a hard, straight-backed chair, sitting upright to commence the maneuver. With the arms hanging loosely by the side to promote relaxation of the thoracic skeletal muscles, he slowly exhales through pursed lips while slowly bending forward and retracting the upper abdomen (Fig. 11-4, A). When properly timed, flexion of the trunk should be complete at the moment of end-expiration. The body is then raised while the patient inhales through the nose, letting the abdomen distend as the lungs fill. When inhalation is completed, the patient should be back in the upright position. To aid exhalation, the forward bending uses

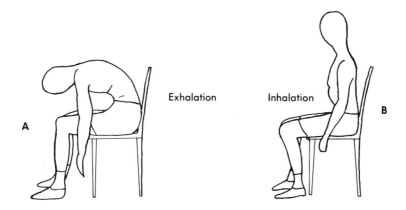

**Fig. 11-4.** Forced-exhalation abdominal breathing, seated. (See text for description.)

the flexion of the trunk to compress the abdomen and elevate the diaphragm. This exercise is especially helpful to the patient when he is troubled with secretions because it enables him to hyperventilate slightly and stimulate the mobility of his secretions for easier cough removal.

*Forced-inhalation abdominal breathing.* In contrast to forced exhalation, the physical effort in forced-inhalation abdominal breathing is directed toward inhalation with exhalation mostly passive. This more closely resembles the normal pattern of breathing. The patient is positioned as for forced exhalation but preferably with a 20-degree head-down tilt, and a weight of 10 to 15 pounds is placed over the mid-abdomen. A set of five fabric bags containing sand or buckshot is helpful, two weighing 5 pounds and three weighing 10 pounds. Since the abdominal weight will make exhalation easy for the patient, his attention is directed to strengthening his inspiratory effort. After letting his air out through pursed lips and terminally contracting his abdominal muscles, the patient is instructed to inhale through his nose, "taking air into the abdomen," with an effort forceful enough to lift the weight visibly. Because of the physical work involved, the initial time tolerated by the patient may be short, but as his performance improves, the exercise may be extended to 30 minutes three to four times daily. The abdominal weight is also increased in increments of 5 pounds and over a period of several weeks may reach 30 pounds. This exercise is especially useful for the patient with paradoxical breathing, since it almost forces him to accept a normal breathing pattern. At the same time the abdominal muscles are strengthened so that he can meet his ventilatory needs by this pattern. The therapist must warn the patient not to overdo the exercise, since soreness of the neglected muscles subjected to the strain of exercise is common and, if severe enough, can impede performance.

*Forced-exhalation with walking.* The primary objective of ventilatory exercise is to increase the patient's tolerance to physical activity, the most important of which is walking. One of his major complaints is his inability to walk comfortably, sometimes even from one room of his home to another, and going out-of-doors may be impossible. Improving his walking tolerance will do more to increase the patient's morale than any other therapeutic benefit. The respiratory therapist will observe that many patients who breathe with ease, resting in bed or chair, will revert to severe thoracic or paradoxical ventilation as soon as they start to walk. The purpose of the present exercise is to coordinate walking, and eventually other exertion, to the rhythm of abdominal breathing, using the prolonged phase of exhalation as the period of maximum effort. This implies that the patient has mastered the act of abdominal breathing and fully understands its purpose.

To prepare for walking exercise, the patient must practice abdominal breathing a few times in the standing position. This position, however, should not be rigidly upright but rather slightly bent forward, and although its esthetic effect may be less than desirable, it will make breathing easier. In a straight position the abdominal muscles are under tension, as the string of a bow, but are relaxed by forward flexion and more available for controlled ventilation. The normal subject exerts and adjusts his ventilation accordingly to supply body oxygen needs, but the patient who is our concern here has limited ventilation and so must adapt his physical activity to it. This makes for an artificial and somewhat awkward relationship between breathing and walking but one that can be mastered profitably with practice. The technique is based on establishing a ratio between a given amount of walking and the phasing of breathing, and experience has shown the following to be practical: The patient is instructed to move and breathe slowly, taking three steps during exhalation and two steps during inhalation. This does two things. It helps the patient to maintain a good ventilatory rhythm whereby exhalation exceeds inhalation, ensuring maximum air clearance of the lung; and it lets the patient perform the most exertion when it is easier, during expiration. Because this exercise is developed so that it can be done smoothly, the patient will find that his walking will consume much less energy than when his breathing was haphazard.

The rationale of this technique can be explained to the patient in the following way so that he will understand the need to persist in what may seem to him at first to be a silly effort: When the normal subject is faced with a strenuous act, he first inhales, closes his glottis to hold his breath, and then contracts the necessary muscles. If the physical action is prolonged, he slowly releases his air, often in short bursts, prolonging exhalation while he continues to strain, and then takes a rapid inspiration and repeats until his effort is finished. The point to note is that maximum physical effort is expended during exhalation, not inhalation. With markedly limited ventilation, it is important that our patient with respiratory insufficiency correlate as much of his effort with exhalation as possible. The patient who learns coordinated walking will find the technique applicable to many other activities. It will greatly help him in climbing stairs, ordinarily one of his most difficult chores, if he develops the habit of managing two or three steps during exhalation and resting during inhalation. Most emphysematous patients become extremely short of breath when bending to pick up an object. This can be made much easier by exhaling slowly through pursed lips while bending and grasping the object, then inhaling while arising and lifting, much in the manner of doing the forward bending exercise in a chair.

**Mobilization of the lower ribs.** The final maneuver to be described is not strictly an abdominal exercise, but it is intended to augment abdominal breathing by utilizing a portion of the thorax that does not hinder ventilation. This consists of expanding and contracting the costal margin, which will give maximum mobility to the diaphragm and increase aeration of the lung bases. At first the exercise needs the help of the therapist, but later it can be self-administered. The patient will best understand the purpose of the exercise if he is introduced to it in the relaxed supine position; but the maneuver can be as well done seated. The therapist places his hands over the costal margins so that they almost cup the lower rib edges, and as the patient exhales through pursed lips, the hands follow the slightly contracting rib margins. Just before the end of exhalation the therapist exerts a forceful crescendo squeeze, holding the pressure firmly. As inhalation begins, the therapist gradually releases his manual pressure but retains some resistance to the expanding ribs. The patient is instructed to "breathe around the waist and push the hands away," to direct his attention to this area. He is also told to make an effort to squeeze in his costal edge himself while he pulls in his abdomen during exhalation. Finally, he is allowed to use his own hands to mobilize the lower ribs, and some therapists recommend the use of a swathe or a belt that the patient can use instead of his hands.

### Graded exercises

Somewhat as the culmination, or end objective, of the breathing exercises just described, a system of graded exercises is used to condition the patient for prolonged activity, principally walking. As the name implies, the patient's effort is built up gradually against controlled resistance, both to minimize injury to him and to monitor his progress with objective data. A patient is ready for this aspect of rehabilitation only after maximum airway patency has been achieved and after he has mastered breath control through abdominal breathing, although it is still frequently necessary to use aerosol therapy, pressure breathing, and postural drainage in conjunction with graded exercise.

Whereas techniques in performing progressive exercises may vary, the general principles are the same. Either a treadmill or an exercising bicycle is used, the resistance of which can be adjusted. Both are satisfactory, but the treadmill has the advantage that it more closely simulates the type of physical activity we are trying to develop—walking—and we will use it in our discussion. Supplemental oxygen is usually given to the patient, at least in the early stage of therapy, so that he can withstand the stress of activity. A loosely fitting plastic mask or nasal cannula is satisfactory. Ventilatory function, blood gas determination, cardiac function, and any other evaluation data are obtained prior to starting the program and are repeated according to the needs of each treatment schedule. The therapist should note that walking on a treadmill is not exactly the same as walking on a stable surface because there is a certain knack to using the legs in a normal manner while the body remains in position and the underfooting moves. This should be explained to the patient and demonstrated by the therapist. The patient should step onto the treadmill mat while it is moving slowly, and although he should be allowed to place his hands gently on the safety railing, he should be instructed not to let the support bear his weight. The first exposure of the patient to exercise is tentative, to judge his response and tolerance and to teach him the proper technique. He is given oxygen and the treadmill adjusted to 0% grade and a rate not to exceed 1 mph. The therapist must give reassurance and encouragement to many patients who are initially apprehensive, and they may be told that they can step off the moving surface at any time. During the first trial the therapist must see that the patient is using his abdomen to breathe, since it is under such conditions of stress that he is likely to revert to thoracic or paradoxical breathing, and this cannot be permitted if the therapy is to be successful. Whatever program is used, graded exercises are given regularly and daily, sometimes for several weeks. The pitch of the walking surface, its speed, and the duration of exercise are increased in increments tailored to each patient; and these are good criteria for evaluating progress. For example, if a patient walks 10 minutes at 0% grade and 1 mph at one time and later walks 15 minutes at 2% grade and 1.5 mph, this represents significant improvement.

Even more important is the gradual reduction in the need for supplemental oxygen as the intensity of the exercise increases. It may seem paradoxical that increasing exercise of a patient with respiratory insufficiency should lower his oxygen requirement, but the physiologic reason for this is the foundation for this aspect of rehabilitation. We must remember that patients with impaired breathing become sedentary, suffering progressive atrophic weakness of their leg muscles from disuse, and the less efficient the work of a muscle the greater is the consumption of oxygen for the energy expended by the muscle. To put it another way, more oxygen must be taken in by the body to supply the needs of a poorly conditioned muscle in performing a given amount of work than is required by a well-conditioned muscle. The clinical improvement from a graded exercise program is attributed to two factors. First, although pulmonary function tests may show little change, ventilatory muscle training improves the patient's pattern of breathing with better pulmonary aeration and an increased ability to satisfy the needs of exertion. Second, the physical conditioning with improved efficiency of ventilatory and leg muscles reduces their oxygen demand. Together, both factors greatly increase the amount of work produced per unit of energy expended. Finally, although strenuous exercise may be contraindicated or must be used with caution in patients with some types of heart disease, cor pulmonale is probably not a contraindication if the heart is not in frank failure. The heart strain is apparently not worsened because of the eventual reduction in metabolic oxygen demand.

The program just described must be carried out in a rehabilitation facility, of course, with elaborate equipment under the constant supervision of trained personnel. It is felt that this is the most desirable management, but there may be instances in which such supervision is not practical or possible. With proper selection many patients can profit from a well-planned home-care program, and one of the many valuable services of the respiratory therapist is the training and follow-up supervision of patients for such programs. The home-care patient must be carefully taught the postural-drainage and breathing-exercise techniques; it is wise also to teach these techniques to a reliable family member who may have to assist the patient. Graded exercises with oxygen can be done at home but should be attempted only if both the patient's attending physician and respiratory therapist consider that the patient is responsible and intelligent enough to follow directions accurately. Home exercise can be provided by an exercise cycle, which is space saving, or by level walking, if space permits. Supportive oxygen, gaseous and liquid, is available in small enough containers to be carried by a shoulder sling. Small gaseous cylinders can be refilled from large cylinders, but there is some potential risk in this and it must be advised with caution. According to the patient's capabilities, a graded schedule of walking can be made for him, but it must be reviewed frequently for modifications and to assess its results. Experience has shown that only an exceptional and unusually motivated patient will persist in a graded exercise program at home, away from professional supervision and encouragement, for long enough periods to realize much gain from it as his primary therapy. As a follow-up to a rehabilitation area course of treatment and after the discontinuance of supportive oxygen, home exercises of the postural and kinetic types not only are valuable but for many patients they must be continued indefinitely.

## OTHER ASPECTS OF REHABILITATION

The rest of our discussion of rehabilitation will not involve the direct technical services of the respiratory therapist, but the therapist should be aware of all the efforts made on the disabled patient's behalf, for each facet of therapy or management has some influence on the others. The more each member of the rehabilitation team knows about the patient, the better able he will be to evaluate the patient's progress and his own role in it.

### Psychosomatic support

The term *psychosomatic* refers to the relationship between the emotional state or outlook of an individual *(psyche)* and the physical responses of the individual's body *(soma)*. Everyday life is full of such relationships, as, for example, the physical fatigue that follows a period of emotional tension, and many of them are considered part of normal human behavior. Some, however, cause or aggravate an existing physical disability; and it is with this aspect of chronic pulmonary insufficiency that we are concerned. It is important for the respiratory therapist to realize that all his skilled technical services, as well as the best pharmacologic therapy, can be negated and a patient driven to a progressively downhill course because of an unfavorable mental attitude. Emotional instability is not unique to patients with respiratory disease alone, of course, for we frequently see severe signs of depression and hostility complicating many acute and chronic diseases. In chronic respiratory disease, however, it may be a double-edged sword, for not only can psychic disturbances affect the general well-being of the patient but they may also directly aggravate the very defects that are responsible for his underlying disability. The ease and frequency with which emotional upsets affect the respiratory function are recognized in such commonly expressed relationships as "holding one's breath in anticipation," or being choked up with emotion." Thus it is not difficult to imagine that a patient with labored breathing could be made much worse by a psychic stimulus affecting his breathing.

The role of emotional and personality problems in the genesis of childhood bronchial asthma is well known and has been extensively recorded in medical literature. It is quite probable that many instances of adult asthma, for which no specific allergic basis can be found, likewise stem from some recent or unresolved emotional conflict. The psychic element in nonasthmatic chronic pulmonary disease is probably of a different nature, although such patients, too, may have preexisting problems. Often the patient with progressive emphysema develops severe anxiety and hostility as a direct consequence of his disability. Because he is fearful of economic loss and death, he develops hostility toward his disease and often toward those with whom he comes into close contact. Patients with chronic respiratory disease are frequently seen to become acutely dyspneic during conversation that touches on subjects arousing fear and hostility.

The therapist should not entertain the impression that all patients chronically ill with pulmonary disability are primarily neurotic or that they imagine their symptoms. From our examinations we know the severe physical impairment of these patients; but we should also recognize that part of their symptomatology may well be due to psychosomatic influences. Unfortunately, proper attention to this side of their disability has been generally neglected, probably for two basic reasons. First, the great spurt of interest in pulmonary disease of the past two decades has centered mostly on the physiology of diseases and physical therapeutic measures. Second, short as are the facilities for chronic physical care and rehabilitation, those for mental rehabilitation have been even shorter, since psychosomatic therapy demands the services of both psychiatrists and clinical psychologists who are especially interested in the chronically disabled respiratory patient. Such therapy has been used in the management of bronchial asthma, and results justify its wider application to nonasthmatic diseases as well. No suggestions are made here as to how to include adequate psychotherapy into the overall rehabilitation program, but it should be an integral part. It is probable that superficial treatment might be satisfactory in the majority of cases, such as could be provided in group therapy. General observation of patients in a respiratory therapy outpatient service suggests that many derive support and encouragement by association with others, but to be most effective, this association should be professionally guided and directed. On the other hand, some would profit most from private care, in which their personal emotional conflicts should be aired and the relationship of such conflicts to their breathing explained to them. It is hoped that, as pulmonary rehabilitation becomes more definitive, some technique of psychotherapy will evolve, directed to the specific needs of the respiratory cripple.

**Occupational retraining and placement**

Many disabled pulmonary patients are in their economically productive years and are anxious to be self-sufficient. For them, occupational retraining and job placement are necessary ingredients of a purposeful rehabilitation program. Such a program should not be on a hit-or-miss basis but on classifiable data, specific for each patient. Much study is yet needed to categorize occupations in terms of their energy requirements of the respiratory system and to derive simple but informative tests of the work of breathing to enable the rehabilitation team to match patients to those jobs in which they would have the greatest chance of success. Not only must the patient's physical status be considered but his education, past experience, and aptitudes as well. Obviously, this is not solely the responsibility of medicine but will require the skills of counselors trained in occupational needs and the cooperation of business and industry in each community. These efforts have already been made in behalf of disability due to such conditions as incapacitating trauma and stroke and could be applied readily to pulmonary disability as soon as the specific needs of the latter have been classified.

**Family counseling**

Family counseling is included not merely to round out the program in a general way but because experience has shown its great importance in therapy. Those of us who treat patients with respiratory diseases daily become familiar with the patterns of their diseases, but among the laity there is still a considerable lack of understanding as to the extent of disability that chronic pulmonary disease can produce. Relatives often consider the patient's cough an unnecessary nuisance to them and his reluctance to be physically active a manifestation of laziness, an impression supported by his frequently healthy appearance in the resting state. The patient is acutely aware of this attitude and is hurt, discouraged, and anxious. So sensitive are many patients with chronic disability to the discrepancy between how they look and how they feel that they react very irritably to simple greetings by their medical attendants of how well they look. It is essential that members of the patient's family fully understand the nature of his disease and the extent of his disability. It must be stressed to them that there are good reasons why he can look comfortable in a chair but may not be able to walk to the next room without assistance. They must also understand the objectives of chronic care and rehabilitation, the duration of treatment, its cost and inconvenience to the family, and the probability of improvement. Because home care is usually an important part of the program, full cooperation of the family is necessary or all efforts will fail.

The first responsibility for educating the family falls to the attending physician, but the follow-up role of the respiratory therapist is equally, if not more, important. His explanation of technique and procedures to both patient and relatives can do much to ensure understanding of and cooperation with the program. Both the social worker and the respiratory-trained visiting nurse can offer valuable services by checking on the home progress and helping to correct unfavorable conditions at home that may be detrimental to the patient. In the latter category, assistance may be offered to relieve the financial problems so often found with long-term illness and advice given on a more efficient arrangement of home facilities and labor-saving techniques.

We can summarize the philosophy of chronic and rehabilitative care of the pulmonary disabled patient by emphasizing the following three points: First, in contrast to the treatment of many other chronic illnesses, respiratory therapy depends to a major degree on a well-trained technical specialist who has often followed the patient through an acute illness into the chronic state and is now available to give long-term care based on first hand knowledge of the patient's present and future needs. The respiratory therapist is a bridge between the acute and chronic phases of the disease and makes possible a valuable continuity of treatment. Second, many of the treatment procedures can be self-administered by the patient, not only relieving the financial burden of his care but also putting on him some of the responsibility for his own welfare and, by such a commitment, helping him to become free of complete dependence on others. Third, for maximum rehabilitation of this evergrowing patient population, the team approach is essential. Only through the cooperative efforts of the many whose services can benefit the respiratory patient will we be able to set up a practical program that will permit us to evaluate him physiologically, socially, and economically and, on the basis of this evaluation, help him to regain optimum well-being and independence.

# Chapter 12

# THE ORGANIZATION, STAFFING, AND SERVICES OF A RESPIRATORY CARE DEPARTMENT

It seems appropriate to close our discussion of the many things we feel a good respiratory therapist should know and be able to do by describing the structure of the unit in which he will work. There can be no blueprint of an ideal respiratory care department that will satisfy the needs of all hospitals, but we will make some suggestions that have been time tested by experience to serve as sort of a skeleton that can be modified for custom use. We will also have an opportunity to summarize the overall services of respiratory therapy in the general hospital and to describe personnel requirements and divisions of labor.

Hospitals have been facing an increasing load of patients with cardiopulmonary diseases over the past several years but often lacking both the physical facilities and technical personnel to provide modern care. The techniques that have evolved for the treatment of these patients require the assistance of skilled technical help, and we have already indicated that they are too detailed for the average attending physician, house physician, or nurse to supervise or administer. It was in response to this need that the technical specialty of respiratory therapy emerged to take its place in the hospital organization. Historically, the predecessor of respiratory therapy was the well-known but little regarded hospital oxygen service. However, the highly skilled offspring bears little resemblance to its humble ancestor, for during his evolution, the respiratory therapist has undergone intensive medically supervised education and training, enabling him to provide skills and services not available from any existing hospital personnel. Because of the large number of patients who can benefit from the well-organized services of respiratory therapy, it is the responsibility of every general hospital that opens its doors to the public to provide such services. The utilization of respiratory therapy services where effective departments operate is remarkable and is ample proof of their acceptance by the medical profession. After observing the growth of this technical specialty for several years and reviewing the experience of several hospitals with active services, we can make the conservative estimate that an efficient department in a busy general hospital will probably provide some form of respiratory therapy to about 20% or more of patients admitted. Let us now comment on the services, structure, operation, and size of a workable respiratory care department.

## SERVICES OF A RESPIRATORY CARE DEPARTMENT

It is not necessary to describe in detail the services offered by respiratory therapy, since we have covered their technical aspects in other chapters, but the outline below summarizes them for us in a bird's-eye view. It can be noted, however, that these services cut across established hospital departmental lines, the administrative implications of which will be mentioned later.

Respiratory therapy services:

A. Therapeutic gases
   1. Oxygen: mask, catheter, cannula, face tent
   2. Helium-oxygen mixtures
   3. Carbon dioxide–oxygen mixtures
B. Aerosols and humidity
   1. Bronchodilators, detergents, mucolytics, proteolytic enzymes, antibiotics, steroids
   2. High humidity, aerosolized water
   3. Procurement of sputum specimens for cytologic and bacterial examination
C. Mechanical ventilation
   1. Inspiratory positive-pressure breathing
      a. Administration of aerosols for airway patency
      b. Prevention of postoperative atelectasis
      c. Treatment of acute pulmonary edema
   2. Assisted ventilation for inadequate spontaneous breathing
      a. Continuous ventilation by pressure-regulated ventilators
      b. Monitoring by blood gas analysis, tidal volume
      c. Maintenance of airway patency by tracheobronchial aspiration
   3. Controlled ventilation for apnea
      a. Continuous ventilation by tank, volume-regulated, flow-regulated, pressure-regulated ventilators
      b. Maintenance of adequate volume, rate, pressure
      c. Maintenance of circulatory stability
D. Physical therapy and rehabilitation
   1. Ambulatory service for aerosol and pressure breathing treatments
   2. Postural drainage
   3. Corrective breathing exercises
   4. Oxygen-supported ambulatory exercises
   5. Integration of treatments into custom-made progressive program for home care: patient instruction, follow-up supervision
E. Pulmonary function testing
   1. Minimum requirement examinations for routine respiratory care
      a. Spirometry
      b. Lung volume measurements
         (1) Nitrogen washout
         (2) Helium equilibration
      c. Arterial or arterialized blood analysis
         (1) pH
         (2) Oxygen tension
         (3) Carbon dioxide tension
   2. Selected examinations
      a. Alveolar ventilation
      b. Dead space volume
      c. Arterial-alveolar carbon dioxide difference
      e. Pulmonary diffusion measurement
      f. Pulmonary compliance measurement
F. Unclassified
   1. Emergency resuscitation
   2. Extracorporeal pump operation
   3. Technical assistance in cardiopulmonary research
   4. Future services yet unexplored

This list is not proposed as total and definitive because the final boundaries of respiratory therapy are far from established, and from hospital to hospital there will be variations in the number and types of services offered. The last item noted above may turn out to be the most important of all as progress in chest medicine continues. It is essential that all departments be developed with a philosophy of flexibility to allow future growth as time may dictate.

## DEPARTMENTAL STRUCTURE:
## ADMINISTRATION AND PERSONNEL

The organization of an effective respiratory care department will include some or all of the following personnel: medical director, technical director, assistant technical director, shift supervisors, area supervisors, staff respiratory therapy technicians, pulmonary laboratory technicians, clinical instructors, aides, and secretary. Certainly, all departments will not have all of these, and there may be other job specialties according to individual hospital needs. Fig. 12-1 outlines a suggested departmental organization, showing the relationship among the components of the department and between the department and the administration. This is presented only as a possible suggestion that is flexible enough to lend itself to the needs of any general hospital.

Note that the administrative outline depicts the respiratory care department in three modules, as a practical method of description. Ideally, it should be an independent administrative unit with its own budget and administrative support stemming from the hospital administration. Thus, in administrative and fiscal matters, the director of the department works directly with the hospital administration. The education module applies primarily to those hospitals that intend to include in their structure a respiratory therapy school or that have departments large enough to maintain a continuing in-service educational program. The medium- to small-sized community hospitals will be primarily interested in the service and laboratory functions of their respiratory care departments. A small hospital may be adequately served by one medical director supervising a service function and a modest pulmonary function laboratory. Where there is a larger demand on the respiratory care department, there may be an effective division of labor, employing two or more associate directors. Here the duties may be divided, with one director responsible for service function and another for the laboratory. In larger hospitals, where the work load may be exceptionally heavy, with much work being done in all three modules, the administrative and professional relationships may be varied again. In some instances it is practical to consider the service function of the respiratory care department, the pulmonary function laboratory, a school or other training and educational facility in respiratory therapy, and an ambulatory clinic for respiratory diseases, all as components of a larger professional unit, a section of respiratory care. Such a facility might have an overall chief of section, and the various subdivisions might have their own individual directors. This arrangement most effectively combines the diagnostic and therapeutic facilities for treatment of cardiopulmonary diseases into a common unit in which administrative work is kept to a

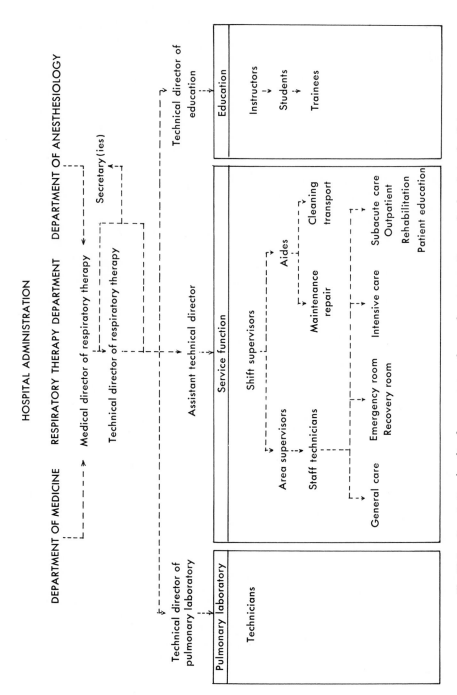

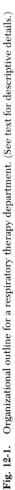

**Fig. 12-1.** Organizational outline for a respiratory therapy department. (See text for descriptive details.)

minimum and the professional cooperation and exchange of ideas make for the highest degree of patient care.

If a respiratory care unit is available, it should be the direct responsibility of the respiratory care department. Its supervision and clinical servicing are assured through the regular departmental personnel and the pulmonary function laboratory. The only nondepartmental service needed is nursing, and this can be provided through an arrangement with the nursing service.

This seems to be a good time and place to describe the current classification of respiratory therapy personnel, the result of some significant changes in the field during the past few years. Definitions of officially recognized levels are as follows:

1. *Respiratory therapist:* A graduate of an American Medical Association (AMA)—approved school designed to qualify the graduate for the Registry Examination of the National Board of Respiratory Therapy. Usually this means a 2-year hospital–community college affiliation granting the graduate an associate degree.
2. *Registered respiratory therapist:* A respiratory therapist who has successfully completed the Registry Examination of the National Board of Respiratory Therapy.
3. *Respiratory therapy technician:* A graduate of an AMA–approved school designed to qualify the graduate for the Technician Certification Examination of the National Board of Respiratory Therapy. Usually this means a 1-year hospital-based program combining a special curriculum of basic sciences with supervised clinical experience.
4. *Certified respiratory therapy technician:* A respiratory therapy technician who has successfully completed the Technician Certification Examination of the National Board of Respiratory Therapy.
5. *Respiratory therapy assistant:* One who has received on-the-job training as part of employment in a hospital respiratory therapy service. For such a program there are no official guidelines or credentials. On-the-job training is gradually being phased out in favor of one of the two formal programs just noted.
6. *Respiratory therapy student:* One who is enrolled in a program that follows AMA–approved guidelines or Essentials.
7. *Respiratory therapy student trainee:* One employed in a hospital respiratory therapy service while engaged in a technical program that follows AMA–approved Essentials. For our purposes the last two categories can be jointly called students.

Generically, the term *respiratory therapist* often refers to anyone involved in technical respiratory care, but there are two basic functioning personnel levels— the respiratory therapist and the respiratory therapy technician. There are many overlaps in their duties and responsibilities, depending on local institutional needs and personnel availability. However, invoking once again a rule of thumb, it can be generalized that by virtue of differences in depth and orientation of therapist and technician educational curriculums, respiratory therapists are given responsibilities for managerial or other high-level administrative supervision, clinical supervision in special areas, supervision of teaching programs, and the development of special projects and research. Respiratory therapy technicians, on the other hand, should be responsible for giving most of the bedside respiratory therapy, low-level super-vision, participation in clinical instruction, and assisting with special projects. The functional relationship between therapist and technician is summarized in Table 12-1. Obviously, this format cannot and should not be applied dogmatically, for in real life the job should go to the one who can do it best. Experience will demonstrate, however, that on the average, administrative and high-level supervisory respon-

**Table 12-1.** *Functions of respiratory therapists and respiratory therapy technicians**

| Therapist | Technician | Therapist | Technician |
|---|---|---|---|
| Administration and supervision | | Resuscitation, emergency | X |
| Diagnostic procedures | | Teaching | |
|   Arterial blood collection | X |   Clinical | X |
|   Blood gas analysis | |   Curriculum development | |
|   Lung volume measurements | |   Preclinical | |
|   Miscellaneous | | Therapy | |
|   Spirometry, bedside | X |   Aerosol and humidity | X |
|   Spirometry, laboratory | |   Gas | X |
| Equipment | |   Pressure breathing | X |
|   Evaluation | | Ventilation, mechanical | |
|   Maintenance | X |   Initiate | |
|   Modification | |   Maintain | X |
| Physiotherapy | | | |
|   Breathing exercises | X | | |
|   Postural drainage | X | | |
|   Rehabilitation | | | |

*Modified from Egan, D. F.: What is inhalation therapy? Clin. Notes Respir. Dis. **11**:3, Fall, 1972.

sibilities will be more easily assumed by the therapist than the technician, while the clinical emphasis of the technician's schooling should direct him naturally into patient care.

The success of any department will be in direct proportion to the efficiency and skill of its personnel, and each member of the department listed in the organizational table will be described, with emphasis on specific duties.

## Medical director

The decision as to whether the departmental directorship should be in the hands of one or more persons or should be full or part time is a matter to be determined by each hospital. Whatever arrangement is made at the start, the hospital can be assured that there will be an increasing amount of time demanded of the director as the department grows, and this must be taken into consideration in planning for the future. Such anticipated growth may necessitate the addition of associate directors as time goes on. The medical director must be a physician who is interested in chest diseases and who has had at least some clinical experience or training in this field. Whether duty hours are full or part time, his responsibility as director of the department will be full time, and he must be reasonably available for consultation and advice for the safe and effective supervision of the department.

The medical director must be a member of the hospital staff and thus will be affiliated with one of the major hospital departments. From a practical point of view, there are only two major departments that lend themselves well to affiliation with respiratory therapy—anesthesiology and internal medicine. Historically, many departments of respiratory care have been organized under the direction of anesthesiologists for two primary reasons: (1) the common foundation of pulmonary physiology underlying both anesthesiology and respiratory therapy and (2) the presence of anesthesiologists in the hospital for extended periods of time. They may be justly credited with much of the development of respiratory therapy into the organized specialty as it now exists. The evolution of respiratory therapy, however, has evoked some subtle changes in its function that affect its relationship to anesthesiology. Whereas the therapist of the early days of the technology performed relatively simple tasks, under the direct guidance of the medical director, the contemporary therapist is permitted a significant degree of exercise of judgment and plays an important role in patient care. Respiratory therapy, as it is now practiced, primarily directs itself to the diagnosis and treatment of medical diseases or medical complications of surgery or trauma; and to realize his full potential, the therapist must be well grounded in many aspects of clinical medicine. It is not sufficient that he merely be skilled in manual techniques, but he must understand cardiopulmonary physiology to a considerable depth and the changes in physiology wrought by disease. Such a view implies a clinical and medical orientation in the teaching and direction of respiratory therapy, most realistically provided by an internist trained in the physiologic and clinical aspect of chest diseases.

Unfortunately, there is still a shortage of clinicians able or willing to undertake the supervision of a respiratory care department, but there is hope for an improved future supply as greater emphasis is placed on postdoctoral training in chest disease. It should also be noted that the availability of the anesthesiologist for management of respiratory therapy is often more apparent than real. Since his first responsibility is to the operating and recovery rooms, as the work load of respiratory therapy grows, he may find himself increasingly unavailable for its supervision; and many anesthesiologists have found the extracurricular demands of the technical field an unwelcome chore. Thus the choice of a medical director depends on the local factor of available personnel and the objectives of respiratory therapy in the individual hospital, but a general recommendation can be made. If the treatment of cardiopulmonary disease in a given hospital is to be completely managed by each attending physician and respiratory therapy is to provide only a skilled technical service of limited scope, supervision and quality control of such services can be performed by either an anesthesiologist or an internist. If, however, respiratory therapy is to function maximally, integrating diagnostic laboratory facilities, professional consultation and referral services, and outpatient and rehabilitation care, a clinically trained internist is preferred as medical director. Where the employment of a full-time department head is not feasible, some hospitals have placed the supervision of respiratory therapy in the hands of a small committee of diversified interests, thus distributing the work and covering different areas of professional responsibility.

Regardless of his disciplinary affiliation, the medical director of the department is professionally responsible for the entire function of the department. Because of this responsibility, he should be afforded considerable authority in establishing the professional policies and practices of respiratory therapy in his hospital, although any major policy involving patient care or relationship between the department and staff physicians should be approved by the hospital medical board. Such a move would ensure understanding of the policy and guarantee maximum cooperation at all levels. The major responsibilities of the medical director include the following: provision or supervision of medical care of patients with respiratory diseases, including consultation and referral, acute respiratory care, ambulatory care, and pulmonary function evaluation; establishment of departmental clinical policies and procedures; supervision of respiratory therapy school and/or in-service training and education; education of medical and nursing staffs; selection and promotion of students, trainees, and therapists; maintenance of personnel and medical records; and preparation of the departmental budget.

In reference to the medical director's involvement in personnel and budgetary matters, it should be emphasized that his nonmedical responsibilities are increasing. The normal, continued growth of respiratory care coupled with the current national economic stress have burdened leadership with administrative problems of major dimensions. A prime challenge to medical and technical directors of respiratory therapy services is to provide increasingly better patient service, but at lower cost. The need for administrative education for medical directors has long been recognized by those active in this work, but only recently has it been given significant exposure in the medical press.[357, 358] Physicians who contemplate assuming medical directorships of respiratory therapy services must be willing and ready to accept administrative responsibilities. It is to be hoped that meaningful exposure to relevant aspects of hospital management and medical economics will one day be part of pulmonary fellowship education.

### Technical director

The efficiency of departmental operation will depend on this key figure. The technical director, an individual who must be well trained in all aspects of respiratory therapy and experienced in its clinical application. He must be thoroughly versed in the techniques of therapy and the function of equipment and must possess leadership qualities and administrative ability. Although his position will probably have more prestige if he is registered by the National Board for Respiratory Therapy, Inc., registration alone is not sufficient, for there are many registered therapists who do not have the other necessary qualities of a technical director. There is no guideline to indicate the depth of experience necessary for this position, but as a generalization, it might be assumed that the average therapist would need a minimum of 3 years of practical experience in the field following his training, to prepare him for the duties of a technical director. His selection for this position must depend on a detailed interview for an appraisal of his background as well as candid references from previous teachers and employers. Whereas the medical director is responsible for the overall policies and professional functioning of the department, the technical director is responsible for the daily operation of this service. His administrative authority must be well understood and completely supported by the medical director, and he is an important link between the medical director and the technical staff. Among the technical director's duties are the scheduling of staff assignments; the maintenance of payroll data on all technical personnel; maintenance of statistical data for reports of departmental activity; the maintenance of an inventory of all expendable equipment and supplies; advice and assistance to technical personnel; assistance in the training of new therapists; and assistance to the medical director on special projects and in preparation of the budget.

## Assistant technical director

One or more assistant technical directors will be needed according to the size of the department. The assistant should possess technical skills similar to those of the director but does not need as much administrative experience. He has a responsible double role. In the absence of the technical director he acts as the director of the department, but in daily operation he is a troubleshooter and may also function as the first shift supervisor. The assistant supervises the service in the respiratory care or intensive care unit and consults with or advises staff therapists in the management of difficult patients, especially when it is necessary to improvise techniques or equipment. He takes an active role in the training and orientation of students and new therapists and evaluates all new or recently repaired equipment.

## Shift supervisor

The three shift supervisors are responsible for the respiratory therapy service function during their segments of the day. Generally, they are directly responsible for the staff technicians and aides on their shifts, although in large hospitals they may have the assistance of, and work through, area supervisors. The shift supervisor reassigns duties of subordinates according to changing needs, assists staff personnel with problems, participates in the work load when necessary, responds to emergency resuscitation calls, and assists in clinical teaching or student supervision. Specific duties of these important people will vary considerably from place to place. The difference in overall hospital activity between the first and third shifts also gives different responsibilities to the respective shift supervisors. For example, whereas the first and second shift supervisors might be primarily concerned with fulfilling request for service, the third shift chief might be responsible for blood gas analysis or clerical work requiring technical knowledge. These supervisors must be flexible and adaptable, as well as mature and experienced.

## Area supervisor

Only where there is a geographical location in the hospital with a high concentration either of work volume or of special services is there need for an area supervisor. Difficult logistics, especially in old hospitals with many additions over the years, may make adequate supervision by a shift supervisor impossible, and quality performance can better be achieved by a locally assigned supervisor. Perhaps more frequently there is need for supervision in specialty areas such as intensive care or respiratory care units, recovery and emergency rooms, and subacute care, rehabilitation, and outpatient areas. Well-trained area supervisors may be a necessity in such locations, overseeing the performance of staff technicians assigned to them and operating educational programs to teach new personnel and to maintain proficiency in the regular staff. The area supervisor, then, is apt to be at least a semispecialist with specific expertise in contrast to the shift supervisor with wider managerial skills.

### Staff respiratory therapy technician

The staff technicians comprise the work force of the department and are expected to know their equipment in detail, including its structure, function, the indications for its use, and its physiologic effect on the patient. They must also know at least the basic maintenance procedures for this equipment. Before a technician is allowed to treat patients, he must understand the physiology of respiration and circulation, both normal and abnormal, as it applies to respiratory therapy, and have a good working knowledge of the diseases to which he will be exposed. He will be responsible for performing all the services listed in Table 12-1 as functions of respiratory care technicians.

Because the respiratory care technician has close and intimate patient contact, it is essential that he be able to establish a good rapport with his patients; this requires a stable personality, a strong motivation to work with the sick, and a personal conservatism in appearance, speech, and manner. He must understand the need for tact and the principles of medical ethics, since patients frequently develop a strong attachment to the technician and often confide in him and ply him with professional questions. The skill of the technician in managing as well as treating his patient is an important factor in the patient's response to therapy. Extreme care and screening are needed in hiring personnel for this important job.

### Pulmonary function laboratory personnel

An experienced and well-trained respiratory therapist is especially well founded to operate a pulmonary function laboratory. His background knowledge of cardiopulmonary physiology as well as of clinical chest diseases makes the purposes of pulmonary function testing more meaningful to him than to a technician without this experience. His insight into laboratory procedures makes him a good judge of the reliability of his results and better able to recognize inaccuracies or laboratory errors or inconsistencies. Also, a pulmonary function laboratory staffed with respiratory therapists and technicians has close technical rapport with the clinical respiratory therapy personnel.

The technical director of the pulmonary function laboratory must know the details and techniques of all the procedures in his laboratory and be able to train or orient students or new employees. He is responsible for supervising the quality of the work done by the other technicians, the scheduling of assignments, the maintenance of laboratory records, and the maintenance of an inventory of supplies. His knowledge of equipment must be sufficient for him to recognize malfunction and know what measures are necessary for repair of equipment. He also assists the director of the department or laboratory with special projects.

The staff technicians of the laboratory must be as well versed in the procedures and techniques as the technical director but without the administrative or supervisory experience or authority. With careful selection of personnel, it is possible to teach nonrespiratory care technicians to perform such specific duties as blood gas analyses for part-time laboratory coverage during the off hours of nights and weekends.

### Technical director of education, and instructor

Wherever respiratory therapy services are available, there should also be an educational program suitable for the size and sophistication of the hospital and its staff. This may vary from a series of in-service demonstrations of respiratory therapy equipment and techniques to a structured school of respiratory therapy. For the former, one therapist should be given its responsibility and designated as technical director of education, assisted by instructors as needed, drawn from the regular staff. In the latter, the responsible therapist is usually referred to as the technical director, or coordinator, of the school, which is a full-time task. Instructors must be well trained and experienced and able to transmit their knowledge to others. The technical instructors are especially valuable in teaching procedures and equipment function and for supervision of the clinical application of respiratory therapy at the bedside, but other subjects may be delegated to them as their qualifications permit. Capable technicians, as well as therapists, should be given teaching roles if they are motivated to participate. An important contribution of the instructor is his evaluation of his student and his recommendation of the degree of independent action that a student can be expected to fulfill. The instructors function directly under the medical director, correlating their material with his overall objectives and reporting their findings and recommendations to him for his final action.

Although not an officially recognized member of respiratory therapy personnel, the aide has been used extensively to great advantage over the years. There are many important tasks to be done in an active respiratory therapy service that do not require the technical knowledge of a therapist or technician. To make the most of valuable manpower, nontechnical personnel can be employed to perform these duties. Such functions as cleaning, sterilizing, and packaging of equipment, pickup and floor delivery of equipment, repair and maintenance, and some clerical work are better done by those other than patient care–oriented therapists or technicians. The use of aides, where safe and practical, is to be encouraged.

## DEPARTMENTAL OPERATION
### Distribution of services

In terms of time coverage and scope of services, local hospital needs and available personnel will be the determining factors. Ideally, all respiratory therapy services should be available 24 hours a day, 7 days a week. However, the very real chronic shortage of trained respiratory therapists makes this an almost impossible task, and most hospitals find it necessary to effect a compromise between demand and supply. Every attempt should be made to complete the maximum work volume during the day shift, and for this the full cooperation of the medical and nursing staffs is essential. Physicians should be urged to order therapy in advance so that it may be scheduled at the start of each day. The technical director always attempts to leave flexibility in assignments to accommodate emergencies, but this requires careful planning of more routine work. Staff nurses are usually too confined with their own responsibilities to take an active role in respiratory therapy, but frequently private-duty nurses can assist their patients by administering therapy under the instruction and supervision of a therapist.

The provision of services during nights and weekends always presents a problem. In general, only emergency cases and patients most acutely ill are serviced during those hours, and since the respiratory therapist is a technical rather than a professional person, it is the responsibility of the attending physician and supervisory nurses to cooperate in determining those patients who need care in off-hours. There is no general rule for the classification of patients according to need for respiratory therapy services, but the following list is offered as a suggested priority scale to help medical, nursing, and respiratory therapy personnel in scheduling work assignments for respiratory therapy services:

1. Emergency resuscitation
2. Continuous mechanical ventilation
3. Any intensive care area
4. Emergency room
5. Postoperative care
6. Oxygen or humidity administration
7. Prescheduled positive-pressure breathing
8. Physical therapy

The grouping represents only a commonsense classification of the patient suffering from acute cardiorespiratory failure as most in need of attention and the patient in a period of convalescence or rehabilitation as least in need. It is emphasized that the objective of such a priority scale is not to restrict the application of respiratory therapy services but rather to enable the department to make the maximum use of them.

Clinical experience has demonstrated the necessity of having pulmonary function evaluation facilities available wherever respiratory therapy is being utilized to its maximum potential. At the current stage of respiratory therapy as a clinical technical specialty, its techniques frequently need some physiologic evaluation to determine proper therapy. This is especially true wherever patients are being maintained on mechanical ventilation. In such circumstances it is mandatory that the physiologic status be monitored by frequent examination of arterial or arterialized blood for pH, carbon dioxide tension, and oxygen tension; and the experienced therapist will use these data along with other criteria to adjust the ventilators accordingly. Since patients in ventilatory failure are as much in need of close supervision during the night and on weekends as at other times, it is necessary that facilities for blood gas monitoring be available. The ease with which this can be accomplished will be determined by the available laboratory facilities and personnel and is another valuable service the respiratory therapist will be able to perform. It is ideal to have full-time laboratory technicians on duty around the clock 7 days a week, but often this is not feasible and a compromise schedule must be established. Sometimes the night supervisor can handle the necessary laboratory work during duty hours, but if this is not sufficient, as indicated earlier, it is frequently practical to employ the part-time services of personnel who are not respiratory therapists. Although they may know little cardiopulmonary physiology, if they are receptive and learn thoroughly, they can be taught techniques of blood gas analysis and free the regular staff for service during the working day. The success of this approach depends on careful selection, meticulous instruction, and close supervision.

## Scheduling of assignments

In the role of a dispatcher, the technical director designates the work areas and assigns patients to the staff technicians or shift supervisors at the beginning of the day. A zone system is usually the most effective, and with experience, most hospitals can be divided into areas according to the average work density. One technician may be designated to circulate, helping in the busy areas, responding to emergencies, and performing such routine duties as monitoring oxygen concentrations, checking tanked gas contents, and examining other operating equipment. At least one therapist should rotate through an equipment-servicing detail, in which he is responsible for cleaning and sterilizing, storage, and maintenance. If local labor supply will permit, hiring nontechnical personnel for this task will free the therapist for patient care or other duties for which he is trained. Arrangements are made to give priority service to intensive care units and the emergency room, and response to floor emergencies is standardized.

Throughout the day all calls for service are submitted to the technical director's office. A written record is executed to include date and time, nature of request, and its disposition, and the record is kept on file. The technical director is responsible for expediting service during the day's operation, shifting personnel and assignments as needed, a difficult but critical task that requires skill and judgment.

Efficiency of communications is an important key to smooth function. Hospital paging systems are at best only partially adequate because most have many "deaf spots," but individual paging or signal units justify their cost in time saved and thus numbers of patients serviced. Since most hospitals with effective departments include a therapist in their resuscitation teams, a radio page will enhance response to emergencies.

## Records and accounts

Each hospital has its own record and accounting system, and only a few comments are indicated. In great vogue now are various types of computerized techniques with memory storage and retrieval capabilities, and the capacity and flexibility of these need no amplification. However, many hospitals must yet rely on manual systems, and every attempt is made to reduce clerical work to a minimum. The use of the portable visible index-type card file enables the therapist and technician to carry with him a record card for each patient for whom he is responsible. All treatments or services for a given day are entered on this card, and at the end of the day charge tickets are executed for each patient and submitted to the accounting office. From the accumulated patient cards, data are obtained for a statistical account of the departmental activity and transferred to a day sheet. The day sheet tabulates such items as the number of patients treated, the patient days of treatment, the numbers of individual services, and patient charges according to type of service. Each month the total of the day sheets is recorded in a monthly statistical report, which is submitted to the hospital administration, the accounting department, and the director of the department, and these reports form the basis for evaluating departmental progress. Many modifications of this system are possible, especially for recall of grouped data, and can be achieved by special filing procedures or the use of punched cards. Because each technician must keep track of service data on patients scattered all over the hospital, it is essential that the system chosen be as simple and error proof as possible.

In addition to accounting records, the respiratory care department must maintain a clinical record in each patient's chart. Simplicity is advised in the format of such a record, and a ruled sheet with a place to note date and time, room for comments, and an initial or signature column is adequate. Following each treatment the therapist is expected to note on the sheet a comment concerning the treatment and the patient and any other information considered relevant. This is an invaluable guide for subsequent therapists.

**Professional supervision**

Reference was made earlier to an important aspect of respiratory therapy when it was noted that the services of respiratory therapy extend into all major hospital divisions. As a hospital service, the department provides facilities available on the order of all staff physicians. At the same time the services so provided are under the control and are the responsibility of another physician, the medical director of the department. Whereas care must be taken to minimize the risk of interference with the autonomy of the attending physician by the medical director, close control of the proper use of respiratory therapy services must be assured by the director. These objectives can easily be attained by willing cooperation among hospital administration, medical staff, and the respiratory care department. Many therapeutic procedures can be classified as "standard," with little ambiguity as to their function and generally complete understanding of their clinical application. Among others, this group might include such services as oxygen administration, aerosols of wide acceptance, and mist therapy. The direct responsibility of the medical director in the application of these services requires little more than ensuring a smooth-running department. In contrast, the safe and effective use of some respiratory therapy techniques requires much experience as well as specific professional and technical knowledge. Especially is this true in the management of the critically ill patient in ventilatory failure, the techniques of rehabilitation and chronic care, and the interpretation of pulmonary function tests.

There are two administrative policies that can be used to handle these sensitive areas, the choice of which will depend on each local hospital situation. First, it can be established that the use of certain specified treatments will require prior official consultation with the medical director, who will follow the patient management with the attending physician. Second, the director can be given the authority to observe closely all patients receiving the services of his department and to interfere with the management at any time his judgment determines that the best interests of a patient are not being served. The degree of sophistication of the medical staff in the management of cardiopulmonary problems will usually be the determinant of the exact supervisory program most suitable. It is strongly suggested that the following philosophic observation be accepted: At the present time, respiratory therapy is still a growing field, and the exact legal and moral responsibilities of a respiratory therapy director toward other physicians and their patients have not been clarified. It must be assumed that he is responsible for the actions of technicians under his jurisdiction and for the safety and efficacy of the procedures of his department. It is only just therefore that being asked to assume responsibility, he also be given authority to control his sphere of responsibility. Further experience will be necessary to delineate more precisely the boundaries of his position.

## SIZE OF RESPIRATORY CARE DEPARTMENT
### Personnel and space

Any opinions concerning number of personnel, size of physical facilities, and type of equipment must be of the most general nature because of the wide variation in individual hospital needs. The following comments are based on the experiences of, and information from, a number of selected hospitals with known active departments. Although there is no statistical significance atttached to the data acquired, they were felt to have general informative value, and analysis of the data revealed better correlation of numbers of personnel and floor space with average yearly admissions than with bed capacity. The range of yearly admissions among the hospitals polled extended from 7000 to 30,000, and the number of therapists thought to be adequate averaged one per 1000 yearly admissions. Despite a wide spread, it is believed that this ratio is a useful guide, especially for hospitals in the initial stages of planning a department. If anything, such a figure is small, since it does not take into account the specialty positions or stratification that inevitably develop. Thus, as a department increases its scope of services, this ratio can be expected to increase.

Data on respiratory therapy floor space yielded an average of about 70 square feet of space per 1000 yearly admissions. However, the breakdown of utilization of space was not available, and it is not known, for example, how much of the reported space was used for general service areas, offices, storage, or treatment rooms. It is strongly advised that hospitals anticipating physical expansion allow extra space above the immediate needs of respiratory therapy, since it can almost be guaranteed that a growing department will find its existing facilities inadequate within 2 to 3 years.

The general service or marshaling area should be large enough to accommodate a generous working space for repair and maintenance of equipment and a convenient area for cleaning and sterilization. The location of bulk storage space is a matter of expediency, but it should be near the general area. Provisions should also be made for separate office space for the medical director, the technical director, and a secretary and a writing area for record-keeping duties of the staff therapists. One of the most important contributions of respiratory therapy will be denied if an adequate ambulatory care room is not provided, preferably immediately adjacent to, but separated from, the general service area. Ideally, the space provided for pulmonary function testing should be isolated from other activities, but this can often be skillfully done by properly placed partitions in the service area or treatment room. The difficulties of incorporating new facilities into existing buildings are well recognized, and makeshift arrangements often must be made. In new construction, however, every attempt should be made to locate the general service room, the laboratory, and the ambulatory service area as close together as possible, and all preferably not far from the intensive or respiratory care units.

## Equipment

The past few years saw a tremendous increase in the use of disposable plastic equipment, presterilized and neatly packaged to save labor costs of cleaning and sterilizing. The convenience of an inventory ready to use from dealer to consumer was another asset. More recently, however, rising costs of disposables and diminishing storage areas have considerably reduced their advantages. As a result, many hospitals are returning, in part at least, to small inventories of recyclable items, effecting savings in more efficient systems of cleaning, sterilizing, and packaging. The choice of disposables versus nondisposables is made on the basis of cost, a task continuously facing all technical directors of busy departments.

Of nonexpendable therapy equipment, the largest and most expensive pieces are the ventilators. It is quite improper here to recommend specific types or brands of such equipment, since these are decisions that should be left to the technical director with the approval of the medical director. Departmental policy will determine whether it is in the best interest of the hospital to strive for maximum uniformity of procedure through the use of a limited variety of types or for greater flexibility with a wide variety. In general, it might be advised that an active respiratory therapy service will be able to use one or two mechanical ventilators per 1000 yearly admissions. The minimum equipment for the pulmonary function laboratory consists of a spirometer with facilities for measurement of lung volumes, available as a single unit if desired, and a blood gas analyzer. Before investing in large numbers of equipment, both the medical and technical directors of a newly developing department would be well advised to visit a few established units to observe utilization and techniques.

## SUMMARY

Respiratory therapy still poses many unsolved problems, some of which have been alluded to in the foregoing text. Paramount among them is the relationship between respiratory therapy and other hospital departments and services. As it has developed, respiratory therapy has admittedly encroached on clinical areas previously in the domains of nursing, physical therapy, clinical laboratory, and even the medical house staff. Such moves have been part of the natural evolution of an emerging clinical field directing itself toward the care of a substantial group of patients who, in the past, have received all too little attention. There is a natural hesitation on the part of physicians to delegate care of their patients to technicians, of whose work the physicians themselves know so little. The medical director of the department may well feel on unsure ground when he supervises the services of his therapists to a patient on whom he has not been asked to consult. Indeed, the matter of legal and moral responsibility of the medical director is still unsettled and will probably require more experience in the field to resolve. In the meantime, cooperation among the respiratory care department, the hospital administration, and the medical and nursing staffs will allow the useful services of respiratory therapy to find its niche in the overall medical care program of the hospital.

Finally, I might indulge in some imaginative speculation as to what the future could hold for respiratory therapy. The rapidly increasing population is straining the ability of currently organized medicine to supply adequate medical care. The problem is not merely a quantitative shortage of personnel, but with the emergence of so many new diagnostic and therapeutic techniques, skills are needed that have not traditionally been part of medicine. This is an era of technical as well as professional specialization, and it seems almost inevitable that delivery of medical care to our society in the near future will depend on the delegation of many responsibilities to highly skilled and finely trained nonphysician specialists. One of the fastest growing segments of medicine is that of cardiopulmonary disease, and it is in this area that the present respiratory therapist may find himself becoming a more committed part of the future medical team. With his background in cardiopulmonary physiology, his participation in laboratory diagnosis, and his intimate patient-care experience, he is a natural subject to expand into related cardiovascular fields, where technology is becoming increasingly important. Perhaps we should already be orienting our education toward the development of *cardiopulmonary technology,* which could formally extend the function of the respiratory therapist beyond his present services. This is being done on scattered individual bases in many centers, and it is quite probable that before long, respiratory therapy will be one facet of the larger technical specialty of cardiopulmonary technology.

# APPENDIXES

## Appendix 1

### SYSTEMS OF MEASUREMENTS AND EQUIVALENTS

I. *Scientific notation*
  A. The purpose of scientific notation is to convert a large or small awkward number from its usual form to an integer between 1 and 10, multiplied by the appropriate power of 10 so its value is unchanged.
  B. Tabulation of the powers of 10:

$10^0 = 1$                              $10^0 = 1$

$10^1 = 10$                         $10^{-1} = {}^1/_{10} = 0.1$

$10^2 = 10 \times 10 = 100$         $10^{-2} = {}^1/_{10^2} = 0.01$

$10^3 = 10 \times 10 \times 10 = 1000$    $10^{-3} = {}^1/_{10^3} = 0.001$

$10^4 = 10 \times 10 \times 10 \times 10 = 10,000$   $10^{-4} = {}^1/_{10^4} = 0.0001$

$10^5 = 10 \times 10 \times 10 \times 10 \times 10 = 100,000$   $10^{-5} = {}^1/_{10^5} = 0.00001$

$10^6 = 10 \times 10 \times 10 \times 10 \times 10 \times 10 = 1,000,000$   $10^{-6} = {}^1/_{10^6} = 0.000001$

  C. General rules for writing scientific notation:
    1. For a number larger than 10: Move the decimal to the position to the right of the first integer, and multiply the new number by 10 raised to the power equal to the number of places the decimal was moved. Zeros to the right of the last integer may be dropped. For example:

$$2655 = 2.655 \times 10^3 \qquad 301,010 = 3.0101 \times 10^5$$
$$54,000 = 5.4 \times 10^4 \qquad 866.67 = 8.6667 \times 10^2$$

    2. For a number smaller than 1: Move the decimal to the position to the right of the first integer, and multiply the new number by 10 raised to a *negative* power equal to the number of places the decimal was moved. For example:

$$0.454 = 4.54 \times 10^{-1} \qquad 0.00000703 = 7.03 \times 10^{-6}$$
$$0.00306 = 3.06 \times 10^{-3} \qquad 0.01010 = 1.01 \times 10^{-2}$$

II. *Metric system*
  A. There are many excellent descriptions of the history of and justification for the metric system so we shall confine ourselves only to a review of its most salient features.[359] There are three basic units of linear, weight, and volume measurement, respectively the *meter* (m), the *gram* (g), and the

*liter* (l), with time,calibrated in *seconds* (s). From its scientific use, especially, these parameters have come to be known as the centimeter-gram-second (cgs) metric system. Even though this system has not yet become popular in the United States, there is a move among many European nations to modernize it because it is old to them. Updated metrecation would comprise the so-called *International System of Units* (SI, for Système International).[360,361] The SI consists of the following seven independent measurable quantities and their respective units: length (meter, m); mass (kilogram, kg); time (second, s); electric current (ampere, A); temperature (Kelvin, K); luminous intensity (candela, cd); and amount of substance (mole, mol). This system is also known as the meter-kilogram-second (MKS) system. We will not describe the SI system in more detail, as it has made little headway so far in the United States, and we will confine ourselves to terms, prefixes, suffixes, and abbreviations of the familiar and useful cgs metric system. Multiples and divisions of cgs units are related to one another as powers of 10. Multiple prefixes are in Greek, and fractional prefixes in Latin.

| deka | da $= 10^1$ | deci | d $= 10^{-1}$ | nano | n $= 10^{-9}$ |
|------|-------------|------|---------------|------|---------------|
| hecto | h $= 10^2$ | centi | c $= 10^{-2}$ | pico | p $= 10^{-12}$ |
| kilo | K $= 10^3$ | milli | m $= 10^{-3}$ | femto | f $= 10^{-15}$ |
| mega | M $= 10^6$ | micro | $\mu^* = 10^{-6}$ | atto | a $= 10^{-18}$ |
| giga | G $= 10^9$ | | | | |
| tera | T $= 10^{12}$ | | | | |

## B. Examples of metric measurement terminology

| Linear | | Weight | | Volume | |
|--------|--|--------|--|--------|--|
| kilometer (km) | m $\times 10^3$ | kilogram (kg) | g $\times 10^3$ | kiloliter | l $\times 10^3$ |
| hectometer | m $\times 10^2$ | hectogram | g $\times 10^2$ | hectoliter | l $\times 10^2$ |
| decameter | m $\times 10$ | decagram | g $\times 10$ | decaliter | l $\times 10$ |
| meter (m) | | gram (g) | | liter ($\ell$) | |
| decimeter | m $\times 10^{-1}$ | decigram | g $\times 10^{-1}$ | deciliter (dl) | l $\times 10^{-1}$ |
| centimeter (cm) | m $\times 10^{-2}$ | centigram | g $\times 10^{-2}$ | centiliter | l $\times 10^{-2}$ |
| millimeter (mm) | m $\times 10^{-3}$ | milligram (mg) | g $\times 10^{-3}$ | milliliter (ml) | l $\times 10^{-3}$ |
| micrometer | m $\times 10^{-6}$ | microgram ($\mu$g) | g $\times 10^{-6}$ | microliter ($\mu$l) | l $\times 10^{-6}$ |
| ($\mu$ or $\mu$m) | | nanogram (ng) | g $\times 10^{-9}$ | nanoliter (nl) | l $\times 10^{-9}$ |

## C. United States customary and metric equivalents

| Linear | | Weight | | Volume | |
|--------|--|--------|--|--------|--|
| inch | 2.54 cm | ounce (oz) | 28.35 g | ounce (fl) | 29.57 ml |
| foot | $3.048 \times 10^{-1}$ m | pound | $4.54 \times 10^{-1}$ kg | quart | $9.463 \times 10^{-1}$ liter |
| mile | 1.609 km | | | gallon | 3.785 liters |
| | | gram | $3.528 \times 10^{-2}$ oz | cubic inch | 16.39 ml |
| micron | $3.937 \times 10^{-5}$ in | kilogram | 2.205 lb | cubic foot | 28.32 liters |
| centimeter | $3.937 \times 10^{-1}$ in | | | | |
| meter | 39.37 in | | | liter | 1.057 qt |
| kilometer | $6.214 \times 10^{-1}$ mi | | | | 61.02 in$^3$ |
| | | | | | $3.532 \times 10^{-2}$ ft$^3$ |

---

*Micro cannot be abbreviated with a small m because of a conflict with milli, and somewhat paradoxically, the Greek letter *mu*, symbolized $\mu$, was chosen to represent it.

D. Equations to convert between Celsius and Fahrenheit temperatures

$$°C = \frac{5 \ (°F - 32)}{9}$$

$$°F = \left[\frac{9 \times °C}{5}\right] + 32$$

# Appendix 2

## PHYSIOLOGIC AND SELECTED PHYSICAL ABBREVIATIONS AND SYMBOLS

*Note:* A small horizontal line over a symbol signifies a mean, or average value; thus ā equals mean arterial value of whatever measurement is being considered. A prime mark following a symbol indicates an end, or terminal value; thus c′ equals end capillary measurement of some variable.

| | |
|---|---|
| a | = (1) Arterial blood |
| | = (2) Acceleration |
| ā | = (1) Mixed arterial blood |
| | = (2) Mean acceleration |
| ATPD<br>ATPD } | = Ambient temperature and pressure, dry |
| ATPS<br>ATPS } | = Ambient temperature and pressure, saturated with water vapor |
| A | = Alveolar gas |
| b | = Blood, generally |
| BTPD<br>BTPD } | = Body temperature, ambient pressure, dry |
| BTPS<br>BTPS } | = Body temperature, ambient pressure, saturated with water vapor |
| B | = Barometric |
| c | = Capillary blood |
| C | = (1) Compliance |
| | = (2) Concentration of gas in blood |
| °C | = Degree of temperature by Celsius scale |
| d | = Distance covered by a moving body |
| dl | = deciliter (0.1 liter) |
| D | = (1) Diffusing capacity |
| | = (2) Density |
| D | = Dead space gas |
| ERV | = Expiratory reserve volume |
| E | = Exhaled gas |
| f | = Respiratory frequency (breaths per minute) |
| F | = (1) Fractional concentration of dry gas |
| | = (2) Force |
| °F | = Degree of temperature by Fahrenheit scale |
| FRC | = Functional residual capacity |
| g | = (1) Acceleration due to the force of gravity |
| | = (2) Gram |
| gfw | = Gram formula weight |

| | |
|---|---|
| gmw | = Gram molecular weight |
| H⁺ | = Ion (hydrogen as an example) |
| [H⁺] | = Molar concentration of ions |
| IC | = Inspiratory capacity |
| IRV | = Inspiratory reserve volume |
| I | = Inhaled gas |
| K | = Constant of a chemical equilibrium (i.e., dissociation constant of a buffer system) |
| °K | = Degree of temperature by Kelvin scale |
| KE | = Kinetic energy |
| ℓ/min<br>or lpm | = liters per minute |
| L | = Lung (pulmonary) |
| mb | = Millibar |
| mM | = Millimole ($M \times 10^{-3}$) |
| M | = Mole(s), molar |
| n | = (1) Number (especially number of molecules) |
| | = (2) nano ($10^{-9}$, i.e., $nM = M \times 10^{-9}$) |
| pH | = Negative common logarithm of molar hydrogen ion concentration |
| pK | = Negative common logarithm of a chemical equilibrium constant (i.e., dissociation constant of a buffer system) |
| psia | = Pounds per square inch, absolute |
| psig | = Pounds per square inch, gauge |
| P | = Gas pressure |
| Q | = Blood volume |
| Q̇ | = Rate of blood flow, volume per time |
| R | = (1) Resistance |
| | = (2) Respiratory exchange ratio ($V_{CO_2}/V_{O_2}$) |
| | = (3) Universal gas constant (0.0820561) |
| °R | = Degree of temperature by Rankine scale |
| RC | = Respiratory center |
| RH | = Relative humidity |
| RV | = Residual volume |

| s | = Distance covered by a moving body |
|---|---|
| S | = Percent saturation of hemoglobin with $O_2$ or CO |
| ST | = Surface tension |
| STPD STPD | = Standard temperature (0° C), standard pressure (760 mm Hg), dry |
| s | = (1) Subscript to show steady state |
|   | = (2) Shunt |
| t | = (1) Temperature generally |
|   | = (2) Time |
|   | = (3) Subscript means total, i.e., $Q_t$ |
| T | = Absolute temperature |
| TLC | = Total lung capacity |
| T | = (1) Tidal gas |
|   | = (2) Thorax |
| v | = (1) Venous blood |
|   | = (2) Velocity |

| $\bar{v}$ | = (1) Mixed venous blood |
|---|---|
|   | = (2) Mean velocity |
| V | = Gas volume |
| VC | = Vital capacity |
| $V_A$ | = Volume of total alveolar space |
| $V_E$ | = Volume of exhaled gas (often used for tidal volume) |
| $V_D$ | = Volume of dead space |
| $V_{D_{alv}}$ | = Volume of alveolar dead space |
| $V_{D_{anat}}$ | = Volume of anatomic dead space |
| $V_{D_{phys}}$ | = Volume of physiologic dead space |
| $V_{RB}$ | = Rebreathed volume |
| $V_T$ | = Tidal volume |
| $\dot{V}$ | = Rate of gas flow, volume per time |
| $\dot{V}_A$ | = Minute alveolar ventilation ($\ell$/min) |
| $\dot{V}_D$ | = Minute dead space ventilation ($\ell$/min) |
| $\dot{V}_E$ | = Volume of exhaled gas per unit of time (usually $\ell$/min, or minute volume) |

# Appendix 3

## ALTITUDE AND DEPTH CHARACTERISTICS OF ATMOSPHERE*

| Feet | t° C | Atm | psi | mm Hg | $P_{O_2}$ | % $O_2$ Equiv | Density |
|---|---|---|---|---|---|---|---|
| 300,000 | − 2.2 | $7.3 \times 10^{-6}$ | $1.1 \times 10^{-4}$ | 0.0055 | $1.1 \times 10^{-4}$ | $1.4 \times 10^{-5}$ | $8.57 \times 10^{-6}$ |
| 200,000 | 33.8 | $3.2 \times 10^{-4}$ | $4.6 \times 10^{-3}$ | 0.24 | $5.0 \times 10^{-2}$ | $6.6 \times 10^{-3}$ | $3.28 \times 10^{-4}$ |
| 100,000 | −55.0 | 0.011 | 0.155 | 8.0 | 1.7 | 0.22 | $1.74 \times 10^{-2}$ |
| 90,000 | −55.0 | 0.017 | 0.250 | 12.9 | 2.7 | 0.36 | $2.80 \times 10^{-2}$ |
| 80,000 | −55.0 | 0.027 | 0.403 | 20.8 | 4.3 | 0.57 | $4.52 \times 10^{-2}$ |
| 70,000 | −55.0 | 0.044 | 0.649 | 33.6 | 7.0 | 0.92 | $7.30 \times 10^{-2}$ |
| 60,000 | −55.0 | 0.071 | 1.05 | 54.1 | 11.3 | 1.49 | $1.18 \times 10^{-1}$ |
| 50,000 | −55.0 | 0.115 | 1.69 | 87.4 | 18.3 | 2.41 | $1.90 \times 10^{-1}$ |
| 40,000 | −55.0 | 0.191 | 2.72 | 140.6 | 29.4 | 3.87 | $3.06 \times 10^{-1}$ |
| 35,000 | −54.3 | 0.236 | 3.46 | 178.6 | 37.4 | 4.92 | $3.87 \times 10^{-1}$ |
| 30,000 | −44.4 | 0.296 | 4.36 | 225.7 | 47.3 | 6.22 | $4.67 \times 10^{-1}$ |
| 25,000 | −34.5 | 0.372 | 5.46 | 282.0 | 59.1 | 7.78 | $5.60 \times 10^{-1}$ |
| 20,000 | −24.6 | 0.460 | 6.76 | 348.8 | 73.1 | 9.62 | $6.66 \times 10^{-1}$ |
| 15,000 | −14.7 | 0.566 | 8.29 | 428.6 | 89.8 | 11.82 | $7.86 \times 10^{-1}$ |
| 10,000 | − 4.8 | 0.690 | 10.11 | 522.9 | 109.5 | 14.41 | $9.22 \times 10^{-1}$ |
| 5000 | 5.1 | 0.835 | 12.23 | 632.3 | 132.5 | 17.43 | 1.08 |
| 0 | 15.0 | 1.000 | 14.70 | 760.0 | 159.0 | 20.95 | 1.25 |
| 33 | | 2.000 | 29.4 | 1520.0 | 318.0 | 41.90 | 2.50 |
| 66 | | 3.000 | 44.1 | 2280.0 | 477.0 | 62.85 | 3.75 |
| 99 | | 4.000 | 58.8 | 3040.0 | 636.0 | 83.80 | 5.00 |
| 132 | | 5.000 | 73.5 | 3800.0 | 795.0 | 104.75 | 6.25 |
| 165 | | 6.000 | 88.2 | 4560.0 | 954.0 | 125.70 | 7.50 |
| 198 | | 7.000 | 102.9 | 5320.0 | 1113.0 | 146.65 | 8.75 |
| 231 | | 8.000 | 117.6 | 6080.0 | 1272.0 | 167.60 | 10.00 |
| 264 | | 9.000 | 132.3 | 6840.0 | 1431.0 | 188.55 | 11.25 |
| 297 | | 10.000 | 147.0 | 7600.0 | 1590.0 | 209.50 | 12.50 |

*Modified from Dittmer, D. S., and Grebe, R. M., editors: Handbook of respiration, Philadelphia, 1958, W. B. Saunders Co.

# Appendix 4

## FACTORS TO CONVERT GAS VOLUMES FROM ATPS TO BTPS*

| Factor to convert volume to 37° C saturated | When gas temperature (°C) is | With water vapor pressure (mm Hg)† of |
|:---:|:---:|:---:|
| 1.102 | 20 | 17.5 |
| 1.096 | 21 | 18.7 |
| 1.091 | 22 | 19.8 |
| 1.085 | 23 | 21.1 |
| 1.080 | 24 | 22.4 |
| 1.075 | 25 | 23.8 |
| 1.068 | 26 | 25.2 |
| 1.063 | 27 | 26.7 |
| 1.057 | 28 | 28.3 |
| 1.051 | 29 | 30.0 |
| 1.045 | 30 | 31.8 |
| 1.039 | 31 | 33.7 |
| 1.032 | 32 | 35.7 |
| 1.026 | 33 | 37.7 |
| 1.020 | 34 | 39.9 |
| 1.014 | 35 | 42.2 |
| 1.007 | 36 | 44.6 |
| 1.000 | 37 | 47.0 |

*Note:* These factors have been calculated only for a barometric pressure of 760 mm Hg. Since factors at 22° C, for example, are 1.0904, 1.0910, and 1.0915, respectively, at barometric pressures of 770, 760, and 750 mm Hg, it is unnecessary to correct for small deviations from standard barometric pressure.

$$\text{Factor} = \frac{[760 - P_{H_2O} \text{ at } t_{amb}] \times 0.435}{[t_{amb} + 273]}$$

*Modified from Comroe, J. H., Jr.: Methods in medical research, Chicago, 1950, Year Book Medical Publishers, Inc., vol 2.

†Water vapor pressures modified from Handbook of chemistry and physics, ed 28, Cleveland, 1944, Chemical Rubber Publishing Co., p. 1802.

# Appendix 5

## TEMPERATURE CORRECTION OF BAROMETRIC READING*

| Temperature (°C) | 730 mm Hg | 740 | 750 | 760 | 770 | 780 |
|---|---|---|---|---|---|---|
| 15.0 | 1.78 | 1.81 | 1.83 | 1.86 | 1.88 | 1.91 |
| 16.0 | 1.90 | 1.93 | 1.96 | 1.98 | 2.01 | 2.03 |
| 17.0 | 2.02 | 2.05 | 2.08 | 2.10 | 2.13 | 2.16 |
| 18.0 | 2.14 | 2.17 | 2.20 | 2.23 | 2.26 | 2.29 |
| 19.0 | 2.26 | 2.29 | 2.32 | 2.35 | 2.38 | 2.41 |
| 20.0 | 2.38 | 2.41 | 2.44 | 2.47 | 2.51 | 2.54 |
| 21.0 | 2.50 | 2.53 | 2.56 | 2.60 | 2.63 | 2.67 |
| 22.0 | 2.61 | 2.65 | 2.69 | 2.72 | 2.76 | 2.79 |
| 23.0 | 2.73 | 2.77 | 2.81 | 2.84 | 2.88 | 2.92 |
| 24.0 | 2.85 | 2.89 | 2.93 | 2.97 | 3.01 | 3.05 |
| 25.0 | 2.97 | 3.01 | 3.05 | 3.09 | 3.13 | 3.17 |
| 26.0 | 3.09 | 3.13 | 3.17 | 3.21 | 3.26 | 3.30 |
| 27.0 | 3.20 | 3.25 | 3.29 | 3.34 | 3.38 | 3.42 |
| 28.0 | 3.32 | 3.37 | 3.41 | 3.46 | 3.51 | 3.55 |
| 29.0 | 3.44 | 3.49 | 3.54 | 3.58 | 3.63 | 3.68 |
| 30.0 | 3.56 | 3.61 | 3.66 | 3.71 | 3.75 | 3.80 |
| 31.0 | 3.68 | 3.73 | 3.78 | 3.83 | 3.88 | 3.93 |
| 32.0 | 3.79 | 3.85 | 3.90 | 3.95 | 4.00 | 4.05 |
| 33.0 | 3.91 | 3.97 | 4.02 | 4.07 | 4.13 | 4.18 |
| 34.0 | 4.03 | 4.09 | 4.14 | 4.20 | 4.25 | 4.31 |
| 35.0 | 4.15 | 4.21 | 4.26 | 4.32 | 4.38 | 4.43 |

*From United States Department of Commerce, Weather Bureau: Barometers and the measurement of atmospheric pressure, Washington, D.C., 1941, Government Printing Office.

# Appendix 6

## FACTORS TO CONVERT GAS VOLUMES FROM ATPS TO STPD

| Observed $P_B$ | 15° | 16° | 17° | 18° | 19° | 20° | 21° | 22° | 23° | 24° | 25° | 26° | 27° | 28° | 29° | 30° | 31° | 32° |
|---|---|---|---|---|---|---|---|---|---|---|---|---|---|---|---|---|---|---|
| 700 | 0.855 | 851 | 847 | 842 | 838 | 834 | 829 | 825 | 821 | 816 | 812 | 807 | 802 | 797 | 793 | 788 | 783 | 778 |
| 702 | 857 | 853 | 849 | 845 | 840 | 836 | 832 | 827 | 823 | 818 | 814 | 809 | 805 | 800 | 795 | 790 | 785 | 780 |
| 704 | 860 | 856 | 852 | 847 | 843 | 839 | 834 | 830 | 825 | 821 | 816 | 812 | 807 | 802 | 797 | 792 | 787 | 783 |
| 706 | 862 | 858 | 854 | 850 | 845 | 841 | 837 | 832 | 828 | 823 | 819 | 814 | 810 | 804 | 800 | 795 | 790 | 785 |
| 708 | 865 | 861 | 856 | 852 | 848 | 843 | 839 | 834 | 830 | 825 | 821 | 816 | 812 | 807 | 802 | 797 | 792 | 787 |
| 710 | 867 | 863 | 859 | 855 | 850 | 846 | 842 | 837 | 833 | 828 | 824 | 819 | 814 | 809 | 804 | 799 | 795 | 790 |
| 712 | 870 | 866 | 861 | 857 | 853 | 848 | 844 | 839 | 836 | 830 | 826 | 821 | 817 | 812 | 807 | 802 | 797 | 792 |
| 714 | 872 | 868 | 864 | 859 | 855 | 851 | 846 | 842 | 837 | 833 | 828 | 824 | 819 | 814 | 809 | 804 | 799 | 794 |
| 716 | 875 | 871 | 866 | 862 | 858 | 853 | 849 | 844 | 840 | 835 | 831 | 826 | 822 | 816 | 812 | 807 | 802 | 797 |
| 718 | 877 | 873 | 869 | 864 | 860 | 856 | 851 | 847 | 842 | 838 | 833 | 828 | 824 | 819 | 814 | 809 | 804 | 799 |
| 720 | 880 | 876 | 871 | 867 | 863 | 858 | 854 | 849 | 845 | 840 | 836 | 831 | 826 | 821 | 816 | 812 | 807 | 802 |
| 722 | 882 | 878 | 874 | 869 | 865 | 861 | 856 | 852 | 847 | 843 | 838 | 833 | 829 | 824 | 819 | 814 | 809 | 804 |
| 724 | 885 | 880 | 876 | 872 | 867 | 863 | 858 | 854 | 849 | 845 | 840 | 835 | 831 | 826 | 821 | 816 | 811 | 806 |
| 726 | 887 | 883 | 879 | 874 | 870 | 866 | 861 | 856 | 852 | 847 | 843 | 838 | 833 | 829 | 825 | 818 | 813 | 808 |
| 728 | 890 | 886 | 881 | 877 | 872 | 868 | 863 | 859 | 854 | 850 | 845 | 840 | 836 | 831 | 826 | 821 | 816 | 811 |
| 730 | 892 | 888 | 884 | 879 | 875 | 870 | 866 | 861 | 857 | 852 | 847 | 843 | 838 | 833 | 828 | 823 | 818 | 813 |
| 732 | 895 | 891 | 886 | 882 | 877 | 873 | 868 | 864 | 859 | 854 | 850 | 845 | 840 | 836 | 831 | 825 | 820 | 815 |
| 734 | 897 | 893 | 889 | 884 | 880 | 875 | 871 | 866 | 862 | 857 | 852 | 847 | 843 | 838 | 833 | 828 | 823 | 818 |
| 736 | 900 | 895 | 891 | 887 | 882 | 878 | 873 | 869 | 864 | 859 | 855 | 850 | 845 | 840 | 835 | 830 | 825 | 820 |
| 738 | 902 | 898 | 894 | 889 | 885 | 880 | 876 | 871 | 866 | 862 | 857 | 852 | 848 | 843 | 838 | 833 | 828 | 822 |
| 740 | 905 | 900 | 896 | 892 | 887 | 883 | 878 | 874 | 869 | 864 | 860 | 855 | 850 | 845 | 840 | 835 | 830 | 825 |
| 742 | 907 | 903 | 898 | 894 | 890 | 885 | 881 | 876 | 871 | 867 | 862 | 857 | 852 | 847 | 842 | 837 | 832 | 827 |
| 744 | 910 | 906 | 901 | 897 | 892 | 888 | 883 | 878 | 874 | 869 | 864 | 859 | 855 | 850 | 845 | 840 | 834 | 829 |
| 746 | 912 | 908 | 903 | 899 | 895 | 890 | 886 | 881 | 876 | 872 | 867 | 862 | 857 | 852 | 847 | 842 | 837 | 832 |
| 748 | 915 | 910 | 906 | 901 | 897 | 892 | 888 | 883 | 879 | 874 | 869 | 864 | 860 | 854 | 850 | 845 | 839 | 834 |
| 750 | 917 | 913 | 908 | 904 | 900 | 895 | 890 | 886 | 881 | 876 | 872 | 867 | 862 | 857 | 852 | 847 | 842 | 837 |
| 752 | 920 | 915 | 911 | 906 | 902 | 897 | 893 | 888 | 883 | 879 | 874 | 869 | 864 | 859 | 854 | 849 | 844 | 839 |
| 754 | 922 | 918 | 913 | 909 | 904 | 900 | 895 | 891 | 886 | 881 | 876 | 872 | 867 | 862 | 857 | 852 | 846 | 841 |
| 756 | 925 | 920 | 916 | 911 | 907 | 902 | 898 | 893 | 888 | 883 | 879 | 874 | 869 | 864 | 859 | 854 | 849 | 844 |
| 758 | 927 | 923 | 918 | 914 | 909 | 905 | 900 | 896 | 891 | 886 | 881 | 876 | 872 | 866 | 861 | 856 | 851 | 846 |
| 760 | 930 | 925 | 921 | 916 | 912 | 907 | 902 | 898 | 893 | 888 | 883 | 879 | 874 | 869 | 864 | 859 | 854 | 848 |
| 762 | 932 | 928 | 923 | 919 | 914 | 910 | 905 | 900 | 896 | 891 | 886 | 881 | 876 | 871 | 866 | 861 | 856 | 851 |
| 764 | 934 | 930 | 926 | 921 | 916 | 912 | 907 | 903 | 898 | 893 | 888 | 884 | 879 | 874 | 869 | 864 | 858 | 853 |
| 766 | 937 | 933 | 928 | 925 | 919 | 915 | 910 | 905 | 900 | 896 | 891 | 886 | 881 | 876 | 871 | 866 | 861 | 855 |
| 768 | 940 | 935 | 931 | 926 | 922 | 917 | 912 | 908 | 903 | 898 | 893 | 888 | 883 | 878 | 873 | 868 | 863 | 858 |
| 770 | 942 | 938 | 933 | 928 | 924 | 919 | 915 | 910 | 905 | 901 | 896 | 891 | 886 | 881 | 876 | 871 | 865 | 860 |
| 772 | 945 | 940 | 936 | 931 | 926 | 922 | 917 | 912 | 908 | 903 | 898 | 893 | 888 | 883 | 878 | 873 | 868 | 862 |
| 774 | 947 | 943 | 938 | 933 | 929 | 924 | 920 | 915 | 910 | 905 | 901 | 896 | 891 | 886 | 880 | 875 | 870 | 865 |
| 776 | 950 | 945 | 941 | 936 | 931 | 927 | 922 | 917 | 912 | 908 | 903 | 898 | 893 | 888 | 883 | 878 | 872 | 867 |
| 778 | 952 | 948 | 943 | 938 | 934 | 929 | 924 | 920 | 915 | 910 | 905 | 900 | 895 | 890 | 885 | 880 | 875 | 869 |
| 780 | 955 | 950 | 945 | 941 | 936 | 932 | 927 | 922 | 917 | 912 | 908 | 903 | 898 | 892 | 887 | 882 | 877 | 872 |

$$\text{Factor} = \frac{[P_{B_{abs}} \text{ corrected for } t_{amg} - P_{H_2O} \text{ at } t_{amb}] \times 0.359}{[t_{amb} + 273]}$$

# Appendix 7

## FACTORS TO CONVERT GAS VOLUMES FROM STPD TO BTPS AT GIVEN BAROMETRIC PRESSURES

| Pressure | Factor | Pressure | Factor | Pressure | Factor | Pressure | Factor |
|---|---|---|---|---|---|---|---|
| 740 | 1.245 | 750 | 1.227 | 760 | 1.211 | 770 | 1.193 |
| 742 | 1.241 | 752 | 1.224 | 762 | 1.208 | 772 | 1.190 |
| 744 | 1.238 | 754 | 1.221 | 764 | 1.203 | 774 | 1.188 |
| 746 | 1.235 | 756 | 1.217 | 766 | 1.200 | 776 | 1.183 |
| 748 | 1.232 | 758 | 1.214 | 768 | 1.196 | 778 | 1.181 |

$$\text{Factor} = \frac{863}{[P_{B_{amb}} - 47]}$$

# Appendix 8

## LOW-TEMPERATURE CHARACTERISTICS OF SELECTED GASES AND WATER

| Substance | Critical temperature | | Critical pressure | Boiling point | | Melting (freezing) point | |
|---|---|---|---|---|---|---|---|
| | °C | °F | atm | °C | °F | °C | °F |
| Acetylene | 36.0 | 96.0 | 62.0 | −88.5 | −119.2 | − 81.8 | −114.6 |
| Air | −140.7 | −221.0 | 37.2 | −194.4 | −317.9 | − | − |
| Ammonia | 132.4 | 270.3 | 111.5 | − 33.4 | − 28.1 | − 77.7 | −108.0 |
| Carbon dioxide | 31.1 | 87.9 | 73.0 | − 78.5 | −109.3 | − 56.6 | − 69.9 |
| Cyclopropane | 124.7 | 256.4 | 54.2 | − 32.9 | − 27.2 | −127.5 | −197.7 |
| Freon-12 | 111.6 | 233.6 | 40.6 | − 29.8 | − 21.6 | −158.0 | −252.4 |
| Freon-14 | − 45.4 | − 49.9 | 36.8 | −128.0 | −198.4 | −184.0 | −299.2 |
| Helium | −267.9 | −450.2 | 2.3 | −268.9 | −452.1 | −272.2 | −455.8 |
| Hydrogen | −239.9 | −399.8 | 12.8 | −252.8 | −423.0 | −259.2 | −434.5 |
| Nitrogen | −147.1 | −232.6 | 33.5 | −195.8 | −320.5 | −209.9 | −345.9 |
| Nitrous oxide | 36.5 | 97.7 | 71.8 | − 88.5 | −127.2 | − 90.8 | −131.6 |
| Oxygen | −118.8 | −181.1 | 49.7 | −183.0 | −297.3 | −218.4 | −361.8 |
| Propane | 95.6 | 206.2 | 43.0 | − 42.2 | − 43.7 | −189.9 | −305.8 |
| Water | 374.0 | 705.0 | 218.0 | 100.0 | 212.0 | 0.0 | 32.0 |

## Appendix 9

### SELECTED ELEMENTS AND RADICALS: SYMBOLS, APPROXIMATE ATOMIC WEIGHTS, VALENCES

| Element | Symbol | Atomic weight | Valence | Element | Symbol | Atomic weight | Valence |
|---|---|---|---|---|---|---|---|
| Aluminum | Al | 27.0 | +3 | Phosphorus | P | 31.0 | +3, 5 |
| Argon | A | 39.9 | 0 | Potassium | K | 39.1 | +1 |
| Arsenic | As | 74.9 | +3, 5 | Silicon | Si | 28.1 | +4, −4 |
| Barium | Ba | 137.4 | +2 | Silver | Ag | 107.9 | +1 |
| Bromine | Br | 79.9 | −1, 3, 5, 7 | Sodium | Na | 23.0 | +1 |
| Calcium | Ca | 40.0 | +2 | Tin | Sn | 118.7 | +2, 4 |
| Carbon | C | 12.0 | +2, 4, −4 | Sulfur | S | 32.0 | ±2, 4, 6 |
| Chlorine | Cl | 35.5 | −1, 3, 5, 7 | Xenon | Xe | 131.3 | 0 |
| Copper | Cu | 63.5 | +1, 2 | Zinc | Zn | 65.4 | +2 |
| Fluorine | F | 19.0 | −1 | | | | |
| Germanium | Ge | 72.6 | +4, −4 | *Radical* | *Symbol* | | *Valence* |
| Helium | He | 4.0 | 0 | Acetate | $CH_3COO$ | | −1 |
| Hydrogen | H | 1.0 | ±1 | Ammonium | $NH_4$ | | −1 |
| Iodine | I | 126.9 | −1, 3, 5, 7 | Bicarbonate | $HCO_3$ | | −1 |
| Iron | Fe | 55.9 | +2, 3 | Borate | $BO_3$ | | −3 |
| Krypton | Kr | 83.8 | 0 | Carbonate | $CO_3$ | | −2 |
| Lead | Pb | 207.2 | +2, 4 | Chlorate | $ClO_3$ | | −1 |
| Magnesium | Mg | 24.3 | +2 | Hydroxyl | $OH$ | | −1 |
| Mercury | Hg | 200.6 | +1, 2 | Nitrate | $NO_3$ | | −1 |
| Neon | Ne | 20.2 | 0 | Nitrite | $NO_2$ | | −1 |
| Nitrogen | N | 14.0 | +3, 5 | Phosphate | $PO_4$ | | −3 |
| Oxygen | O | 16.0 | −2 | Sulfate | $SO_4$ | | −2 |

## Appendix 10

### CALCULATION OF $P_{CO_2}$ FROM H-H EQUATION

$$pH = 6.1 + \log\left[\frac{HCO_3}{\text{Dissolved } CO_2}\right]$$

$$pH = 6.1 + \log\left[\frac{\text{Total } CO_2 - 0.03\, P_{CO_2}}{0.03\, P_{CO_2}}\right]$$

$$pH - 6.1 = \log\left[\frac{\text{Total } CO_2}{0.03\, P_{CO_2}} - 1\right]$$

$$\text{antilog}\,(pH - 6.1) = \frac{\text{Total } CO_2}{0.03\, P_{CO_2}} - 1$$

$$\text{antilog}\,(pH - 6.1) + 1 = \frac{\text{Total } CO_2}{0.03\, P_{CO_2}}$$

$$P_{CO_2} = \frac{\text{Total } CO_2}{0.03 \times [1 + \text{antilog}\,(pH - 6.1)]}$$

# Appendix 11

## RELATION OF ARTERIAL OXYGEN SATURATION TO CAPILLARY UNSATURATION

With 15 g/dl of hemoglobin and an arterial-venous oxygen content difference of 5.0 vol%, the a-v oxygen saturation difference is 24%. The arterial oxygen saturation required to produce a specific concentration, in grams per deciliter, of unsaturated capillary blood hemoglobin can be computed by the following formula, derived below:

$$S_{a_{O_2}} = \frac{16.8 - y}{15}$$

(1) Mean capillary unsaturation = $\dfrac{\text{Arterial unsaturation} + \text{Venous unsaturation}}{2}$

(2) $x = S_{a_{O_2}}$ thus $(1.00 - x) = $ Arterial unsaturation
$(x - 0.24) = S_{v_{O_2}}$
$(1.00 - [x - 0.24]) = $ Venous unsaturation
$y = $ g/dl unsaturated hemoglobin in capillary blood

(3) Substituting in (1) above:

$$\frac{15\,(1.00 - x) + 15\,(1.00 - [x - 0.24])}{2} = y$$

(4) $15 - 15x + 15 - 15x + 3.60 = 2y$

(5) $-30x + 33.6 = 2y$

(6) $x = \dfrac{16.8 - y}{15}$

## Appendix 12

### ALVEOLAR AIR EQUATION

Accurate measurement of alveolar oxygen tension by direct analysis of alveolar air samples is difficult because of the inability to obtain reliable samples that are representative of all lung areas. The alveolar air equation permits calculation of a close estimation of $P_{A_{O_2}}$ if the $F_{I_{O_2}}$, $P_{a_{CO_2}}$, and respiratory exchange ratio ($\dot{V}_{CO_2}/\dot{V}_{O_2}$) are known. Its derivation is well explained by Comroe,* and need not be repeated here, but its application will be demonstrated by two examples. The equation is stated as follows:

$$P_{A_{O_2}} = F_{I_{O_2}}(713) - P_{a_{CO_2}}\left(F_{I_{O_2}} + \frac{1 - F_{I_{O_2}}}{R}\right)$$

*Example 1.* Calculate $P_{A_{O_2}}$ breathing room air, when $P_{a_{CO_2}} = 40$ mm Hg, and $R = 0.8$:

$$P_{A_{O_2}} = 0.21(713) - 40\left(0.21 + \frac{1 - 0.21}{0.8}\right)$$

$$= 149.73 - 40(1.198)$$
$$= 149.73 - 47.92$$
$$= 101.8 \text{ mm Hg}$$

*Example 2.* Calculate $P_{A_{O_2}}$ breathing 40% oxygen, when $P_{a_{CO_2}} = 5$ mm Hg, and $R = 0.9$:

$$P_{A_{O_2}} = 0.40(713) - 55\left(0.40 + \frac{1 - 0.40}{0.9}\right)$$

$$= 285.2 - 55(1.07)$$
$$= 285.2 - 58.85$$
$$= 226.4 \text{ mm Hg}$$

---

*Modified from Comroe, J. H., Jr., et al.: The lung, Chicago, 1962, Year Book Medical Publishers, Inc.

# Appendix 13

## BREATHING NOMOGRAM*

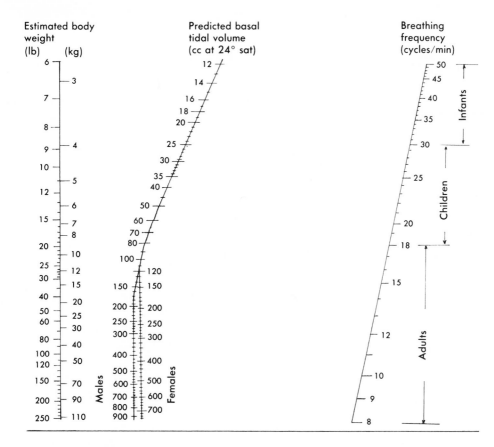

Estimated body weight (lb) (kg)

Predicted basal tidal volume (cc at 24° sat)

Breathing frequency (cycles/min)

Corrections of predicted basal tidal volumes.
 For patients not in coma: add 10%
 Fever: add 5% for each °F above 99 (rectal)
        add 9% for each °C above 37 (rectal)
 Altitude add 5% for each 2000 feet above sea level
         add 8% for each 1000 meters above sea level
 Intubation: subtract volume equal to one half body weight in pounds
           subtract 1 cc/kg of body weight
 Dead space: add equipment dead space

*Modified from Radford, E. P., Jr.: Ventilation standards for use in artificial respiration, J. Appl. Physiol. 7:451, 1955.

# ANSWERS TO EXERCISES

Exercise 1-1
  (a) 1.161 g/$\ell$  (f) 1.455
  (b) 0.759  (g) 0.429
  (c) 4.65  (h) 0.554
  (d) 1.250  (i) 2.120
  (e) 2.857  (j) 1.445

Exercise 1-2
  (a) 1023.1 g/cm$^2$
  (b) 15.4 lb/in$^2$
  (c) 14.8 lb/in$^2$
  (d) 982.1 g/cm$^2$
  (e) 34.8 ft $H_2O$
  (f) 751.2 mm Hg
  (g) 30.9 in Hg
  (h) 11.0 mm Hg
  (i) 763.0 mm Hg
  (j) 1022.0 mb

Exercise 1-3
  (a) 157.5 mm Hg
  (b) 167.7 mm Hg
  (c) 668.3 mm Hg
  (d) 400.4 mm Hg
  (e) 124.5 ft

Exercise 1-4
  (a) $P_2 = P_1 V_1 T_2 / V_2 T_1$
  (b) $T_1 = P_1 V_1 T_2 / P_2 V_2$
  (c) $V_1 = P_2 V_2 T_1 / P_1 T_2$
  (d) $T_2 = P_2 V_2 T_1 / P_1 V_1$

Exercise 1-5
  (a) 137 ml
  (b) 2.55 liters
  (c) 348 ml
  (d) 20.9 liters
  (e) 94.4 ml

Exercise 1-6
  (a) 251.6 ml
  (b) 1.896 liters
  (c) 59.72 ml
  (d) 358.2 ml
  (e) 2.370 liters

Exercise 1-7
  (a) $V_1 \times 726.4 \times 303/694.6 \times 303$
  (b) $V_1 \times 724.7 \times 297/734.6 \times 297$
  (c) $V_1 \times 724.1 \times 298/741.0 \times 293$
  (d) $V_1 \times 754.2 \times 295/715.6 \times 288$
  (e) $V_1 \times 763.0 \times 303/734.4 \times 297$

Exercise 2-1
  (a) 80.9 g  (f) 56.1 g
  (b) 32.7 g  (g) 49.7 g
  (c) 47 g  (h) 26 g
  (d) 47.3 g  (i) 35 g
  (e) 17 g  (j) 29.15 g

Exercise 2-2
  (a) 31.15 g
  (b) 55.5 g
  (c) 54.7 g
  (d) 51.7 g
  (e) Al = 32.2 g; OH = 48.3 g; Cl = 96.5 g

Exercise 2-3
  (a) 1.99 gEw
  (b) 0.9 gEw
  (c) 2.19 gEw
  (d) 0.193 gEw
  (e) 22.3 gEw

Exercise 2-4
  (a) 100 mEq
  (b) 0.1 mEq
  (c) 17.8 mEq
  (d) 204.5 mg
  (e) 1.614 g

Exercise 2-5
  (a) 129 mEq/$\ell$
  (b) 291 mg/d$\ell$
  (c) 5.9 mEq/$\ell$
  (d) 4.5 mEq/$\ell$
  (e) 159 mg/d$\ell$

Exercise 2-6
  (a) 9 g  (d) 249.5 g
  (b) 1 ml  (e) 2.5 M
  (c) 25 g : 225 g  (f) 500 ml

  (g) 51.3 g  (i) 100 ml
  (h) 0.5 N  (j) 114 mg

Exercise 2-7
  (a) 22.5 ml
  (b) 13 ml
  (c) 10.14%
  (d) 0.8 ml
  (e) 1.5 N

Exercise 2-8
  (a) $6.42 \times 10^{-5}$
  (b) $1.84 \times 10^{-5}$

Exercise 2-9
  (a) 4.12
  (b) 1.52
  (c) 11.29
  (d) 7.99
  (e) 9.06

Exercise 2-10
  (a) $6.17 \times 10^{-4}$
  (b) $1.21 \times 10^{-9}$
  (c) $9.77 \times 10^{-6}$
  (d) $5.50 \times 10^{-11}$
  (e) $2.19 \times 10^{-7}$

Exercise 3-1
  (a) 13.6 cm $H_2O$
  (b) $2.33 \times 10^{-2}$ cm (233 $\mu$)

Exercise 3-2
  $C_T = 0.18$ $\ell$/cm $H_2O$

Exercise 4-1
  2.01 times as diffusible

Exercise 4-2
  (a) 7.49
  (b) 7.32
  (c) 6.82
  (d) 53.2
  (e) 22.6
  (f) 23.9
  (g) 35.3  33.7
  (h) 31.1  29.9
  (i) 13.1  12.4

# REFERENCES

1. Williams, A. L., et al.: Introduction to chemistry, Reading, Mass., 1973, Addison-Wesley Publishing Co., Inc.
2. Saunders, F. A.: A survey of physics for college students, New York, 1936, Henry Holt & Co.
3. Quagliano, J. V.: Chemistry, Englewood Cliffs, N.J., 1964, Prentice-Hall, Inc.
4. Armstrong, H.G.: Aerospace medicine, Baltimore, 1961, The Williams & Wilkins Co.
5. List, R. J., editor: Smithsonian meteorological tables, Washington, D.C., 1958, Smithsonian Institution.
6. Campbell, E. J. M.: The respiratory muscles and the mechanics of breathing, London, 1958, Lloyd-Luke, Ltd.
7. Sinclair, J. D.: In Licht, S., editor: Electrodiagnosis and electromyography, New Haven, Conn., 1961, Elizabeth Licht, Publisher.
8. Agostoni, E.: In Howell, J. B. L., and Campbell, E. J. M., editors: International Symposium on Breathlessness, Oxford, 1966, Blackwell Scientific Publications.
9. Best, C. H., and Taylor, N. B.: The physiological basis of medical practice, Baltimore, 1943, The Williams & Wilkins Co.
10. McDonald, J. E.: The shape of raindrops, Sci. Am. **190**:64, 1954.
11. Clements, J. A.: Surface tension in lungs, Sci. Am. **207**:121, 1962.
12. Avery, M. E., and Clements, J. A.: Pulmonary surfactants and atelectasis, Physiology, vol 1, March, 1963.
13. Scarpelli, E. M.: The surfactant system of the lung, Philadelphia, 1968, Lea & Febiger.
14. Clements, J. A.: In Liebow, A. A., et al., editors: The lung, Baltimore, 1968, The Williams & Wilkins Co.
15. Rahn, H., Otis, A. B., Chadwick, L. E., and Fenn, W. O.: The pressure-volume diagram of the thorax and lung, Am. J. Physiol. **146**:161, 1946.
16. Fenn, W. O.: Mechanics of respiration, Am. J. Med. **10**:79, 1951.
17. Comroe, J. H., Jr., et al.: The lung, Chicago 1962, Year Book Medical Publishers, Inc.
18. Black, N. H.: An introductory course in college physics, New York, 1956, The Macmillan Co.
19. Mead, J.: Mechanical properties of the lung, Physiol. Rev. **41**:281, 1961.
20. Bates, D. V., and Christie, R. V.: Respiratory function in disease, Philadelphia, 1964, W. B. Saunders Co.
21. Cherniak, R. M., and Cherniak, L.: Respiration in health and disease, Philadelphia, 1962, W. B. Saunders Co.
22. Divertie, M. B., and Brown, A. L., Jr.: The fine structure of the normal alveolocapillary membrane, J.A.M.A. **187**:938, 1964.
23. Dittmer, D. S., and Grebe, R. M., editors: Handbook of respiration, Philadelphia, 1958, W. B. Saunders Co.
24. Roughton, F. J. W.: The average time spent by the blood in the human lung capillary, and its relation to the rates of carbon monoxide uptake and elimination in man, Am. J. Physiol. **143**:621, 1945.
25. Nunn, J. F. Applied respiratory physiology, London, 1969, Butterworth & Co. (Publishers), Ltd.
26. Benesch, R., and Benesch, R. E.: Intracellular organic phosphates as regulators of oxygen release by haemoglobin, Nature **221**:618, 1969.
27. Astrup, P.: Red-cell pH and oxygen affinity of hemoglobin, N. Engl. J. Med. **283**:202, 1970.
28. Oski, F. A., et al.: Red-cell 2,3-diphosphoglycerate levels in subjects with chronic hypoxemia, N. Engl. J. Med. **280**:1165, 1969.
29. Torrance, J., et al.: Intraerythrocyte adaptation to anemia, N. Engl. J. Med. **283**:165, 1970.
30. Lichtman, M. A., et al.: Reduced red cell glycolysis, 2,3-diphosphoglycerate and adenosine triphosphate concentration, and increased hemo-

globin-oxygen affinity caused by hypophosphatemia, Ann. Intern. Med. **74**:562, 1971.

31. Klocke, R. A.: Oxygen transport and 2,3-diphosphoglycerate (DPG), Chest **62**(suppl.):79s, 1972.

31a. Peters, J. P., and Van Slyke, D. D.: Quantitative clinical chemistry, Baltimore, 1931, The Williams & Wilkins Co., vol. 2.

32. ACCP-ATS Joint Committee on Pulmonary Nomenclature: Pulmonary terms and symbols, Chest **67**:583, 1975.

33. Dejours, P.: Respiration, New York, 1966, Oxford University Press, Inc.

34. Winterstein, H.: Chemical control of pulmonary ventilation, N. Engl. J. Med. **255**:331, 1956.

35. Winterstein, H.: Chemical control of pulmonary ventilation, N. Engl. J. Med. **255**:216, 1956.

36. Peters, R. M.: The mechanical basis of respiration. Boston, 1969, Little, Brown & Co.

37. Lugliani, R., et al.: Effect of bilateral carotid-body resection on ventilatory control at rest and during exercise in man, N. Engl. J. Med. **285**:1105, 1971.

38. Dorland's illustrated medical dictionary, ed. 25, Philadelphia, 1974, W. B. Saunders Co.

39. Refsum, H. E.: Acid-base disturbances in chronic pulmonary disease, Ann. N.Y. Acad. Sci. **133**:142, 1966.

40. Petty, T. L., and Neff, T. A.: Renal function in respiratory failure, J.A.M.A. **217**:82, 1971.

41. Snively, W. D., et al.: Systematic approach to fluid balance, Part 1, G.P. **13**:74, Jan., 1956.

42. Snively, W. D., et al.: Systematic approach to fluid balance, Part 2, G. P. **13**:74, Feb., 1956.

43. Fordham, C. C., III, and Relman, A. J.: Mixed respiratory and metabolic acidosis, N. Engl. J. Med. **256**:698, 1957.

44. Robin, E. D.: Abnormalities of acid-base regulation in chronic pulmonary disease, with special reference to hypercapnia and extracellular alkalosis, N. Engl. J. Med. **268**:917, 1963.

45. Scher, A. M.: The electrocardiogram, Sci. Am. **205**:137, 1961.

46. Bjurstedt, H.: In Luisada, A., editor: Cardiovascular functions, New York, 1962, McGraw-Hill Book Co.

47. Visscher, M. B., et al.: The physiology and pharmacology of lung edema, Pharmacol. Rev. **8**:389, 1956.

48. Egan, D. F.: Management of acute pulmonary edema, Hosp. Med. **2**:20, 1966.

49. Ferrer, M. I., and Harvey, R. M.: In Adams, W. R., and Vieth, I., editors: Pulmonary circulation: an international symposium, New York, 1959, Grune & Stratton, Inc.

50. Steinborn, K. E., et al.: Chronic cor pulmonale in the respiratory poliomyelitis patient, Arch. Intern. Med. **110**:249, 1962.

51. Stuart-Harris, C. H.: Pulmonary hypertension and chronic obstructive bronchitis, Am. Rev. Respir. Dis. **97**:9, 1968.

52. Rushmer, R. F., et al.: In Bock, K. D., editor: Essential hypertension symposium on shock, Berlin, 1962, Springer-Verlag.

53. Friedberg, C. H.: Diseases of the heart, Philadelphia, 1956, W. B. Saunders Co.

54. Bordicks, K. J.: Patterns of shock, New York, 1965, The Macmillan Co.

55. Warren, R.: Surgery, Philadelphia, 1963, W. B. Saunders Co.

56. Editorial: Central venous monitoring in shock, Conn. Med. **32**:79, 1968.

57. Jernigan, W. R., et al.: The internal jugular vein for access to the central venous system, J.A.M.A. **218**:97, 1971.

58. Goldman, R. H., et al.: The use of central venous oxygen saturation measurements in a coronary care unit, Ann. Intern. Med. **68**:1280, 1968.

59. Hutter, A. M., Jr., and Moss, A. J.: Central venous oxygen saturation, J.A.M.A. **212**:299, 1970.

60. Swan, H. J. C., and Ganz, W.: Catheterization of the heart in man with the use of a flow-directed balloon-tipped catheter, N. Engl. J. Med. **283**: 447, 1970.

61. Bolognini, V.: The Swan-Ganz pulmonary artery catheter: implications for nursing, Heart Lung **3**:976, 1974.

62. Rackley, C. E., et al.: Left ventricular function in acute myocardial infarction, and its clinical significance, Circulation **45**:231, 1972.

63. Forrester, J. S., et al.: Filling pressures in the right and left sides of the heart in acute myocardial infarction, N. Engl. J. Med. **285**:190, 1971.

64. Smith, R. E.: In Watson, C. J., editor: Outlines of internal medicine, Dubuque, Iowa, 1958, William C. Brown Co.

65. Rushmer, R. F.: Cardiac diagnosis, Philadelphia, 1955, W. B. Saunders Co.

66. Price, H. L.: Effects of carbon dioxide on the cardiovascular system, Anesthesiology **21**:652, 1960.

67. Hoffman, B. F., et al.: Physiological basis of cardiac arrhythmias, Mod. Concepts Cardiovasc. Dis. **35**:103, 1966.

68. Cherniak, R. M., and Cherniak, L.: Respiration in health and disease, Philadelphia, 1962, W. B. Saunders Co.

69. Williams, M. H., Jr.: Clinical applications of cardiopulmonary physiology, New York, 1960, Paul B. Hoeber, Inc., Medical Book Division, Harper & Row, Publishers.

70. Editorial: Hypoxemia vs. hypoxia, N. Engl. J. Med. **274**:908, 1966.

71. Barcroft, J.: Anoxemia, Lancet **2**:485, 1920.

72. Van Liere, E. J., and Stickney, J. C.: Hypoxia, Chicago, 1963, University of Chicago Press.

73. Campbell, E. J. M.: The management of acute respiratory failure in chronic bronchitis and emphysema, Am. Rev. Respir. Dis. **96**:626, 1967.

74. Cherniak, R. M., and Cherniak, L.: Respiration in health and disease, Philadelphia, 1962, W. B. Saunders Co.

75. Shaw, D. B., and Simpson, T.: Polycythemia in emphysema, Q. J. Med. **30**:135, 1961.

76. Comroe, J. H., Jr.: Physiology of respiration, Chicago, 1966, Year Book Medical Publishers, Inc.

77. Filley, G. F.: Pulmonary insufficiency and respiratory failure, Philadelphia, 1967, Lea & Febiger.

78. Shulman, L. E.: Hypertrophic osteoarthropathy, Bull. Rheum. Dis. **7**:135, 1957.

79. Lipman, B. S., and Massie, E.: Signs and symptoms, Philadelphia, 1957, J. B. Lippincott Co.

80. Field, A. S., Jr., and Gray, F. D., Jr.: The width of the nail fold capillary stream in clubbing, Dis. Chest **41**:631, 1962.

81. Kenney, J. (Carney Hospital, Dorchester, Maine): Personal communication.

82. Tappan, V., and Zalar, V.: Pathophysiology of bronchial mucus, Ann. N.Y. Acad. Sci. **106**:722, 1963.

83. Pratt, P. C., and Klugh, G. A.: Chronic expiratory air-flow obstruction—cause or effect of centrilobular emphysema? Dis. Chest **52**:342 1967.

84. Bouhuys, A.: Lung volumes and breathing patterns in wind instrument players, J. Appl. Physiol. **19**:967, 1964.

85. Colp, C., et al.: Diffuse emphysema as a result of non-obstructive interstitial pulmonary disease, Am. Rev. Respir. Dis. **96**:788, 1967.

86. Gray, F. D., Jr.: Ventilation-perfusion ratios in cardiopulmonary diseases, Conn. Med. **31**:338, 1967.

87. Shibel, E. M., et al.: Inhalation lung scanning evaluation—radioaerosol versus radioxenon techniques, Chest **56**:284, 1969.

88. DeNardo, G. L., et al.: The ventilatory scan in the diagnosis of pulmonary embolism, N. Engl. J. Med. **282**:1334, 1970.

89. Dittrich, F. A., and Goodman, D. A.: Early recognition of airway disease by the [133]Xe lung scan, J.A.M.A. **220**:1120, 1972.

90. Krumholz, R. A., et al.: Lung scan utilization in the diagnosis of pulmonary disease, Chest **62**:4, 1972.

91. McNeill, B. J., et al.: The scintographic definition of pulmonary embolism, J.A.M.A. **227**:753, 1974.

92. Shoop, J. D.: Why do a lung scan? J.A.M.A. **229**:567, 1974.

93. Dittmer, D. S., and Grebe, R. M., editors: Hand-

book of respiration, Philadelphia, 1958, W. B. Saunders Co.

94. Ayers, L. N.: A guide to the interpretation of pulmonary function tests, New York, 1974, Projects in Health, Inc.

95. West, J. B.: Ventilation/blood flow and gas exchange, Oxford, 1965, Blackwell Scientific Publications.

96. Neuberger, H.: Condensation nuclei: their significance in atmospheric pollution, Mechanical Engineering **70**:221, 1948.

97. Goetz, A.: The physicochemical behavior of submicron aerosols, Am. Rev. Respir. Dis. **83**:410, 1961.

98. Brown, J. H., et al.: The retention of particulate matter in the human lung, Am. J. Public Health **40**:450, 1960.

99. Lovejoy, F. W., Jr., and Morrow, P. E.: Aerosols, bronchodilators, and mucolytic agents, Anesthesiology **23**:460, 1962.

100. Hatch, T. F., and Gross, P.: Pulmonary deposition and retention of inhaled aerosols, New York, 1964, Academic Press, Inc.

101. Altshuler, B., et al.: Aerosol deposition in the human respiratory tract, Arch. Industr. Health **15**: 293, 1957.

102. Dautrebande, L., et al.: Lung deposition of fine dust particles, Arch. Industr. Health **16**:179, 1957.

103. Hayek, A.: Cellular structure and mucus activity in the bronchial tree and alveoli, Ciba Foundation symposium on pulmonary structure and function, Boston, 1962, Little, Brown & Co.

104. Hatch, T. F., and Gross, P.: Pulmonary deposition and retention of inhaled aerosols, New York, 1964, Academic Press, Inc.

105. Hatch, T. F.: Distribution and deposition of inhaled particles in the respiratory tract, Bacteriol. Rev. **25**:237, 1961.

106. Dautrebande, L.: Microaerosols, New York, 1962, Academic Press, Inc.

107. Mercer, T. T., et al.: Output characteristics of several commercial nebulizers, Ann. Allergy **23**:314, 1965.

108. Muir, D. C. F.: Distribution of aerosol particles in exhaled air, J. Appl. Physiol. **23**:210, 1967.

109. Patton, D. M.: The evidence for different types of beta-adrenergic receptors, Am. Heart J. **77**: 707, 1969.

110. Lands, A. M., et al.: Differentiation of receptor systems activated by sympathomimetic amines, Nature **214**:597, 1967.

111. Santa Cruz, R., et al.: Tracheal mucous velocity in normal man and patients with obstructive lung disease: effects of terbutaline, Am. Rev. Respir. Dis. **109**:458, 1974.

112. Keighley, J. F.: Iatrogenic asthma associated with

adrenergic aerosols, Ann. Intern. Med. **65**:985, 1966.

113. Editorial: Sympathomimetic bronchodilators, Lancet **1**:535, 1971.

114. Sollman, T.: A manual of pharmacology, Philadelphia, 1957, W. B. Saunders Co.

115. Lands, A. M., et al.: The pharmacologic actions of the bronchodilator drug isoetharine J. Am. Pharm. Assoc. **47**:744, 1958.

116. Shulman, M., et al.: Cardiovascular effects of isoetharine administered to surgical patients during cyclopropane anesthesia, Br. J. Anaesth. **42**:439, 1970.

117. El-Shaboury, A. H.: Controlled study of a new inhalant in asthma and bronchitis, Br. Med. J. **5416**:1037, 1964.

117a. Kelman, G. R., et al.: Cardiovascular effects of solbutamol, Nature **221**:1251, 1969.

118. Eisenstadt, W. S., and Nichols, S. S.: Adverse effects of adrenergic aerosols in bronchial asthma, Ann. Allergy **27**:283, 1969.

119. Cohen, A. A., and Hale, F. C.: Comparative effects of isoproterenol aerosols on airway resistance in obstructive pulmonary disease, Am. J. Med. Sci. **249**:309, 1965.

120. Davison, F. R.: Handbook of materia medica, toxicology, and pharmacology, St. Louis, 1949, The C. V. Mosby Co.

121. Nadel, J. A., and Widdicombe, J. G.: Mechanism of bronchoconstriction with dust inhalation, Clin. Res. **10**:91, 1962.

122. Dautrebrande, L., et al.: Effects of atropine microaerosols on airway resistance in man, Arch. Int. Pharmacodyn. **139**:198, 1962.

123. Chamberlain, D. A., et al.: Atropine methonitrate and isoprenaline in bronchial asthma, Lancet **2**:1019, 1962.

124. Storms, W. W., et al.: Aerosol Sch 1000, Am. Rev. Respir. Dis. **111**:419, 1975.

125. Gross, N. J.: Sch 1000: a new anticholinergic bronchodilator, Am. Rev. Respir. Dis. **112**:823, 1975.

126. Davidson. M. B.: Reaction to intravenous aminophylline, N. Engl. J. Med. **285**:689, 1971.

127. Segal, M. S.: Advances in inhalation therapy, with particular reference to cardiorespiratory disease, N. Engl. J. Med. **231**:553, 1944.

128. Prigol, S. J., et al.: The treatment of asthma by inhalation of aerosol of aminophylline, J. Allerg. **18**:16, 1947.

129. Horton, G. E.: The value and safety of nebulized aminophylline in acute bronchial asthma, J. Tenn. Med. Assoc. **59**:239, 1966.

130. Forsham, P. H.: The adrenal gland, Clin. Symp. **15**:3, 1963.

131. Kleiner, I. S., and Orten, J. M.: Biochemistry, St. Louis, 1962, The C. V. Mosby Co.

132. Williams, R. H., editor: Textbook of endocrinology, Philadelphia, 1962, W. B. Saunders Co.

133. Norman, P. S., et al.: Adrenal function during the use of dexamethasone aerosols in the treatment of ragweed hay fever, J. Allerg. **40**:57, 1967.

134. Fisch, B. R., and Grater, W. C.: Dexamethasone aerosol in respiratory tract disease, J. New Drugs **2**:298, 1962.

135. Crepea, S. B.: Inhalation corticosteroid (dexamethasone) management of chronically asthmatic children, J. Allerg. **34**:119, 1963.

136. Novey, H. S., and Beall, G.: Aerosolized steroids and induced Cushing's syndrome, Arch. Intern. Med. **115**:602, 1965.

137. Linder, W. R.: Adrenal suppression by aerosol steroid inhalation, Arch. Intern. Med. **113**:655, 1964.

138. Cohen, B.: Acute bronchodilator properties of a steroid microaerosol, Curr. Ther. Res. **6**:73, 1964.

139. Mathison, D. A., et al.: Cromolyn treatment of asthma, J.A.M.A. **216**:1454, 1971.

140. Nikano, J.: Prostaglandins and the circulation, Mod. Concepts Cardiovasc. Dis. **40**:49, 1971.

141. Parker, C. W., and Snider, D. E.: Prostaglandins in asthma, Ann. Intern. Med. **78**:963, 1973.

142. Katz, R. L., and Katz, G. J.: Prostaglandins— basic and clinical considerations, Anesthesiology **40**:471, 1974.

143. Said, S. I., et al.: Pulmonary alveolar hypoxia: release of prostaglandins and other humoral mediators, Science **185**:1180, 1974.

144. Tainter, M. L., et al.: Alevaire as a mucolytic agent, N. Engl. J. Med. **253**:764, 1955.

145. Miller, J. B., et al.: Alevaire inhalations for eliminating secretions in asthma, sinusitis, and bronchiectasis of adults, Ann. Allergy **12**:611, 1954.

146. Sadove, M. S., and Miller, C. E.: Postoperative aerosol therapy, J.A.M.A. **156**:759, 1954.

147. Denton, R.: Continuous nebulization therapy, Pediatr. Clin. North Am. **1**:625, 1954.

148. Palmer, K. N. V.: The effect of an aerosol detergent in chronic bronchitis, Lancet **272-1**:611, 1957.

149. Sheffner, A. L.: The mucolytic activity, mechanisms of action, and metabolism of acetylcysteine, Pharmacotherapy **1**:47, 1964.

150. Hirsch, S. R., and Kory, R. C.: An evaluation of the effect of nebulized N-acetylcysteine on sputum consistency, J. Allerg. **39**:265, 1967.

151. Moser, K. M., and Rhodes, P. G.: Acute effects of aerosolized acetylcysteine upon spirometric measurements in subjects with and without obstructive pulmonary disease, Dis. Chest **49**:370, 1966.

152. Thomas, P. A., and Treasure, R. I.: Effect of

N-acetyl-L-cysteine on pulmonary surface activity, Am. Rev. Respir. Dis. **94**:175, 1966.

153. Webb, W. R.: New mucolytic agents for sputum liquefaction, Postgrad. Med. **36**:449, 1964.

154. Mucolytic agent, Br. Med. J. **2**:603, Sept, 1966.

155. Anderson, G.: A clinical trial of a mucolytic agent —acetylcysteine— in chronic bronchitis, Br. J. Dis. Chest **60**:101, 1966.

156. Denton, R., et al.: N-acetylcysteine in cystic fibrosis, Am. Rev. Respir. Dis. **95**:643, 1967.

157. Luisada, A. A., et al.: Alcohol vapor by inhalation in the treatment of acute pulmonary edema, Circulation **5**:363, 1952.

158. Cosentino, A. M.: Queries and comments, Inhal. Ther. **15**:95, 1970.

159. Finley, T. M.: Pulmonary surface activity and the problems of atelectasis, wetting, foaming, and detergency in the lung, Anesth. Analg. **42**:35, 1963.

160. Modell, J. H., et al.: The effect of wetting and antifoaming agents on pulmonary surfactant, Anesthesiology **30**:164, 1969.

161. Limber, C. R., et al.: Enzymatic lysis of respiratory secretions by aerosol trypsin, J.A.M.A. **149**:816, 1952.

162. Unger, L., and Unger, A. H.: Trypsin inhalations in respiratory conditions with thick sputum, J.A.M.A. **152**:1109, 1953.

163. Prince, H. E., et al.: Aerosol trypsin in the treatment of asthma, Ann. Allergy **12**:25, 1954.

164. Salomon, A., et al.: Aerosols of pancreatic dornase in bronchopulmonary disease, Ann. Allergy **12**:71, 1954.

165. Sherry, S., et al.: Presence and significance of desoxyribose nucleotide in purulent exudate, Proc. Soc. Exp. Biol. Med. **68**:179, 1948.

166. Meunster, J. J., et al.: Treatment of unresolved pneumonia with streptokinase and streptodornase, Am. J. Med. **12**:367, 1952.

167. Craven, J. F.: Treatment of obstructive atelectasis by aerosol administration of proteolytic enzymes, J. Pediatr. **42**:228, 1953.

168. Cliffton, E. E.: Pancreatic dornase aerosol in pulmonary, endotracheal, and endobronchial disease, Dis. Chest **30**:1, 1956.

169. Lyons, H. A.: Use of therapeutic aerosols, Am. J. Cardiol. **12**:461, 1963.

170. Miller, W. F.: Antibiotic aerosols. In Kagan, B. M., editor: Antimicrobial therapy, Philadelphia, 1970, W. B. Saunders Co.

171. Olsen, A. M.: Streptomycin aerosol in the treatment of chronic bronchiectasis: preliminary report, Proc. Staff Meet. Mayo Clin. **21**:53, 1946.

172. Garthwaite, B., and Barach, A. L.: Penicillin aerosol therapy in bronchiectasis, lung abscess, and chronic bronchitis, Am. J. Med. **3**:261, 1947.

173. Eastlake, C., Jr.: Aerosol therapy in sinusitis, bronchiectasis, and lung abscess, Bull. N.Y. Acad. Med. **26**:423, 1950.

174. Christie, H. E., et al.: Aerosol therapy for lung abscess, Can. Med. Assoc. J. **62**:478, 1950.

175. Melica, A., et al.: Oxytetracycline inhalation in the treatment of acute and chronic bronchial infection, G. Clin. Med. **47**:416, 1962.

176. Naumov, G. P.: Pathologic changes in upper respiratory passages and lungs following use of antibiotic electroaerosols, Fed. Proc. **25**:654, 1966.

177. Pines, A., et al.: Gentamicin and colistin in chronic purulent bronchial infections, Br. Med. J. **2**:543, 1967.

178. Bilodeau, M., et al.: Studies of absorption of kanamycin by aerosol, Ann. N.Y. Acad. Sci. **132**:870, 1966.

179. Spier, R., et al.: Aerosolized pancreatic dornase and antibiotics in pulmonary infection, J.A.M.A. **178**:878, 1961.

180. Egan, D.: Humidity and water aerosol therapy, Conn. Med. **31**:353, 1967.

181. Cushing, I. E., and Miller, W. F.: Consideration in humidification by nebulization, Dis. Chest, vol. 34, Oct., 1958.

182. Yue, W. Y., and Cohen, S. S.: Sputum induction by newer inhalation methods in patients with pulmonary tuberculosis, Dis. Chest **51**:611, 1967.

183. Cohen, B. M., and Crandall, C.: Physiologic benefits of "thermo-fog" as a bronchodilator vehicle: acute ventilation responses of 93 patients, Am. J. Med. Sci. **247**:57, 1964.

184. Tomashefski, J. F., et al.: An environmental contamination control unit for use during aerosol administration, Am. Rev. Respir. Dis. **96**:1246, 1967.

185. Hensler, N., et al.: The use of hypertonic aerosol in production of sputum for diagnosis of tuberculosis, Dis. Chest **40**:639, 1961.

186. Lillehei, J. P.: Sputum induction with heated aerosol inhalations for the diagnosis of tuberculosis, Am. Rev. Respir. Dis. **84**:276, 1961.

187. Umiker, W. O.: A new vista in pulmonary cytology: aerosol induction of sputum, Dis. Chest **39**:512, 1961.

188. Johnson, J. R., et al.: Aerosol-induced sputum: an effective, inexpensive method for nebulization of a super-heated mixture of 40 percent propylene glycol in isotonic saline, Dis. Chest **42**:251, 1962.

189. Robillard, E., et al.: Microaerosol administration of synthetic dipalmitoyl-lecithin in the respiratory distress syndrome: a preliminary report, Can. Med. Assoc. J. **90**:55, 1964.

190. Rosner, S. W.: Heparin administration as an aerosol, Vasc. Dis. **2**:131, 1965.

191. Smith, G. M., and Armen, R. N.: Pulmonary moniliasis treated by brilliant green aerosol: re-

port of a case, Ann. Intern. Med. 43:1302, 1955.

192. Kass, I., et al.: Treatment of bronchopulmonary moniliasis by dye inhalation, Dis. Chest 21:205, 1952.

193. Egan, D. F.: Humidity and water aerosol therapy, Conn. Med. 31:353, 1967.

194. Dautrebande, L.: Microaerosols, New York, 1962, Academic Press, Inc.

195. Taylor, G. J., IV, and Harris, W. S.: Cardiac toxicity of aerosol propellants, J.A.M.A. 214:81, 1970.

196. Silverglade, A.: Cardiac toxicity of aerosol propellants, J.A.M.A. 222:827, 1972.

197. Harris, W.: Aerosol propellants are toxic to the heart, J.A.M.A. 223:1508, 1973.

198. Chiov, W. L.: Aerosol propellants: cardiac toxicity and long biological half-life, J.A.M.A. 227:658, 1974.

199. Silverglade, A.: Aerosol propellants, J.A.M.A. 231:136, 1975.

200. Tovell, R. M., and Little, D. M., Jr.: The utilization of fog as a therapeutic agent, Anesthesiology 18:470, 1957.

201. Cushing, I. E., and Miller, W. F.: Considerations in humidification by nebulization, Dis. Chest 34:388, 1958.

202. Welts, R. E., et al.: Humidification of oxygen during inhalational therapy, N. Engl. J. Med. 268:644, 1963.

203. Litt, M., and Swift, D. F.: The Babington nebulizer: a new principle for generation of therapeutic aerosols, Am. Rev. Respir. Dis. 105:308, 1972.

204. Klein, E. F., et al.: Performance characteristics of conventional and prototype humidifiers and nebulizers, Chest 64:690, 1973.

205. Andrews, A. H., Jr.: Ultrasonic aerosol generator, Presbyt. St. Luke Hosp. Med. Bull. 3:155, 1964.

206. Proceedings of the First Conference on Clinical Application of the Ultrasonic Nebulizer, Somerset, Pa., 1966, DeVilbiss Co.

207. Boucher, R. M. G., and Kreuter, J.: Ultrasonic nebulization, Ann. Allergy 26:591, 1968.

208. Gauthier, W. D.: Operational characteristics of the ultrasonic nebulizer, Proceedings of the First Conference on Clinical Application of the Ultrasonic Nebulizer, Somerset, Pa., 1966, De Vilbiss Co.

209. Stevens, H. R., and Albregt, H. B.: Assessment of ultrasonic nebulization, Anesthesiology 27:648, 1966.

210. Modell, J. H., et al.: Effect of ultrasonic nebulized suspensions on pulmonary surfactant, Dis. Chest 50:627, 1966.

211. Modell, J. H., et al.: Effect of chronic exposure to ultrasonic aerosols on the lungs, Anesthesiology 28:680, 1967.

212. Allan, D.: Artificial humidification, Med. Sci. 17:41, Jan., 1966.

213. Doershuk, C. F., and Matthews, L. W.: Cystic fibrosis, Postgrad. Med. 40:550, 1966.

214. Boucher, R. G. M., and Kreuter, J.: Fundamentals of the ultrasonic atomization of medicated solutions, Ann. Allergy 26:591, 1968.

215. Glick, R. V.: Drug reconcentration in aerosol generators, Inhal. Ther. 15:179, 1970.

216. National Fire Protection Association, 470 Atlantic Ave., Boston, Mass., 02210, Pamphlet nos. 565, 566

217. Compressed Gas Association, 500 Fifth Ave., New York, N.Y. 10036, Pamphlet P-2, Characteristics and safe handling of medical gases.

218. Compressed Gas Association, 500 Fifth Ave., New York, N.Y. 10036, Pamphlet V-1, American Standard Compressed Gas Cylinder Valve Outlet and Inlet Connections.

219. Compressed Gas Association, 500 Fifth Ave., New York, N.Y. 10036, Pamphlet V-5, Diameter Index Safety System.

220. Dole, M.: The natural history of oxygen, J. Gen. Physiol. 49(supp.):5, 1965.

221. Clamann, H. G.: Fire hazards, Ann. N.Y. Acad. Sci. 117:814, 1965.

222. Cullen, J. H., and Kaemmerlen, J. T.: Effect of oxygen administration at low rates of flow in hypercapnic patients, Am. Rev. Respir. Dis. 95:116, 1967.

223. Massaro, D. J., et al.: Effect of various modes of oxygen administration on the arterial gas values in patients with respiratory acidosis, Br. Med. J. 2:627, 1962.

224. Hutchison, D. C. S., et al.: Controlled oxygen therapy in respiratory failure, Br. Med. J. 2:1157, 1964.

225. Arnold, W. H., Jr., and Grant, J. L.: Oxygen-induced hypoventilation, Am. Rev. Respir. Dis. 95:255, 1967.

226. Fine, J., Banks, B., and Hermanson, L.: The treatment of gaseous distention of the intestine by inhalation of 95% oxygen, Ann. Surg. 103:375, 1936.

227. Dole, M.: The natural history of oxygen. (Source unknown.)

228. Welch, B. E., et al.: Time-concentration effects in relation to oxygen toxicity in man, Fed. Proc. 22:1053, 1963.

229. Doleval, V.: Voluntary tolerance of 100% oxygen, Rev. Med. Aeron. 25:219, 1962.

230. Laurenzi, G. A., et al.: Adverse effect of oxygen on tracheal mucus flow, N. Engl. J. Med. 279:333, 1968.

231. Caldwell, P. R. B., et al.: Effect of oxygen breathing at one atmosphere on the surface activity of lung extracts in dogs, Ann. N.Y. Acad. Sci. 121:823, 1965.

232. Hyde, R. W., and Rawson, A. J.: Unintentional iatrogenic oxygen pneumonitis—response to therapy, Ann. Intern. Med. **71**:517, 1969.

233. Northway, W. H., Jr., and Rosan, R. C.: Oxygen therapy hazards in the neonate, Hosp. Practice, Jan., 1969.

234. Nash, G., et al.: Pulmonary lesions associated with oxygen therapy and artificial ventilation, N. Engl. J. Med. **276**:368, 1967.

235. Pratt, P. C.: Pulmonary capillary proliferation induced by oxygen inhalation, Am. J. Pathol. **34**:1033, 1958.

236. Bruns, P. D., and Shields, L. V.: High oxygen and hyaline-like membranes, Am. J. Obstet. Gynecol. **67**:1224, 1954.

237. Shanklin, D. R., and Wolfson, S. L.: Therapeutic oxygen as a possible cause of pulmonary hemorrhage in premature infants, N. Engl. J. Med. **277**:833, 1967.

238. Patz, A.: Oxygen administration to the premature infant, Am. J. Ophthalmol. **63**:351, 1967.

239. Kobayashi, T., and Murakami, S.: Blindness of an adult caused by oxygen, J.A.M.A. **219**:741, 1972.

239a. Fridovich, I.: Oxygen: boon and bane, Am. Sci. **63**:54, 1975.

239b. Crapo, J. D.: Superoxide dismutase and tolerance to pulmonary oxygen toxicity, Chest **67** (suppl.):39s, 1975.

239c. McCord, J. M., and Fridovich, I.: Superoxide dismutase, J. Biol. Chem. **244**:6049, 1969.

240. Babior, B. M., et al.: The production by leukocytes of superoxide: a potential bactericidal agent, J. Clin. Invest. **52**:741, 1973.

241. Curvette, J. T., et al.: Defect in pyridine nucleotide dependent superoxide production by a particulate fraction from the granulocytes of patients with chronic granulomatous diseases, N. Engl. J. Med. **293**:628, 1975.

242. Lee, C. J., et al.: Cardiovascular and metabolic responses to spontaneous and positive-pressure breathing of 100% oxygen at one atmosphere, J. Thorac. Cardiovasc. Surg. **53**:770, 1967.

243. Wright, R., et al.: Risk of mortality in interrupted exposure to 100% oxygen: role of air vs. lowered oxygen tension, Am. J. Physiol. **210**:1015, 1966.

244. Collis, J. M., and Bethune, D. W.: Oxygen by face mask and nasal catheter, Lancet **1**:787, 1967.

245. Hedley-Whyte, J., and Winter, P. M.: Oxygen therapy, Clin. Pharmacol. Ther. **8**:696, 1967.

246. Buck, J. B., and McCormack, W. C.: A nasal mask for premature infants, J. Pediatr. **66**:123, 1965.

247. Committee on Public Health: A report: effective administration of inhalational therapy with special reference to ambulatory and emergency oxygen treatment, Bull. N.Y. Acad. Med. **38**:135, 1962.

248. Kory, R. C., et al.: Comparative evaluation of oxygen therapy techniques, J.A.M.A. **179**:767, 1962.

249. McPherson, S. P.: Oxygen percentage accuracy of air-entrainment masks, Respir. Care **19**:658, 1974.

250. Glick, R. V., and Benner, J. N.: Arterial oxygen tension during oxygen breathing, Inhal. Ther. **13**:31, 1968.

251. Jahn, R. E.: An examination of oxygen and carbon dioxide concentrations in adult oxygen tents, Br. J. Anaesth. **25**:188, 1953.

252. Plano, R. J.: Tests evaluate fire hazards of static sparks, Mod. Hosp. **95**:154, Sept., 1960.

253. Guest, P. G.: Oily fibers may increase oxygen tent fire hazard, Mod. Hosp. **104**:180, May, 1965.

254. Berry, R. C.: Safe practices in handling oxygen equipment, Hospitals **37**:376, 1963.

255. Campbell, E. J. M., and Gebbie, T.: Masks and tent for providing controlled oxygen concentrations, Lancet **1**:468, 1966.

256. Levine, B. E., et al.: The role of long-term continuous oxygen administration in patients with chronic airway obstruction with hypercapnia, Ann. Intern. Med. **66**:639, 1967.

257. Eldridge, F., and Gherman, C.: Studies of oxygen administration in respiratory failure, Ann. Intern. Med. **68**:569, 1968.

258. Egan, D. F.: Therapeutic uses of helium, Conn. Med. **31**:355, 1967.

259. Ishikawa, S., and Segal, M. S.: Re-appraisal of helium-oxygen therapy on patients with chronic lung disease, Ann. Allergy **31**:536, 1973.

260. Souadjian, J., and Cain, J.: Intractable hiccup, Postgrad. Med. **43**:72, 1968.

261. Fishman, A. P.: The roads to respiratory insufficiency, Ann. N.Y. Acad. Med. **121**:657, 1965.

262. Weiss, E. B., and Dulfano, M. J.: Controlled ventilation with intermittent positive-pressure breathing in the management of acute ventilatory failure associated with chronic obstructive pulmonary disease, Ann. Intern. Med. **67**:556, 1967.

263. Mushin, W. W., et al.: Automatic ventilation of the lungs, Oxford, 1959, Blackwell Scientific Publications.

264. Mapleson, W. W.: The effect of changes of lung characteristics on the functioning of automatic ventilators, Anaesthesia **17**:300, 1962.

265. Rattenborg, C., and de Borde, R.: Lung ventilators: function and principles, Inhal. Ther. **12**:48, 1967.

266. Drinker, P., and McKhann, C.: The use of a new

apparatus for prolonged administration of artificial respiration, J.A.M.A. **92**:1658, 1929.

267. Sheldon, G. P.: Pressure breathing in chronic obstructive lung disease, Medicine **42**:197, 1963.

268. Bird Corporation, Richmond, Calif, form no. 8.101 (rev. 1).

269. Edwards, W. L., and Sappenfield, R. S.: Pressure-cycled ventilators and flow-rate control, Anesth. Analg. **47**:77, 1968.

270. Glick, R. V., and Woods, R. H.: The importance of measuring inspired oxygen concentrations during mechanical pulmonary ventilation, Inhal. Ther. **11**:7, 1966.

271. Bennett Respiration Products, Inc.: Bennett PR-2 respiration unit, instruction manual, form 2131 (12-64).

272. Bennett Respiration Products, Inc.: Bennett PR-2 respiration unit, trainer's script, form EA-110TS.

273. Torres, G. E., et al.: The effects of IPPB on intrapulmonary distribution of inspired air, Am. J. Med. **29**:946, 1960.

274. Ayers, S. M., and Giannelli, S., Jr.: Oxygen consumption and alveolar ventilation during intermittent positive pressure breathing, Dis. Chest **50**:409, 1966.

275. Gray, F. D., Jr., and MacIver, S.: The use of inspiratory positive pressure breathing in cardiopulmonary diseases, Dis. Chest, Jan., 1958.

276. Motley, H. L.: Intermittent positive pressure breathing therapy, Inhal. Ther. vol. 7, Feb., 1962.

277. Werko, L.: Influence of positive pressure breathing on the circulation in man, Acta. Med. Scand. (Suppl. 193), 1947.

278. Opie, L. H., et al.: Intrathoracic pressure during intermittent positive-pressure respiration, Lancet **1**:911, 1961.

279. Coonse, G. K., and Aufrance, O. E.: The relation of the intrapleural pressure to the mechanics of the circulation, Am. Heart J. **9**:347, 1934.

280. Printzmetal, M., and Kounts, W. B.: Intrapleural pressure in health and disease and its influence on body function, Medicine **14**:457, 1935.

281. Christie, R. V., and McIntosh, C. A.: The measurement of intrapleural pressure in man, and its significance, J. Clin. Invest. **13**:279, 1934.

282. Kilburn, K. H., and Sicker, H. O.: Hemodynamic effects of continuous positive and negative pressure breathing in normal man, Circ. Res. **8**:660, 1960.

283. Bashour, F. A., et al.: Effect of intermittent positive pressure breathing on the cardiac output and the splanchnic blood flow, Inhal. Ther. **13**:47, 1968.

284. Ashbaugh, D. G., et al.: Acute respiratory distress in adults, Lancet **2**:319, 1967.

285. Sladen, A., et al.: Pulmonary complications and water retention in prolonged mechanical ventilation, N. Engl. J. Med. **279**:448, 1968.

286. Murdaugh, H. V., et al.: Effect of altered intrathoracic pressure on renal hemodynamics, electrolyte excretion, and water clearance, J. Clin. Invest. **38**:834, 1959.

287. Drury, D. R., et al.: The effects of continuous pressure breathing on kidney function, J. Clin. Invest. **26**:945, 1947.

288. Henry, J. P., and Pierce, J. W.: Possible role of cardiac atrial stretch receptors in induction of changes in urine flow, J. Physiol. **131**:572, 1956.

289. Weg, J. G.: Prolonged endotracheal intubation in respiratory failure, Arch. Intern. Med. **120**: 679, 1967.

290. Kuner, J., and Goldman, A.: Prolonged nasotracheal intubation in adults versus tracheostomy, Dis. Chest **51**:270, 1967.

291. Garzon, A. A., et al.: Influence of cannula size on resistance to breathing through tracheostomies, Surg. Forum **14**:219, 1963.

292. Greene, N. M.: Fatal cardiovascular and respiratory failure associated with tracheotomy, N. Engl. J. Med. **261**:846, 1959.

293. Yanagisawa, E., and Kirchner, J. A.: The cuffed tracheotomy tube, Arch. Otolaryngol. **79**:80, 1964.

294. Meyer, J. A.: Tracheotomy care, Int. Anesthesiol. Clin. **4**:675, 1966.

295. Gunn, I. P., et al.: Expiratory resistance of oxygen catheters in patients with tracheostomies, J.A.M.A. **193**:737, 1965.

296. Decancq, H. G., Jr.: Tissue "snowplowing": a post-tracheostomy complication, Am. J. Dis. Child. **108**:94, 1964.

297. Bendixen, H. H., et al.: Respiratory care, St. Louis, 1965, The C. V. Mosby Co.

298. Cooper, J. D., and Grillo, H. C.: The evolution of tracheal injury due to ventilatory assistance through a cuffed tube, Ann. Surg. **169**:334, 1969.

299. Dane, T. E. B., and King, E. G.: A prospective study of complications after tracheostomy for assisted ventilation, Chest **67**:398, 1975.

300. Head, J. M.: Tracheostomy in the management of respiratory problems, N. Engl. J. Med. **264**: 587, 1961.

301. Nelson, T. G., and Bowers, W. T.: Tracheostomy —indications, advantages, techniques, complications, and results, J.A.M.A. **164**:1530, 1957.

302. Cullen, J. H.: An evaluation of tracheostomy in pulmonary emphysema, Ann. Intern. Med. **58**: 953, 1963.

303. Feldman, S. A., editor: Tracheostomy and arti-

ficial ventilation, London, 1967, Edward Arnold (Publishers) Ltd.

304. Engström, C., and Herzog, P.: Ventilation nomogram for practical use with the Engström respirator, Acta Chir. Scand. (Suppl. 245), 1959.

305. Engström, C., et al.: Ventilation nomogram for the newborn and small children to be used with the Engström respirator, Acta Anaesthiol. Scand. 6:175, 1962.

306. Radford, E. P., Jr.: Ventilation standards for use in artificial respiration, J. Appl. Physiol. 7:451, 1955.

307. Merck manual of therapeutics and materia medica, Rahway, N.J., 1940, Merck & Co., Inc.

308. Dittmer, D. S., and Grebe, R. M., editors: Handbook of respiration, Philadelphia, 1958, W. B. Saunders Co.

309. Growth charts used by Children's Hospital Medical Center, Boston, Mass. Courtesy H. C. Stuart, Department of Maternal and Child Health, Harvard School of Public Health, Boston.

310. Avery, M. E.: The lung and its disorders in the newborn infant, Philadelphia, 1964, W. B. Saunders Co.

311. Holt, L. E., Jr., and McIntosh, R.: Diseases of infancy and children, New York, 1940, D. Appleton-Century Co.

312. Cooke, R. J.: The biologic basis of pediatric practice, New York, 1968, McGraw-Hill Book Co.

313. Bendixen, H. H., et al.: Impaired oxygenation in surgical patients during general anesthesia with controlled ventilation, N. Engl. J. Med. 269:991, 1963.

314. Egan, D. F.: Personal experience.

315. Breivik, H., et al.: Normalizing low arterial $CO_2$ tension during mechanical ventilation, Chest 63:525, 1973.

316. DeSautels, D. A., and Bartlett, J. L.: Methods of administering intermittent mandatory ventilation, Respir. Care 19:187, 1974.

317. Civetta, J. M., et al.: "Optimal PEEP" and intermittent mandatory ventilation in the treatment of acute respiratory failure, Respir. Care 20:551, 1975.

318. Greenhouse, B. B.: Muscle relaxants and some problems with their use, Conn. Med. 34:723, 1970.

319. Thomas, E. T.: Circulatory collapse following succinylcholine, Anesth. Analg. 48:333, 1969.

320. Smith, J. P., et al.: Acute respiratory failure in chronic lung disease, Am. Rev. Respir. Dis. 97:791, 1968.

321. Kettel, L. J., et al.: Treatment of acute respiratory acidosis in chronic obstructive lung disease, J.A.M.A. 217:1503, 1971.

322. Anderson, E. F., and Rosenthal, M. H.: Pan-

curonium bromide and tachyarrhythmias, Crit. Care Med. 3:13, 1975.

323. Cherniak, R. M., and Hakimpour, K.: The rational use of oxygen in respiratory insufficiency, J.A.M.A. 199:178, 1967.

324. Mithoefer, J. C., et al.: Oxygen therapy in respiratory failure, N. Engl. J. Med. 277:947, 1967.

325. Drinker, P., et al.: A constant ratio air-oxygen mixer, J.A.M.A. 202:531, 1967.

326. Cheney, F. W.: The effect of respiratory resistance on the blood gas tensions of anesthetized patients, Anesthesiology 28:670, 1967.

327. Ashbaugh, D. G., et al.: Continuous positive pressure breathing (CPPB) in adult respiratory distress syndrome, J. Thorac. Cardiovasc. Surg. 57:31, 1969.

328. Kumar, A., et al.: Continuous positive-pressure ventilation in acute respiratory failure, N. Engl. J. Med. 283:1430, 1970.

329. Gregory, G. A., et al.: Treatment of the idiopathic respiratory-distress syndrome with continuous positive airway pressure, N. Engl. J. Med. 284:1333, 1971.

330. Trinkle, J. K.: A simple modification of existing respirators to provide constant positive-pressure breathing, J. Thorac. Cardiovasc. Surg. 61:617, 1971.

331. Editorial: The difference between PEEP, CPPB, and CPAP, Respir. Care 19:14, 1974.

332. Kirby, R. R., et al.: High level positive end-expiratory pressure (PEEP) in acute respiratory insufficiency, Chest 67:156, 1975.

333. Suter, P. M., et al.: Optimum end-expiratory airway pressure in patients with acute pulmonary failure, N. Engl. J. Med. 292:284, 1975.

334. Demers, R. R., and Saklad, M.: "Assisted PEEP" —assisted mechanical ventilation with positive end-expiratory pressure, Respir. Care 19:435, 1974.

335. Gjerde, G. E.: IMV with PEEP versus MV with PEEP, Respir. Care 20:894, 1975.

336. Ayers, S. M.: Assisted PEEP: helpful or disastrous? Respir. Care 19:410, 1974.

337. Civetta, J. M., et al.: A simple and effective method of employing spontaneous positive pressure ventilation, J. Thorac. Cardiovasc. Surg. 63:312, 1972.

338. Hamilton, F. N., and Singer, M. M.: A breathing circuit for continuous positive airway pressure (CPAP), Crit. Care. Med. 2:86, 1974.

339. Gjerde, G. E.: A method for spontaneous breathing with expiratory positive pressure, Respir. Care 20:839, 1975.

340. Sheely, R. B., and Boudria, C.: More on spontaneous breathing with EPP, Respir. Care 20: 1116, 1975.

341. Kenney, F.: Mechanical ventilation and CPPB with modified Ohio 560 ventilator, Respir. Care **20:**655, 1975.

342. Gregory, G. A., et al.: Treatment of the idiopathic respiratory distress syndrome with continuous positive airway pressure, N. Engl. J. Med. **284:**1333, 1971.

343. Smith, A. C.: Effect of mechanical ventilation on the circulation, Ann. N.Y. Acad. Sci. **121:**742, 1965.

344. Stamm, S. J.: Reliability of capillary blood for the measurement of $P_{O_2}$ and $O_2$ saturation, Dis. Chest **52:**191, 1967.

345. Begin, R., et al.: Value of capillary blood gas analysis in the management of acute respiratory distress, Am. Rev. Respir. Dis. **112:**879, 1975.

346. Downs, J. B., et al.: Intermittent mandatory ventilation: a new approach to weaning patients from mechanical ventilators, Chest **64:**331, 1973.

347. McPherson, S. P., et al.: A circuit that combines ventilator weaning methods using continuous flow ventilation (CFV), Respir. Care **20:**261, 1975.

348. Modell, J. H.: Weaning patients from mechanical ventilation, Respir. Care **20:**373, 1975.

349. Feeley, T. W., and Hedley-Whyte, J.: Weaning from controlled ventilation and supplemental oxygen, N. Engl. J. Med. **292:**903, 1975.

350. Bowser, M. A., et al.: A systematic approach to ventilator weaning, Respir. Care **20:**959, 1975.

351. Thacker, E. W.: Postural drainage and respiratory control, London, 1963, Lloyd-Luke, Ltd.

352. Physiotherapy Department, Brompton Hospital, London: Physiotherapy for medical and surgical thoracic conditions, 1967.

353. Department of Physical Medicine and Rehabilitation, University of Minnesota Medical School, Minneapolis: Techniques of bronchial drainage, 1967.

354. Heimlich, H. J.: A life-saving maneuver to prevent food-choking, J.A.M.A. **234:**398, 1975.

355. Visintine, R. E., and Choong, H. B.: Ruptured stomach after Heimlich maneuver, J.A.M.A. **234:**415, 1975.

356. Editorial: Statement on the "Heimlich maneuver," J.A.M.A. **234:**416, 1975.

357. Yanda, R. L.: The need for leadership in hospital respiratory services, Chest **68:**81, 1975.

358. Egan, D. F.: The stethoscope and the ledger, Chest **68:**1, 1975.

359. United States Department of Commerce, National Bureaus of Standards: The English and metric systems of measurement, special Pub. 304A, rev. ed., 1970.

360. Vawter, S. M., and DeForest, R. E.: The international metric system and medicine, J.A.M.A. **218:**723, 1971.

361. Young, D. S.: Standardized reporting of laboratory data, N. Engl. J. Med. **290:**368, 1974.

# INDEX

## A

A; *see* Ambient temperature or pressure
A-a$_{O_2}$ gradient; *see* Alveolar-arterial oxygen tension gradient
Abbreviations, 506–507
Abdomen
  mechanical ventilation and, 450
  muscles of, 89, 477–482
  negative-pressure breathing and, 385
  vascular reservoirs and, 378
Abdominal breathing, 477–482
Abdominal distention, 201
  mechanical ventilation and, 450
  oxygen and, 293, 308
Abdominal rectus muscle, 89
Abdominal splinting, 201
Abscesses, pulmonary, 240, 461, 471
A-C membrane; *see* Alveolar-capillary membrane
Accessory muscles of ventilation, 87–89
Acetic acid, 69
Acetylcholine, 223–224, 229
Acetylcholinesterase, 224
Acetylcysteine, 236–237
  induced sputum specimen and, 246
  tracheobronchial aspiration and, 410
  ultrasonic nebulizers and, 267–268
Acid salt, 72–73
Acid-base balance; *see* Blood gases and acid-base balance; pH
Acid-base map, 154, 155
Acidemia, 137, 148
  mechanical ventilation and, 332
Acidity, 77–78; *see also* pH
Acidosis, 147–149
  buffers and, 427–428
  metabolic, 148, 152–154
    hyperventilation and, 145
    and respiratory acidosis, 427–428
    treatment of, 424, 425
    oxygen dissociation curves and, 129
  respiratory, 148, 149–151
    buffers in, 424, 425

Acidosis—cont'd
  respiratory—cont'd
    and metabolic acidosis, 427–428
    ventilators and, 422–423
Acids
  equivalent weight of, 51
  ions and, 70–71
ACTH; *see* Adrenocorticotropic hormone
Active transport, 145
Activity, exercises and, 480
Adenosine triphosphate, 130, 296
ADH; *see* Antidiuretic hormone
Administration of respiratory care department; *see* Respiratory care department
Adrenal glands, 223, 231
Adrenaline; *see* Epinephrine
Adrenergic bronchodilators, 224–228
Adrenergic nerves, 224–225
Adrenocorticosteroids, 231–235, 298
Adrenocorticotropic hormone, 232–233
Aerosol and humidity therapy, 213–268; *see also* Aerosols
  adrenocorticosteroids and, 231–235
  antibiotics and, 240–242
  autonomic-active bronchodilators and, 221–230; *see also* Bronchodilators
  for bronchospasm and mucosal edema, 221
  generators in, 248–268
    bubble-diffusion humidifier in, 262
    Hydro-Sphere nebulizer-humidifier in, 260–261
    impeller nebulizer in, 262
    jet aerosol-humidifier in, 249–260
    oxygen tents and, 311
    pass-over humidifier in, 261
    ultrasonic nebulizer in, 262–268
  for humidification of respiratory tract, 242–248
  mobilization of bronchial secretions and, 235–240
  xanthine and, 230–231
Aerosol mask, 255
Aerosols; *see also* Aerosol and humidity therapy
  airway obstruction and, 197

Aerosols—cont'd
  atmospheric, 213–215
  bland, 245
  bronchodilator, abdominal breathing exercises and, 477
  clearance of, 215, 219–220
  definition of, 213
  diffusion of, 216
  drug toxicity and, 267
  inspiratory positive-pressure breathing and, 461
  instability of, 214
  penetration and deposition of, 215–218
  physical properties of, 213–220
  pulmonary distention and, 200
  retention of, 215
  stability of, 214
  term of, 243
  warming of, 249, 258
  water, 244–248, 255
Agglomerate, 214
Agitated patient, 379–380
Aides, 497
Air entrainment, 250
Air-mix venturi, 352–360
Air pressure, 9–13
Air trapping, 114, 195, 475–476
  controlled ventilation and, 350
  cough control and, 474–475
  inspiratory positive-pressure breathing and, 464
  monitoring and, 455
  negative expiratory pressure and, 383–384
  patent airways and, 389
  pursed-lip breathing and, 477
Airflow patterns, 108–114
  Bird ventilator and, 353–355
Airway
  collapse of, positive end-expiratory pressure and, 440–441
  obstruction of; *see* Airway obstruction
  patent, 388–410
    bronchoscopy and, 389–390
    intubation and, 390–406
    tracheobronchial aspiration and, 407–410
  restriction of, gas flows and pressure and, 109–112; *see also* Airway resistance
  size of, 107–108
  status of, 389
Airway obstruction, 192–197, 388–410; *see also* Ventilatory failure
  carbon dioxide therapy and, 321
  epigastric compressions and, 476
  helium therapy and, 316–319
  inspiratory/expiratory ratio and, 420
  oxygen administration and, 293
  oxygen masks and, 301
  pulmonary distention and, 197
  sputum induction and, 247, 255

Airway obstruction—cont'd
  tracheostomy and, 403–405
  ventilation and, 196, 420–421
  Wright respirometer and, 455
Airway resistance, 104–114
  compliance, ventilatory frequency, and flow, 112–114
  to exhalation, 114–115
  gas flow, and pressure, 104–105
  normal, 105
Alcohol, ethyl, 237–239, 467
Alevaire; *see* Tyloxapol
Alkalemia, 137, 148
  mechanical ventilation and, 323
Alkaline reserve, 133, 150
Alkalinity, 77–78; *see also* pH
Alkalis, 72
Alkalosis, 147–149
  induced, 425–426
  metabolic, 148, 154–155
  oxygen dissociation curves and, 129
  ventilators and, 422
Allergies, 233, 234
Alpha adrenergic receptors, 224–225
Altitudes, 507
  hypoxia and, 187–188
Aludrine; *see* Isoproterenol
Alupent; *see* Metaproterenol sulfate
Alveolar air, 120
  equation for, 123, 514
Alveolar-arterial oxygen tension gradient, 120–121, 207–212
  hypoxia and, 183
  pulmonary edema and, 466
  weaning from ventilator and, 457
Alveolar-capillary block, 184
Alveolar-capillary diffusion, impaired, 184
Alveolar-capillary membrane, 118
  oxygen toxicity and, 297–298
Alveolar dead space, 81; *see also* Dead space
Alveolar gas tensions, 121–122
Alveolar minute volume, reduction in, 82
Alveolar rinsing, ineffective minute, 322
Alveolar walls
  emphysema and, 197–198
  oxygen toxicity and, 296
Alveoli
  bronchopulmonary dysplasia and, 297
  collapse of
    positive end-expiratory pressure and, 440–441
    pulmonary surfactant and, 100
  diffusion and, 117–119
  hyperventilation of, 151
  hypoventilation of
    mechanical ventilation and, 322–323
    respiratory acidosis and, 149
  hypoxia and, 184

Alveoli—cont'd
  oxygen administration and, 293
  plateau pressure of, 439
  respiratory/exchange ratios and, 204–212
  superoxide dismutase and, 299–300
  surface tension and, 100
  ventilation of, 81
    inspiratory positive-pressure breathing and, 461
    mechanical ventilation and, 322–323, 369–372
Ambient chamber, 347
  backflows into, 359
Ambient temperature or pressure, 17
Ambulatory care room, 502
American standard connections, 286–287
Amine oxidase, 224
Aminophylline, 230–231, 466
Ammeter, 313
Ammonia, 71
Amphotericin, 241
Analyzers, oxygen, 312–314
Anatomic dead space, 80; *see also* Dead Space
Anectine; *see* Succinylcholine
Anemia
  cyanosis and, 187
  DPG and, 131
  hypoxia and, 184
  oxygen administration and, 300
Aneroid barometer, 11
Anesthesiology, 492–493
Anesthetic gases, 270
Angina pectoris, 168
Anions, 45, 152, 153
Antibiotics, 220, 240–242, 267
Anticholinergic bronchodilators, 228–230
Antidiuretic hormone, 386
Aortic bodies, 143–146
Apneustic center, 146
ARDS; *see* Respiratory distress syndrome, adult
Area supervisor, 495–496
Arrhythmias, cardiac, 175–180
Arterial blood
  carbon dioxide in, 136; *see also* Carbon dioxide tension
  gas partial pressures in, 120
    weaning from ventilator and, 456–457
  oxygen in, 127; *see also* Oxygen tension
  pH of, 128
    mechanical ventilation and, 324, 371
  sampling of, 453–455
Arterial carbon dioxide tension; *see* Carbon dioxide tension
Arterial oxygen saturation; *see* Oxygen saturation
Arterial oxygen tension; *see* Oxygen tension
Arterial-venous difference, 127, 129
Arterialized capillary blood, 454
Arthritis, 200

Ascites, 171, 201
Aspiration
  airway obstruction and, 196–197
  of blood, tracheostomy and, 405
  inspiratory/expiratory ratio and, 419
  tracheobronchial, 407–410
Asthma
  airway obstruction and, 192, 193
  aminophylline and, 230–231
  beclamethasone dipropionate and, 234
  chronic care and rehabilitation and; *see* Chronic care and rehabilitation
  cromolyn sodium and, 234
  dexamethasone and, 233
  epinephrine and, 226
  psychosomatic support and, 484, 485
  pulmonary distention and, 197
ata; *see* Atmospheres, absolute
Atelectasis
  bronchial secretions and, 194
  bronchoscopy and, 390
  inspiratory positive-pressure breathing and, 461
  oxygen administration and, 293
  physiological shunt hypoxia and, 438
  postoperative, 320
  prolonged artificial ventilation and, 421
  pulmonary surfactant and, 100
  tracheostomy and, 404
atg; *see* Atmospheres, gauge
Atmosphere
  aerosols in, 213–215
  composition of, 8–9
  depth characteristics of, 507
  pressure of, 9–13
    oxygen partial pressure and, 13–14
Atmospheres
  absolute, 270
  gauge, 270
Atomic numbers, 42, 43
Atomic weights, 512
Atomization, 243
Atoms, 1, 39–45
  bonding of, 45–49
ATP; *see* Adenosine triphosphate
ATPS, 17
  BTPS and, 26, 508
  STPD and, 26, 510
Atria, 178, 374
Atrioventricular block, 179–180
Atrioventricular bundle, 158
Atrioventricular node, 157–158
Atropine, 228–230
Auscultation of chest, 451
Autonomic nervous system, 156, 157, 221–224, 229
  sinus arrhythmia and, 176
a-v difference; *see* Arterial-venous difference
A-V node; *see* Atrioventricular node

Avogadro's law and number, 5

**B**

*Bacillus pyocyaneus,* 242
Bacitracin, 241
Bacterial contamination, 249
Bacteriologic sputum examination, 246
Baking soda; *see* Bicarbonate sodium
Bar, 12
Barometer, 10, 11, 12
  correction of readings of, 24–25, 509
Barotrauma, 444
Barrel chest, 115, 199
Barye, 12
Bases
  combined carbon dioxide and, 139
  equivalent weight of, 51
  ions and, 71–72
  nonhydroxide, 71
Basic salt, 73
Beclamethasone dipropionate, 233–234
Bennett ventilators, 325, 326–327, 340–342, 360–369
  adjustable, variable, and fixed functions of, 412, 421
  choice of, 415
  inspiratory/expiratory ratio and, 418–419
  leak in delivery system of, 365
  negative pressure and, 366–367
  peak flow and, 365–366
  sigh and, 422
  terminal flow and, 364–365
  timing accumulators and, 367–369
Bernoulli effect, 109–112
  flowmeters and, 283, 285
  helium therapy and, 316–317
  jet aerosol-humidifier and, 249, 250
Beta adrenergic receptors, 224–225
Bicarbonate, 137–142
  in acidosis, 427–428
  blood-brain barrier and, 145
  carbon dioxide bound as, 133, 139
  excess of, 425–426
  ventilators and, 422–424
Bicarbonate sodium, 239
  in acidosis, 424, 425
  buffer system and, 137–142
  and tyloxapol, 235
Bicycle, exercising, 482
Bigeminy, 177
Biopsy, 389
Biot's respiration, 116
Bird ventilators, 325, 326–327, 346–360
  adjustable, variable, and fixed functions of, 412
  air-mix venturi of, 352–360
  choice of, 415

Bird ventilators—cont'd
  cycling mechanism of, 347–349
  exhalation valve and, 349–350
  expiratory timer of, 351–352
  inspiratory/expiratory ratio and, 419
  nebulizer of, 350
  negative pressure of, 350–351
Bistable fluidic device, 342, 343
Bite block, 393
Bleeding, 396, 405
Blood
  arterial; *see* Arterial blood
  aspiration of, 405
  carbon dioxide in, 131–136; *see also* Carbon dioxide tension
  coronary, 167–168
  oxygen in, 122–131; *see also* Oxygen tension
  pH of; *see* pH
  plasma; *see* Plasma
  pulmonary, 165–167
  shock and volume of, 172, 173
  systemic, 162–165
  venous; *see* Venous blood
Blood-brain barrier, 145
Blood buffers; *see* Buffers
Blood gases and acid-base balance, 117–155; *see also* Carbon dioxide tension; Oxygen tension
  acid-base balance in, 136–142; *see also* pH
    oxygen administration and, 315–316
    tracheotomy and, 397
    ventilators and, 422–426, 453
  analyses of
    laboratory for, 498–499
    personnel and, 496–497
  carbon dioxide transportation in, 131–136
  clinical states in, 147–155
  diffusion gradients in, 119–122
  diffusion mechanics in, 117–119
  hypoxia and, 183
  oxygen transportation in, 122–131
  ventilation control in, 142–147
  weaning from ventilator and, 456–457
Blood pressure, 163–164
  carbon dioxide therapy and, 319, 321
  glucocorticoids and, 232
  mechanical ventilation and, 452
  shock and, 172
Body plethysmograph, 106
Body respirator, negative-pressure, 413
Bohr effect, 128
Boiling point, 34, 58
Boiling, solutes and, 63–64
Bone calcium, 232
bone diseases, 200
Bourdon flow gauge, 280, 281, 282, 283
Bourns ventilators, 325, 326–327, 339–340
  adjustable, variable, and fixed functions of, 412

Boyle's law, 19
  moisture in gas volumes and, 22–23
Brain
  hypoxia and, 185–186
  ischemia of, 423
Breathing; *see* Respiration
Breathing head assembly, 349
Breathing nomogram, 515
Brilliant green, 248
British thermal unit, 29
Bronchial asthma; *see* Asthma
Bronchial collateral flow, 166
Bronchial infections, 245
Bronchial secretions
  aerosols and humidity and, 220, 221–230,
    235–240, 265
  airway obstruction and, 193–194
  atropine and, 229
  chest percussion and, 473
  collecting bottle for, 407, 408
  postural drainage and, 470–473
Bronchial spasm; *see* Bronchospasm
Bronchial suctioning, 407–410
Bronchial toilet, 407
Bronchial venous blood, 125–126, 166
Bronchiectasis
  antibiotics and, 240
  bronchial collateral flow and, 166
  bronchiolar collapse and, 195
  dornase and, 240
  inspiratory positive-pressure breathing and, 461
  postural drainage and, 471
Bronchiolar collapse, 194–196
Bronchitis, 170–171
  acetylcysteine and, 237
  inspiratory positive-pressure breathing and, 461
  postural drainage and, 471
Bronchodilators, 221–230
  abdominal breathing exercises and, 477
  airway obstruction and, 197
  antibiotics and, 242
  anticholinergic, 228–230
  atropine and, 229–230
  bland aerosols and, 245
Bronchopneumonia, 264–265
Bronchopulmonary dysplasia, 297
Bronchoscopy, 389–390
  airway obstruction and, 196
Bronchospasm, 192–193, 197
  aerosols and humidity and, 220, 221
  inspiratory/expiratory ratio and, 419
  inspiratory positive-pressure breathing and,
    461
  *d*-tubocurarine and, 434
Brownian movement, 2
  aerosols and, 216
BT; *see* Temperature of body

BTPS, 17
  ATPS and, 26, 508
  STPD and, 27, 511
Bubble diffusion humidifier, 262
Bubbles
  in clumps, 99
  in liquid mass, 97, 98, 99
Budget, 494
Buffalo hump, 232
Buffers, 137–139, 152, 153
  negative log of equilibrium constant of acid com-
    ponent and, 139
  in respiratory acidosis, 424, 425
  in respiratory failure, 427–428
  ventilators and, 423–424
Bundle branches, 158
Bundle of His, 158

**C**

$C_L$; *see* Compliance
$C_{LT}$; *see* Lung-thorax compliance
$C_T$; *see* Compliance
c-a; *see* Carbonic-anhydrase
Caffeine, 230
Calcium, bone, 232
Calorie, 29
Calorimeter, 29
*Candida albicans,* 248
Cannulas
  oxygen, 307–309
  tracheostomy and, 397, 401, 404
Canopy tents, 259
Capillaries
  oxygen toxicity and, 296
  unsaturation of, 186, 187, 513
Capillary tufting, 297
Carbamino compound, 133
Carbamino-hemoglobin, 133
Carbenicillin, 241
Carbon, helium and, 290
Carbon dioxide, 131–136, 139; *see also* Hypercapnia;
    Hypocapnia
  with air-oxygen inspired gas mixture, 426–427
  arrhythmias and, 180
  bound, 131, 136, 139
  combined, 139
  in cylinders, 270, 274
  diffusibility of, 119
  dissolved, 133, 136, 139
  metabolic acidosis and, 424
  in therapy, 319–321
Carbon dioxide dissociation curves, 134
Carbon dioxide mixer, 426–427
Carbon dioxide tension, 120
  arterial, 120
    inspiratory positive-pressure breathing and,
      461

Carbon dioxide tension—cont'd
  arterial—cont'd
    mechanical ventilation and, 324, 371, 372,
      415, 422, 453
    oxygen induced hypoventilation and, 292
    calculation of, from H-H equation, 512
    converted to millimoles per liter, 139–140
    inspiratory positive-pressure breathing and, 461
Carbon monoxide, 119, 300
Carbonates, 71–72
Carbonic acid
  buffer system and, 137–142
  carbon dioxide as, 133–136
Carbonic-anhydrase, 133
Cardiac action, shock and, 172, 173
Cardiac arrest
  fluorocarbon-induced, 252
  tracheobronchial aspiration and, 409
  tracheotomy and, 396
Cardiac arrhythmias, 175–180
Cardiac cycle, 156–159; *see also* Heart
Cardiac decompensation, 168
Cardiac failure, 169–171, 466
Cardiac output, 163
  circulatory failure and, 163, 171–175
  inspiratory positive-pressure breathing and, 461
  mechanical ventilators and, 372–378, 383
Cardiac rate; *see* Heart rate
Cardiopulmonary technology, 503
Cardiovascular system, 156–181
  airway obstruction and, 192–197
  arrhythmias and, 175–180
  carbon dioxide therapy and, 319
  cardiac cycle in, 156–159
  congenital heart disease and, 181
  coronary blood flow and, 167–168
  electrophysiology and, 159–162
  failure of, 168–175
  hypoxia and, 182–191
  mechanical ventilation and, 372–385, 452
  peripheral, 163, 172, 173
  positive end-expiratory pressure and, 444
  pulmonary blood flow and, 165–167
  pulmonary distention and, 197–200
  pulmonary edema and, 466
  pulmonary restriction and, 200–202
  succinylcholine and, 435
  systemic blood flow and, 162–165
  tracheotomy and, 396–397
  ventilation-perfusion imbalance and, 202–212
Carina, 404
Carotid bodies, 143–146
Cascade humidifier, 262, 402
Catecholamines, 223
Catheters
  central venous, 455
  oxygen, 307–309

Catheters—cont'd
  Swan-Ganz, 174–175, 445, 455
  for tracheobronchial aspiration, 407
Cations, 45, 152, 153
Celsius temperatures, 506
Centerbody, 347
Central nervous system
  carbon dioxide therapy and, 319–321
  hypoxia and, 185–186
Central tendon, 84
Central venous catheter, 445
Central venous oxygen saturation, 174
Central venous pressure, 173–174, 175
Ceramic cylinder, 347–348
Cerebral blood flow, 320, 423
Cerebrospinal fluid, 145
Certified respiratory therapy technician, 491
Change of state, 30–38
Charles' law, 19
Charts of patients, 500
Chemical bonds, 45–49
Chemical equivalents, 50
Chemical reaction, reversible, 67
Chemoreceptors, 142–146
  inactivation of, 433
  metabolic acidosis and, 145
  oxygen administration and, 292
Chest; *see also* Thorax
  auscultation of, 451
  compression of, acute, 475–476
  percussion of, 473–474
  vibration and, 474
Chest respirator, 331–332, 413
  adjustable, variable, and fixed functions of, 412
Chest wall, 379
Cheyne-Stokes respiration, 116
Chloramphenicol, 241
Chloride shift, 134
Cholinergic nerves, 224
Chronic care and rehabilitation, 468–486
  family counseling and, 485–486
  objectives of, 468–469
  occupational retraining and placement and, 485
  psychosomatic support and, 484–485
  respiratory therapy and, 470–484; *see also*
    Respiratory therapy
Cilia, 296
Ciliary mucus clearance, 219
Circulation; *see* Cardiovascular system
Clapping, 473
Climbing stairs, 481
Clinical records, 500
Clubbing, 189–191
Clutch plate, 348
Cold spots, 203
Cold steam, 243, 255
Collecting bottle for bronchial secretions, 407, 408

Colloids, 63
Color code for gas cylinders, 272, 273
Colymycin-M, 241
Combustion, 291
Common cold, 192, 193
Compensation
    cardiac, 169
    concept of, 148–149
Compensatory pause, 177
Compliance, 101–103
    adult respiratory distress syndrome and, 386
    inspiratory/expiratory ratio and, 420
    left heart failure and, 170
    mechanical ventilation and, 379, 413
    monitoring and, 455
    positive end-expiratory pressure and, 440–441
    pulmonary restriction and, 200
    static, 440
    ventilatory frequency, flow, and airway resistance
        and, 112–114
    ventilatory pattern and, 417
Compound, 39
Compression
    of chest, 475–476
    of costal margins, 476
    heat of, 5
Compressor-bellows, 340–342
Condensation nuclei, 213
Conduction system of heart, 156–157
Congenital heart disease, 181
Congestion, pulmonary, 169–170, 175, 201; *see
        also* Pulmonary edema
Congestive heart failure, 169–171
Connector systems, 285–289
Connectors
    for tracheobronchial aspiration, 407
    from ventilator to inner cannula, 401
Constant positive airway pressure, 448
Constant positive pressure breathing, 448
Constant pressure and volume of gas, 30
Continuous positive airway pressure, 448
Continuous positive pressure breathing, 448
Continuous positive pressure ventilation, 441
Cooling of expansion, 5
Cooling unit of oxygen tent, 310
Cor pulmonale, 166, 170–171, 189
Coramine; *see* Nikethamide
Coronary blood flow, 167–168
Coronary occlusion, 168
Cortisol, 231
Cortisone, 231
Costal margins
    compression of, 476
    mobilization of, 481–482
Cough, 474–475
    carbon dioxide therapy and, 320
    after intubation, 394

Cough—cont'd
    postural drainage and, 473
    after tracheostomy removal, 458
Counseling, family, 485–486
Couplant, 263
Covalent bonding, 46–49
Covalent electrolytes, 66–69
Covalent molecules, polarization of, 47
Covalent solutions, polar, 65–68
CPAP; *see* Constant positive airway pressure
CPPB; *see* Constant positive pressure breathing
CPPV; *see* Continuous positive pressure ventilation
Critical Care Ventilator, 340–342
Critical point, 31, 35
Critical pressure, 35
Critical temperature, 35
Cromylyn sodium, 234
Croup
    humidification and, 245, 256, 266, 312
    ventilation and, 196
Croup tent, 312
Crystals, 46, 64
Cuffs
    for intubation, 391, 392
    tracheostomy; *see* Tracheostomy tubes and cuffs
Cuirass, 331
Cultures, tissue, 295–296
Cushing's syndrome, 231
CVP; *see* Central venous pressure
$CVS_{O_2}$; *see* Central venous oxygen saturation
Cyanosis
    congenital heart disease and, 181
    hypoxia and, 186, 187, 189
    mechanical ventilation and, 450
    polycythemia and, 187, 188–189
Cycling mechanism, 347–349
Cyclopropane, 270, 274
Cylinders, gas; *see* Gas cylinders
Cystic fibrosis, 265–266
    acetylcysteine and, 237
    bronchiolar collapse and, 195
    dornase and, 240
    humidification and, 245
    sodium bicarbonate and, 239
Cytologic sputum examination, 245–246

**D**

D; *see* Dry gas
$D_L$; *see* Diffusion capacity of lung
Dalton's law of partial pressure, 13
Dead space, 79–81, 210
    oxygen masks and, 301–302
    pathologic increase in, 82
    weaning from ventilator and, 457
Decompensation, cardiac, 168
Decongestants, 197, 221
Demand valves, 346

Deoxyribonucleic acid
dornase and, 240
oxygen toxicity and, 296
sputum and, 193
Detergents, 235–236
Dew point, 16–17
Dexamethasone sodium phosphate, 233
Diameter-Index Safety System, 287–288
Diaphragm, 84–86
hypercapnia and, 321
low position of, 198–199
paralysis of, 86
Diastole, 158, 159, 164
mechanical ventilation and, 380–381
Diffusion
mechanics of, 117–119
rates of, for gases, 317, 318
Diffusion capacity of lung, 119
Diffusion coefficient, 119, 216
Diffusion defect, 184
for oxygen, 170
venous admixture and, 207–209
Diffusion deposition, 216, 217
Diffusion gradients, 119–122
Diffusion head, 261, 262
Diffusion separation, 9
Digitalis, 176, 179, 466
Dilabron; *see* Isoetharine
Dilution calculations, 62
Dipalmitoyl-lecithin, 247–248
2,3-Diphosphoglycerate, 130–131
Dipoles, 49
Dispersions, 63
Disposable equipment, 502
DISS; *see* Diameter-Index Safety System
Dissociation, 46, 64
degree of, 73–75
Distention
abdominal; *see* Abdominal distention
pulmonary, 197–200
Diuretics, 444, 466
DNA; *see* Deoxyribonucleic acid
Dornase, 240, 242, 246
Dornavac; *see* Dornase
Double-circuit positive-pressure ventilator, 336–338
Double-gradient study, 209
DPG; *see* 2,3-Diphosphoglycerate
Drainage, postural, 197, 470–473
Drinker ventilators, 325, 326–327, 330–332
Drug nebulizers, 267
Drug reconcentration, 267–268
Dry gas, 17
breathing of, 244
Dusts, 213
Dynamic inspiratory period, 338
Dyne, 11–12
Dyspnea, 116

**E**

Ectopic foci, 176
Edema
laryngeal, 393, 394
airway obstruction and, 192
humidification and, 256
left ventricular failure and, 169–170
mucosal, 192, 220, 221
pulmonary; *see* Pulmonary edema
right ventricular failure and, 171
Education, technical director of, 497
Effective static compliance, 440
Effector organs or cells, 223
Elastic resistance to ventilation, 101–103
exhalation mechanics and, 114–115
Elasticity of lungs, 114, 197, 198
Electric analyzers, 312–313
Electrical sparks, 314
Electrocardiogram, 161, 162
Electrolytes
balance between fixed and buffer, 153
equilibrium of, 73
and ions, 63–69
measurement of activity of, 73–77
Electron orbits, 40–43
Electronic monitors, 455
Electrons, 39, 40
distribution of, 42, 43
valence, 43
Electrovalent bonding, 45–46
Electrovalent solutions, 64–65
Elements, 39
equivalent weight of, 50–51
symbols, weights, and valences of, 512
Embolism, pulmonary, 211
Emergencies, 498
Emerson ventilators, 325, 326–327, 332, 335–336
adjustable, variable, and fixed functions of, 412
inspiratory/expiratory ratio and, 418
Emivan; *see* Ethamivan
Emphysema, 197–198
acetylcysteine and, 237
air trapping and, 115, 475
bronchiolar collapse and, 195
chest compression and, 475
chronic care and rehabilitation in; *see* Chronic care and rehabilitation
inspiratory positive-pressure breathing and, 461
and obstructive bronchitis, 170–171
positive end-expiratory pressure and, 444, 445
postural drainage and, 471
psychosomatic support and, 484
pursed-lip breathing and, 477
respiratory acidosis and, 150
senile, 198
subcutaneous, 396, 405, 444
tracheotomy and, 406

Encapsulation of particles, 219
End-expiratory position, 90
End-expiratory pressure, *see* Positive end-expiratory
    pressure
End-tidal carbon dioxide, 211
Endotracheal tube, 392–394
    airway obstruction and, 196
    helium therapy and, 318
    neuromuscular blocking agents and, 434
    removal of, 458
    too low, 451
Energy
    levels of, principal, 40
    mechanical ventilation and, 371–372
    in moving fluid, 110
Engström ventilators, 325, 326–327, 336–338
    adjustable, variable, and fixed functions of, 412
    inspiratory/expiratory ratio and, 418
    tidal volumes and rates and, 416
Enzymes, oxygen and, 296
Ephedrine, 225, 226–227
Epigastric compressions, 476
Epiglottal reflexes or paralysis, 308
Epinephrine, 223–224, 225, 226
    oxygen toxicity and, 296
    ventricular fibrillation and, 179
Epinephrine-fast, 226
Equilibrium constant, 73
    calculation of, 76
    negative log of, of acid component of buffer
        system, 139
    of water, 76–77
Equivalent weights, 50–56, 504–506
ERV; *see* Expiratory reserve volume
Erythrocytes
    carbon dioxide in, 131, 132, 133–136
    hypoxia and, 188–189
Ethamivan, 466
Ethanol; *see* Ethyl alcohol
Ethyl alcohol, 237–239, 467
Ethylene, 270, 274
Evaporation, 14, 15, 32
Exercises, graded, 482–484
Exhalation, 79, 114–115
    air composition and, 120
    mechanical ventilation and, 380–381
    passive, 338
Exhalation valve, 349–350
Exosphere, 9
Expansion, cooling of, 5
Expiratory pressure, shock and, 452; *see also*
    Positive end-expiratory pressure
Expiratory reserve volume, 93
Expiratory retard, 464
Expiratory timer, 351–352
External oblique muscles, 89
Extubation, 458

**F**

f; *see* Frequency of breathing
Face mask, 391
Face tent, 314
Fahrenheit temperatures, 506
Family counseling, 485–486
Fats, 232
Fenestrated tracheostomy tube, 458–459
Fiberoptic bronchoscopy, 390
Fibromyositis, 200
Fibrosis
    diffuse myocardial, 168
    of lung, 201
Fibrous tissue deposits, 219
Filling density, 273–274
Finger stick, 454
Fire hazard, 313–314
First rib, 83, 84
Flammability of gases, 270
Flip-flop, 342, 343
Flow and velocity, terms of, 110
Flow-adjustable ventilator, 346–360
    choice of, 414, 415
Flow generators, 355–357
Flow-sensitive valve, 362–364
Flow-sensitive ventilators, 360–369
Flow sensitivity, 357
Flowmeters
    back pressure and, 282–283
    Bourdon gauge, 280, 281, 282, 283
    compensated, 284–285
    helium therapy and, 318–319
    pressure compensation and, 282–285
    Thorpe-tube, 279, 280, 282
    uncompensated, 283–284
Fluid-controlled ventilators, 342
Fluid logic units, 342
Fluidic devices, 342
Fluidity, 2
Fluorocarbons, 252
Fog, 243
Fog nebulizers, 267
Force, surface area and, 9–10
Forced-exhalation
    abdominal breathing and, 478–480
    with walking, 480–481
Forced-inhalation abdominal breathing, 480
FRC; *see* Functional residual capacity
Free radicals, 295
Freezing, 32, 58
    sodium chloride and, 74
    solutes and, 63–64
Freon 11, 252
Frequency of breathing, 79
    aerosol deposition and, 218
    flow, airway resistance and compliance, 112–114

Friction
  aerosol deposition and, 218
  ventilation and, 103–104
Fuel cell analyzers, 312, 313
Functional residual capacity, 93
  mechanical ventilation and, 370
  positive end-expiratory pressure and, 440–441
  pulmonary distention and, 197, 199

**G**

Galvanic electrochemical sensing, 312, 313
Galvanometer, 162
Gas, term of, 35; *see also* Gases
Gas bubbles
  in clumps, 99
  in liquid mass, 97, 98, 99
Gas cylinders, 270–276
  estimating duration of flow and, 275–276
  filling of, 273–274
  high-pressure regulators and, 279–282
  for liquid oxygen, 278–279
  measuring contents of, 274–275
  pressures and volumes of, 276
Gas flow
  airway resistance, and pressure, 104–105
  pressure, and air passage restriction, 109–112
  regulation of, 279–289
  ultrasonic nebulizers and, 265
Gas laws, 17–20
  combined, 20–21
Gas regulators
  high pressure, 279–282
  low pressure, 282
Gas therapy, 269–321
  carbon dioxide and, 319–321
  helium and, 316–319
  medical gases in, 269–289
    bulk oxygen in, 276–279
    cylinder gases in, 270–276; *see also* Gas
      cylinders
    regulation of flow in, 279–289
  oxygen therapy in, 289–316; *see also* Oxygen
    therapy
Gases
  aerosol deposition and, 216–217
  anesthetic, 270
  blood; *see* Blood gases and acid-base balance
  breathing of dry, 244
  compressibility of, 4, 5
  cylinder; *see* Gas cylinders
  density of, 6–8, 27–28, 317, 318
  diffusion rates of, 317, 318
  flammability of, 270
  flow of; *see* Gas flow
  inert, 44
  mobility of, 1–2
  oxygen in bulk and, 276–279

Gases—cont'd
  permanent, 35
  pressure of, 3–5, 104–105, 109–112
    Bennett ventilator and, 360, 361
    constant, 30
    extreme, 28–38
    flow-sensitive ventilator and, 360, 361
    inspiratory positive pressure and, 345
    for liquid state at room temperature, 36
    partial, in venous and arterial blood, 120; *see
      also* Carbon dioxide tension; Oxygen tension
    ranges of, in therapy, 271, 273
  temperature of, 3–5
    extreme, 28–38
    low, 511
  tension of, 3
  in therapy; *see* Gas therapy
  ventilators and, 342, 353
    Bennett, 360
  viscosity of, 106–107
  volume of
    calculations of, 25–27
    constant, 30
    conversion of, 273, 508, 510, 511
    correction of, 21–24
    molar, 5–6
Gastric acidity, 232
Gastric distention; *see* Abdominal distention
Gastric rupture, 308
Gate spring, 350, 358–359
Gay-Lussac's law, 19–20
Gel/sol relationship, 296
Gels, 63
Generators, flow and pressure, 355–357; *see also*
  Aerosol and humidity therapy
Gentamicin, 241, 242
gfw; *see* Gram formula weight
Globin, 123
Glucocorticoids, 231, 232
Glucose, 232
Glycerine and tyloxapol, 235
gmw; *see* Gram molecular weight
Goblet cells, 219
Graded exercises, 482–484
Graham's law, 119
  helium therapy and, 316–317
Gram equivalent weight, 50–53
Gram formula weight, 1
Gram molecular weight, 1
Grams per liter, 7
Granulation tissue, 404
Gravity, 215–216
Group therapy, 485

**H**

Haldane effect, 134, 135
Hamburger phenomenon, 134

Hand nebulizer, 254
Hb; *see* Hemoglobin
Head tent, 314–315
Heart; *see also* Cardiovascular system
　arrest of, 252, 396, 409
　arrhythmias and, 175–180
　cycles of, 156–159
　electrophysiology of, 159–162
　hypoxia and, 186
　output of; *see* Cardiac output
　shock and, 172, 173
Heart block, 158, 179–180
Heart disease, congenital, 181
Heart failure, 168–175, 466
Heart rate, 157, 158–159
　carbon dioxide therapy and, 319, 321
　mechanical ventilation and, 379, 380, 383, 452
Heat
　of compression, 5
　of fusion, 32, 33
　nebulizers and, 249, 258
　specific, 30
　of sublimation, 37
　units of, 29–30
　of vaporization, 34
Heimlich maneuver, 476
Helium, 270
　atomic structure of, 40
　and oxygen, 437
　in therapy, 316–319
　transformation of, to carbon, 290
Hematocrit, 188–189
Hematopoiesis, 188
Heme, 123
Hemoglobin, 123–125
　carbon dioxide with, 133
　cyanosis and, 186
　hypoxia and, 184
　oxygen saturation and, 183
Hemoglobinemia, 123
Hemolysis, 123
Hemorrhage, 396, 405
Henderson-Hasselbalch equation, 137–139
　application of, 139–142
　metabolic acidosis and, 424, 425
　in $P_{CO_2}$ calculation, 512
Henry's law, 118
Heparin, 248
Hepatomegaly, 171
Hering-Breuer reflexes, 146, 147
Hiccups, 320
High-pressure cylinder gas regulators, 279–282
Histamine, 234, 434
Histotoxins, 185
Home care, 483, 486
Homeostasis, 222

Hormones
　adrenocorticotropic, 232–233
　antidiuretic, 386
Humidification; *see also* Aerosol and humidity therapy; Humidity
　intubation and, 402
　nasal oxygen and, 308
　of respiratory tract, 220, 242–248
　tracheobronchial aspiration and, 409
　ultrasonic nebulizers and, 265
Humidifiers, 249; *see also* Aerosol and humidity therapy
　bubble-diffusion, 262
　cascade, 262, 402
　helium and, 319
　Hydro-Sphere, 260–261
　jet aerosol, 259–260
　pass-over, 261
Humidity, 14–17; *see also* Humidification
　absolute, 16, 243
　oxygen tents and, 310, 311
　percent body, 243
　relative, 16, 243
Humidity deficit, 244
Hyaline membrane, 438
Hyaline membrane disease, 298; *see also* Respiratory distress syndrome
Hydrated ion, 65
Hydration, 65
　ultrasonic nebulizers and 266
Hydrogen
　atomic structure of, 40
　ionizable, 70
Hydrogen chloride, 66
Hydrogen ions, 70, 77
　of blood; *see* pH, blood
Hydronium ion, 66
Hydro-Sphere nebulizer-humidifier, 260–261
Hydrothorax, 170
Hydroxides, 71
Hydroxyl free radicals, 295
Hygrometers, 16
Hyperbaric chamber, 449
Hyperbarism, 13–14
Hyperbasemia, 148
Hypercapnia, 117, 148
　chemoreceptors and, 146
　chronic, 433
　correction of, 422–423
　diaphragm and, 321
　mechanical ventilation and, 322
　oxygen administration and, 292
Hypercarbia; *see* Hypercapnia
Hyperkalemia, 435
Hyperoxemia, 117
Hyperoxia, 117
Hypertonic solution, 62

Hyperventilation, 83
  hazards of, 422–428
  mechanical ventilation and, 323, 421–428
  metabolic acidosis and, 145
  respiratory alkalosis and, 151
Hypobarism, 13–14, 184
Hypobasemia, 184
Hypocapnia, 117, 148
  augmented ventilation and, 292
  inspiratory positive-pressure breathing and, 464
  mechanical ventilation and, 323
Hypocarbia; *see* Hypocapnia
Hypokalemia, 422
Hypopharynx, obstruction in, 476
Hypophase, 97
Hypotension, 434, 445
Hypothermia, 130
Hypotonic solution, 62
Hypoventilation, 82–83
  carbon dioxide and, 320
  chronic, 146
  hypoxia and, 435–437
  mechanical ventilation and, 322–323
  oxygen and, 291–293
  respiratory acidosis and, 149, 151
Hypovolemia, 172
Hypoxemia, 117, 182–183
  adult respiratory distress syndrome and, 386
  chemoreceptors and, 146
  mechanical ventilation and, 322, 323
  positive end-expiratory pressure and, 440, 441, 445
Hypoxia, 117, 182–191
  acute, 185–187
  arrhythmias and, 180
  chronic, 171, 187–191
  classification of, 184–185
  DPG and, 131
  hypoventilation and, 435–437
  mechanical ventilation and, 323, 435–449
  oxygen administration and, 292–293
    acid-base balance and, 315–316
  physiological shunt, 437–440
    mechanical ventilation and, 323
    positive end-expiratory pressure and, 440
  pulmonary edema and, 466–467
  tissue, 171–175
  tracheobronchial aspiration and, 409
  ventilation/perfusion ratio and, 323
Hypoxic drive, 150

**I**

[133]I; *see* Iodine, radioactive
[133]I MAA; *see* Microaggregated albumin labeled
    with radioactive iodine
IC; *see* Inspiratory capacity
Immunologic response, 232

Impeller nebulizer, 262
IMV; *see* Intermittent mandatory ventilation
[113]In; *see* Indium particles
Incubators, 299, 311–312
Indium particles, 203
Inert gas-powered nebulizers, 252–260
Inert gases, 44
Inertia, 7
  impaction of particles and, 217–218
Infants
  blood sampling in, 454
  Bournes ventilator and, 339–340
  incubators and, 299, 311–312
  premature, tidal volumes of, 417
  respiratory distress syndrome and; *see* Respiratory distress syndrome
  ultrasonic nebulizers and, 265–266
Infarction, myocardial, 168
Infection, 240–242, 245, 249
  tracheostomy and, 405–406
  weaning from ventilator and, 457
Inflammatory response, 232
Inflation hold, 438–440
Inflation reflexes, 146, 147
Inhalation, 79; *see also* Respiration
In-service, 497
Inspiratory capacity, 94
  pulmonary distention and, 198
Inspiratory/expiratory ratio, 418–420
  Bennett ventilator and, 341, 361
    timing accumulators and, 368
  Bourns ventilator and, 339
  Engström ventilator and, 336, 338
  pressure-time curve and, 382, 383
Inspiratory positive-pressure breathing, 329, 460–467
  postural drainage and, 470–471
  pulmonary edema and, 465–467
  ventilators and, 344–369
    helium therapy and, 318
Inspiratory pressure
  mechanical ventilation and, 380–381
  weaning from ventilator and, 457
Inspiratory reserve volume, 94
Inspiratory time, patent airways and, 389
Inspired air
  composition of, 120
  distribution of, 199, 200
  water vapor and, 243–244
Inspired gas, mechanical ventilation and, 370–371
Instructor, 497
Intensive care unit, 410
Intercostal muscles, 86–87
Intermembranous space, 118
Intermittent mandatory ventilation, 428–432
  positive end-expiratory pressure and, 442
  weaning with, 460

Intermittent nebulizers, 253–255
Intermittent positive-pressure breathing; *see* Inspiratory positive-pressure breathing
Internal oblique muscle, 89
Interrupter valve, 350–351
Interstitial space, 118
Intestinal distention, 293; *see also* Abdominal distention
Intra-alveolar pressures, 91
  mechanical ventilation and, 373
Intrabronchial catheter, 407
Intracardiac shunts, 181
Intracranial pressure, 473
Intrapleural pressure, 91, 92, 102
Intrapleural space, 90
  break in, 94, 95
Intrapulmonary pressure
  Bird ventilator and, 348
  controlled-positive end-expiratory pressure and, 443, 444, 449
  pulmonary edema and, 467
Intrapulmonary vascular congestion, 201
Intrathoracic pressure, 91
  cough and, 475
  intermittent mandatory ventilation and, 431
  mechanical ventilation and, 372–385
  postural drainage and, 473
  pulmonary edema and, 467
  shock and, 173
  venous return to heart and, 164–165
Intubation, 390–406
  endotracheal; *see* Endotracheal tube
  local anesthesia for, 393
  nasotracheal, 394–395, 451, 458
  too low, 451
  tracheostomy, 395–406
  ventilators and, 332
Inventory of equipment, 495
Iodine, radioactive, 203
Ionic bonding, 45–46
Ionic compounds, 1
Ionic dissociation, 64
Ionic solutions, 64–65
Ionizable hydrogen, 70
Ionization, 65, 73–75
  of strong polar covalent electrolyte, 66–67
  of water, 68, 69
  of weak polar covalent electrolyte, 67–68, 69
Ionization constant, 73, 76
  of water, 76–77
Ionosphere, 9
Ions, 45; *see also* Solutions and ions
  acids, bases, and salts and, 70–73
  electrolytes and, 63–69
  formation of, 64–69
    polar covalent compounds and, 49
  hydrated, 65

Ions—cont'd
  hydronium, 66
  spectator, 70
IPPB; *see* Inspiratory positive-pressure breathing
Iris, 449
Iron lung, 330
IRV; *see* Inspiratory reserve volume
Ischemia of brain, 423
Isoelectric line, 161
Isoetharine, 225, 227–228
N-Isopropyl nortropine, 230
Isoproterenol, 225, 227
  and atropine, 230
  dexamethasone sodium phosphate and, 233
  metabolic products of, 228
  oxygen toxicity and, 296
Isotonic solution, 61
Isuprel; *see* Isoproterenol

**J**

Jet aerosol-humidifier, 249–260
Job placement, 485

**K**

Kanamycin, 241
Kelvin scale, 3
Kidney
  circulation in, 386
  electrolytes and, 149–150, 151
  hypoxia and, 186
  mechanical ventilation and, 386
Kinetic activity, 2
  aerosol deposition and, 216–217
  in moving fluid, 110
Kistner tracheostomy tubes, 458
Kyphoscoliosis, 200

**L**

Laboratory, pulmonary function, 496–499
Laminar flow, 108
LaPlace's law, 96, 97
Laryngeal croup; *see* Croup
Laryngitis, 255
Laryngoscope, 393
Laryngotracheobronchitis, 256
Larynx
  edema of, 192, 256, 393, 394
  obstruction in; *see also* Airway obstruction
    epigastric compressions and, 476
    ventilation and, 196
  spasm of, 393, 394
Latent heat, 34
Laws
  Boyle's, 19, 22–23
  Charles', 19
  Dalton's, of partial pressure, 13

Laws—cont'd
  gas, 17–20
    combined, 20–21
  Gay-Lussac's, 19–20
  Graham's, 119, 316–317
  Henry's, 118
  LaPlace's, 96, 97
  Poiseuille's, 107, 108
  Stoke's, of sedimentation, 215–216
Leaks
  Bennett ventilator and, 365
  tracheostomy cuffs and, 402
Left ventricular failure, 169–170
Left ventricular systolic pressure, 163
Leg muscles, 483
Levallorphan tartrate, 466
Levarterenol, 223–224, 225, 227
Liquefacients, 197
Liquid
  to solids, 32
  to vapor, 32–37
Liquid filtration nebulizers, 252
Load resistor, 313
Lorfan; *see* Levallorphan tartrate
Lung abscess, 240, 461, 471
Lung compliance; *see* Compliance
Lung photo scanning, 203
Lung-thorax compliance, 101, 102; *see also* Compliance
Lung-thorax relationship, 90–95, 101, 102
Lungs
  air distribution in, 200
  blood flow in, 165–167, 466
  capacities of, 93–94
  congestion of, 169–170, 175, 201; *see also* Pulmonary edema
  distention of, 197–200
  drainage of, 471, 472, 473
  elasticity of, 114, 197, 198
  fibrosis or scarring of, 201
  hyperinflation of, 445
  mechanical ventilation and, 379–380
  normal, ventilating patients with, 331, 413
  positive end-expiratory pressure and, 444
  pressure-controlled inflation of, 467
  scarring of, 201
  surfactant of, 99–100, 293, 296–297, 438
  volumes of, 93–94
    hypoxia and, 188

**M**

MA-1 respirator unit, 340–342
Macromolecules, 46
Mainstream nebulization, 257–259
Manometer, positive end-expiratory pressure and, 442
Manual sighing, 422
Mask pressure, 376

Masks
  for helium, 318
  oxygen, 301–307
  tracheostomy, 403
  venturi, 305–307, 436
Mass, 6–7
Matter, state of, 30–38
Mean free path, 2
Mean negativity, 377
Mean positivity, 378
Mean pressure, 375–376
Measurements and equivalents, 504–506
Mechanical ventilation, 322–387
  atelectasis and, 421
  monitoring of, 449–456
    laboratory findings in, 452–456
  physiologic effect of, 369–387
    on circulation, 372–385
    on metabolism, 385–387
    on ventilation, 369–372
  pressure in, oxygen concentration and, 358–360
  prolonged, 385–387
  ventilators in, 325–369; *see also* Ventilators
  weakness after, 474–475
  work energy and, 371–372
Mediastinal emphysema, 396
Mediator, 223
Medical director, 492–494
Medical gases, 269–289; *see also* Gas therapy
Medullary center, 142–143
Medullary chemoreceptors, 143–146
Melting point, 32
Membranes
  alveolar, 118, 297–298
  semipermeable, 61
Mental attitude
  rehabilitation and, 484
  weaning from ventilator and, 457
Metabolic acidosis; *see* Acidosis, metabolic
Metabolic alkalosis, 148, 154–155
Metabolism, 385–387
Metaprel; *see* Metaproterenol sulfate
Metaproterenol sulfate, 225, 228
Methemoglobin, 184–185
Methylene blue, 248
Metric system, 504–505
Microaerosols, 252
Microaggregated albumin
  labeled with radioactive iodine, 203
  labeled with radioactive technetium, 203
Microatelectasis, 438
Millibar, 12
Milliequivalent, 50, 53–54
  per liter, 55
Milligram equivalent weight, 50, 53–54
Milliliters of gas per milliters of plasma, 123
Millimole, 5
  per liter, 136

Minimal air, 94, 95
Minute volume, 79, 81
  mechanical ventilation and, 370
  systemic blood flow and, 162–163
Mist, 243
Mist tent, 256, 259
Mixed acid-base states, 155
Mixing valves, 437
Molal solution, 58
Molar gas constant, 28
Molar solution, 58–59
Molar volume of gases, 5–6
Mole, 5
Molecular water, 14
Molecules, 1, 46
  covalent, polarization of, 47
  force of mass attraction between liquid, 95
  of gas, aerosol deposition and, 216–217; *see also*
    Gases
  giant, 46
Monaghan ventilators, 325, 326–327, 331, 342–
    344, 412
Moniliasis, 248
Monitoring of mechanical ventilation, 449–
    456
Monostable fluidic device, 343, 344
Moon face, 232
Moore buttons, 458
Morphine, 433–434, 466
Morphine antagonists, 466
Motor nerve impulses, blocking of, 434–435
Mountain sickness, 184
Mouth pressure, 376, 439
Mucociliary action, 296
Mucoevacuants, 235
Mucolytics, 235–239
Mucomyst; *see* Acetylcysteine
Mucopolysaccharides, 193
Mucosa
  crusting of, 244
  edema of, 192, 220, 221
  trauma to, 404, 408–409
Mucoviscidosis, pulmonary, 265–266; *see also*
    Cystic fibrosis
Mucus, 219
Multiple-stage regulator, 282
Muscles
  abdominal, 89
  diaphragm as, 84–86
  intercostal, 86–87
  pectoralis major, 88–89
  scalene, 87–88
  sternomastoid, 88
  training of, 483
  ventilatory, 83–90, 450
    accessory, 87–89
    paralysis of, 200
Myasthenia gravis, 200

*Mycobacterium tuberculosis*, 247
Mycostatin, 241
Myocardial fibrosis, diffuse, 168
Myocardial infarction, 168
Myocardium, refractory period of, 158

**N**

N-acetylcysteine; *see* Acetylcysteine
Nalline; *see* Nalorphine
Nalorphine, 466
Nanomoles per liter of [H$^+$], 77
Nasal catheter or cannula, 307–309
Nasotracheal tube, 394–395
  removal of, 458
  too low, 451
Nebulizers, 243, 249
  Bennett ventilator and, 361
  Bird ventilator and, 350
  concentration of inspired gas and, 359
  continuous use of, 256
  drug, 267
  fog, 267
  hand, 254
  Hydro-Sphere, 260–261
  impeller, 262
  inert gas-powered, 252–260
  intermittent, 253–255
  liquid filtration, 252
  mainstream, 257–259
  power source for, 255, 266–267
  prolonged use of, 255–256
  reservoir, 255–260
  sidestream, 257–259
  tubing of, vapor temperature and, 258
  ultrasonic, 262–268
    prolonged humidification and, 256
Negative log of equilibrium constant of acid com-
    ponent of buffer system, 139
Negative pressure
  double-circuit positive-pressure ventilator and,
    336
  during exhalation, 383
  intrathoracic pressure and, 384–385
    cardiac output and, 372–378
  positive-pressure, pressure-cycled, pneumatic
    assistor-controller ventilator and, 346
  shock and, 452
  ventilators and, 328
    Bennett, 361, 366–367
    Bird, 350–351
    time-cycled, 330–332
Neomycin, 241
Neostigmine methylsulfate, 434
Nerves; *see also* Nervous system
  adrenergic, 224
  cholinergic, 224
  parasympathetic, 157, 176, 222, 229
  phrenic, 84, 320

Nerves—cont'd
sympathetic, 156, 157, 222
vagus; *see* Vagus nerve
Nervous system; *see also* Nerves
autonomic, 156, 157, 221–224, 229
sinus arrhythmia and, 176
central
carbon dioxide therapy and, 319–321
hypoxia and, 185–186
parasympathetic, 157, 176, 222, 229
sympathetic, 156, 157, 222
Neuroeffector junction, 223
Neuromuscular blocking agents, 434–435
Neutral particles, 213
Neutrons, 40
Nikethamide, 466
Nitrogen, 270, 293
Nitrogen partial pressure, 121
Nitrous oxide, 270, 274
Nomograms
breathing, 515
for tidal volumes and rates, 416
Nonelastic resistance to ventilation, 103–104
Nonelectrolytes, 69
Nonpolar covalent bonding, 47, 48
Nonpolar covalent solutions, 68–69
Norepinephrine, 223–224, 225, 227
Norisodrine; *see* Isoproterenol
Normal saline, 72, 245, 255, 266
Normal solution, 59
Nucleus of atom, 39
Nurses, 411

**O**

Obesity, 463
Oblique muscles, 89
Obstruction of airway; *see* Airway obstruction
Obstructive disease
inspiratory/expiratory ratio and, 419
postural drainage and, 471
ventilators and, 414
Obturator, 397
Occupational retraining and placement, 485
Ohio Critical Care Ventilator, 340–342
Ohio 550 ventilators, 342–344
Operculum, 83
Oral endotracheal intubation; *see* Endotracheal
tube
Orbitals, 42
Organization of respiratory care department; *see*
Respiratory care department
Oropharyngeal catheter, 307–309
Oscilloscope, 162
Osmotic pressure, 60–62
Osteoarthropathy, hypertrophic, 189–191
Osteoporosis, 232
Overhydration, 266

Oxidation, 45
Oxidation number, 44–45
Oxidizing agent, 45
Oximeter, 311
Oxygen, 290–291; *see also* Hypoxemia; Hypoxia
in alveoli, reduced, 184
in arterial and venous blood, 127
bulk, 276–279
carotid bodies and, 146
combined, 123–131
concentration of; *see* Oxygen concentration
diffusion, 119, 170
dissolved, 123
hypoventilation and, 291–293
liquid bulk, 277–279
partial pressure of, 126–127; *see also* Oxygen
tension
suppression of breathing and, 433
in therapy; *see* Oxygen therapy
tolerance to, 299
toxicity of, 293–301
transportation of, 122–132
ventilatory effects of, 291–293
Oxygen cannulas and catheters, 307–309
Oxygen capacity, 125
Oxygen concentration
Bennett ventilator and, 360–361
Bird ventilator and, 358
compressed air and, 437
control of, 436–437
face tent and, 314
incubators and, 299
masks and, 303, 305
nasal catheter or cannula and, 308–309
nebulizers and, 259–260
tents and, 310
Oxygen dissociation curves, 126–127
blood partial pressure and, 183
body temperature and, 130
pH ranges and, 128–129
Oxygen-limiter, 311–312
Oxygen masks, 301–307
Oxygen pneumonia, 297
Oxygen saturation
arterial
capillary unsaturation and, 513
hydrogen ion concentration and, 127–130
hypoxia and, 183
inspiratory positive-pressure breathing and,
461
and partial pressure of oxygen, 126–127
carbon dioxide dissociation curves and, 134
hemoglobin, 183
Oxygen tension, 120
arterial, 120
hypoxia and, 183

Oxygen tension—cont'd
  arterial—cont'd
    mechanical ventilation and, 324, 371, 415, 453
    oxygen administration and, 315
    oxygen saturation and, 126–127
    oxygen unsupported by mechanical ventilation
      and, 436
    positive end-expiratory pressure and, 445
   atmospheric pressure and, 13–14
   low ambient, hypoxia and, 184
   in plasma, 123
   pulmonary edema and, 466
Oxygen tents, 309–314
Oxygen therapy, 270, 289–316
  equipment and techniques in, 301–315
   cannulas and catheters in, 307–309
   face and head tents in, 314–315
   masks in, 301–307
   tents in, 309–314
  exercises and, 482, 483
  hazards in, 291–301
   toxicity and, 293–301
   ventilation and, 291–293
  humidification and, 256
  hypoxia and, 191; *see also* Hypoxia
  indiscriminate use of, 151
  intubated patient and, 402–403
  oxygen characteristics and, 290–291
  pulmonary edema and, 467
  shock and, 173
  tracheobronchial aspiration and, 409
  unsupported by mechanical ventilation, 436
Oxygen uptake, average, 127
Oxyhemoglobin, 124

**P**

$P_{50}$; *see* Partial pressure of blood oxygen that half
  saturates hemoglobin
$P_{CO_2}$; *see* Carbon dioxide tension
$P_{O_2}$; *see* Oxygen tension
P wave, 162
Pacemaker, 157
  electronic, 179–180
Pallor, 450
Pancreatic deoxyribonuclease, 240
Pancreatic dornase, 240, 410
Pancuronium bromide, 435
Paradoxical breathing, 199, 450, 477
Paralysis
  of diaphragm, 86
  epiglottal, 308
  of ventilatory muscles, 200
Paramagnetic susceptibility, 312–313
Parasympathetic nerves, 157, 222, 229
  sinus arrhythmia and, 176
Paresthesias, 152
Paroxysmal tachycardia, 177–178

Partial pressure; *see also* Carbon dioxide tension;
  Oxygen tension
  of blood oxygen that half saturates hemoglobin,
   129–130
  Dalton's law of, 13
  nitrogen, 121
Particles, 39
  aerosol deposition and, 218
  neutral, 213
  size of
   penetration and, 215
   pulmonary tissue clearance and, 219–220
   ultrasonic nebulizers and, 264
  submicronic, 252
Pass-over humidifier, 261
Pavulon; *see* Pancuronium bromide
PCW; *see* Pulmonary capillary wedge pressure
Peak flow; 365–366
Peak flow control, 362
Peak inflation hold, 438–439
Pectoralis major muscle, 88–89
Pediatrics, ultrasonic nebulizers and, 265–266; *see
  also* Infants
PEEP; *see* Positive end-expiratory pressure
Percent body humidity, 243
Percent solution, 58
Percussion, chest, 473–474
Perfusion scan, 203
Perhydroxyl free radicals, 295
Periodic breathing, 116
Periodic sigh, 421–422
Peripheral cardiovascular collapse, 383; *see also*
  Cardiovascular system
Peripheral chemoreceptors, 143–146
Peripheral vasculature
  resistance of, 163
  shock and, 172, 173
Permeability, selective, 62
Personnel, number of 501–502; *see also* Respira-
  tory care department
pH, 78; *see also* Blood gases and acid-base balance
  bicarbonate therapy and, 427–428
  blood, 127–130
   acid-base balance and, 136–142
   DPG and, 131
   mechanical ventilation and, 324, 371
   oxygen unsupported by mechanical ventilation
    and, 436
  ventilators and, 324, 371, 415, 422, 423, 453
  weaning from, 456–457
Phagocytes, 219
Phlebotomy, 191, 466–467
Phosphates, organic, 130–131
Photosynthesis, 290, 294
Phrenic nerves, 84, 320
Physical activity, exercises and, 480
Physical analyzers, 312, 313

Physicians
 as medical directors, 492–494
 professional supervision and, 500–501
 ventilated patient and, 411
Physiologic compensation, 149
Physiologic dead space, 81; *see also* Dead space
Physiotherapy, 469–470
Piezoelectric transducer, 262–263
Pilot balloon, 391, 399
Pin-Index Safety System, 288–289
PISS; *see* Pin-Index Safety System
Piston, linear-drive, single-circuit ventilator, 339–340
Pituitary gland, 232
pK, 139
Plasma
 carbon dioxide in, 131, 132, 133
 dissolved oxygen and, 123
 electrolytic balance in, 153
Plateau alveolar pressure, 439
Plateau inflation hold, 439–440
Plethysmograph, body, 106
Pleural cavity, fluid in, 201
Pleural space, 90, 94, 95
Pleural traction, 94
Pleurisy, 200
Pneumatic clutch, 353–355, 357
Pneumocytes, 296, 299–300
Pneumonia
 antibiotics and, 240
 dornase and, 240
 inspiratory positive-pressure breathing and, 461
 oxygen and, 297
 postural drainage and, 471
 tracheostomy and, 405
Pneumotachograph, 106
Pneumotaxic center, 146, 147
Pneumothorax, 444
Poiseuille's law, 107, 108
Polar, term of, 47
Polar covalent bonding, 48, 49
Polar covalent electrolytes, 66–69
Polar covalent solutions, 65
Polarization of covalent molecules, 47
Poliomyelitis, 200, 330–332
Polycythemia, 187, 188–189
Polymyxin, 241
Polyphloretin phosphate, 235
Portable respirator, 331–332
Positive end-expiratory pressure, 440–449
 arteriovenous shunting and, 440
 assisted, 446
 Bennett ventilator and, 340
 best, 445
 contraindications to, 444–445
 controlled, 442–446

Positive end-expiratory pressure—cont'd
 hazards of, 444
 indications for, 444–445
 initiating and discontinuing, 445–446
 intermittent mandatory ventilation and, 442
 optimal, 445
 spontaneous, 446–449
 terminology and, 441
 with unassisted spontaneous ventilation, 446–449
Positive pressure
 intrathoracic pressure and cardiac output and, 372–378
 lung-thorax compliance and, 102
Positive-pressure ventilators, 328
 helium therapy and, 318
 pressure-cycled, pneumatic assistor-controller, 344–369
  flow-adjustable, 346–360
  flow-sensitive, 360–369
 restrictive lung disease and, 413
 shock and, 173
 tissue emphysema and, 405
 volume-cycled
  electric, 333–342
  pneumatic, 342–344
Postoperative atelectasis, 320
Postoperative cough control, 474–475
Postural drainage, 197, 470–473
Potassium, 40, 435
 ventilators and, 422
Potassium hydroxide, 313
Potential energy in moving fluid, 110
Pounds per square inch, 269, 270
P-R interval, 162
PR-2 respiration unit, 360
Prednisone, 233
Preinspiratory level, 90
Premature contractions, 176–177
Premature infants
 Bournes ventilator and, 339–340
 tidal volumes of, 417
Preset regulator, 279–280
Pressure
 airway resistance, and gas flow, 104–105, 109–112
 atmosphere of, 11
 atmospheric, oxygen partial pressure and, 13–14
 blood; *see* Blood pressure
 critical, 35
 end-expiratory; *see* Positive end-expiratory pressure
 gas cylinders and, 274, 275, 276
 of gases; *see* Gases, pressure of
 intra-alveolar, 373
 intracranial, 473
 intrapleural, 91, 92, 102

Pressure—cont'd
  intrapulmonary
    Bird ventilator and, 348
    controlled-positive end-expiratory pressure
      and, 443, 444, 449
    pulmonary edema and, 467
  intrathoracic; *see* Intrathoracic pressure
  moving fluid and, 110
  negative; *see* Negative pressure
  osmotic, 60–62
  partial; *see* Carbon dioxide tension; Oxygen
    tension; Partial pressure
  pulmonary; *see* Pulmonary pressure
  transairway, 104–105
  vaporization and, 15
  venous
    central, 173–174, 175
    measurement of, 165
  ventilation and, 91–92
  water vapor, 16–17
Pressure compensation, flowmeters and, 282–
  285
Pressure-control magnet, 348
Pressure-cycling of ventilator; *see* Ventilators
Pressure generators, 355–357
Pressure gradient, 91, 96
Pressure-time relationship, 375–376
  mechanical ventilation and, 380–385
Professional supervision, 500–501
Proportionality constant, 18–19
Propylene glycol, 228
  in normal saline, 245, 255
  tuberculosis and, 246–247
  ultrasonic nebulizers and, 267
Prostaglandins, 234–235
Protein, 133, 232
Proteolytics, 239–240
Protons, 39, 70
*Pseudomonas aeruginosa*, 242, 406
psi; *see* Pounds per square inch
Psychosomatic support, 484–485
Psychotherapy, 485
Pulmonary abscess, 240, 461, 471
Pulmonary air distribution, 200
Pulmonary artery pressure, 165–166
Pulmonary blood flow, 165–167
  reduction of, 466
Pulmonary capillary wedge pressure, 175
Pulmonary compliance; *see* Compliance
Pulmonary congestion, 169–170, 175, 201; *see also*
  Pulmonary edema
Pulmonary distention, 197–200
Pulmonary edema
  acute, 166–167, 465–467
  capillary wedge pressure and, 175
  ethyl alcohol and, 238
  mechanical ventilation and, 386

Pulmonary edema—cont'd
  negative expiratory pressure and, 383–384
Pulmonary embolism, 211
Pulmonary emphysema; *see* Emphysema
Pulmonary function laboratory, 496–499
Pulmonary hyperinflation, 445
Pulmonary insufficiency, chronic; *see* Chronic care
  and rehabilitation
Pulmonary pressure; *see also* Intrapulmonary pres-
  sure
  arterial, 165–166
  Bird ventilator and, 348
  congenital heart disease and, 181
Pulmonary restriction, 200–202
  postoperative or posttraumatic, 474–475
Pulmonary surfactant, 99–100, 438
  oxygen and, 293, 296–297
Pulmonary tissue clearance, 219–220
Pulmonary veins, 166
Pulse deficit, 178
Purkinje fibers, 158
Pursed-lip breathing, 196, 476–477

**Q**

QRS complex, 162
QT time, 162

**R**

R; *see* Resistance; Respiratory/exchange ratio
Radford nomogram, 416
Radicals
  equivalent weight of, 50–51
  free, 295
  symbols, weights, and valences of, 512
Radioactive substances, 203
Rales, 167, 196
Rankine scale, 5
Ratio solution, 58
RDS; *see* Respiratory distress syndrome
Rebreathed volume, 79–81
  added to patient tubing, 426
Receptors
  adrenergic, 224–225
  organs or cells as, 223
Records, 499–500
Red cells, 188–189
Reduced hemoglobin, 124
Reduction, 45
Reflexes
  epiglottal, 308
  Hering-Breuer, 146, 147
  inflation, 146, 147
  stretch, 146, 147
Registered respiratory therapist, 491
Regulator-diluter, 360
Regulators, 279–282
Rehabilitation, 468–486
  family counseling and, 485–486

Rehabilitation—cont'd
   objectives of, 468–469
   occupational retraining and placement and, 485
   psychosomatic support and, 484–485
   respiratory therapy in, 470–484; *see also* Respiratory therapy, rehabilitation and
Relaxation-pressure curve, 102
Reservoir bag, 303, 429, 442
Reservoir nebulizers, 255–260
Residual volume, 93
   mechanical ventilation and, 370
Resistance
   compliance, ventilatory frequency, and flow, 112–114
   to exhalation, 114–115
   gas flow, and pressure, 104–105
   normal, 105
   to pulmonary flow, 165–166
Respiration; *see also* Ventilation
   abdominal, 477–482
   carbon dioxide therapy and, 319, 320
   dry gas and, 244
   paradoxical, 199, 450, 477
   periodic, 116
   pursed-lip, 476–477
   rate of, 79
      aerosol deposition and, 218
   spontaneous
      ventilators and, 418, 428–432
      weaning from ventilator and, 457, 460
   suppression of, 432–435
   term of, 79
   thoracic, exercises and, 477
   transition from controlled to independent, 430–431
Respirator shock, 378, 383, 385; *see also* Ventilators
Respiratory acidosis; *see* Acidosis, respiratory
Respiratory alkalosis, 148, 151–152
   ventilators and, 422
Respiratory care department, 487–503
   administration and personnel of, 489–497
   components of, 489
   operation of, 497–501
   organizational outline of, 489, 490
   services of, 488–489
      distribution of, 497–499
   size of, 501–502
Respiratory center, 142–146
   carbon dioxide therapy and, 320
   intermittent mandatory ventilation and, 431
Respiratory distress syndrome, 298
   adult, 173, 386
   of infants, 448–449
   positive end-expiratory pressure and, 440, 448–449

Respiratory equilibrium, 292
Respiratory/exchange ratio, 202
   high, 210–212
   low, 204–210
Respiratory failure; *see* Ventilatory failure
Respiratory infections, acute, 240
Respiratory mucosa
   edema of, 192, 220, 221
   induration of, 192
Respiratory quotient, 202
Respiratory therapist, 491, 492
Respiratory therapy
   of chronic care; *see* Chronic care and rehabilitation
   functions of, 493
   rehabilitation and, 470–484
      abdominal breathing in, 477–482
      acute chest compression and, 475–476
      chest percussion in, 473–474
      chest vibration in, 474
      cough control and, 474–475
      graded exercises in, 482–484
      postural drainage in, 470–473
      pursed-lip breathing and, 476–477
   school of, 497
Respiratory therapy assistant, 491
Respiratory therapy student, 491
Respiratory therapy student trainee, 491
Respiratory therapy technician, 491, 492, 496
Respiratory tract, perfusion of, 80
Retard of airflow, pursed-lip, 477
Retard cap, 464
Retrolental fibroplasia, 298–299
Reversible reaction, 67
RH; *see* Humidity, relative
Rhinitis, 192
Rhonchi, 196
Ribonucleic acid, 193, 296
Ribs, 83–84
   lower, mobilization of, 481–482
Right-to-left shunts, 125, 210
Right ventricular failure, 170–171
Ringer's solution, 56
RNA; *see* Ribonucleic acid
Rotary drive, 333
Rotating tourniquets, 467
RQ; *see* Respiratory quotient
Rule of three, 186
RV; *see* Residual volume

**S**

S; *see* Saturated gas
Safety indexed connector systems, 285–289
Safety pressure release valves, 260
Saline; *see also* Sodium chloride
   inspiratory positive-pressure breathing and, 461

Saline—cont'd
  normal, 72, 245, 255, 266
  prolonged intermittent use of aerosol, 255
  tracheobronchial aspiration and, 410
Salt, equivalent weight of, 51–52; *see also* Saline;
    Sodium chloride
Salts, ions and, 72–73
Saturated with water vapor, 15
Saturated gas, 17
Saturated solutions, 56–57
Saturation
  hemoglobin, 125
  oxygen; *see* Oxygen saturation
Scalene muscles, 87–88
Scanning, 203–204
Sch 1000; *see* N-Isopropyl nortropine
Scheduling
  of assignments, 495, 499
  of personnel, 495
  of services, 497–499
School of respiratory therapy, 497
Scleroderma, 200
Secretions
  bronchial; *see* Bronchial secretions
  bronchoscopy and, 390
  inspiratory/expiratory ratio and, 419
  inspiratory positive-pressure breathing and, 461
  intubated patient and, 402, 403
Sedimentation, Stoke's law of, 215–216
Selective permeability, 62
Semipermeable membrane, 60
Sensitivity control, 348
Sepsis
  tracheostomy and, 405–406
  weaning from ventilator and, 457
Shift supervisor, 495
Shock, 172
  negative expiratory pressure and, 452
  phlebotomy and, 467
  pulmonary edema and, 466
  respirator, 378, 383, 385
  tank, 331, 385
Shock lung, 173
Shunts, 125–126
  hypoxia and, 184, 437–440
    mechanical ventilation and, 323
    positive end-expiratory pressure and, 440–441
  intracardiac, 181
  physiologic venous-arterial, 204–210, 437–440
  right-to-left, estimation of, 210
Sidestream nebulization, 257–259
Sideways slip, 217
Sighs, 421–422
Sine curve, 333–335
Single-circuit positive-pressure ventilator, 335–336
Singulation, 320–321

Sinoatrial node, 157
Sinus arrest, 180
Sinus arrhythmia, 176
Sinus node, 157
Skeletal muscles, blocking innervation of, 434–435
Slow-reacting substance of anaphylaxis, 234
Slow spaces, 438
Smog, 17, 214
Snowplow effect, 404
SOD; *see* Superoxide dismutase
Sodium bicarbonate; *see* Bicarbonate sodium
Sodium chloride, 51–52; *see also* Saline
  freezing and, 74
  induced sputum specimen and, 246, 247
  water and, 65
Solbutamol, 225, 228
Solids
  to liquids, 32
  to vapor, 37–38
Solubility, 56
Solubility coefficient, 118
Solute, 56
  freezing and boiling and, 63–64
Solutions, 56–58
  dilute, 56
  and ions, 39–78
    acidity and alkalinity in, 77–78
    acids, bases, and salts in, 70–73
    atomic bonding and, 45–49
    atomic structure and, 39–45
    colloids in, 63
    dilution calculations and, 62
    electrolytes and, 63–69
    electrolytic activity in, 73–77
    equivalent weights and, 50–56
    osmotic pressure and, 60–62
    suspensions and, 63
  nonpolar covalent, 68–69
  quantitative classification of, 58–60
  saturated, 56–57
  standard, 59
  supersaturated, 57
  tonicity of, 61–62
Solvent, 56
Sparks, 313–314
Specific gravity, 7
Specific heat, 30
Specimens, laboratory, 245–246, 255, 265
Spectator ions, 70
Spine, diseases of, 200
Spirometers, 455
Splinting, abdominal, 201
Splitter, 343
Spontaneous breathing, ventilators and, 418, 428–432
  weaning and, 457, 460

Spring-loaded gate, 357
Spring-loaded plunger, 351–352
Sputum
    mucoid and purulent, 193–194
    specimens of, 245–246, 265
        induced, 246, 255, 265
SRS-A; *see* Slow-reacting substance of anaphylaxis
ST; *see* Surface tension
S-T interval, 162
Staffing of respiratory care department; *see* Respiratory care department
Standard solutions, 59
Standard temperature and pressure, 17
Static compliance, 440
Static pressure period, 338
Static sparks, 313–314
Static volume, 370
Sternomastoid muscle, 88
Steroids, 231–235
Stoke's law of sedimentation, 215–216
Stokes-Adams syncope, 179
Stoma, residual, 458
STP; *see* Standard temperature and pressure
STPD, 17
    ATPS and, 26, 510
    BTPS and, 27, 511
Stratosphere, 9
Streptococcal deoxyribonuclease, 240
Streptococcal fibrinolysin, 240
Streptodornase, 240
Streptokinase, 240
Streptokinase-streptodornase, 240
Streptomycin, 241
Stretch reflex, 146, 147
Stridor, 196
Stroke volume, 159, 162
Stylus, 162
Subcutaneous emphysema, 396, 405, 444
Subdiaphragmatic compression, external, 476
Sublimation, 31, 37
    heat of, 37
Submicronic particles, 252
Subshells, 41–42
Succinylcholine, 434–435
Suctioning, bronchial, 407–410
Sulfhydryl groups, 296
Sulfur dioxide, 246
Superinone; *see* Tyloxapol
Superoxide dismutase, 299–300
Superoxide free radicals, 295
Supersaturated solutions, 57
Supervision, professional, 500–501
Supervisors, 495–496
Suprarenin; *see* Epinephrine
Surface area, force and, 9–10
Surface tension, 95–100
    ultrasonic nebulizers and, 264

Surfactants, 99–110, 438
    oxygen and, 293, 296–297
Suspensions, 63
Swan-Ganz catheter, 174–175, 445, 455
Symbols, 506–507, 512
Sympathetic nerves, 156, 157, 222
Sympathomimetics, 226
Syncope, Stokes-Adams, 179
Syndromes
    Cushing's, 231
    respiratory distress; *see* Respiratory distress syndrome
Systemic blood flow, 162–165
Systole, 158, 159, 163, 164

**T**

T wave, 162
Tachycardia, 159
    paroxysmal, 177–178
Tank shock, 331, 385
Tank ventilator, 412, 413
Tapping, 473
$^{99m}$Tc; *see* Technetium, radioactive
$^{99m}$Tc-iron hydroxide; *see* Technetium-iron hydroxide aggregates
$^{99m}$Tc MAA; *see* Microaggregated albumin labeled with radioactive technetium
Technetium, radioactive, 203
Technetium albuminate, 203
Technetium-iron hydroxide aggregates, 203
Technical director, 494–495
    assistant, 495
    of education, 497
Teflon membrane, 313
Temperature
    absolute, 3
    barometric reading correction and, 509
    of body, 17, 130
    conversion of Celsius and Fahrenheit, 506
    critical, 35
    gas cylinders and, 274
    of gases; *see* Gases, temperature of
    of oxygen tent, 310
    vapor, tubing and, 258
    vaporization and, 15
Temperature inversion, 17
Tendons, central, 84
Tension of gas, 3
Tents
    nebulizer and, 259
    oxygen, 309–314
Terbutaline, 225
Terminal flow, 364–365
Tetany, 422
Thebesian venous drainage, 125
Theobromine, 230
Theophylline, 230

Thermal conductivity, 312–313
Thoracic breathing, 477
Thoracic cage movements, 83–84
Thoracic compliance; *see* Compliance
Thoracic pressure; *see* Intrathoracic pressure
Thoracic resting position, 94
Thorax; *see also* Chest
  bone disease of, 200
  normal, ventilators and, 413
  venous return to heart and, 164–165
Thorax-lung relationship, 90–95, 101, 102; *see also* Compliance
Thorpe-tube flowmeter, 279, 280, 282
Thromboses
  atrial fibrillation and, 178
  coronary blood flow and, 168
  polycythemia and, 189
Tidal volumes, 79, 416–417
  aerosol deposition and, 218
  induced alkalosis and, 425–426
  lung capacity and, 93
  mechanical ventilation and, 370, 415
Tilt-table, 471
Time cycling, 329–330
Timing accumulators, 367–369
Tipping, 470
Tissue cultures, 295–296
Tissue emphysema, 396, 405, 444
TLC; *see* Total lung capacity
Tolerance to physical activity, 480
Tone, 224
Tonicity, 61
Total lung capacity, 94
Tourniquets, 467
Toxicity, drug, 267
Tracheal obstruction, epigastric compressions and, 476
Trachael stenosis, 404–405
Tracheal tube, too low, 451; *see also* Intubation
Tracheal wall, perforation of, 405
Tracheobronchial aspiration, 407–410
Tracheobronchial flow, 108, 112–114
Tracheomalacia, 404
Tracheostomy, 395–406
  airway obstruction and, 196
  breath sounds and, 404
  complications of, 396–397, 403–406
  humidification and, 255, 256
  nasotracheal intubation and, 394
  patient management and, 401–403
  tracheotomy and, 395–397
Tracheostomy mask, 403
Tracheostomy tubes and cuffs, 397–401, 458–459
  definition of, 395
  deflation of, 401–402
  fenestrated, 458–459
  helium therapy and, 318

Tracheostomy tubes and cuffs—cont'd
  inflation of, 400
  Kistner, 458
  obstruction and, 403
  plugging of, 459–460
  removal of, 458
  too low, 451
Tracheotomy, 395–397
  incision for, 396
    bleeding from, 405
  mortality and, 396, 406
  oral intubation prior to, 394
Transairway pressure, 104–105
Transducer, piezoelectric, 262–263
Transport, active, 145
Transverse abdominal muscle, 89
Trauma
  aspiration and, 408–409
  pulmonary restriction and, 200
Treadmill, 482
Triamcinolone acetonide, 233
Triple point, 31, 33
Trophosphere, 8–9
Trypsin, 239
Tuberculosis, 246–247; *see also* Chronic care and rehabilitation
Tubes
  for intubation, cuffed, 391, 392
  of nebulizers, vapor temperature and, 258
  tracheostomy; *see* Tracheostomy tubes and cuffs
*d*-Tubocurarine, 434
Turbulent flow, 108–112
Tyloxapol, 235–236

**U**

U-Cyclit chest respirator, 332
Ultrasonic nebulizer, 262–268
  children and, 265–266
  power source of, 266–267
  prolonged humidification and, 256
Unit regulator, 361
Univalent reduction, 295
Unsaturation, 125
  of capillary blood perfusing body surfaces, 186
  of hemoglobin, 186
Urinary output, 444

**V**

$V_A$; *see* Alveolar ventilation
$V_A/Q_c$; *see* Respiratory/exchange ratio
$V_D$; *see* Dead space
$V_D$ alv; *see* Alveolar dead space
$V_D$ ant; *see* Anatomic dead space
$V_D$ phys; *see* Physiologic dead space
$V_E$; *see* Minute volume
$V_{RB}$; *see* Rebreathed volume
$V_T$; *see* Tidal volumes

Vagus nerve, 156, 157, 229
  paroxysmal tachycardia and, 177
  physical manipulation of body and, 180
  sinus arrest and, 180
  sinus arrhythmia and, 176
Valence electrons, 43
Valences, 44–45, 512
Valves
  cylinder, 271–272
  demand, 346
  exhalation, 349–350
  flow-sensitive, 362–364
  interrupter, 350–351
van der Waals force, 28
Vapor, 35, 243
  to liquid, 32–37
  to solid, 37–38
  temperature of, tubing and, 258
Vapor pressure, 14, 57
Vaporization, 14–15, 32
  heat of, 34
Vaporizer, liquid oxygen and, 279
Varidase; *see* Streptokinase-streptodornase
Vascular congestion, intrapulmonary, 201
Vascular reservoirs, 378
Vasculature, peripheral, 163, 172, 173
VC; *see* Vital capacity
Veins, pulmonary, 166; *see also* Venous blood
  congestion of, 169–170, 175, 201
Velocity
  and flow, terms of, 110
  gas particle, 3
  gas pressure and, 109–112
Venous admixture, 125, 204–210
  and diffusion defect, 207–209
  positive end-expiratory pressure and, 440
Venous-arterial shunt; *see* Shunts
Venous blood
  bronchial, 125–126, 166
  carbon dioxide in, 120, 136
  gas partial pressures in, 120; *see also* Carbon
    dioxide tension; Oxygen tension
  to heart, thorax and, 164–165
  mechanical ventilators and, 378, 383
  monitoring and, 454
  negative-pressure breathing and, 385
  oxygen in, 120, 127
  pH and, 128
  pulmonary edema and, 466–467
Venous pressure
  central, 173–174, 175
  measurement of, 165
Ventilation, 79–116; *see also* Respiration
  aerosol deposition and, 218
  airway obstruction and, 196
  airway resistance to, 104–114
  assisted, 324

Ventilation—cont'd
  classification of, 81–83
  control of, 142–147
  controlled, 324–325
  dead space and; *see* Dead space
  elastic resistance to, 101–103
  exhalation mechanics and, 114–115
  instituting and maintaining, 415–456
    correcting hypoxia and, 435–449
    establishing ventilatory pattern and, 417–432;
      *see also* Ventilatory pattern, mechanical
      ventilation and
    monitoring mechanical ventilation and, 449–
      456
    suppressing ventilation and, 432–435
    tidal volume and rate and, 415–417
  intermittent mandatory; *see* Intermittent manda-
    tory ventilation
  lung-thorax relationship and, 90–95, 101, 102;
    *see also* Compliance
  mechanical; *see* Mechanical ventilation
  minute, weaning from ventilator and, 457
  muscle action and, 83–90, 450
  nonelastic resistance to, 103–104
  normal, 82
  of obstructed airways, 420–421
  oxygen and, 291–293
  paradoxical, 199, 450, 477
  positive-pressure, tissue emphysema and, 405;
    *see also* Positive end-expiratory pressure
  pulmonary distention and, 198–199, 200
  pulmonary restriction and, 201
  semi-controlled, 418
  surface tension and, 95–100
  term of, 79
  total, 81
    inspiratory positive-pressure breathing and,
      461
  wasted, 211
Ventilation/perfusion ratio, 125, 126
  hypoxia and, 185, 202–212
  mechanical ventilation and, 323, 370–371
  in scattered areas of lung, 438
Ventilation scan, 203–204
Ventilation setup, simple, 429
Ventilator-induced alkalosis, 422
Ventilators; *see also* Mechanical ventilation
  adjustable, variable, and fixed functions of, 412
  assistor-controller, 328
  attachment of, to tracheostomy tube, 401
  choice of, 411–415
  control modes of, 329–330
  controller, 328
  costs of, 415
  dependence on, 456
  flow, pressure, time and frequency and, 419
  helium therapy and, 318

Ventilators—cont'd
  negative-pressure; *see* Negative pressure, venti-
    lators and
  number of, 502
  positive-pressure; *see* Positive-pressure ventila-
    tors
  pressure cycling in, 329–330, 344–369
    oxygen concentration and, 437
  pulmonary distention and, 200
  restrictive lung disease and, 413, 414
  term of, 328–329
  time cycling and, 329–330
  volume cycling in; *see* Volume-cycled ventilators
  weaning from 456–460
Ventilatory failure, 388–467; *see also* Airway ob-
    struction
  chronic, respiratory acidosis and, 151
  chronic care and rehabilitation and; *see* Chronic
    care and rehabilitation
  guidelines of, 324
  inspiratory positive-pressure breathing and, 460–
    467
  mechanical ventilation and, 323–324; *see also*
    Mechanical ventilation; Ventilators
  oxygen and, 292
  patent airways and; *see* Airway, patent
  patient management and, 410–460
    instituting and maintaining ventilation in, 415–
      456; *see also* Ventilation, instituting and
      maintaining
    ventilator choice and, 411–415
    weaning from ventilator and, 456–460
Ventilatory muscles, 83–90, 450
  paralysis of, 200
Ventilatory pattern, mechanical ventilation and,
    380–385, 417–432
  inspiratory/expiratory ratio and, 418–420
  intermittent mandatory ventilation and, 428–432
  obstructed airways and, 420–421
  periodic hyperventilation and, 421–422
  pressure, rate, and volume and, 417–418
  sustained hyperventilation and, 422–428
Ventricular fibrillation, 179
Venturi, 109–110
  air-mix, 352–360
  Bennett ventilator and, 360–361
  negative-pressure
    Bennett ventilator and, 366–367
    Bird ventilator and, 350–351

Venturi gate, 358–359
Venturi mask, 305–307, 436
Vertebrochondral ribs, 83, 84
Vertebrosternal ribs, 83, 84
Vibration, chest, 474
Viscosity, 106–107
Vital capacity, 93–94, 201
Volume-cycled ventilators, 329–330, 333–344
  intermittent mandatory ventilation and, 429
  restrictive lung disease and, 413, 414
Volume percent, 123
  of oxygen in plasma, 123

**W**

Walking, exercises and, 482
Water
  in aerosols, 244–248
    airway obstruction and, 197
    prolonged intermittent use of, 255
  induced sputum specimen and, 246
  ionization of, 68, 69
  ionization constant of, 76–77
  low temperature characteristics of, 511
  as solvent, 64–65
Water vapor, 243–244
  pressure of, 16–17
Weaning from ventilator, 456–460
Weight per volume solution, 58
Weight density, 7
Weights, 7
  of elements and radicals, 512
  equivalent, 50–56
  gram, equivalent weight and, 52–53
Wetting agents, 235–236
Wheatstone bridge, 312, 313
Wheezes, 196
Wright respirometer, 455
W/V solution; *see* Weight per volume solution

**X**

Xanthine, 230–231
$^{133}$Xe; *see* Xenon gas, radioactive
Xenon gas, radioactive, 203–204

**Y**

Yoke connector, 271